THE MAST CELL IN HEALTH AND DISEASE

LUNG BIOLOGY IN HEALTH AND DISEASE

Executive Editor

Claude Lenfant
Director, National Heart, Lung, and Blood Institute
National Institutes of Health
Bethesda, Maryland

1. Immunologic and Infectious Reactions in the Lung, *edited by Charles H. Kirkpatrick and Herbert Y. Reynolds*
2. The Biochemical Basis of Pulmonary Function, *edited by Ronald G. Crystal*
3. Bioengineering Aspects of the Lung, *edited by John B. West*
4. Metabolic Functions of the Lung, *edited by Y. S. Bakhle and John R. Vane*
5. Respiratory Defense Mechanisms (in two parts), *edited by Joseph D. Brain, Donald F. Proctor, and Lynne M. Reid*
6. Development of the Lung, *edited by W. Alan Hodson*
7. Lung Water and Solute Exchange, *edited by Norman C. Staub*
8. Extrapulmonary Manifestations of Respiratory Disease, *edited by Eugene Debs Robin*
9. Chronic Obstructive Pulmonary Disease, *edited by Thomas L. Petty*
10. Pathogenesis and Therapy of Lung Cancer, *edited by Curtis C. Harris*
11. Genetic Determinants of Pulmonary Disease, *edited by Stephen D. Litwin*
12. The Lung in the Transition Between Health and Disease, *edited by Peter T. Macklem and Solbert Permutt*
13. Evolution of Respiratory Processes: A Comparative Approach, *edited by Stephen C. Wood and Claude Lenfant*
14. Pulmonary Vascular Diseases, *edited by Kenneth M. Moser*
15. Physiology and Pharmacology of the Airways, *edited by Jay A. Nadel*
16. Diagnostic Techniques in Pulmonary Disease (in two parts), *edited by Marvin A. Sackner*
17. Regulation of Breathing (in two parts), *edited by Thomas F. Hornbein*
18. Occupational Lung Diseases: Research Approaches and Methods, *edited by Hans Weill and Margaret Turner-Warwick*
19. Immunopharmacology of the Lung, *edited by Harold H. Newball*
20. Sarcoidosis and Other Granulomatous Diseases of the Lung, *edited by Barry L. Fanburg*
21. Sleep and Breathing, *edited by Nicholas A. Saunders and Colin E. Sullivan*

22. *Pneumocystis carinii* Pneumonia: Pathogenesis, Diagnosis, and Treatment, *edited by Lowell S. Young*
23. Pulmonary Nuclear Medicine: Techniques in Diagnosis of Lung Disease, *edited by Harold L. Atkins*
24. Acute Respiratory Failure, *edited by Warren M. Zapol and Konrad J. Falke*
25. Gas Mixing and Distribution in the Lung, *edited by Ludwig A. Engel and Manuel Paiva*
26. High-Frequency Ventilation in Intensive Care and During Surgery, *edited by Graziano Carlon and William S. Howland*
27. Pulmonary Development: Transition from Intrauterine to Extrauterine Life, *edited by George H. Nelson*
28. Chronic Obstructive Pulmonary Disease: Second Edition, Revised and Expanded, *edited by Thomas L. Petty*
29. The Thorax (in two parts), *edited by Charis Roussos and Peter T. Macklem*
30. The Pleura in Health and Disease, *edited by Jacques Chrétien, Jean Bignon, and Albert Hirsch*
31. Drug Therapy for Asthma: Research and Clinical Practice, *edited by John W. Jenne and Shirley Murphy*
32. Pulmonary Endothelium in Health and Disease, *edited by Una S. Ryan*
33. The Airways: Neural Control in Health and Disease, *edited by Michael A. Kaliner and Peter J. Barnes*
34. Pathophysiology and Treatment of Inhalation Injuries, *edited by Jacob Loke*
35. Respiratory Function of the Upper Airway, *edited by Oommen P. Mathew and Giuseppe Sant'Ambrogio*
36. Chronic Obstructive Pulmonary Disease: A Behavioral Perspective, *edited by A. John McSweeny and Igor Grant*
37. Biology of Lung Cancer: Diagnosis and Treatment, *edited by Steven T. Rosen, James L. Mulshine, Frank Cuttitta, and Paul G. Abrams*
38. Pulmonary Vascular Physiology and Pathophysiology, *edited by E. Kenneth Weir and John T. Reeves*
39. Comparative Pulmonary Physiology: Current Concepts, *edited by Stephen C. Wood*
40. Respiratory Physiology: An Analytical Approach, *edited by H. K. Chang and Manuel Paiva*
41. Lung Cell Biology, *edited by Donald Massaro*
42. Heart–Lung Interactions in Health and Disease, *edited by Steven M. Scharf and Sharon S. Cassidy*
43. Clinical Epidemiology of Chronic Obstructive Pulmonary Disease, *edited by Michael J. Hensley and Nicholas A. Saunders*
44. Surgical Pathology of Lung Neoplasms, *edited by Alberto M. Marchevsky*
45. The Lung in Rheumatic Diseases, *edited by Grant W. Cannon and Guy A. Zimmerman*

46. Diagnostic Imaging of the Lung, *edited by Charles E. Putman*
47. Models of Lung Disease: Microscopy and Structural Methods, *edited by Joan Gil*
48. Electron Microscopy of the Lung, *edited by Dean E. Schraufnagel*
49. Asthma: Its Pathology and Treatment, *edited by Michael A. Kaliner, Peter J. Barnes, and Carl G. A. Persson*
50. Acute Respiratory Failure: Second Edition, *edited by Warren M. Zapol and Francois Lemaire*
51. Lung Disease in the Tropics, *edited by Om P. Sharma*
52. Exercise: Pulmonary Physiology and Pathophysiology, *edited by Brian J. Whipp and Karlman Wasserman*
53. Developmental Neurobiology of Breathing, *edited by Gabriel G. Haddad and Jay P. Farber*
54. Mediators of Pulmonary Inflammation, *edited by Michael A. Bray and Wayne H. Anderson*
55. The Airway Epithelium, *edited by Stephen G. Farmer and Douglas Hay*
56. Physiological Adaptations in Vertebrates: Respiration, Circulation, and Metabolism, *edited by Stephen C. Wood, Roy E. Weber, Alan R. Hargens, and Ronald W. Millard*
57. The Bronchial Circulation, *edited by John Butler*
58. Lung Cancer Differentiation: Implications for Diagnosis and Treatment, *edited by Samuel D. Bernal and Paul J. Hesketh*
59. Pulmonary Complications of Systemic Disease, *edited by John F. Murray*
60. Lung Vascular Injury: Molecular and Cellular Response, *edited by Arnold Johnson and Thomas J. Ferro*
61. Cytokines of the Lung, *edited by Jason Kelley*
62. The Mast Cell in Health and Disease, *edited by Michael A. Kaliner and Dean D. Metcalfe*
63. Pulmonary Disease in the Elderly Patient, *edited by Donald A. Mahler*

ADDITIONAL VOLUMES IN PREPARATION

Cystic Fibrosis, *edited by Pamela B. Davis*

Signal Transduction in Lung Cells, *edited by Jerome Brody, David M. Center, and Vsevolod Tkachuk*

Pharmacology of the Respiratory Tract: Experimental and Clinical Research, *edited by K. Fan Chung and Peter J. Barnes*

Fluid Solute Transport in the Airspaces of the Lungs, *edited by Richard Effros and H. K. Chang*

Prevention of Respiratory Diseases, *edited by Albert Hirsch, Marcel Goldberg, and J. P. Martin*

Tuberculosis: A Comprehensive International Approach, *edited by Lee Reichman and Earl Hershfield*

THE MAST CELL IN HEALTH AND DISEASE

Edited by

Michael A. Kaliner
Dean D. Metcalfe

National Institute of Allergy and Infectious Diseases
National Institutes of Health
Bethesda, Maryland

Marcel Dekker, Inc. **New York • Basel • Hong Kong**

Library of Congress Cataloging-in-Publication Data

The mast cell in health and disease / edited by Michael A. Kaliner, Dean D. Metcalfe.
p. cm. -- (Lung biology in health and disease ; v. 62)
Includes bibliographical references and indexes.
ISBN 0-8247-8732-3 (alk. paper)
1. Mast cells. 2. Mast cell disease. I. Kaliner, Michael A. II. Metcalfe, Dean D. III. Series.
[DNLM: 1. Mast Cells--congresses. W1 LU62 v. 62 / QS 532.5.C7 M42295]
QR185.8.M35M364 1992
616.07'9--dc20
DNLM/DLC
for Library of Congress 92-49151
CIP

Views expressed in this book are the opinions of the authors and do not constitute official National Institutes of Health opinions.

This book is printed on acid-free paper.

MARCEL DEKKER, INC.
270 Madison Avenue, New York, New York 10016

Current printing (last digit):
10 9 8 7 6 5 4 3 2 1

PRINTED IN THE UNITED STATES OF AMERICA

INTRODUCTION

Mastzellen *(well fed cells), mastocytes, mast cells . . . heparinocytes . . . !*

The mast cells as producers of heparin, histamine, hyaluronic acid, 5-HT . . . !

The "riddle of the mastocytes," mast cell heterogeneity . . . !

It is little wonder that in the Foreword of his book *The Mast Cells* (1965) Hans Selye made the comment: "Ever since its discovery almost a century ago, the mast cell (MC) has excited the curiosity of morphologists and physiologists; more recently it has also acquired interest for pharmacologists, biochemists and clinicians."

Then later he asked, "What is a mast cell?"

Undoubtedly, many before Selye, and many since, have asked this question. Truly, few cells have attracted so much attention for so long. Yet, despite the tremendous amount of scientific investigation that mast cells have generated, the "riddle of the mastocytes" is still not resolved.

In the Preface of this book, *The Mast Cell in Health and Disease,* Drs. Kaliner and Metcalfe underscore the remarkable "momentum of the research in mast cells and their related disorders." Thus, it is exciting and timely that they bring together the latest information available on the biology of these elusive—and always surprising—cells.

This volume is a little different from other monographs of the Lung Biology in Health and Disease series in that it was developed from the proceedings of a workshop held some time back. Thus, each chapter has benefited from open and thoughtful discussion among the participants at that meeting. This has added to the breadth of each contribution as well as to the breadth of the volume as a whole. A review of the Contents confirms this: Topics range from basic biology and pharmacology to disease and its treatment.

Although this volume could have been part of another series of monographs concerned with allergy, I am pleased to have it included in this series for the benefit of those readers with an interest in allergic and pulmonary diseases as well as pulmonary biology. This monograph represents an important building block to ensure that this series is as comprehensive as possible. As such, it should be of great interest to all the readership.

Editors and authors are to be commended for their efforts on behalf of this volume. As the Executive Editor of the series, I am grateful to all of them, but particularly to Dr. Kaliner, who has contributed so much to this entire series.

Claude Lenfant, M.D.
Bethesda, Maryland

PREFACE

About 10 years ago, we wrote a comprehensive review of mast cells that we hoped would provide a lasting reference for the field (Metcalfe, 1981). We underestimated the momentum of the research in mast cells and their related disorders. In the past decade, enormous strides have been taken in recognizing mast cell heterogeneity, the conditions required to culture mast cells, and the influence of lymphocyte-derived cytokines on mast cell differentiation and survival—all topics that did not exist at the time of our review. The receptor for IgE was only a concept in 1981, while it has now been cloned and expressed. The ability to examine mast cell–deficient mice, which were recognized in the last decade, has led to the discovery of a major growth factor for mast cells—the c-kit ligand (stem cell factor), an insight certain to lead to further delineation of the regulation of the growth and differentiation of mast cells. These and other achievements led us to develop a new and more comprehensive book covering mast cell biology. The development of this book was greatly facilitated by the generous assistance of Cedric Grigg of the Fisons Corporation, who supported a meeting held in Florida in December 1990. From that meeting, attended by more than 30 highly select scientists, *The Mast Cell in Health and Disease* was generated. This work was designed to comprehensively review the latest understanding of the mast cell and related diseases. The intention was to write a book that provided scientists with a state-of-the-art review and clinicians with both a reference and a clinical text of mast cell diseases.

Each area of scientific achievement relating to mast cells has been examined. The elucidation of the biochemistry of mast cell activation has kept pace with that of the 1970s with the intriguing new data on the role of phospholipids, G proteins, cyclophilins, and tyrosine phosphorylation in mast cell secretion. The participation of mast cells in the inflammation associated with allergic diseases involves not only activation of mediator release through IgE interacting with allergen, but also histamine releasing factors and cytokines. The latest understanding of the biology of these factors is reviewed. Studies of mast cell mediators have led to recognition of their diversity, the molecular controls of mediator synthesis and secretion, and amazing progress in defining the importance of these mediators clinically. SRS-A has been defined as a related set of sulfido-peptide leukotrienes that may be inhibited in humans in vivo with chemicals now entering clinical trials. PAF has been characterized and has also generated sufficient interest for clinically testable inhibitors to be examined in asthmatics. Histamine receptor antagonists are still the major mediator antagonist used clinically, and in addition to the generation of nonsedating antihistamines, a third receptor, the H-3 receptor, has been discovered. Kinins have received renewed interest due to their elaboration in allergic and inflammatory diseases, including the common cold.

Of course, the major advance in the past decade relates to lymphocyte biology, with the appreciation of the various cytokines. Mast cells also generate and release cytokines. The roles of the cytokines in relationship to allergic diseases are currently being defined and are reviewed in this text.

Mast cell–related diseases include asthma, rhinitis, anaphylaxis, urticaria, and food allergy. Knowledge regarding each of these diseases has advanced enormously in the past decade, and a chapter devoted to each has been included in this book. The major therapeutic advances in the treatment of mast cell diseases have been summarized and updated.

We believe this to be a timely and comprehensive book devoted to the biology of the mast cell, and we hope it will be a standard for the foreseeable future. We have attempted to capture the advances in our knowledge of this subject from the 1980s and early 1990s and place them in a clinical context whenever possible. We hope and judge that we have succeeded and that this reference book will prove useful to clinicians and scientists alike.

Michael A. Kaliner
Dean D. Metcalfe

Reference

Metcalfe, D. D., Donlon, M., and Kaliner, M.: The mast cell. *CRC Crit. Rev. Immunol.* 3:23–74, 1981.

CONTRIBUTORS

Jonathan P. Arm, M.A., M.B.B.S., M.R.C.P., M.D. Lecturer in Medicine, Department of Allergy and Allied Respiratory Diseases, Guy's Hospital, London, England

K. Frank Austen, M.D. Theodore B. Bayles Professor of Medicine, Harvard Medical School, and Chairman, Department of Rheumatology and Immunology, Brigham and Women's Hospital, Boston, Massachusetts

J. Bienenstock, M.D., F.R.C.P.(C.), M.R.C.P., M.B.B.S. Professor, Department of Pathology and Medicine, McMaster University, Hamilton, Ontario, Canada

Parris R. Burd, Ph.D. Senior Staff Fellow, National Institute of Allergy and Infectious Diseases, National Institutes of Health, Bethesda, Maryland

Joseph H. Butterfield, M.D. Consultant, Department of Allergy and Immunology, Mayo Clinic, Rochester, Minnesota

Thomas B. Casale, M. D. Associate Professor of Internal Medicine and Acting Director of the Division of Allergy and Immunology, University of Iowa College of Medicine, Iowa City, Iowa

Diana K. Cavanah, M.D. Fellow, Division of Allergy and Immunology, Department of Internal Medicine, University of Iowa College of Medicine, Iowa City, Iowa

Pandora E. Christie, M.B., M.R.C.P. Research Assistant, Department of Allergy and Allied Respiratory Diseases, Guy's Hospital, London, England

Henry N. Claman Professor, Departments of Medicine and Microbiology/ Immunology, University of Colorado, Denver, Colorado

John J. Costa, M.D. Instructor, Department of Pathology, Beth Israel Hospital and Harvard Medical School, Boston, Massachusetts

Judah A. Denburg, M.D. Professor, Department of Medicine, McMaster University, Hamilton, Ontario, Canada

Barbara L. Deuell, M.D. Instructor, Department of Internal Medicine, University of Virginia, Charlottesville, Virginia

Ratko Djukanović, M.D. Department of Medicine, University of Southampton, Southampton, England

Jerry Dolovich, M.D. Professor, Department of Pediatrics, McMaster University, Hamilton, Ontario, Canada

Ann M. Dvorak, M.D. Professor and Senior Pathologist, Department of Pathology, Harvard Medical School and Beth Israel Hospital, Boston, Massachusetts

Susetta Finotto, Ph.D. Department of Pathology, McMaster University, Hamilton, Ontario, Canada

Takuma Furitsu, M.D. Post-Doctoral Fellow, Division of Allergy, La Jolla Institute for Allergy and Immunology, La Jolla, California

Stephen J. Galli, M.D. Director, Division of Experimental Pathology, Department of Pathology, Beth Israel Hospital, and Associate Professor of Pathology, Harvard Medical School, Boston, Massachusetts

Edwin N. Geissler, Ph.D. Research Associate, Department of Pathology, Beth Israel Hospital, and Assistant Professor of Pathology, Harvard Medical School, Boston, Massachusetts

Lawrence E. Gelber, M.D. Fellow in Allergy, Department of Internal Medicine, University of Virginia, Charlottesville, Virginia

Julie P. Goff Reseach Associate, Division of Virology and Immunology, Department of Microbiology, Georgetown University Medical Center, Rockville, Maryland

Sanford M. Goldstein, M.D. Assistant Clinical Professor, Department of Dermatology, University of California, San Francisco, California

John R. Gordon, Ph.D. Associate Professor, Department of Veterinary Microbiology, Western College of Veterinary Medicine, University of Saskatchewan, Saskatoon, Saskatchewan, Canada

Ilan Hammel, D.Sc. Senior Lecturer, Department of Pathology, Sackler School of Medicine, Tel-Aviv University, Tel-Aviv, Israel

Jon M. Hanifin, M.D. Professor, Department of Dermatology, Oregon Health Sciences University, Portland, Oregon

Mary L. Hayden, R.N., M.S. Research Nurse, Department of Internal Medicine, University of Virginia, Charlottesville, Virginia

Robert J. Hohman, Ph.D. Allergic Diseases Section, National Institute of Allergy and Infectious Diseases, National Institutes of Health, Bethesda, Maryland

Stephen T. Holgate, D.Sc. Department of Medicine, University of Southampton, Southampton, England

Thomas Hultsch, M.D. Allergic Diseases Section, National Institute of Allergy and Infectious Diseases, National Institutes of Health, Bethesda, Maryland

Naoki Inagaki, Ph.D. Postdoctoral Fellow, Division of Allergy, La Jolla Institute for Allergy and Immunology, La Jolla, California

Teruko Ishizaka, M.D., Ph.D. Member and Head, Division of Allergy, La Jolla Institute of Allergy and Immunology, La Jolla, California

Manel Jordana, M.D., Ph.D. Associate Professor, Department of Pathology, McMaster University, Hamilton, Ontario, Canada

Michael A. Kaliner, M.D. Head, Allergic Disease Section, National Institute of Allergy and Infectious Diseases, National Institutes of Health, Bethesda, Maryland

Allen P. Kaplan, M.D. Professor and Chairman, Department of Medicine, State University of New York, Stony Brook, New York

Shin-Ichi Kawabori, M.D. Department of Otolaryngology, Asahikawa Medical School, Asahikawa, Hokkaido, Japan

Donald Kennerly, M.D., Ph.D. Associate Professor, Allergy Division, Department of Internal Medicine, University of Texas Southwestern Medical Center at Dallas, Dallas, Texas

Arnold S. Kirshenbaum, M.D. Assistant Professor, Department of Pediatrics, Johns Hopkins University Hospital, Baltimore, and Director, Allergy Division, Homewood Hospital, Baltimore, and Laboratory of Clinical Investigation, National Institute of Allergy and Infectious Diseases, National Institutes of Health, Bethesda, Maryland

Tak H. Lee, M.D. Department of Allergy, Guy's Hospital, London, England

Chin-Yang Li, M.D. Head, Section of Hematopathology, Department of Laboratory Medicine and Pathology, Mayo Clinic, Rochester, Minnesota

Lawrence M. Lichtenstein, M.D., Ph.D. Professor, Division of Clinical Immunology, Department of Medicine, The Johns Hopkins University School of Medicine, Baltimore, Maryland

Daniel G. Malone, M.D. Associate Professor, Section of Rheumatology, Department of Medicine, University of Wisconsin, Madison, Wisconsin

Jean S. Marshall, Ph.D. Assistant Professor, Department of Pathology, McMaster University, Hamilton, Ontario, Canada

Dean D. Metcalfe, M.D. Head, Mast Cell Physiology Section, National Institute of Allergy and Infectious Diseases, National Institutes of Health, Bethesda, Maryland

Thomas B. Nutman, M.D. Senior Clinical Investigator, Laboratory of Parasitic Diseases, National Institute of Allergy and Infectious Diseases, National Institutes of Health, Bethesda, Maryland

Thomas A. E. Platts-Mills, M.D., Ph.D., F.R.C.P. Professor of Medicine and Microbiology, and Head, Division of Allergy and Clinical Immunology, Department of Medicine, University of Virginia, Charlottesville, Virginia

David Proud, Ph.D. Associate Professor of Medicine, The Johns Hopkins Asthma and Allergy Center, The Johns Hopkins University School of Medicine, Baltimore, Maryland

Dale S. Reynolds, M.D., Ph.D. Harvard Medical School and Brigham and Women's Hospital, Boston, Massachusetts

Juan Rivera, Ph.D. Senior Staff Fellow, Arthritis and Rheumatism Branch, National Institute of Arthritis, Musculoskeletal, and Skin Diseases, National Institutes of Health, Bethesda, Maryland

Menachem Rottem, M.D. Visiting Associate, Laboratory and Clinical Investigation, National Institute of Allergy and Infectious Diseases, National Institutes of Health, Bethesda, Maryland

Hugh A. Sampson, M.D. Professor, Division of Allergy and Immunology, Department of Pediatrics, The Johns Hopkins University School of Medicine, Baltimore, Maryland

Robert P. Schleimer, Ph.D. Associate Professor of Medicine, The Johns Hopkins Asthma and Allergy Center, The Johns Hopkins University School of Medicine, Baltimore, Maryland

Lawrence B. Schwartz, M.D., Ph.D. Charles and Evelyn Thomas Professor of Medicine, Medical College of Virginia, Richmond, Virginia

Thomas Scott, M.D. Medical Staff Fellow, Allergy Diseases Section, Laboratory of Clinical Investigation, National Institute of Allergy and Infectious Disease, National Institutes of Health, Bethesda, Maryland

William E. Serafin, M.D. Assistant Professor, Department of Medicine and Pharmacology, Vanderbilt University School of Medicine, Nashville, Tennessee

R. H. Stead, Ph.D. Assistant Professor, Department of Pathology, McMaster University, Hamilton, Ontario, Canada

Richard L. Stevens, Ph.D. Associate Professor, Department of Medicine, Harvard Medical School, Boston, Massachusetts

Timothy J. Sullivan, M.D. Head, Division of Allergy and Immunology, Department of Internal Medicine and Microbiology, University of Texas Southwestern Medical Center, Dallas, Texas

Yutaka Tagaya, M.D., Ph.D. Research Associate, Division of Immunobiology, La Jolla Institute for Allergy and Immunology, La Jolla, California

Helen L. Thompson, Ph.D. Fogarty Visiting Scientist, Mast Cell Physiology Section, Laboratory of Clinical Investigation, National Institute of Allergy and Infectious Diseases, National Institutes of Health, Bethesda, Maryland

Alkis G. Togias, M.D. Assistant Professor in Medicine, Division of Clinical Immunology, The Johns Hopkins University School of Medicine, Baltimore, Maryland

William D. Travis, M.D. Laboratory of Pathology, National Cancer Institute, National Institutes of Health, Bethesda, Maryland

Mindy Tsai, B.D.S., D.M.Sc. Post-Doctoral Research Fellow, Department of Pathology, Beth Israel Hospital, Boston, Massachusetts

George W. Ward, Jr., Ph.D. Associate Professor, Department of Internal Medicine, University of Virginia, Charlottesville, Virginia

Barry K. Wershil, M.D. Clinical Associate in Pediatrics, Massachusetts General Hospital, and Research Associate, Department of Pathology, and Assistant Professor, Department of Pediatrics, Harvard Medical School, Boston, Massachusetts

Martha V. White, Ph.D. Senior Staff Fellow, Department of Allergic Diseases, National Institute of Allergy and Infectious Diseases, National Institutes of Health, Bethesda, Maryland

Bruce U. Wintroub, M.D. Professor and Chairman, Department of Dermatology, University of California, San Francisco, California

CONTENTS

1

Human Mast Cells

Ultrastructural Observations of In Situ, Ex Vivo, and In Vitro Sites, Sources, and Systems

ANN M. DVORAK

Harvard Medical School
and Beth Israel Hospital
Boston, Massachusetts

I. Introduction

Morphology-oriented investigators have been fascinated with human mast cells since their original description based on the affinity of their cytoplasmic granules to metachromatic dyes (Ehrlich, 1877). The apparent wide distribution of mast cells and their unique ultrastructural granule patterns have similarly fascinated ultrastructural investigators (reviewed in Dvorak AM, 1989c, 1991a). Although difficulties may arise in the identification/delineation of mast cells from cells of different lineages, the ultrastructural anatomy of human mast cells is sufficiently unique that they may be identified with certainty by specific ultrastructural criteria in various in situ, ex vivo, and in vitro sites, sources, and systems (Table 1). In this review, we present our ultrastructural observations based on examination of human mast cells in these various circumstances. The major disease entities in which we have studied human mast cells, often as a by-product of other ongoing investigations, are listed in Table 2. These diseases span an extensive range of human affliction, including the following pathological processes: acute and chronic inflammation, cell injury, lysosomal storage diseases, delayed hypersensitivity, neoplasia, graft rejection, arthritis, and various inflammatory and fibrotic diseases of uncertain origin (e.g., bullous pemphigoid,

Table 1 In Situ, Ex Vivo, and In Vitro Sites, Sources, and Systems upon Which Ultrastructural Observations of Human Mast Cells Are Based

Site	Source	System	In Vivo	Ex Vivo	In Vitro	References
Kidney			+			Colvin et al., 1974; Dvorak, A. M. and Monahan, 1985
Skin			+			Cable et al., 1982; Dickersin et al., 1980; Dienstag et al., 1978; Dvorak, A. M., 1988b; Dvorak, A. M., 1989c; Dvorak, A. M., 1991; Dvorak, A.M., 1992; Dvorak, A. M. and Kissell, 1991; Dvorak, A. M. et al., 1976; Dvorak, A. M. et al., 1980b; Dvorak, A. M. et al., 1981; Dvorak, A. M. et al., 1982; Dvorak, H. F. et al., 1974; Dvorak, H. F. et al., 1976; Dvorak, H. F. et al., 1980a; Dvorak, H. F. et al., 1986; Galli et al., 1984; Schnitt et al., 1986
Skin		Grafts	+			Dvorak, H. F. et al., 1979; Dvorak, H. F., et al. 1980b
Skin		Wound healing	+			Dvorak, A. M. and Kissell, 1991
	Skin			+		Dvorak, A. M. et al., 1991c
Gastrointestinal			+			Dvorak, A. M., 1979; Dvorak, A. M., 1988b; Dvorak, A. M., 1988c; Dvorak, A. M., 1988d; Dvorak, A. M., 1989a; Dvorak, A. M., 1989b; Dvorak, A. M., 1989c; Dvorak, A. M., 1989d; Dvorak, A. M., 1989f; Dvorak, A. M., 1991a; Dvorak, A. M., 1991b; Dvorak, A. M., 1992; Dvorak, A. M. and Dickersin, 1979; Dvorak, A. M. and Monohan, 1983; Dvorak, A. M. and Monahan, 1984a; Dvorak, A. M. and Monahan, 1984b; Dvorak, A. M. and Silen, 1985; Dvorak, A. M. et al., 1978; Dvorak, A. M. et al., 1980c; Dvorak, A. M. et al., 1992a; Dvorak, A. M. et al., 1992b; Dvorak, A. M. et al., 1992c; Dvorak, A. M. et al.,1992d; Galli et al., 1984; Galli et al., 1990
		Colon		+		Dvorak, A. M., 1989c; Fox et al., 1985
Breast			+			Dvorak, A. M., 1989c; Dvorak, A. M., 1989d; Dvorak, A. M., 1991a; Dvorak, A. M., 1992; Dvorak, A. M. and Kissell, 1991, Dvorak, H. F. et al., 1981

Multiple		Benign tumors and primary and metastatic malignant tumors	+			Dvorak, A. M., 1987; Dvorak, A. M., 1989b; Dvorak, A. M., 1989d; Dvorak and Kissell, 1991; Dvorak, A. M. and Monahan, 1982; Dvorak, A. M. and Monahan-Earley, 1985; Dvorak, A. M. and Monahan-Earley, 1986; Dvorak, A. M. and Monahan-Earley, R. A., 1992; Dvorak, A. M. et al., 1980b; Dvorak, A. M. et al., 1992a; A. M. Dvorak et al., 1992b; Dvorak, H. F. et al., 1981; Harris et al., 1982; Peters et al., 1989; Schnitt et al., 1986
Lymph Node			+			Dvorak, A. M., 1987; Dvorak, A. M. and Monahan-Earley, 1986; Harris et al., 1982
Lung			+			Dvorak, A. M., 1989c; Dvorak, A. M., 1991a; Dvorak, A. M., 1992; Dvorak, A. M. and Monahan-Earley, 1985; Peters et al., 1989
	Lung			+		Dvorak, A. M., 1986b; Dvorak, A. M., 1988b; Dvorak, A. M., 1989c; Dvorak, A. M., 1989e; Dvorak, A. M., 1991a; Dvorak, A. M., 1992; Dvorak, A. M. et al., 1983a; Dvorak, A. M. et al., 1983b; Dvorak, A. M. et al., 1983c; Dvorak, A. M. et al., 1984; Dvorak, A. M. et al., 1985b; Dvorak, A. M. et al., 1986; Dvorak, A. M. et al., 1987; Dvorak, A. M. et al., 1988; Galli et al., 1984; Galli et al., 1985; Hammel et al., 1985; Peters et al., 1987; Peters et al., 1989
	Lung	Isolated mast cells cocultured with 3T3 fibroblasts			+	Dvorak, A. M. and Ishizaka, T., 1992; Dvorak, A. M. et al., 1991d
Heart			+			Dvorak, A. M., 1986a
Synovium			+			Dvorak, A. M., unpublished data
	Synovium			+		Kopicky-Burd et al., 1988
	Uterus			+		Massey et al., 1991
	Cord blood cells	Cocultured with 3T3 fibroblasts			+	Furitsu et al., 1989; Dvorak, A. M. and Ishizaka T, 1992; Dvorak et al., 1992e

Table 2 Human Diseases upon Which Ultrastructural Observations of Human Mast Cells Are Based

Disease	Reference
Chronic glomerulonephritis	Colvin et al., 1974
Contact allergy	Dvorak, A. M., 1988b; Dvorak, A. M., 1989c; Dvorak, A. M., 1991a; Dvorak, A. M., 1992; Dvorak, A. M. et al., 1976; Dvorak, H. F. et al., 1974; Dvorak, H. F. et al., 1976; Dvorak, H. F. et al., 1980a; Dvorak, H. F. et al., 1986; Galli et al., 1984
Primary benign and malignant tumors; metastatic tumors	Dvorak, A. M., 1987; Dvorak, A. M., 1989b; Dvorak, A. M., 1989d; Dvorak, A. M., 1992; Dvorak, A. M. and Kissell, 1991; Dvorak, A. M. and Monahan, 1982; Dvorak, A. M. and Monahan, 1985; Dvorak, A. M. and Monahan-Early, 1985; Dvorak, A. M. and Monahan-Earley, 1986; Dvorak, A. M. and Monahan-Earley, R. A., 1992; Dvorak, A. M. et al., 1980b; Dvorak, A. M. et al., 1992a; Dvorak, H. F. et al., 1981; Harris et al., 1982; Peters et al., 1989; Schnitt et al., 1986
Uticaria associated with acute viral hepatitis type B	Dienstag et al., 1978
Graft rejection	Dvorak, H. F. et al., 1979; Dvorak, H. F. et al., 1980b
Mannosidosis	Dickersin et al., 1980
Fabry's disease	Cable et al., 1982; Dvorak, A. M. et al., 1981
Crohn's disease	Dvorak, A. M., 1979; Dvorak, A. M., 1988c; Dvorak, A. M., 1988d; Dvorak, A. M., 1989a; Dvorak, A. M., 1991b; Dvorak, A. M. and Dickersin, 1979; Dvorak, A. M. and Monahan, 1983; Dvorak, A. M. and Monahan, 1984a; Dvorak, A. M. and Silen, 1985; Dvorak, A. M. et al., 1978; Dvorak, A. M. et al., 1980c; Dvorak, A. M. et al., 1992a; Dvorak, A. M. et al., 1992b
Whipple's disease	Dvorak, A. M., 1989f; Dvorak, A. M. and Monahan, 1984b
Ulcerative colitis	Dvorak, A. M. and Silen, 1985; Dvorak, A. M. et al., 1992a; Dvorak, A. M. et al., 1992b

Table 2 Continued

Disease	Reference
Familial polyposis syndrome	Dvorak, A. M. et al., 1992a; Dvorak, A. M. et al., 1992b
Scleroderma lung disease	Dvorak, A. M. and Monahan-Earley, 1985
Interstitial fibrosis of the lung	Dvorak, A. M. and Monahan-Earley, 1985; Peters et al., 1989; Dvorak, A. M., unpublished data
Rheumatoid arthritis	Kopicky-Burd et al., 1988; Dvorak, A. M., unpublished data
Osteoarthritis	Kopicky-Burd et al., 1988
Sclerosing hemangioma of the lung	Dvorak, A. M., unpublished data
Amyloidosis	Dvorak, A. M., unpublished data

Crohn's disease, ulcerative colitis, Whipple's disease, scleroderma, interstitial lung fibrosis). In all these investigations, clinically and pathologically normal tissues adjacent to the diseased areas were also examined. In addition, biopsy samples of nondiseased tissues were regularly available to our diagnostic unit, as resection margins and other specimens were submitted for examination. We present ultrastructural criteria for the identification of human mast cells and, of equal importance, criteria for the identification of other cell lineages with which mast cells have been confused (Table 3). Even when mast cells, partly or completely devoid of granules or their contents, are present, they can be reliably distinguished from other lineages by the absence of key features (or a constellation of features) that facilitate positive cellular identifications in ultrastructural samples. We have organized this review of our experience by organ or tissue sites with which we have sufficient experience to adduce the status of mast cells contained therein. Thus, we discuss human lung mast cells first, followed by mast cells of the gastrointestinal system, heart, synovium, skin, and uterus. Our observations include those of in situ biopsies (often obtained for diagnostic purposes), those related to purified mast cell suspensions from various sites (lung, skin, colon, synovium, uterus), and mast cells in two culture systems–lung mast cells maintained on 3T3 feeder layers and mast cells developing from cord blood cells cultured on 3T3 cells. In some instances, such as in the latter system, our studies are quite preliminary (Dvorak AM and Ishizaka T, unpublished data; Furitsu et al., 1989).

Ultrastructural studies of human mast cells provide not only the necessary means of definitive cell lineage identifications, but also windows of insight into mast cell biological mechanisms. We present our observations regarding the possible role of a specific cellular organelle—the lipid body—in arachidonic acid metabolic cellular affairs (Tables 4 and 5) and the widespread ultrastructural

Table 3 Key Ultrastructural Cellular Criteria That Are Important for Identification of Human Mast Cells and Subsequent Differentiation of Mast Cells from Cells with Which They Have Been Confused

Cell	Criteria	References
Mast cell	Narrow surface folds, lipid bodies, monolobed nucleus; scroll, crystal, particle, and mixed granules; free ribosomes > membrane-bound ribosomes; extensive cytoplasmic filaments	Dvorak, A. M., 1986b; Dvorak, A. M., 1988a; Dvorak, A. M., 1988b; Dvorak, A. M., 1989c; Dvorak, A. M., 1991a; Dvorak, A. M., 1992; Dvorak, A. M. and Kissell, S. 1991; Dvorak, A. M. et al., 1983a; Dvorak, A. M. et al., 1984; Furitsu et al., 1989
Mature basophil	Polylobed granulocyte nucleus, particle granules, intragranular, multiple dense membranes, Charcot-Leyden crystals, broad surface processes, glycogen	Dvorak, A. M., 1978; Dvorak, A. M., 1986b; Dvorak, A. M., 1988a; Dvorak, A. M., 1988b; Dvorak, A. M., 1989c; Dvorak, A. M., 1991a; Dvorak, A. M., 1992; Dvorak, A. M. et al., 1983a; Dvorak, A. M. et al., 1985a; Dvorak, A. M. et al., 1989; Ishizaka et al., 1985
Basophylic myelocyte	Monolobed, lobular nucleus with partly dispersed chromatin, rough endoplasmic reticulum (RER) with dilated, full cisterns, immature, large particle granules, active Golgi area	Dvorak, A. M., 1986b; Dvorak, A. M., 1987; Dvorak, A. M., 1988a; Dvorak, A. M., 1988b; Dvorak, A. M., 1991a; Dvorak, A. M., 1992; Dvorak, A. M. et al., 1983a; Dvorak, A. M. et al., 1985a
Eosinophilic myelocyte	Monolobed, lobular nucleus with partly dispersed chromatin, RER with dilated, full cisterns, large, immature, homogeneously dense granules, endogenous peroxidase in immature granules, and cisterns of RER and perinuclear area, active Golgi area	Dvorak, A. M., 1987; Dvorak, A. M., 1988a; Dvorak, A. M. et al., 1985a; Dvorak, A. M. et al., 1991a; Saito et al., 1988
Macrophage	Active surface and cytoplasmic endocytotic-vacuolar structures, lysosomes, nondilated RER, lobular, single nucleus with partly condensed chromatin, lipid bodies	Ciano et al., 1986; Dvorak, A. M., 1987; Dvorak, A. M. et al., 1980a; Dvorak, A. M. et al., 1983b; Dvorak, A. M. et al., 1989; Dvorak, A. M. et al., 1990; Dvorak, A. M. et al., 1991b; Lanir et al., 1988; Monahan et al., 1981
Fibroblasts	Extensive dilated, full cisterns of RER, lipid bodies, active Golgi area, lysosomes, stellate to spindle-shaped cells	Brown et al., 1992; Dvorak, A. M., 1987; Dvorak, A. M., and Monahan-Earley, 1992; Dvorak, A. M. et al., 1979; Hammond et al., 1974

Table 4 Cell Types Within Which Electron Microscopic Autoradiography Has Localized [^{3}H] Arachidonic Acid to Lipid Bodies

Cell	Species	Reference
Mast cell	Human	Dvorak, A. M. et al., 1983b; Dvorak, A. M. et al., 1984; Dvorak, A. M. et al., 1992f; Galli et al., 1985
Macrophage	Human, guinea pig, mouse	Dvorak, A. M. et al., 1983b; Dvorak, A. M. et al., 1992f; Gali et al., 1985
Eosinophil	Human	Weller and Dvorak, A. M., 1985; Weller et al., 1991a
Line 10 hepatocarcinoma	Guinea pig	Galli et al., 1985
Ciliated respiratory epithelium	Human	Galli et al., 1985
Lymphocyte	Mouse	Galli et al., 1985
Reproductive system	*Brugia malayi*	Longworth et al., 1988
Neutrophil	Human	Weller et al., 1989; Weller et al., 1991b

Table 5 Lipid Bodies in Human Mast Cells from Individual Organ Sites or Sources

Site	Circumstance	Lipid bodies
Skin	In situ biopsy	Virtually never present
Skin	Ex vivo cells	Small numbers present
Lung	In situ biopsy	Present
Lung	Ex vivo cells	Present
Lung	Anti-IgE-stimulated anaphylactic degranulation (AND)	Decreased, early
Lung	Recovery from AND	Increased, late
Lung	In vitro (isolated mast cells cocultured with 3T3 cells)	Present
Intestine	In situ biopsy	Present
Intestine	Ex vivo cells	Present; numerous round lucencies within dense structure
Synovium	Ex vivo cells	Rare
Uterus	Ex vivo cells	Present in large numbers; large and small round lucencies within dense structure
Heart	In situ biopsy	Rare
Cord blood cells	In vitro (cocultured with 3T3 cells)	Rare

Table 6 Ultrastructural Identification of Piecemeal and Anaphylactic Degranulation of Human Mast Cells in Unstimulated Biopsy Samples

Degranulation morphotype	Organ	Disease	Reference
Anaphylactic degranulation	Intestine	Crohn's disease	Dvorak, A. M. et al., 1992b
Anaphylactic degranulation	Intestine	Ulcerative colitis	Dvorak, A. M. et al., 1992b
Anaphylactic degranulation	Heart		Dvorak, A. M., 1986a
Piecemeal degranulation	Kidney	Chronic glomerulonephritis	Colvin et al., 1974
Piecemeal degranulation	Skin	Allergic contact dermatitis	Dvorak, A. M. et al., 1976; Dvorak, H. F. et al., 1976
Piecemeal degranulation	Skin	Allograft rejection	Dvorak, A. M., 1978; Dvorak, A. M., unpublished data
Piecemeal degranulation	Intestine	Crohn's disease	Dvorak, A. M., 1988c; Dvorak, A. M. and Dickersin, 1979; Dvorak, A. M. and Silen, 1985; Dvorak, A. M. et al., 1980c; Dvorak, A. M. et al., 1992b
Piecemeal degranulation	Intestine	Ulcerative colitis	Dvorak, A. M. et al., 1992b
Piecemeal degranulation	Skin	Melanoma	Dvorak, A. M., et al., 1980b
Piecemeal degranulation	Skin	Bullous pemphigoid	Dvorak, A. M. and Kissell, 1991; Dvorak, A. M. et al., 1982
Piecemeal degranulation	Kidney	Adenoma	Dvorak, A. M. and Monahan, 1985
Piecemeal degranulation	Lung	Interstitial fibrosis	Dvorak, A. M., unpublished data
Piecemeal degranulation	Intestine	Whipple's disease	Dvorak, A. M. and Monahan, 1984b
Piecemeal degranulation	Multiple	Multiple neoplastic lesions	Dvorak, A. M., 1992; Dvorak, A. M., unpublished data

presence of piecemeal degranulation in tissue mast cells in disease (Table 6). These observations provide the necessary background for subsequent functional and biochemical analyses of human mast cell populations in or from individual organ sites in health and disease.

II. Human Lung Mast Cells

A. In Situ

Ultrastructural biopsy material from human lungs includes tissue from a wide variety of primary and metastatic malignant tumors, benign neoplastic tumors, mast-cell-rich, so-called sclerosing hemangiomas, and pulmonary interstitial fibrosis of variable etiologies (Dvorak AM, unpublished data). In one case, biopsy material from pulmonary fibrosis accompanying scleroderma lung disease and widespread bronchioloalveolar carcinoma was examined (Dvorak AM and Monahan-Earley, 1985). Human lung mast cells (HLMC) in these settings contain a majority of scroll-filled granules (Kawanami et al., 1979; Peters et al.,

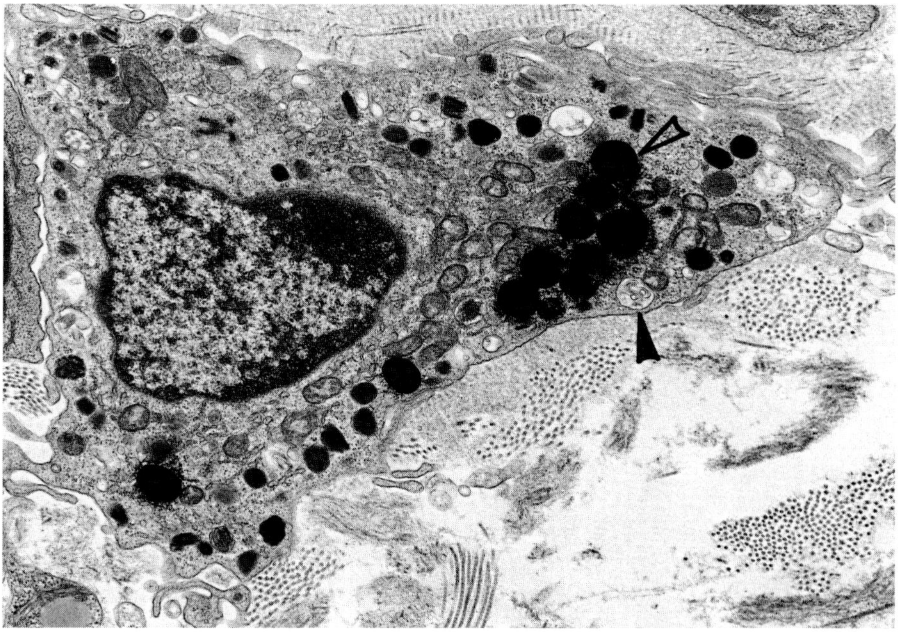

Figure 1 HLMC in situ in alveolar cell carcinoma of lung shows primarily scroll granules and a cluster of large, round, dense lipid bodies (open arrowhead). Some granules show PMD, partial or complete losses from granule containers (closed arrowhead). ×11,000.

1989; Warton et al., 1986), numerous lipid bodies, and variable ultrastructural evidence of piecemeal degranulation (PMD) (Fig. 1). Certain features of cellular immaturity, such as large nuclei with dispersed chromatin and large nucleoli, diminished numbers of granules, expanded Golgi areas, and free and membrane-bound ribosomes, can also be found in mast cells within this material. In addition to the scroll granules, HLMC have granules containing homogeneously dense material, particles, crystalline arrays of several periodicities and orientations, and mixtures of these patterns (Kawanami et al., 1979; Peters et al., 1989; Warton et al., 1986). Some granules contain thickened, irregular, or concentric threads; other granules display homogeneously dense central nucleoids, a feature we note more frequently in immature cells than in fully granulated mature cells (Dvorak AM et al., 1976; Dvorak AM et al., 1992a; Dvorak AM et al., 1992e; Dvorak HF et al., 1974, 1976, 1979, 1980b). While some individual mast cells contain granule patterns that are all generally alike, other mast cells display individual granules that are filled with either scrolls, crystals, particles, or homogeneously dense material; and yet other mast cells display individual granules with mixtures of these patterns. Thus, remarkable morphologic diversity exists in lung mast cells in situ.

B. Ex Vivo

The morphological diversity of HLMC noted in situ extends to these cells when they are removed from excised human lungs containing malignant tumors and partially purified by a variety of established methods (Schulman et al., 1982) (Figs. 2–6). Despite the described variability, human mast cells prepared from this source express mostly scroll granules and numerous lipid bodies (Dvorak AM et al., 1983b; Dvorak AM et al., 1984) as in in situ samples (Haslam et al., 1987; Kawanami et al., 1979; Peters et al., 1989) (Figs. 2, 6). Initially, we examined these purified mast cell preparations after each step in the isolation procedures: i.e., mechanical and enzymatic dispersion, separation using an IgE-mediated affinity technique, countercurrent centrifugation elutriation, centrifugation over discontinuous Percoll gradients, overnight culture, and periodic culture intervals over a 48-hr period (Dvorak AM, 1989e; Dvorak AM et al., 1984, 1985b). These studies validated this model for future studies of stimulated release and recovery reactions. Examination of the ex vivo mast cells from human lung revealed well-preserved cells that showed progressively less evidence of individual granule swelling with time after the initial separation from lung parenchyma (Dvorak AM et al., 1985b). Particularly, we noted that ≈5% of the granules so affected completely resolved following overnight culture (Dvorak AM, 1989e). Granule fusions, degranulation channels, and granule extrusion were not present in control isolated cells. Therefore, it is clear that the isolation procedures did not induce the morphology associated with anaphylactic degranulation (AND), and it is also clear that the isolation-induced granule

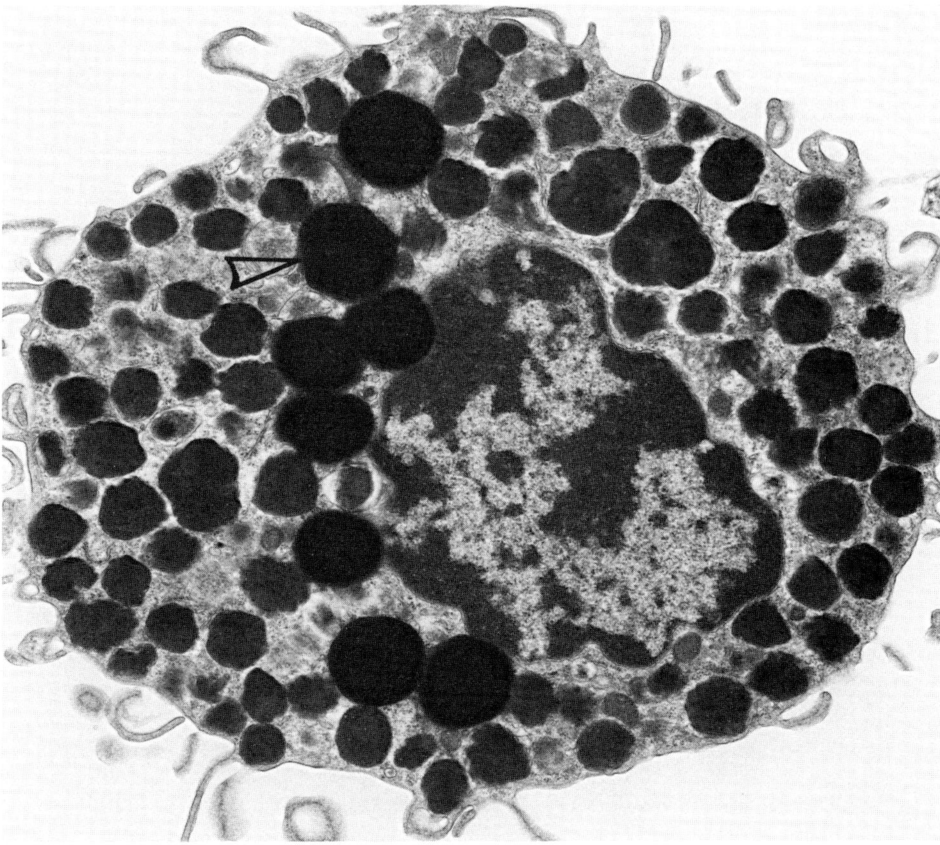

Figure 2 HLMC ex vivo shows numerous dense scroll granules, larger dense lipid bodies (arrowhead), a monolobed nucleus, and narrow surface folds. ×15,000. (From Dvorak, A. M., 1989e, with permission.)

swelling is reversible. Thus, human mast cell granules can individually expand and condense their granule contents in samples showing small, spontaneous histamine release values (Dvorak AM, 1989e; Dvorak AM et al., 1984, 1985b).

We used isolated HLMC to examine their IgE-mediated release and recovery reactions (Dvorak AM, 1989e; Dvorak AM et al., 1984, 1985b, 1986, 1987, 1988). In this setting, we found that HLMCs generally developed a sequence of granule swelling, matrix alterations, and membrane fusions to form intracytoplasmic degranulation chambers within which granules solubilized prior to their release (Fig. 7). Similar findings in part were presented by Caulfield et al. (1980) using isolated HLMCs. We also noted release of arachidonic acid-rich lipid bodies into degranulation chambers (Dvorak AM et al., 1983b, 1984). The

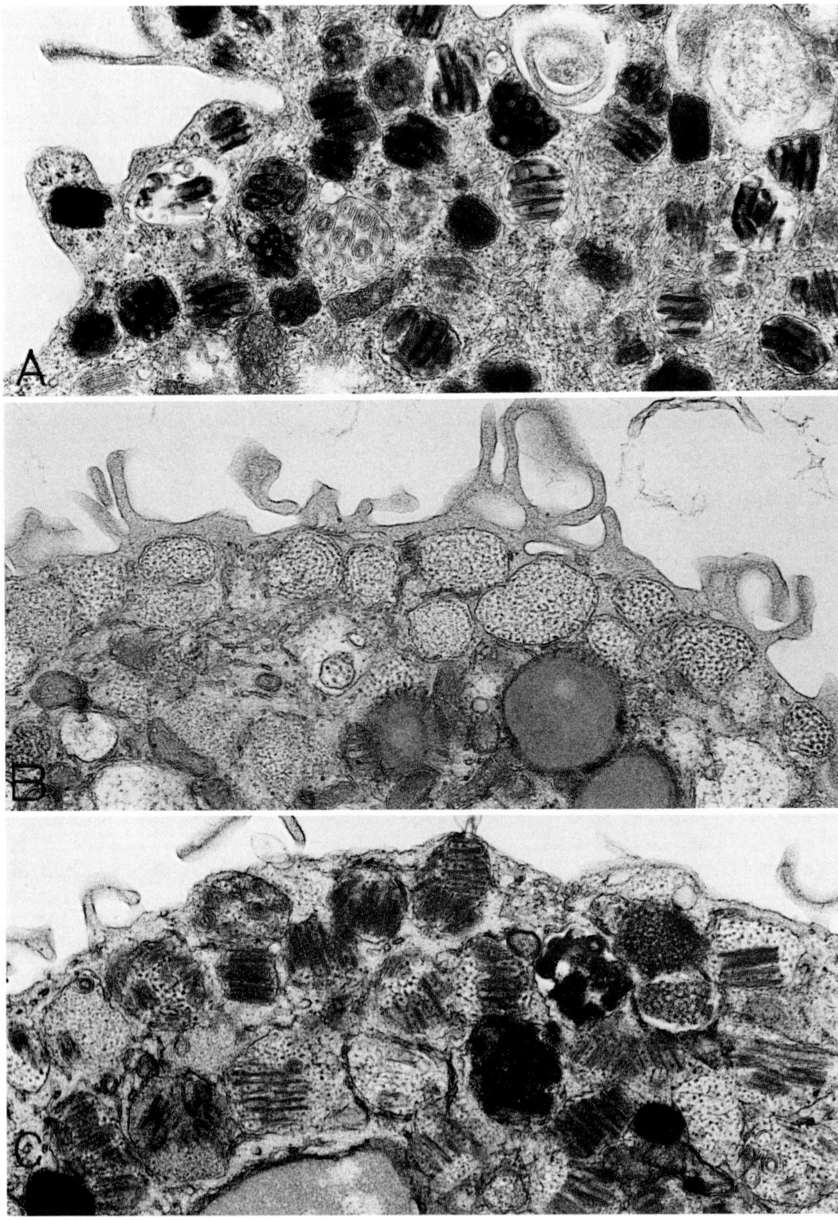

Figure 3 HLMCs ex vivo show basic granule patterns: scrolls (A), particles (B), and mixed scrolls and particles (C). (A) ×21,000; (B) ×23,500; (C) ×23,000. (A, C, From Dvorak, A. M., 1989c, with permission; B, from Dvorak, A. M., 1988a, with permission.)

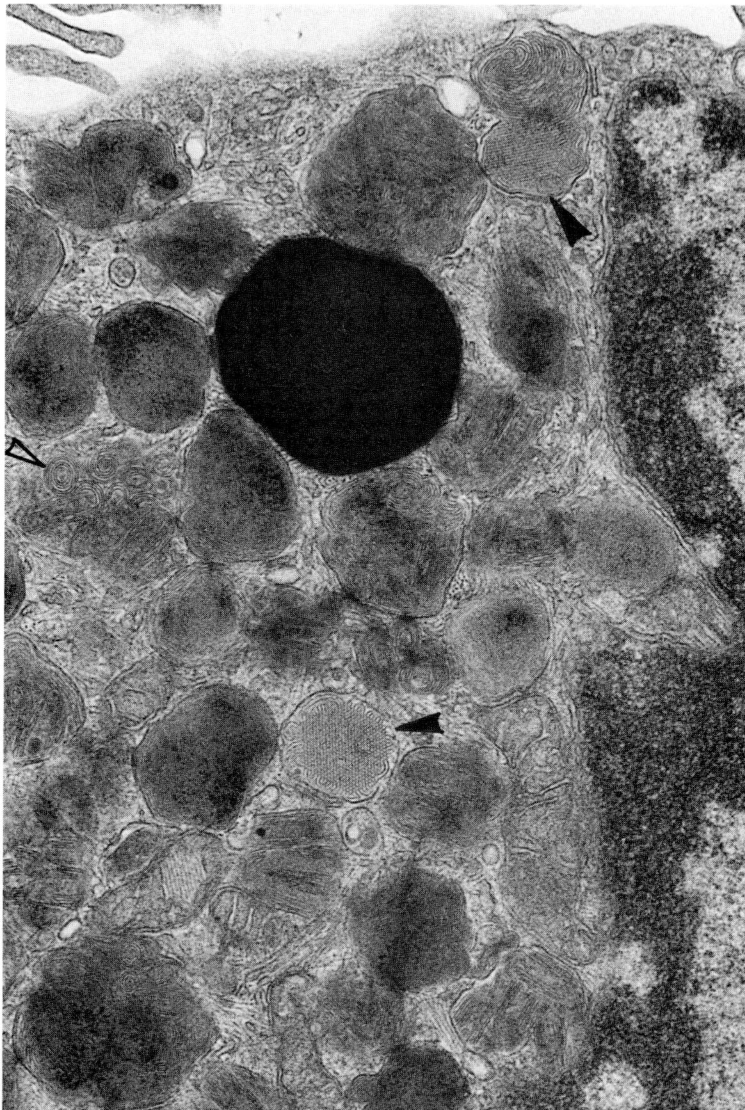

Figure 4 HLMC ex vivo, cultured and recovered 18 hr after anaphylactic degranulation, shows a single, large, round, dense lipid body and numerous crystal (closed arrowheads) or scroll (open arrowhead) granules. ×54,500. (From Dvorak, A. M., 1991a, with permission.)

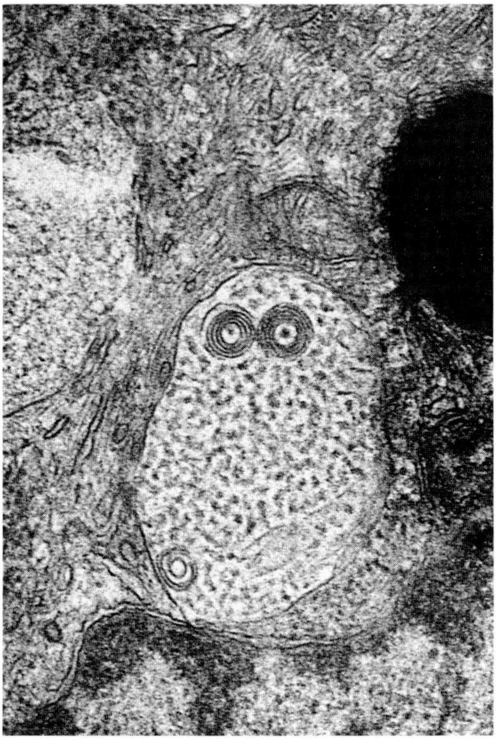

Figure 5 HLMC ex vivo, cultured for 18 hr after isolation, shows a mixed granule containing particles and scrolls adjacent to an osmiophilic lipid body enmeshed in cytoplasmic filaments. ×49,000. (From Dvorak, A. M., 1991a, with permission.)

incidence of this event was small, however. In one kinetic experiment, we noted direct extrusion of membrane-free, altered granule matrices through plasma membrane pores to the exterior (Fig. 8). Thus, this route for granule release was minor in the kinetic experiments we did with isolated HLMCs. Extensive amplification of HLMC surfaces accompanied AND, and some cells shed membranes and processes with their associated, altered granules as intracytoplasmic degranulation channels were exteriorized (Fig. 8).

We followed the recovery of HLMCs from these stimulated release reactions in short-term cultures (Dvorak AM, 1989e; Dvorak AM et al., 1986, 1987, 1988). By 48 hr after AND, a majority of the cells in recovering samples were fully granulated. This occurred in the absence of mitosis, cell death, and, in this closed ex vivo system, recruitment of immature, granule-free precursors. We noted three major morphological processes contributing to the recovery of HLMCs: (1) conservation of degranulation chamber membranes and contents as

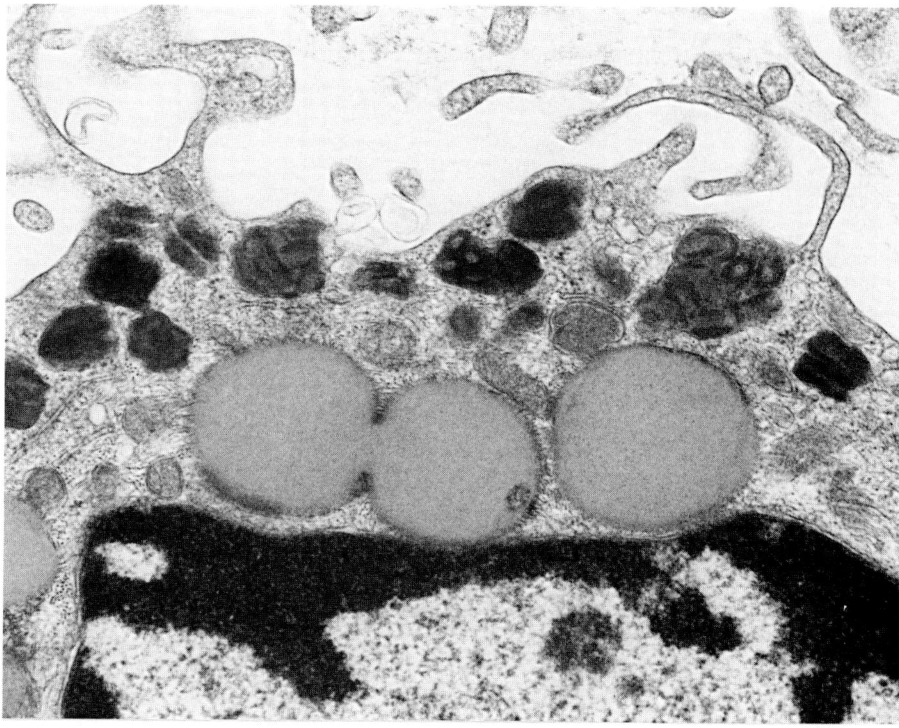

Figure 6 HLMC ex vivo shows peripheral scroll granules and fused, lightly dense lipid bodies adjacent to the nucleus. ×32,000. (From Dvorak, A. M., 1991a, with permission.)

crystallization, condensation, and separation contributed to new granule domains (Dvorak AM et al., 1986) (Figs. 9–15); (2) synthesis of new granules (Dvorak AM et al., 1988) (Fig. 16); (3) blastogenesis of small, granule-poor, immature mast cells to produce a continuum of mast cells that were enlarging in size and granule contents (Dvorak AM, 1989e; Dvorak AM et al., 1987) (Fig. 17). As this process developed, extraordinary numbers of lipid bodies were present in the cytoplasm (Fig. 18). Thus, HLMCs use these multiple morphological mechanisms to effect their recovery from the explosive release reaction induced by crosslinking IgE receptors on their surfaces.

C. In Vitro

Isolated, enriched HLMCs cocultured with 3T3 fibroblasts display excellent viability (Dvorak AM and Ishizaka T, 1992; Dvorak AM et al., 1991d; Levi-Schaffer et al., 1987). In one study, biochemical information was accrued on

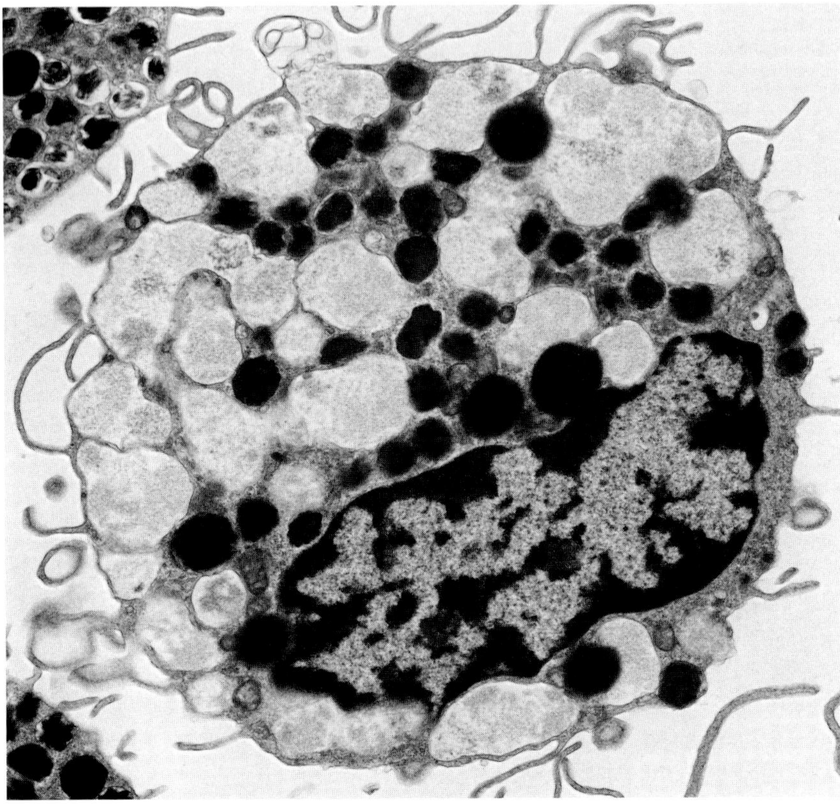

Figure 7 HLMC ex vivo, 5 min after stimulation with anti-IgE, shows degranulation channels filled with altered granule matrix materials. Some granules are unaltered. Larger lipid bodies are adjacent to degranulation channels. ×10,000. (From Dvorak, A. M., 1989e, with permission.)

HLMCs maintained in cultures up to 13 days after isolation from lung; ultrastructural analysis was done on HLMCs recovered at 7 days after coculture with 3T3 cells (Levi-Schaffer et al., 1987). These studies showed that HLMCs, cocultured in this manner, released histamine and generated and released arachidonic acid metabolites when stimulated with antihuman IgE. In contrast to freshly isolated HLMCs, the cocultured mast cells generated LTC_4 and LTB_4 by the 5-lipoxygenase pathway and considerably increased the amount of PGD_2 generated and released by the cyclooxygenase pathway over freshly isolated cells. Ultrastructural studies showed that the cultured HLMCs resembled mast cells in vivo and displayed scroll granules (Levi-Schaffer et al., 1987).

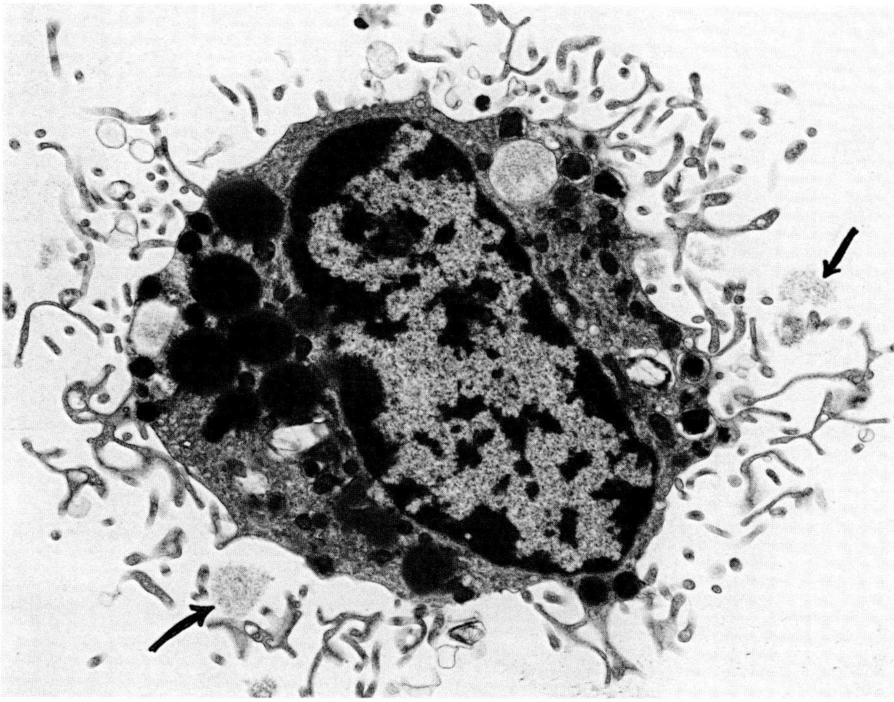

Figure 8 HLMC ex vivo, fixed 20 min after exposure to anti-IgE, shows extruded, membrane-free, swollen granules (arrows) among markedly elongated and shed surface folds. ×7,000. (From Dvorak, A. M., 1988b, with permission.)

We also examined isolated HLMCs cocultured with 3T3 fibroblasts or alone for extended periods of time by electron microscopy (Dvorak AM and Ishizaka T, 1992; Dvorak AM et al., 1991d). In this case, we recovered mast cells cultured for 4 weeks in either the presence or absence of mouse 3T3 cells and prepared them for electron microscopy. The cells were 95% viable in both cases by trypan blue dye exclusion; 32% of the nonadherent cells were mast cells in cultures without 3T3 fibroblasts, and 49% were mast cells in cocultures with 3T3 cells. By ultrastructural criteria, HLMCs retained excellent viability in each culture instance and retained the principal morphotype of HLMCs in vivo, whether cultured with (Fig. 19) or without 3T3 cells (Fig. 20). For example, the predominant granule pattern contained scrolls (Fig. 21); the next most frequent pattern contained particles (Fig. 22), and crystal granules were rare. Individual cells with both scroll and particle granules were present (Fig. 22); cells with scroll and crystal granules were infrequent. In both types of long-term cultures of

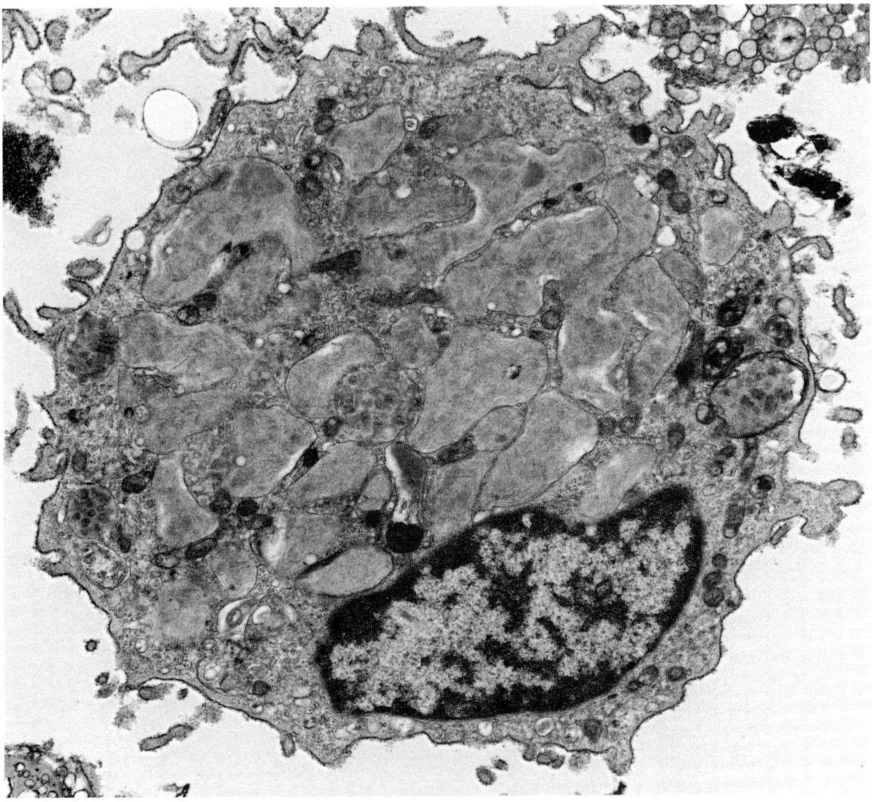

Figure 9 HLMC ex vivo, recovered 12 hr after stimulation with anti-IgE, shows conservation of channel containers as degranulation channels are partitioned into new granule domains. All channel-granule contents have condensed, and scroll patterns have emerged. ×11,000. (From Dvorak, A. M. et al., 1986, with permission.)

HLMCs, well-preserved mast cells contained large numbers of lipid bodies (Figs. 19, 20, 23) and a full complement of granules that showed no evidence of granule content swelling, alteration, or losses (Figs. 19–21, 24). Thus, the ultrastructural data show that isolated HLMCs have the capacity to thrive in long-term cultures (of ≈1 month) with or without added mouse 3T3 cells and to retain the in vivo morphotype of lung mast cells. Further, these cultured HLMCs show no evidence of granule losses, granule perturbation (swelling), or piecemeal losses of contents (Dvorak AM and Ishizaka T, 1992; Dvorak AM et al., 1991d). Biochemical studies of HLMCs cultured for 2 weeks with 3T3 cells showed normal and enhanced functional capacities (Levi-Schaffer et al., 1987), supporting the ultrastructural analysis of cellular preservation (Dvorak AM and Ishizaka T, 1992; Dvorak AM et al., 1991d).

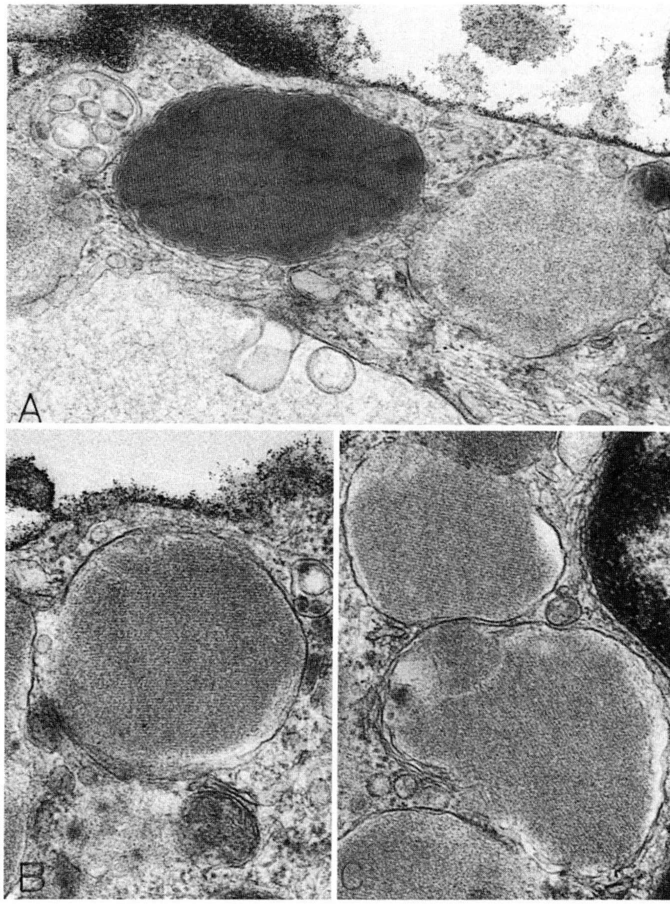

Figure 10 HLMCs ex vivo, recovered 12 hr (B,C) and 24 h (A) after exposure to anti-IgE, show newly formed crystal granules. (A) ×45,000; (B,C) ×48,000. (A, From Dvorak, A. M. et al., 1986, with permission; B,C, from Dvorak, A. M., 1989c, with permission.)

III. Human Gastrointestinal System Mast Cells

A. In Situ

Ultrastructural material for these observations includes examination of material rapidly obtained from ileocolectomy specimens (Dvorak AM, 1979; Dvorak AM and Dickersin, 1979; Dvorak AM and Monahan, 1983, 1984a; Dvorak AM et al., 1978, 1980c) and biopsy samples from a wide variety of disorders (Dvorak

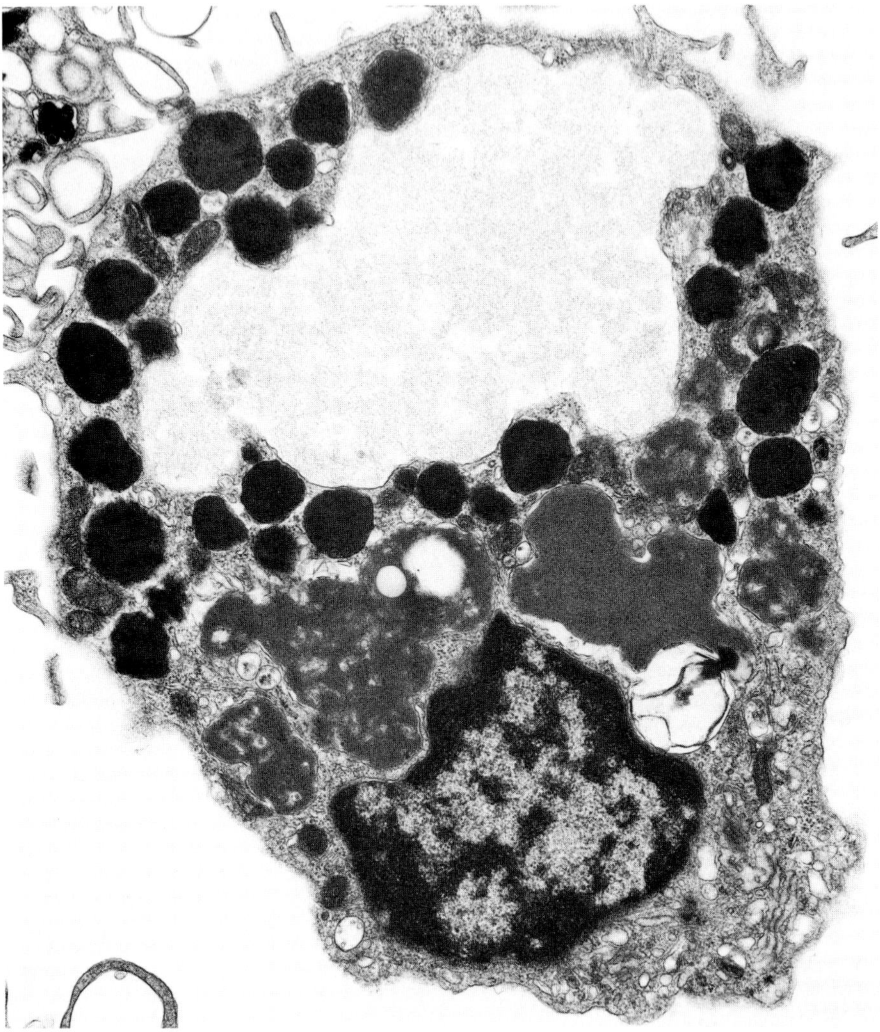

Figure 11 HLMC ex vivo, 24 hr after anti-IgE, shows progressive condensation of channel contents and separation of new granule domains with variably condensed contents. ×15,500. (From Dvorak, A. M., 1989c, with permission.)

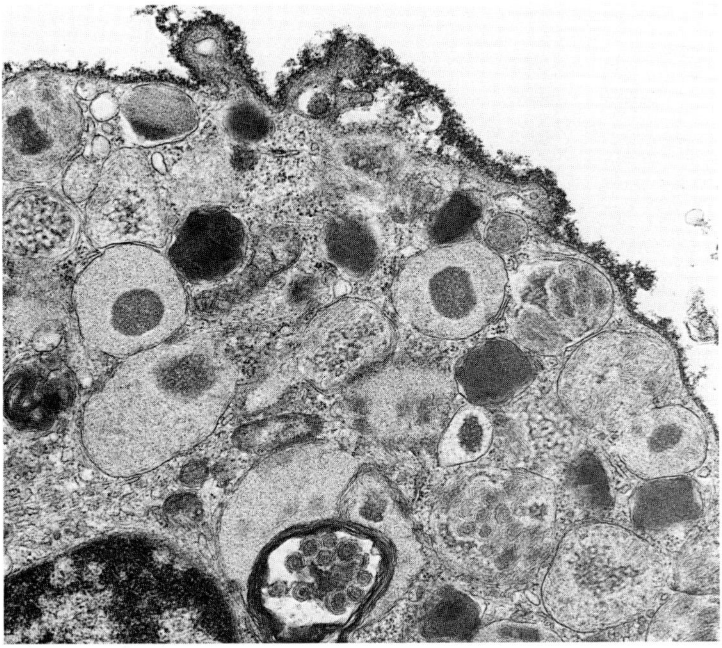

Figure 12 HLMC ex vivo, 24 hr after anti-IgE, shows condensing central foci of scrolls, crystals, particles, and homogeneous dense material within the central areas of less dense material in reforming granule spaces. Cationized ferritin stains the plasma membranes but not the granule membranes, indicating that they are not open at this time. ×24,500. (From Dvorak, A. M., 1989c, with permission.)

AM, 1987, 1988c,d, Dvorak AM, 1989a,b,d,f, 1991b; Dvorak AM and Monahan, 1984b; Dvorak AM and Monahan-Earley, 1986; Dvorakam and Monahan-Earley RA, 1992; Dvorak AM and Silen, 1985; Dvorak AM et al., 1992a,b,c,d; McLeod et al., 1992; Onderdonk et al., 1992). These samples include large amounts of material from patients with Crohn's disease and ulcerative colitis. A smaller number of biopsies from many conditions include various inflammatory and neoplastic disorders. Most of the latter are by-products of samples submitted to the ultrastructural pathology laboratory for diagnosis. In addition, we have recently completed a multi-institutional study of 117 encoded intestinal biopsies from which observations regarding human intestinal mast cells have been made (Dvorak AM et al., 1992a,b,c,d; McLeod et al., 1992; Onderdonk et al., 1992) (Fig. 25). Human gastrointestinal system mast cells (HGMC) in these settings generally contain a majority of scroll granules (Fig. 26A). Particle-filled granules (Fig. 26C) are also present, particularly in intraepithelial mast cells in

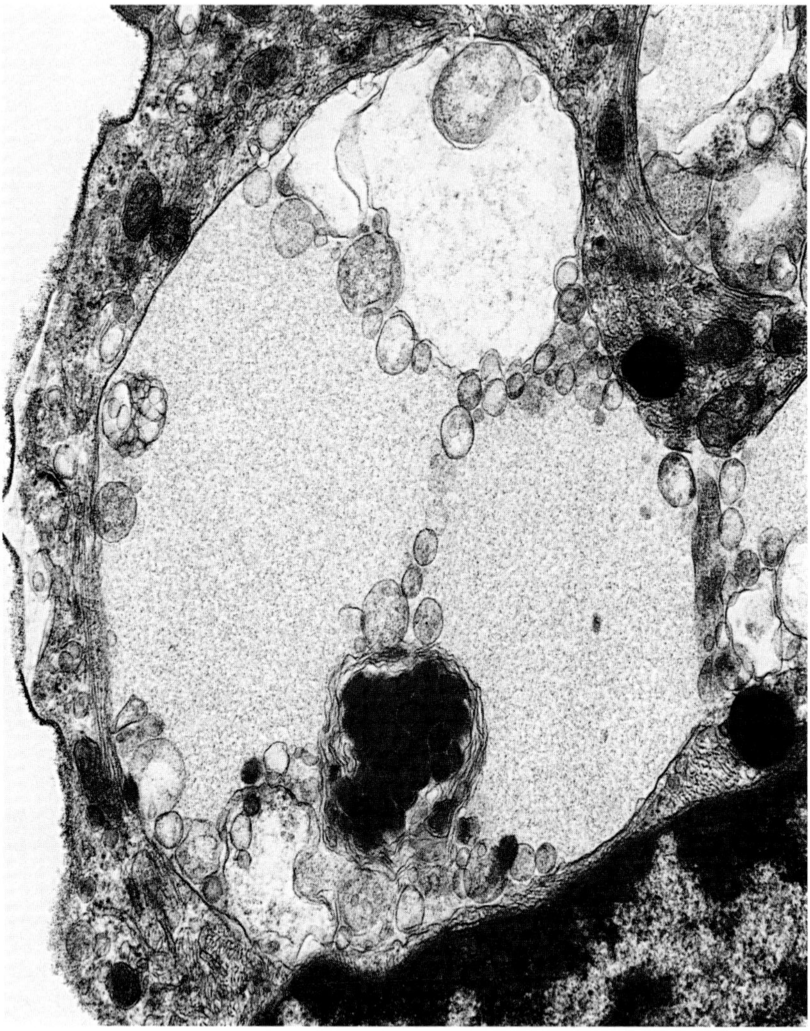

Figure 13 HLMC ex vivo, 24 hr after anti-IgE, shows granule domains within a recovering degranulation channel that are demarcated by rows of vesicles. ×27,000. (From Dvorak, A. M. et al., 1986, with permission.)

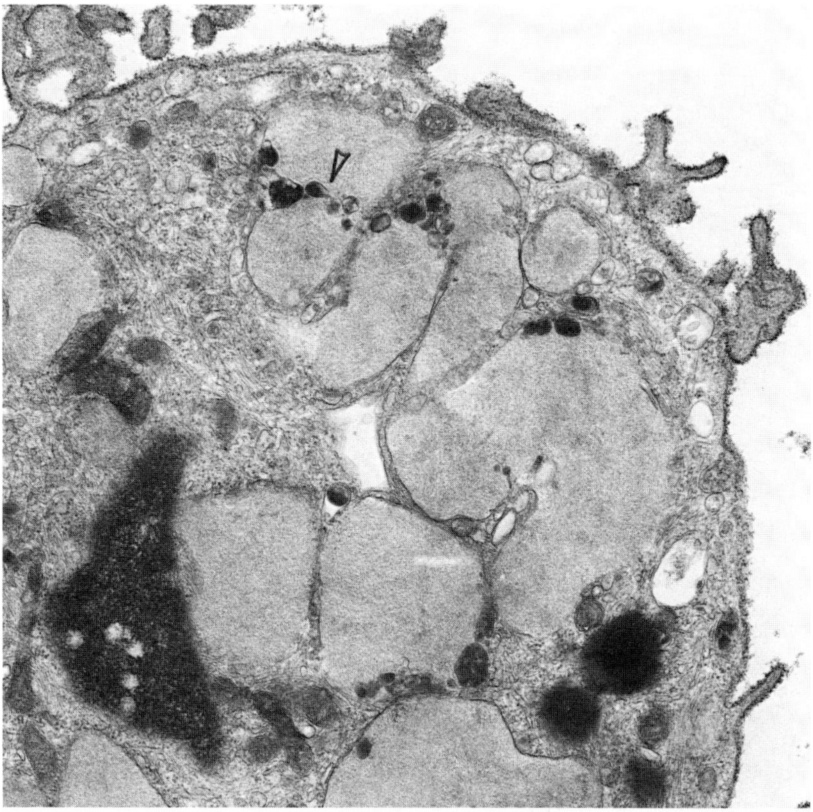

Figure 14 HLMC ex vivo, 48 hr after anti-IgE, shows granule domains within recovering degranulation channels that are closely associated with strings of small, intrachannel lipid bodies at separation points (arrowhead). ×20,000. (From Dvorak, A. M., 1989c, with permission.)

ulcerative colitis samples (Dvorak AM et al., 1992a) (Fig. 27). Crystal granules are rare; mast cells with mixed granules are present. Generally, these are scroll-particle combinations (Fig. 26B). All reported ultrastructural granule patterns can, however, be found in gastrointestinal tissues. Of all tissue locations that we regularly examine, we find particle granules more frequently in gastrointestinal tissues than in other locations. Particle granules have been regularly described when human mast cells migrate into the epithelial layer of tissues, as we have seen in ulcerative colitis (Dvorak AM et al., 1992a). For example, mast cells within bronchiolar epithelium of lung (Haslam et al., 1987; Kawanami et al., 1979), respiratory epithelium of maxillary sinus (Dvorak AM and

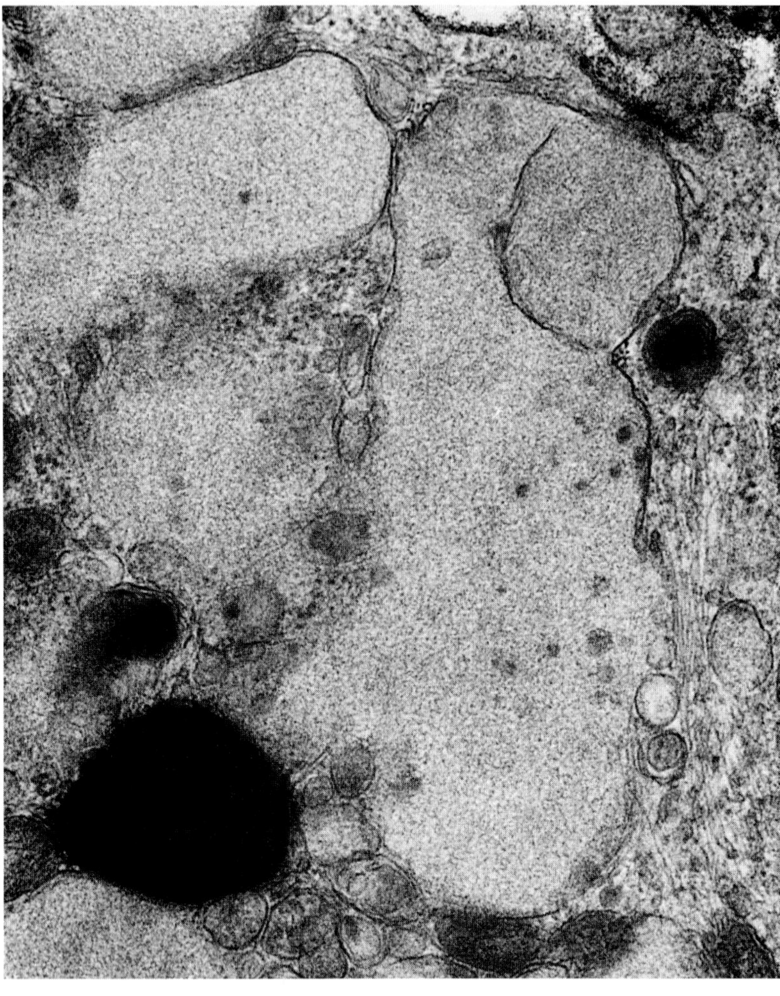

Figure 15 HLMC ex vivo, 48 hr after anti IgE, shows nearly complete membrane delineation of new granule domain in a recovering degranulation channel. ×42,500. (From Dvorak, A. M. et al., 1986, with permission.)

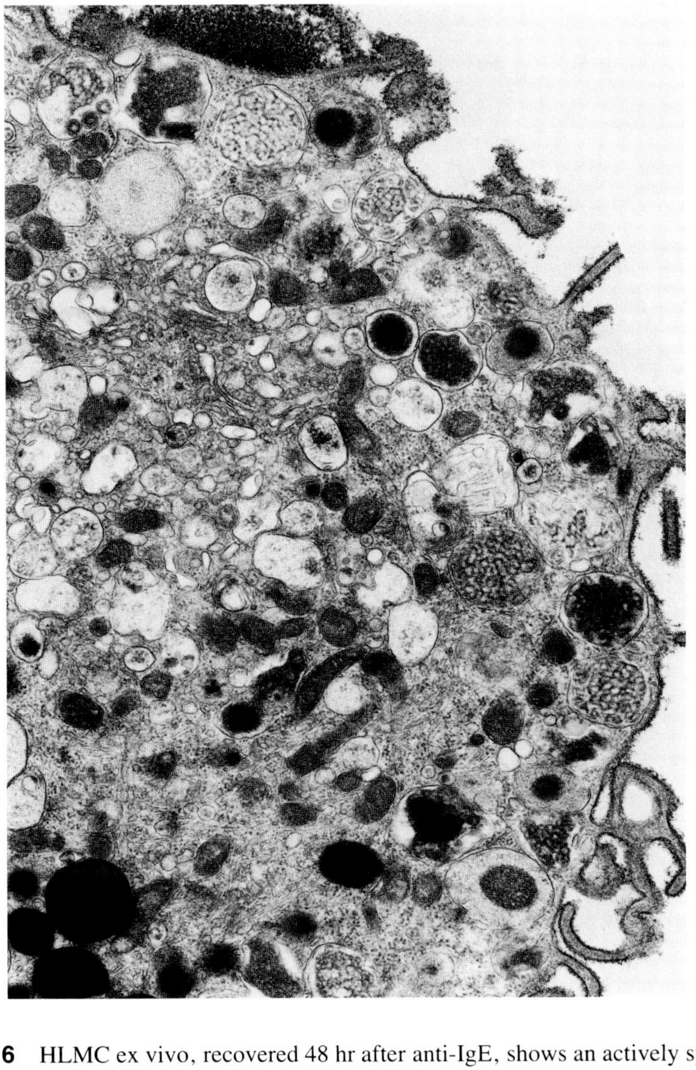

Figure 16 HLMC ex vivo, recovered 48 hr after anti-IgE, shows an actively synthesizing Golgi area filled with numerous particle-filled progranules. Larger granules in the peripheral cytoplasm contain particles, scrolls, and mixed patterns. ×23,500. (From Dvorak, A. M. et al., 1988, with permission.)

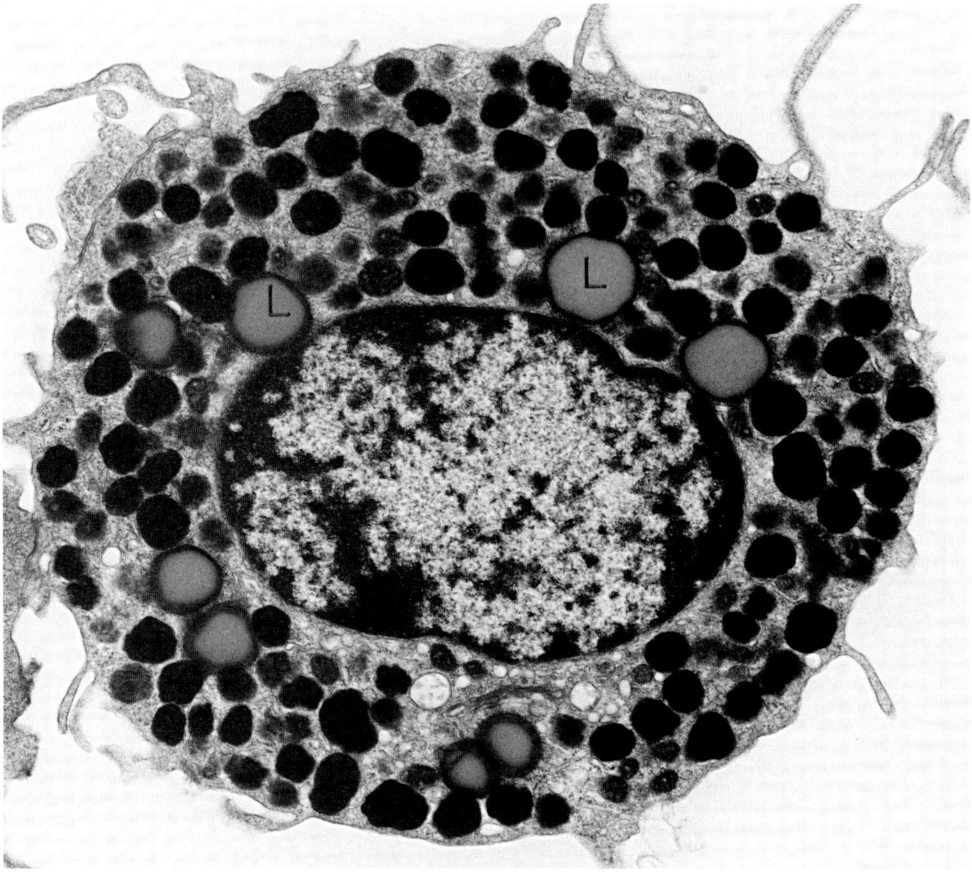

Figure 19 HLMC in vitro, cocultured for 1 month with 3T3 mouse skin fibroblasts, shows excellent preservation. Note large lipid bodies (L) and the fact that all granules are completely filled. Most granules are scroll granules as in HLMCs in situ. ×12,500.

Kissell S., 1991), and tubular epithelium of kidney (Colvin et al., 1974) all show an increased incidence of particle granules. While scroll granules are present in HGMC of all locations, crystal granules are more generally found in mast cells within the gastrointestinal system submucosa and the underlying muscle layers.

HGMCs frequently display increased numbers of lipid bodies (Fig. 28), as do lung mast cells (Dvorak AM et al., 1983b, 1984; Peters et al., 1989), in contrast to skin mast cells (Dvorak AM and Kissell S., 1991; Dvorak AM et al.,

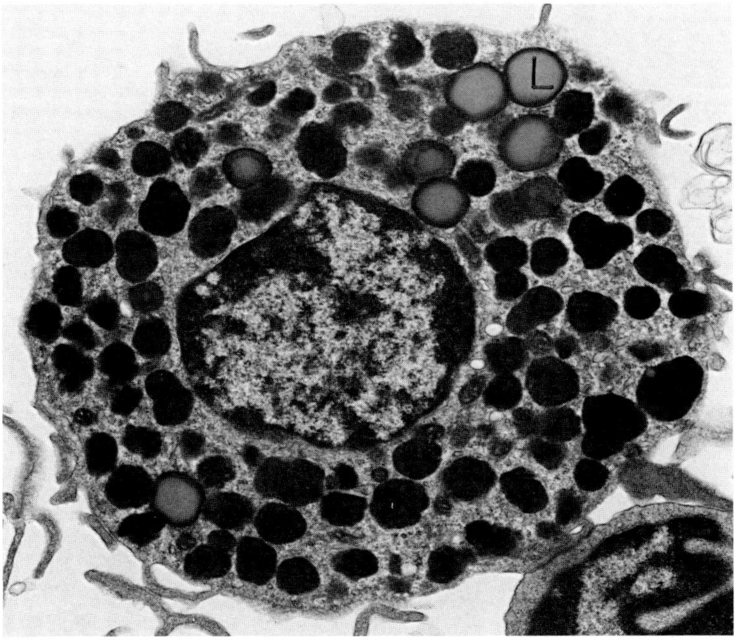

Figure 20 HLMC in vitro, cultured for 1 month alone, also shows excellent preservation with numerous completely filled, dense scroll granules and several lipid bodies (L). ×11,000.

1991c), which do not. Lipid bodies are increased in completely granulated cells (Fig. 28); some lipid bodies display centrally located, round, lucent structures containing densities within them. Others have fused, and some display large, focal lucent areas within them (Figs. 28, 29). Closely associated cytoplasmic filaments encase HGMC lipid bodies, as is also seen in HLMCs (Dvorak AM et al., 1983b). HGMCs are present in all layers of the gastrointestinal system as well as near vessels and nerves (Dvorak AM, 1991b; Dvorak AM et al., 1980c,d, 1992a,b). We have not detected mitosis in any mast cells examined in human gastrointestinal tissues. Mast cells are rounded or markedly elongated, with numerous narrow surface folds. Mast cells of variable degrees of immaturity can be found in the gastrointestinal system (Fig. 29) (Dvorak AM et al., 1992a). The morphological criteria for immature cells include nuclear and cytoplasmic changes like those seen in lung tissues. Morphological criteria for both PMD and AND are present in HGMCs in certain settings (see later) (Dvorak AM, 1979, 1988c; Dvorak AM et al., 1978, 1980c, 1992b).

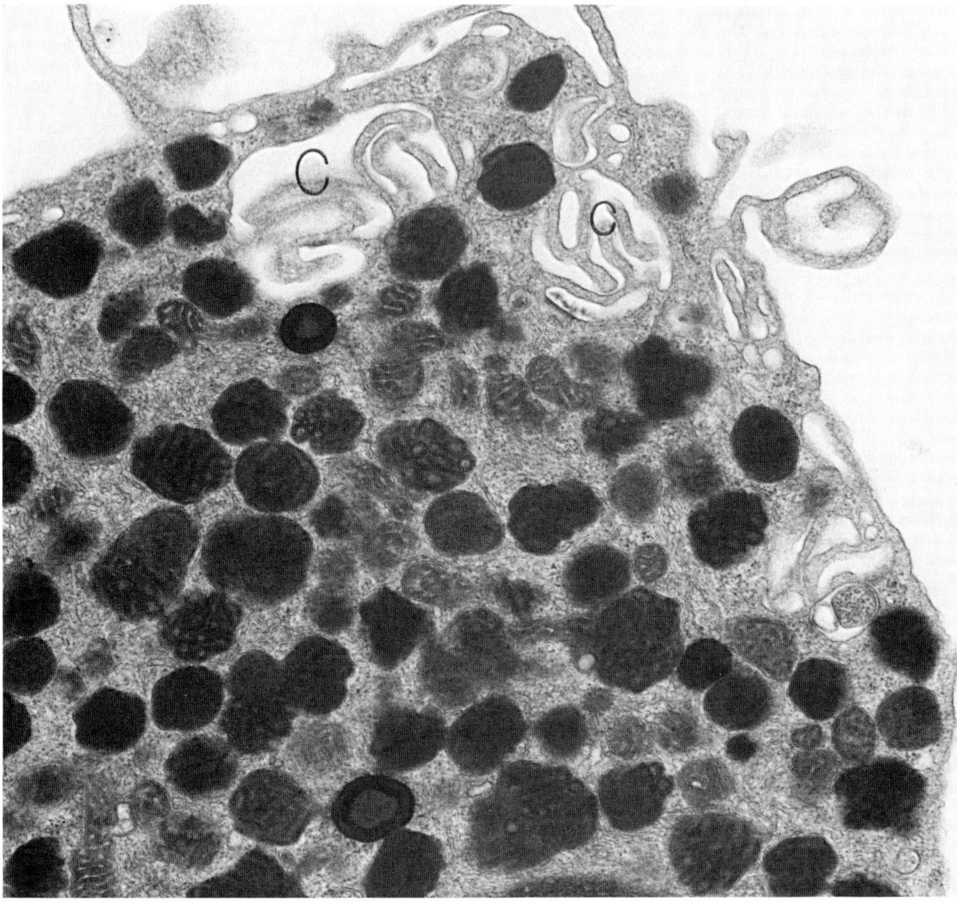

Figure 21 HLMC in vitro, cultured for 1 month, retains the in situ phenotype. Note numerous scroll granules. Two canaliculi (C) with enclosed surface folds are also present. ×24,500.

Crohn's Disease

HGMCs are increased in intestinal tissues obtained from patients with Crohn's disease (CD) (Cook and Turnbull, 1975; Dvorak AM and Monahan, 1983; Ranlöv et al., 1972; Rao, 1973). We initially noted this in ileocolectomy samples (Dvorak AM and Monahan, 1983; Dvorak AM et al., 1980c). Mast cells in CD are plentiful in the mucosa, the submucosa, and particularly the large muscle layers beneath the submucosa (Dvorak AM and Monahan, 1983). Mast cells in perivascular locations, in areas of increased and abnormal fibrosis, and associ-

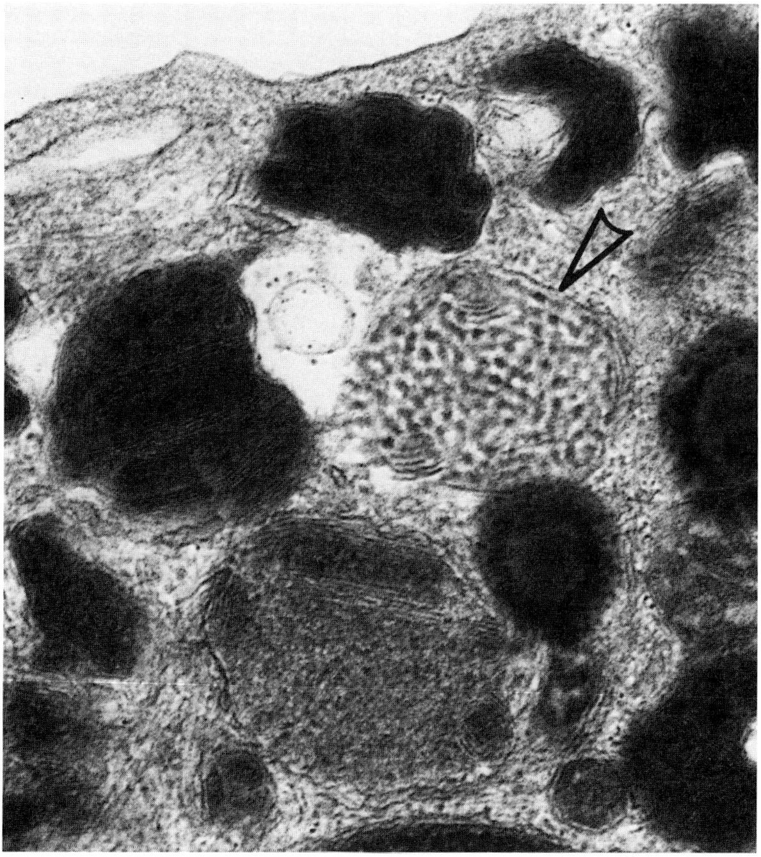

Figure 22 HLMC in vitro, cultured for 1 month, shows scroll, particle (arrowhead), and mixed granules. ×58,000.

ated with the enteric nerves were evident in studies of ileocolectomy samples (Dvorak AM and Monahan, 1983; Dvorak AM et al., 1980c,d). Intraepithelial mast cells were not present in any of the material examined from patients with CD. Axonal necrosis regularly occurs in CD samples (Dvorak AM, 1988d, 1989a; Dvorak AM and Silen, 1985; Dvorak AM et al., 1980d). We noted also that normal and degranulated mast cells were often closely associated with these damaged enteric nerves (Dvorak AM and Silen, 1985; Dvorak AM et al., 1980c,d). Mast cells are increased in CD samples taken from grossly diseased areas as well as in grossly and microscopically uninvolved resection margins (Dvorak AM and Monahan, 1983). Additionally, we have found increased mast

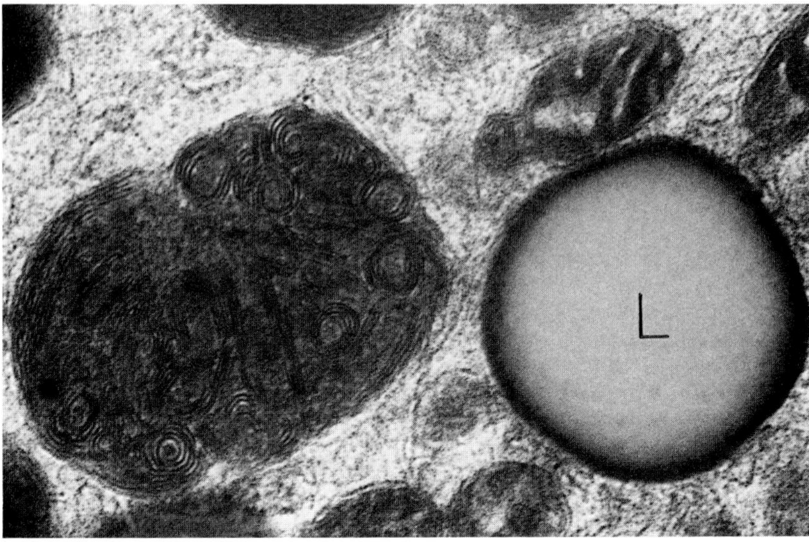

Figure 23 HLMC in vitro, cultured for 1 month, shows a typical scroll granule and a lipid body (L) at high magnification. Note that the lipid body has a dense outer shell and is only moderately dense centrally. ×76,500. (From Dvorak, A. M. and Ishizaka, T., 1992, with permission.)

cells in duodenal and jejunal biopsies of patients with radiologically documented ileal disease only (Dvorak AM and Silen, 1985). When we examined biopsies taken from conventional ileostomies of patients from whom all disease was previously excised, we also found increased numbers of mast cells (Dvorak AM and Silen, 1985; Dvorak AM et al., 1992a), and recently, we have documented a high degree of degranulation in the mast cells in this location (Dvorak AM et al., 1992b). Generally, the degranulation was of the piecemeal type (Fig. 30) (Dvorak AM, 1991a, 1992; Dvorak HF and Dvorak AM, 1975; Galli et al., 1984), but degranulation channel formation, alteration and swelling of intrachannel granules, and extrusion of visible, altered granules to the cells' exterior through plasma membrane pores have also been found (Dvorak AM, 1991b; Dvorak AM et al., 1992b). Thus, HGMCs in this setting display both PMD and AND (Dvorak AM et al., 1992b). In an encoded study of biopsy samples from a subset of 19 patients with CD, within a larger study of intestinal biopsies, we found that 68% of the samples displayed morphological evidence of degranulation of HGMCs (Dvorak AM et al., 1992b). Recently, patients with CD have been shown to have elevated levels of histamine in jejunal luminal contents (Knutson et al., 1990). These levels were shown to be highest in

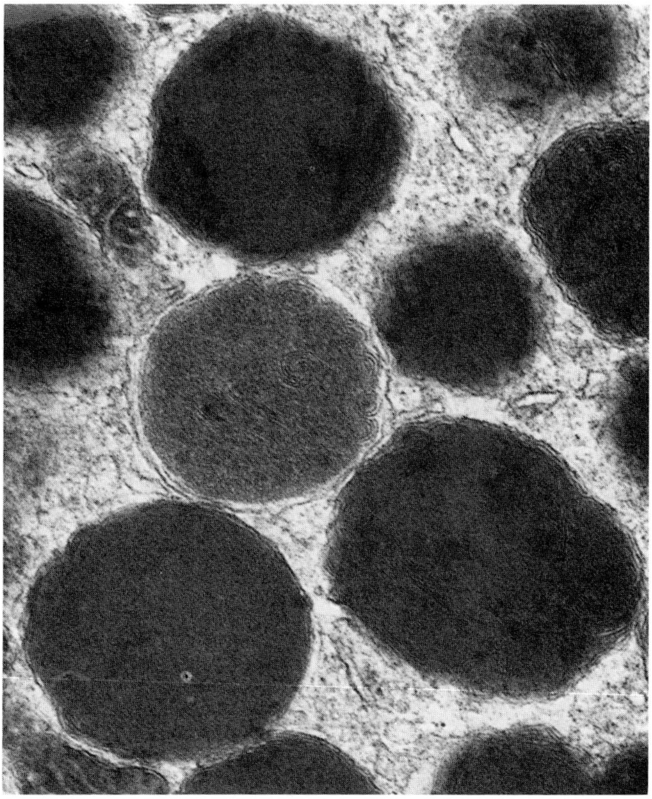

Figure 24 HLMC in vitro for 1 month. Many granules are completely filled with homogeneous dense material with superimposed central and peripheral scrolls. ×59,500.

patients with clinically active disease, yet those with clinically inactive disease had significantly higher histamine levels than did control individuals (Knutson et al., 1990). These data, in conjunction with the regularly identified ultrastructural evidence of noncytotoxic mast cell secretion (Dvorak AM et al., 1992b), document a significant role for release of mast cell mediators in CD, an inflammatory bowel disorder of uncertain etiology.

Ulcerative Colitis

HGMCs are also increased in intestinal tissues obtained from patients with ulcerative colitis (UC), another inflammatory bowel disease of unknown etiology (Dvorak AM et al., 1992a; McAuley and Sommers, 1961; Sommers, 1966). In an encoded sample of 81 intestinal biopsies from patients with UC, within a

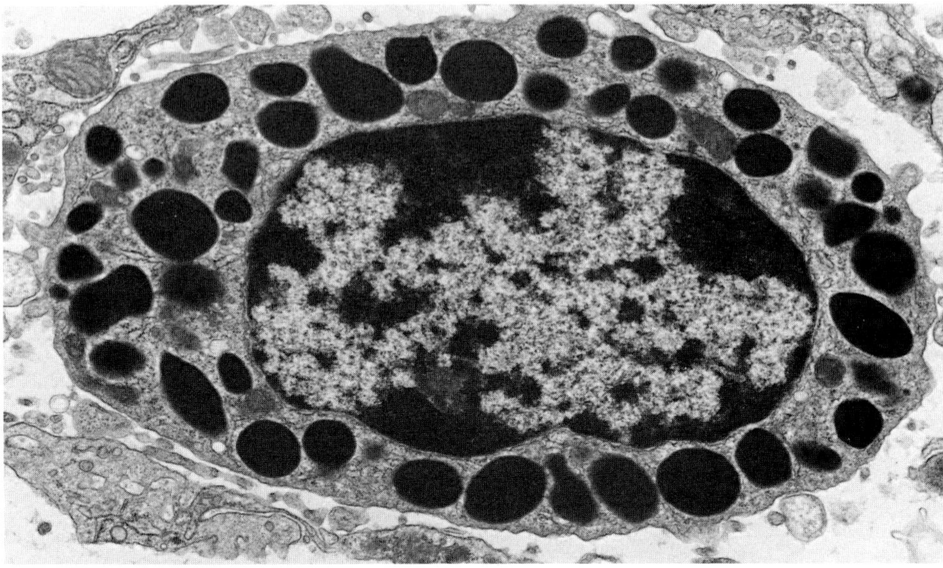

Figure 25 HGMC in situ. Biopsy of ileal continent pouch in patient with familial polyposis shows mononuclear mast cell in the lamina propia. Note that all granules are completely filled with homogeneous dense contents. ×12,500.

larger number of intestinal biopsies, we found a high rate of morphologically degranulated mast cells (56%) (Dvorak AM et al., 1992b). Again, the entire continuum of PMD (Fig. 31) to AND (Fig. 32) was identifiable in these degranulating HGMCs, many of which were closely associated with enteric nerves. The ultrastructural morphology of HGMCs in UC tissues did not differ from that found in CD tissues. Thus, we also found the rank order of identifiable granule patterns to be scrolls > particles > crystals, as well as increased numbers of cytoplasmic lipid bodies in fully granulated and degranulating mast cells (Dvorak AM et al., 1992a, 1992b).

Familial Polyposis

The material we examined was all obtained from either conventional ileostomies or continent ileal pouches constructed in these patients after ileocolectomies were done (Dvorak AM et al., 1992a,b). Fourteen encoded biopsies within a large group of intestinal biopsies revealed 71% degranulation of HGMCs associated with familial polyposis (FP) tissues. The number of lipid bodies and the rank order of observed granule patterns in HGMCs in FP were similar to those in CD

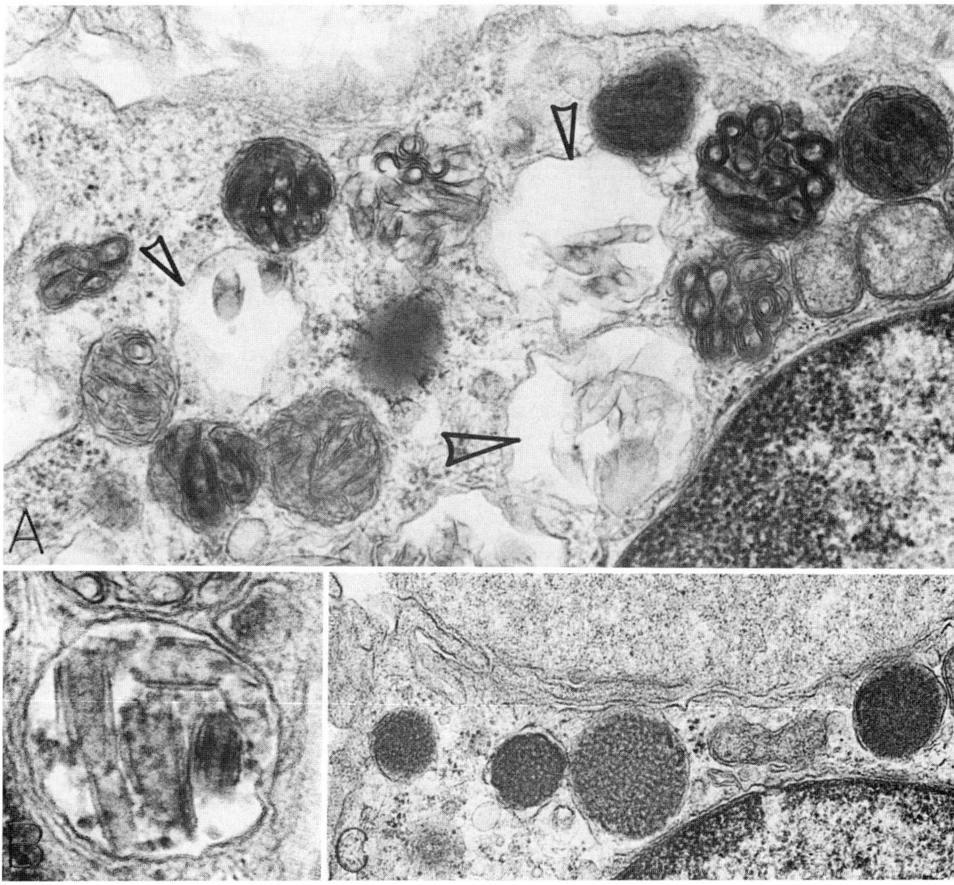

Figure 26 HGMCs in situ from small intestinal biopsy of patient with gluten enteropathy (A,B) and ileostomy biopsy of patient with UC (C). Typical scroll granules (A) and particle granules (C) are illustrated. Note (B) high magnification view of mixed scroll-particle granule from cell illustrated in (A). (A) also shows residual scrolls in three empty granules, characteristic of PMD (arrowheads). (A) ×32,500; (B) ×64,500; (C) ×32,000.

and UC. As in biopsies of inflammatory bowel disease patients, FP biopsies showed both PMD (Fig. 33) and AND (Fig. 34A) of mast cells. Cytoplasmic canaliculi with enclosed surface folds, a mechanism for membrane recovery after AND (Dvorak AM, 1989e; Dvorak AM et al., 1988), were also present in mast cells (Fig. 34B).

Histamine levels, determined for jejunal contents, as in CD (Knutson et al., 1990), have not been determined for patients with UC or the preneoplastic

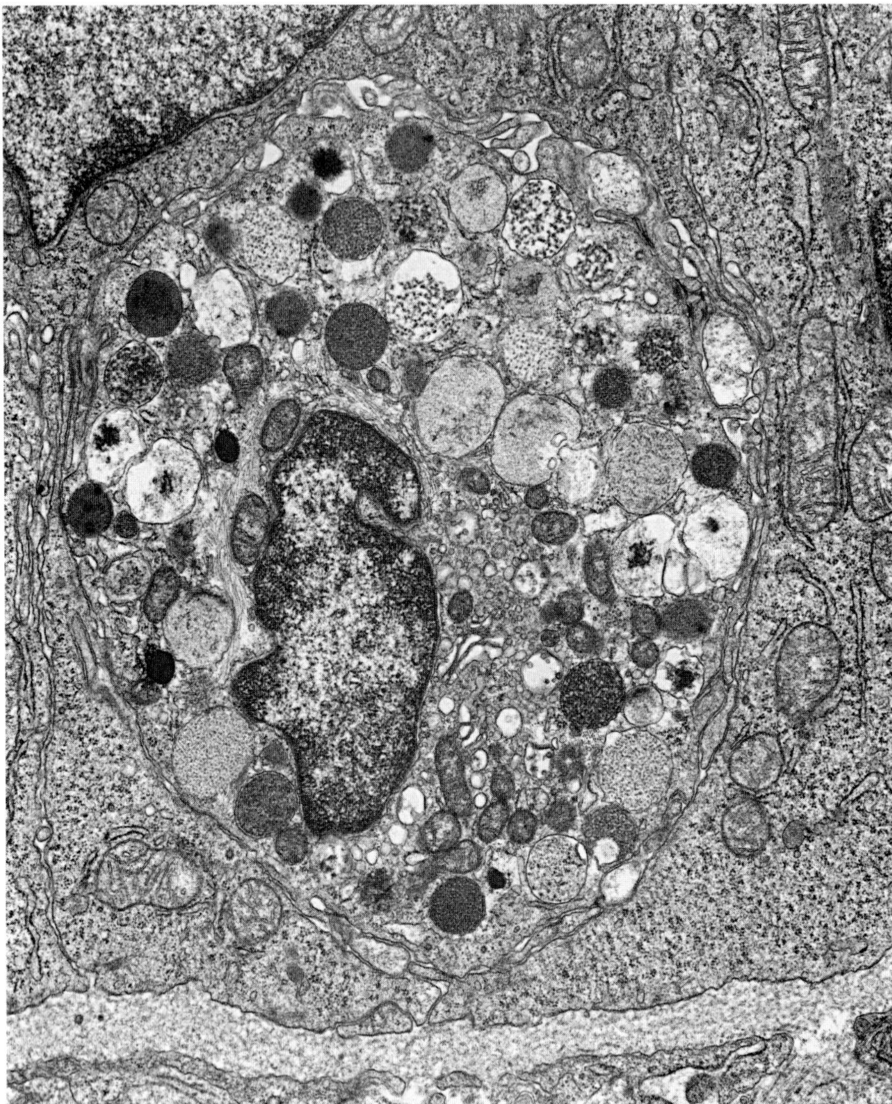

Figure 27 HGMC in situ from continent ileal pouch biopsy of a patient with UC shows an intraepithelial mast cell undergoing PMD. Note that all granules are of the particle type. ×16,500.

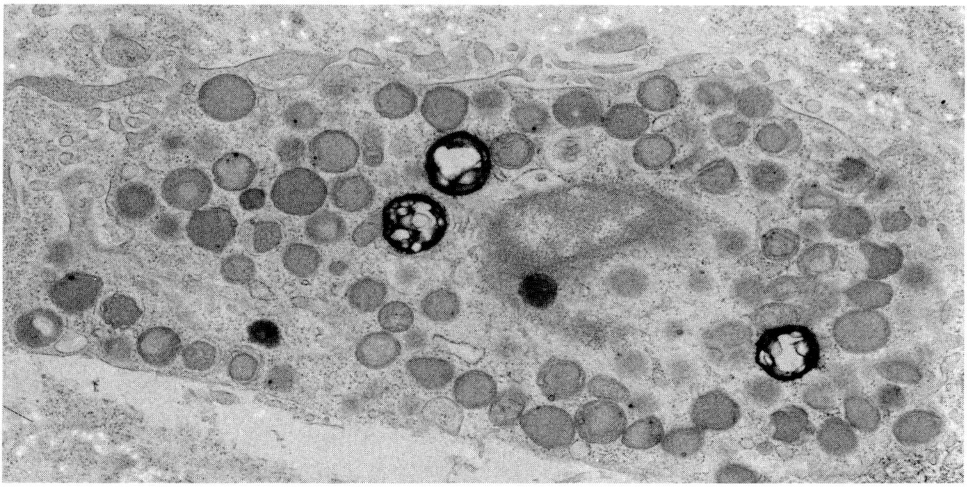

Figure 28 HGMC in situ from ileal biopsy of a patient with Crohn's disease, prepared cytochemically to demonstrate peroxidase activity, shows large, peroxidase-positive lipid bodies displaying focal areas of no activity, in a mast cell filled with granules. ×14,000. (From Dvorak, A. M., 1991a, with permission.)

syndrome, FP. We think these studies would be of interest in view of the high rate of mast cell degranulation we observed in patients with UC or FP. The morphological findings regarding HGMCs in human intestinal biopsies are currently being further analyzed in relationship to a number of parallel studies conducted on these same biopsy samples (Dvorak AM et al., 1992a,b,c,d; McLeod et al., 1992; Onderdonk et al., 1992).

B. Ex Vivo

We examined isolated mast cells, prepared by mechanical and enzymatic dispersion of cells obtained from colons resected for carcinoma, with the electron microscope (Fox et al., 1985). These mast cells were functionally intact, as assessed by short-term culture, low spontaneous histamine release, and appropriate IgE-mediated histamine release (Fox et al., 1985). They were morphologically well preserved and resembled their in situ counterparts in gastrointestinal tissues (Fig. 35). Functional and morphological analyses, including histamine content, kinetics of IgE-mediated histamine release, unresponsiveness to f-Met peptide, production of arachidonic acid metabolites PGD_2 and LTC_4, and ultrastructural granule patterns and lipid body content, revealed human mast cells from this intestinal source to be similar to HLMCs (Fox et al., 1985). We have

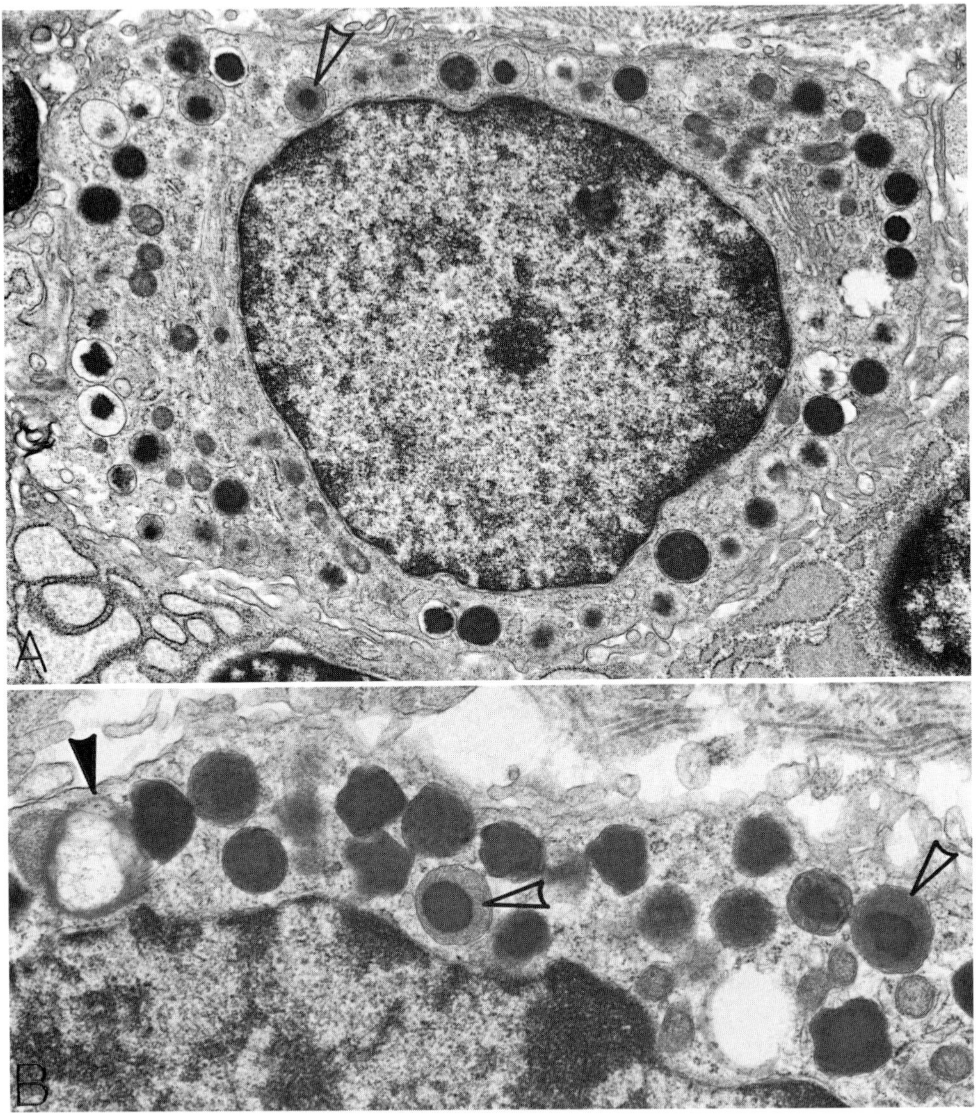

Figure 29 HGMCs in situ from continent ileal pouch biopsy of a patient with UC show central, dense nucleoids condensing within granules (open arrowheads) of immature mast cells. Focal lucencies within lipid bodies (closed arrowhead) are also seen in (B). (A) ×14,000; (B) ×23,000.

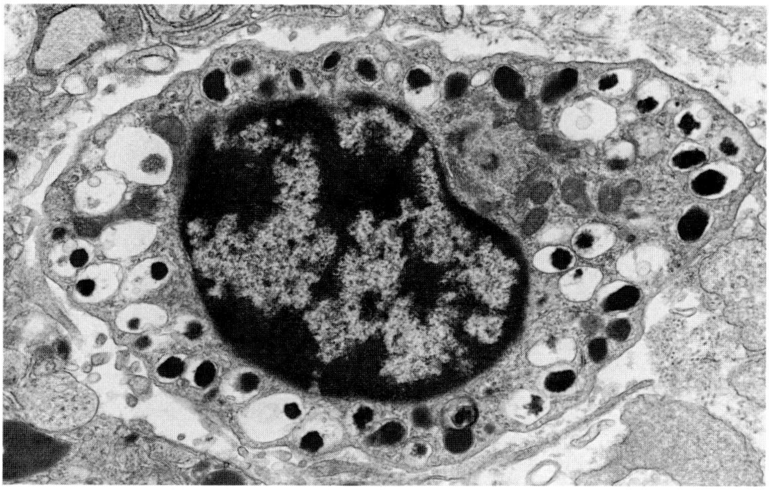

Figure 30 HGMC in situ from continent ileal pouch biopsy of a patient with CD shows PMD. Note that nonfused granule chambers are partly empty. ×14,000.

not yet examined the morphology of stimulated release and recovery reactions of isolated human colonic mast cells.

IV. Human Heart Mast Cells

A. In Situ

Mast cells have been implicated in the pathogenesis of cardiac disease (Estensen, 1984; Ginsburg et al., 1981; Kalsner and Richards, 1984; Levi et al., 1985; Michelassi et al., 1982; Triggiani et al., 1985). We regularly examine cardiac biopsies by electron microscopy for diagnostic purposes, a series that now totals 140 samples. Mast cells occur infrequently in electron microscopic sections of these biopsies, but those which we have examined generally contain scroll granules, mixed granules, and infrequent lipid bodies. A larger sample of cells is required to be certain that other granule patterns do or do not occur in this location. We identified AND of human heart mast cells (HHMCs) (Fig. 36) accompanied by massive interstitial edema in two patients in the first 70 biopsies examined by electron microscopy (Dvorak AM, 1986a). In both cases, the heart disease was of uncertain etiology but was characterized by hypokinetic ventricles in the absence of cardiac valvular or coronary vessel disease. These human cardiac mast cells displayed a combination of degranulation channel formation within which altered granules resided, as well as extrusion of membrane-free

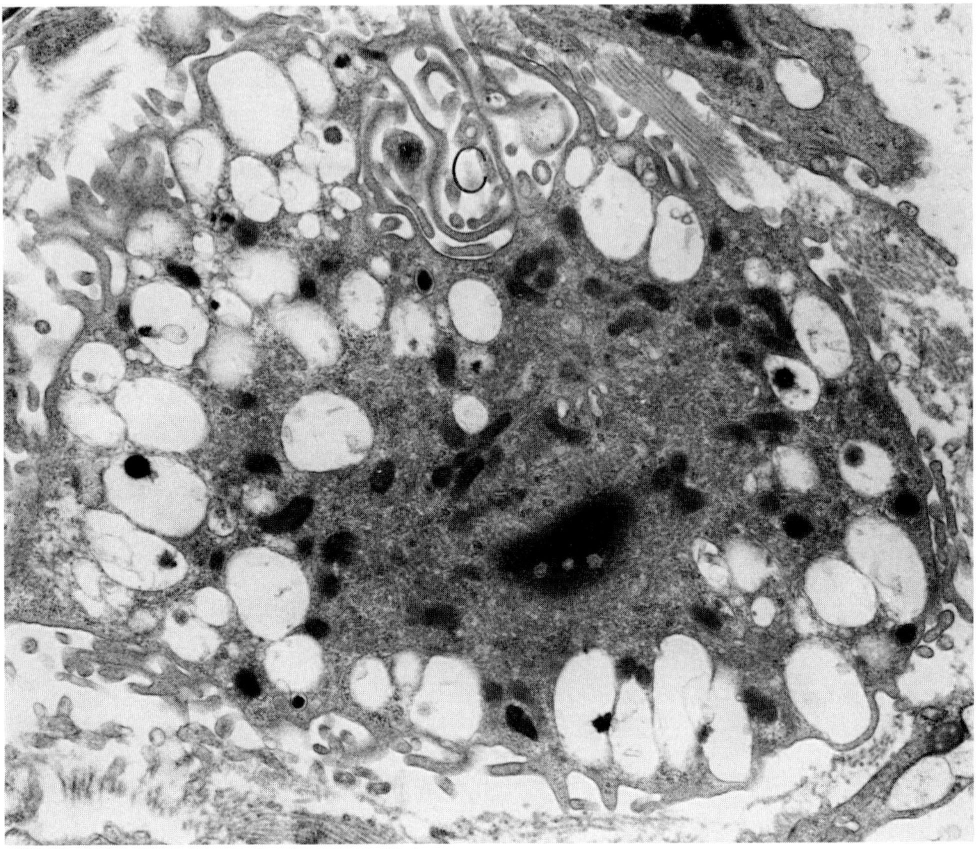

Figure 31 HGMC in situ from continent ileal pouch biopsy of a patient with UC shows extensive PMD. Note a canaliculus (C) filled with cell surface folds. ×15,000.

altered granules through plasma membrane pores to the extracellular milieu (Dvorak AM, 1986a). These two cases document the unequivocal occurrence of AND of mast cells in human heart tissues in vivo. The degranulation mechanism included the extrusion of altered granules as well as intacytoplasmic solubilization of granules within degranulation channels (Fig. 36). These are difficult images to capture in in vivo tissues. In ex vivo studies of isolated lung (Dvorak AM et al., 1984; Dvorak AM et al., 1985b) and skin (Dvorak AM et al., 1991c) mast cells, these morphological events are clearly associated with the rapid release of histamine. The precise triggering mechanism, among the many possible ones for human mast cells, cannot be determined by morphological analysis. The identification of AND in these settings, however, suggests a role

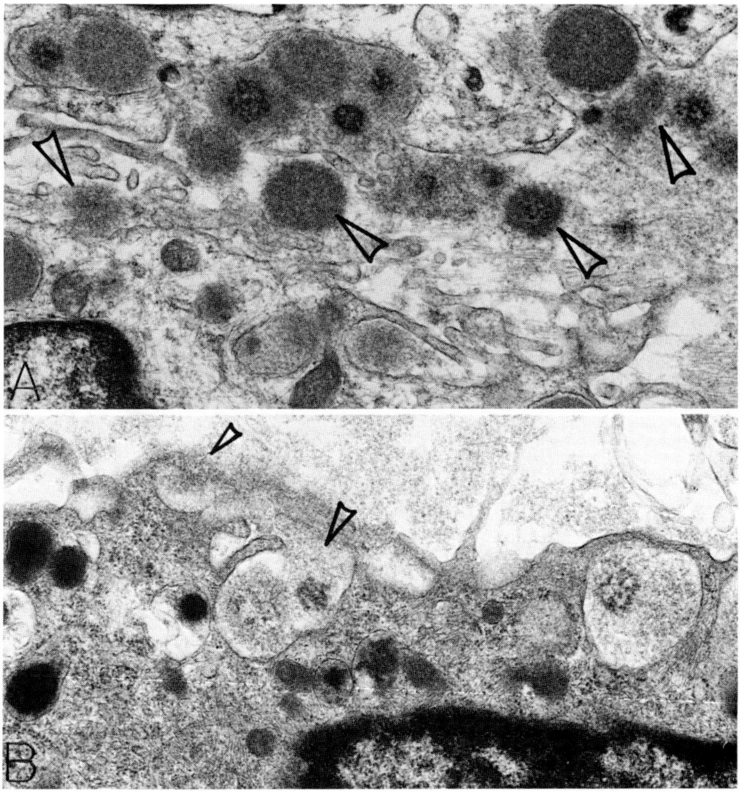

Figure 32 HGMCs in situ from continent ileal pouch biopsy of a patient with UC show extrusion of membrane-free granules (arrowheads) to the exterior, typical of AND. (A) ×19,000; (B) ×24,000.

for mast cells and their release reactions in the pathogenesis of otherwise unexplained cardiac disorders.

V. Human Synovial Mast Cells

A. In Situ

Our ultrastructural experience of in situ biopsy material is confined to the examination of synovial tissues in juvenile rheumatoid arthritis. Increased numbers of well-preserved mast cells, with ultrastructural features similar to those of lung and intestinal mast cells, are present in this setting. More extensively

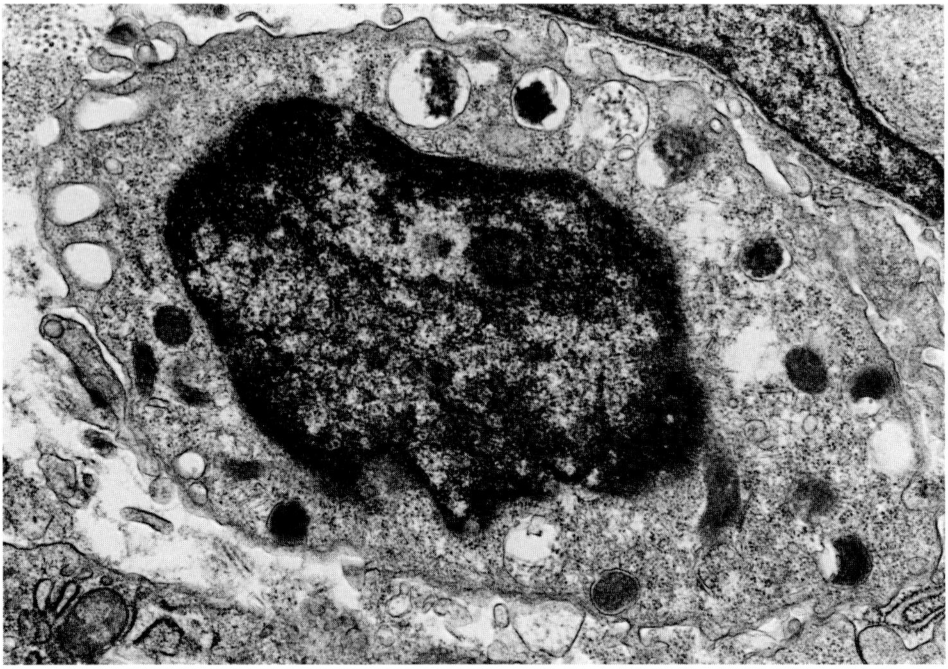

Figure 33 HGMC in situ from continent ileal pouch biopsy of a patient with familial polyposis shows PMD. ×19,000.

sampled material is necessary for us to make further morphological statements regarding mast cells in synovial tissues in situ.

B. Ex Vivo

Human synovia, obtained at arthroplasty from patients with rheumatoid arthritis and osteoarthritis, were the source for preparation of isolated human synovial mast cells (HSYMCs) using enzymatic digestion and overnight cultures (Kopicky-Burd et al., 1988). These preparations were assessed functionally and by light and electron microscopy. Mast cell numbers were elevated in synovial tissues obtained from either arthritic disorder, and by functional and morphological criteria, HSYMCs did not differ from HLMCs or HGMCs (Kopicky-Burd et al., 1988). Thus, HSYMCs released histamine, PGD_2, and LTC_4 when appropriately stimulated with anti-IgE but did not respond to compound 48/80, f-Met peptide, or bradykinin (Kopicky-Burd et al., 1988). By electron microscopy, HSYMCs were rounded cells filled with cytoplasmic granules (Fig. 37).

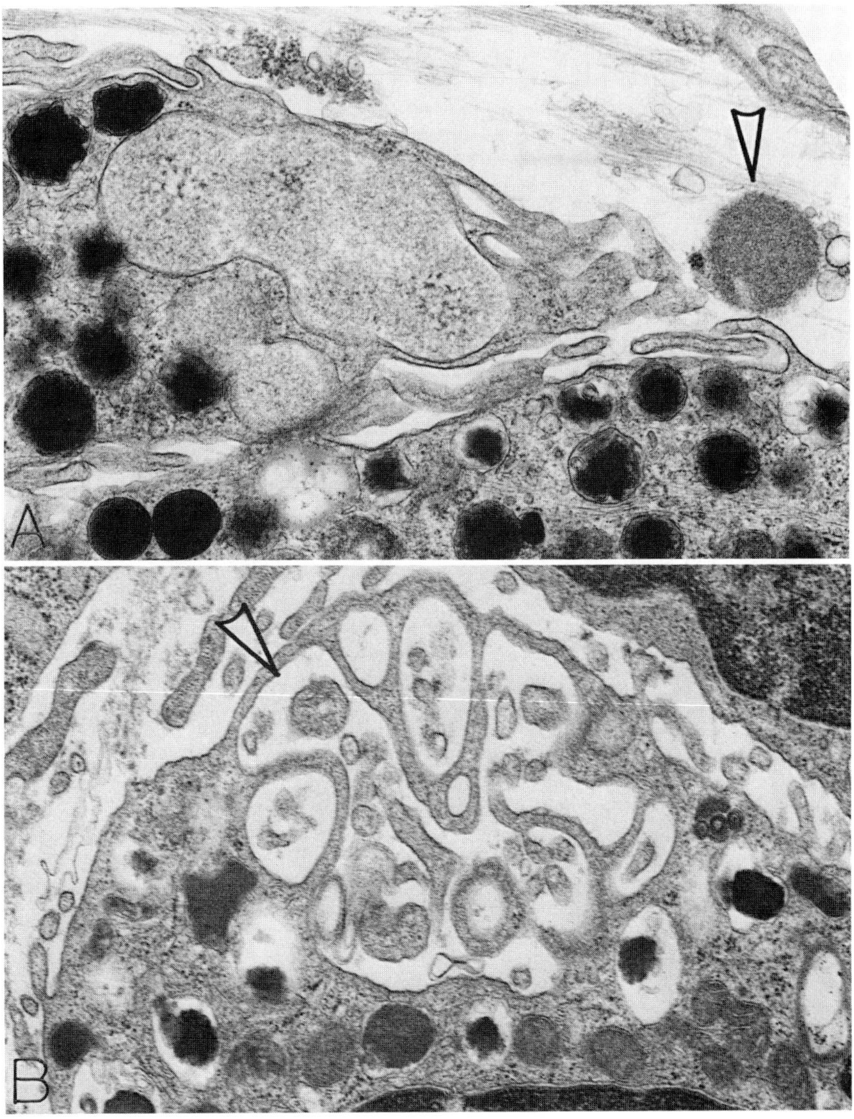

Figure 34 HGMCs in situ from continent ileal pouch biopsies of patients with familial polyposis (A,B) show AND with granule extrusion (arrowhead, A) and canaliculi formation (arrowhead, B), structures that facilitate membrane recovery following AND. (A,B) ×27,000.

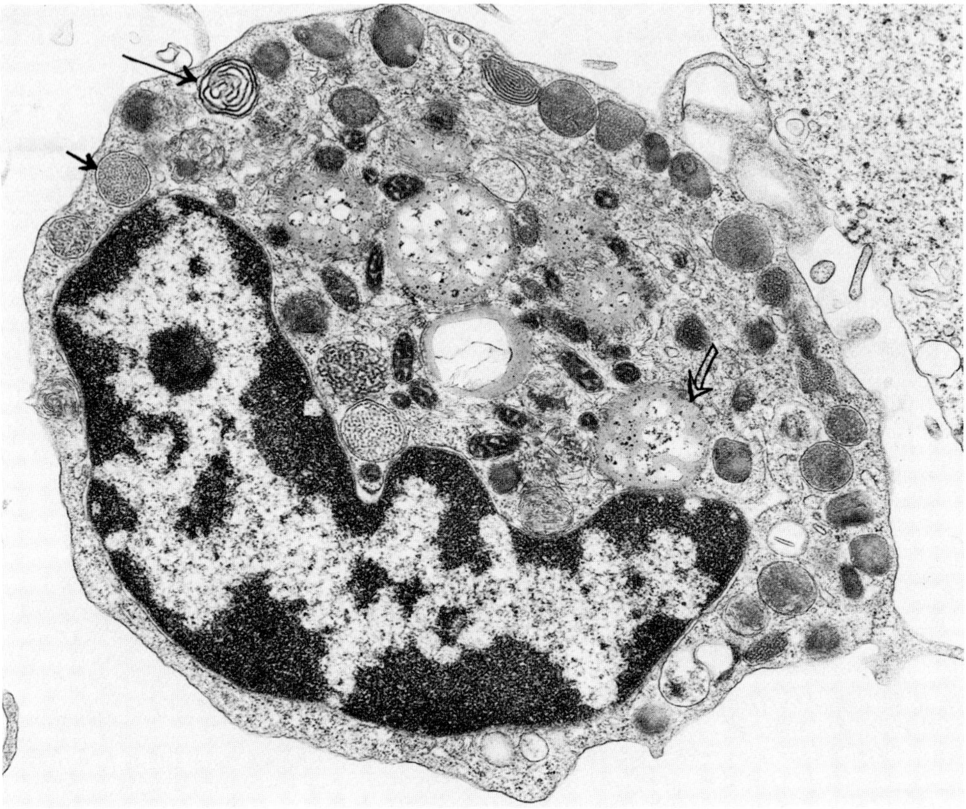

Figure 35 HGMC ex vivo is filled with particle granules (short arrow). Several granules contain beaded threads in a reticular array (long arrow). Lipid bodies are moderately dense and contain central vesicles and densities (open arrow). ×21,500. (From Fox et al., 1985, with permission.)

The surfaces of HSYMCs displayed many short, narrow surface folds (Kopicky-Burd et al., 1988). Lipid bodies were also present in moderate numbers. These highly osmiophilic structures sometimes contained central, rounded lucencies, as we previously noted in HGMCs (Fox et al., 1985). Mature HSYMCs did not have active Golgi areas. Cytoplasmic granules displayed scrolls (Fig. 37) most commonly, as in HLMCs (Dvorak AM et al., 1984; Peters et al., 1989) and HGMCs (Dvorak AM et al., 1992a,b; Fox et al., 1985); crystal granules, like those regularly present in HSMCs (Dvorak AM and Kissell S, 1991; Dvorak AM et al., 1991c), were less commonly present in HSYMCs. Crystal granules

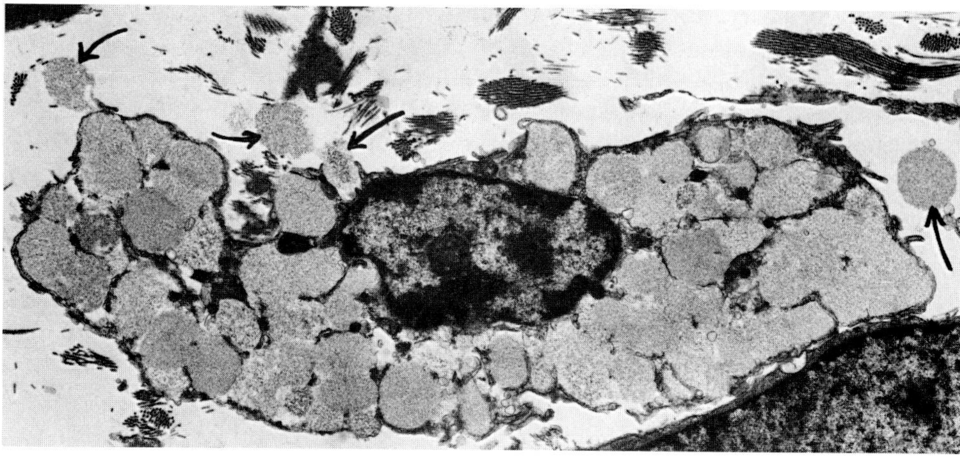

Figure 36 HHMC in situ shows AND characterized by degranulation channel formation filled with altered granules and granule extrusion (arrows). ×8,000. (From Dvorak, A. M., 1986a, with permission.)

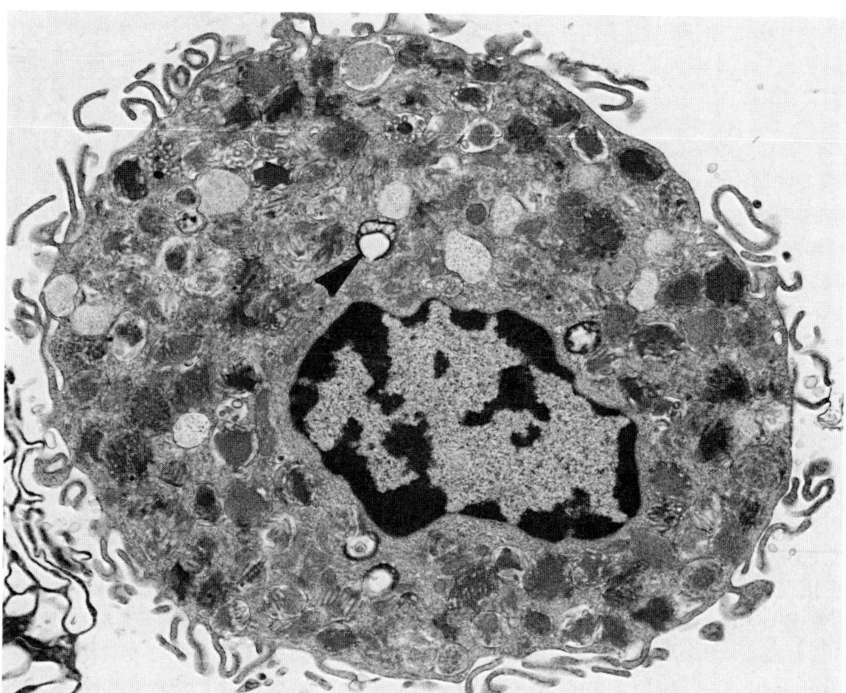

Figure 37 HSYMC ex vivo shows scroll granules, focal lucencies in lipid bodies (arrowhead), and PMD. ×12,000.

displayed regular arrays oriented in multiple directions. Mixed granules primarily contained scrolls and crystals; particle granules, in contrast to HGMCs, were rarely evident in HSYMCs (Kopicky-Burd et al., 1988).

We noted morphological evidence of antecedent release and recovery events in some osteoarthritis samples of synovium (Kopicky-Burd et al., 1988). Low yields of mast cells from rheumatoid arthritis synovial samples, prepared for electron microscopy, may have precluded us from gaining evidence for similar events in this arthritis. At any rate, HSYMCs revealed closed, recovering degranulation channels filled with amorphous, altered granule contents, as in HLMCs recovering from AND stimulated ex vivo (Dvorak AM et al., 1986). Since the HSYMC samples we examined were not similarly stimulated, these images might reflect antecedent degranulation events that occurred prior to cell isolation (Kopicky-Burd et al., 1988). We also noted that some HSYMCs contained nearly empty, nonfused granule chambers, typical of PMD (Fig. 37)—again, perhaps, reflecting antecedent events in vivo (Kopicky-Burd et al., 1988). Morphologically immature mast cells were present in synovial mast cell preparations. These cells showed considerable size variation, expanded Golgi structures, numerous cytoplasmic vesicles, and immature granules (Kopicky-Burd et al., 1988). Many of the latter contained central condensations of dense granule materials. Immature mast cells also displayed typical nuclear criteria for immaturity. We have noted similar morphological features in many HLMCs recovering from AND ex vivo (Dvorak AM et al., 1987, 1988). In the case of HLMCs degranulated and recovered ex vivo, recruitment of immature precursors is not possible in the closed ex vivo system. The immature mast cells in isolated, unstimulated human synovial preparations could have resulted from recovery from antecedent degranulation in vivo, by recruitment of immature precursors in vivo, or by a combination of these events.

VI. Human Skin Mast Cells

A. In Situ

Our light and electron microscopic studies of human skin mast cells (HSMC) began in 1971 when we initiated several large studies of newly stimulated, sequentially biopsied contact allergy skin reactions (Dvorak AM et al., 1976; Dvorak HF et al., 1974, 1976, 1980a, 1986) and, later, sequential biopsies of freshly transplanted human skin grafts (Dvorak HF et al., 1979, 1980b). Subsequently, we have conducted untrastructural studies of involved areas of skin as well as adjacent, clinically uninvolved skin in a wide variety of circumstances (Tables 1, 2). Most of this material was regularly submitted to us for diagnostic purposes. Among the diseases and conditions we have studied are the following: contact allergy (Dvorak AM et al., 1976), primary benign and malignant tumors

(Dvorak AM, unpublished data), metastatic tumors (Dvorak AM, unpublished data), superficial spreading melanomas (Dvorak AM et al., 1980b), halo nevi (Dvorak AM and Kwan T, unpublished data), wound healing (Dvorak AM and Kissell S, 1991), bullous pemphigoid (Dvorak AM and Kissell S, 1991; Dvorak AM et al., 1982), mannosidosis (Dickersin et al., 1980), Fabry's disease (Cable et al., 1982; Dvorak AM et al., 1981), dermatographism (Glovsky et al., 1987), amyloidosis (Dvorak AM, unpublished data), benign vascular proliferation of unclassified origin (Dvorak AM and Kissell S, 1991), urticaria associated with acute viral hepatitis B (Dienstag et al., 1978). We recently summarized some of this experience and much of the ultrastructural human mast cell morphological literature prior to 1987 (Dvorak AM, 1988b, 1989c, 1991a).

HSMCs have been examined by electron microscopists for years (Asboe-Hansen, 1971; Barnett, 1975; Bowyer, 1968; Burns and Hoak, 1975; Dvorak AM and Kissell S, 1991; Dvorak AM et al., 1976, 1980b, 1982, 1991c; Fedorko and Hirsch, 1965; Fujita et al., 1969, 1972; Hashimoto et al., 1966; Hibbs et al., 1960; Kobayasi and Asboe-Hansen, 1969a,b; Moriyasu and Yamura, 1973; Naveh et al., 1975; Orr, 1977; Pasyk et al., 1983; Tharp et al., 1988a,b; Trotter and Orr, 1974; Yancey et al., 1985; reviewed in Dvorak AM, 1989c), and these studies are generally in agreement regarding their ultrastructural features. HSMCs are often elongated, frequently perivascular granulated cells in normal skin samples. Their surfaces display regularly spaced, narrow, short surface folds, even when encased in interstitial collagen (Fig. 38). They are mononuclear cells with partly condensed nuclear chromatin. Large nucleoli are absent. Cytoplasmic organelle content is similar to that of mast cells of other locations, with two main exceptions. While lipid bodies do occur, they are rare in normal skin mast cells in situ (Dvorak AM and Kissell S, 1991). While all granule substructural patterns exist in HSMCs, crystal granules generally prevail (Dvorak AM and Kissell S, 1991) (Fig. 39). These granules are readily recognized by extremely regular arrays with basically two periodicities, measuring 12 nm and 6 nm (Asboe-Hansen, 1971). These parallel structures can be oriented in several different directions in individual granules. When seen in cross-section, they present a hexagonal array. These are the crystalline structures originally referred to by Fedorko and Hirsch in human mast cells (Fedorko and Hirsch, 1965). Individual HSMCs may contain mixtures of granule types as well as mixed granules. While these mixtures are variable, we regularly found the presence of crystals and scrolls in mast cells of skin origin (Dvorak AM and Kissell S, 1991; Dvorak AM et al., 1991c).

In certain pathological states, HSMCs undergo PMD characterized by partial or complete losses of their dense granule contents (Dvorak AM and Kissell S, 1991; Dvorak AM et al., 1982). These losses are clearly evident in high-magnification electron micrographs, where focal, ragged alteration of and loss of density to granules are well visualized (Dvorak AM and Kissell S, 1991)

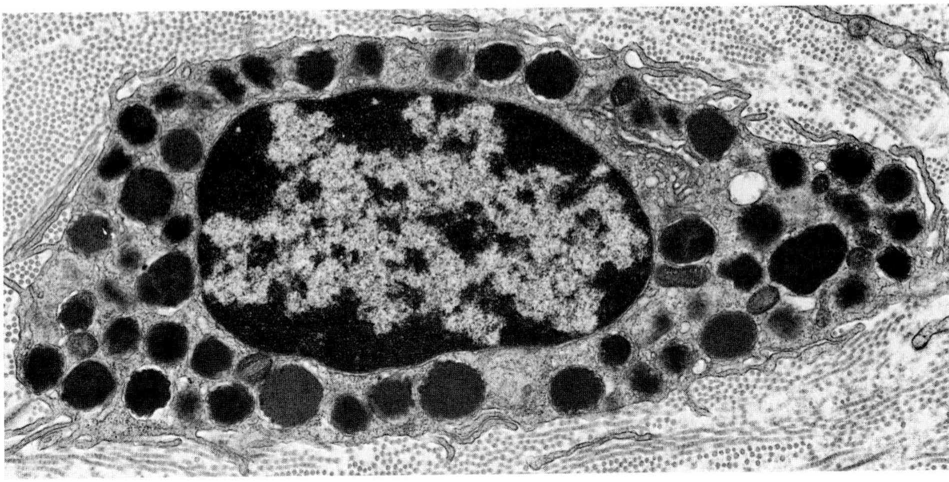

Figure 38 HSMC in situ in breast biopsy of a patient with fibroadenoma shows monolobed nucleus with partially condensed chromatin, small Golgi area, numerous membrane-bound, homogeneously dense granules with peripheral scrolls, mitochondria, and narrow surface folds. The entire cell is encased in interstitial collagen. ×16,500. (From Dvorak A and Kissell S; 1991, with permission.)

(Fig. 40). We recently examined PMD of HSMCs in bullous pemphigoid skin lesions at high magnification and found that focal, geographic losses of granule contents were uniquely associated with crystalline portions of mixed granules (Dvorak AM and Kissell S, 1991). Additionally, perigranular cytoplasmic smooth vesicles were prominent in cells participating in PMD (Dvorak AM and Kissell S, 1991) (Fig. 40). These structures were either empty or contained granule-like dense materials and were free in the cytoplasm or attached to granules (Fig. 40). Similarly, we have identified granule losses associated with PMD in HSMCs participating in the host response to superficial spreading melanoma (Dvorak AM et al., 1980b), in graft rejection (Dvorak HF et al., 1979; Dvorak HF et al., 1980b), and in contact allergy (Dvorak AM et al., 1976; Dvorak HF et al., 1974, 1976). Other investigators have described either focal or complete losses of granule contents in HSMCs in the absence of granule extrusion (Asboe-Hansen, 1971; Murphy et al., 1987). While different terms have been used to indicate this event, we believe that these also represent the process of PMD in situ by HSMCs.

Since it is now apparent that HLMCs have the capacity to reconstitute their granules by several mechanisms following AND in ex vivo samples (Dvorak AM et al., 1986, 1987, 1988) and since HSMCs undergoing PMD are not damaged

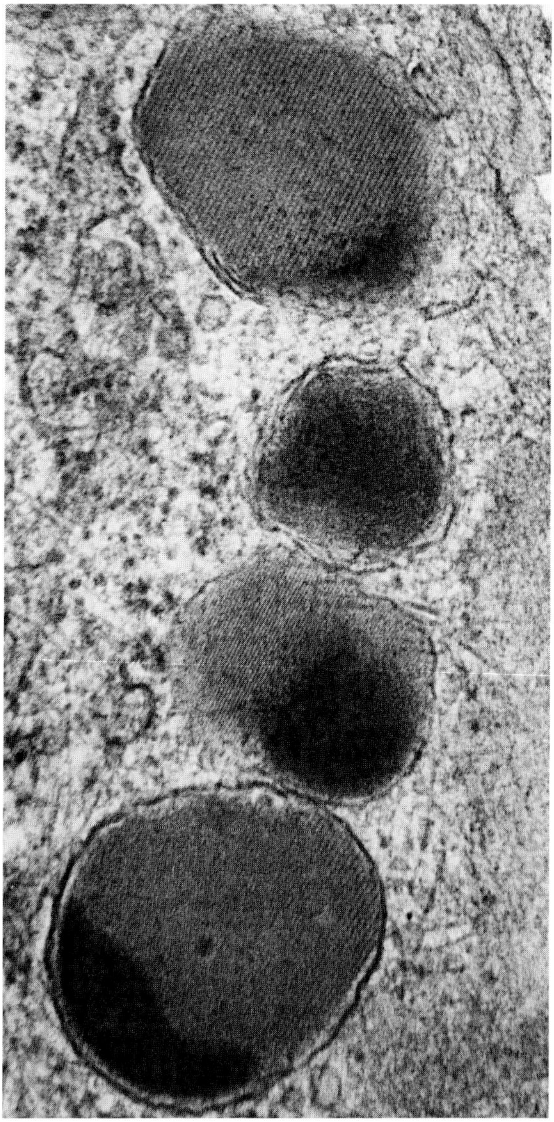

Figure 39 HSMC in situ in skin biopsy of patient with bullous pemphigoid shows four granules. These crystal granules express several periodicities, sometimes within the same granule, and focal areas of dense homogeneous contents. ×90,000. (From Dvorak, A. M. and Kissell S, 1991, with permission.)

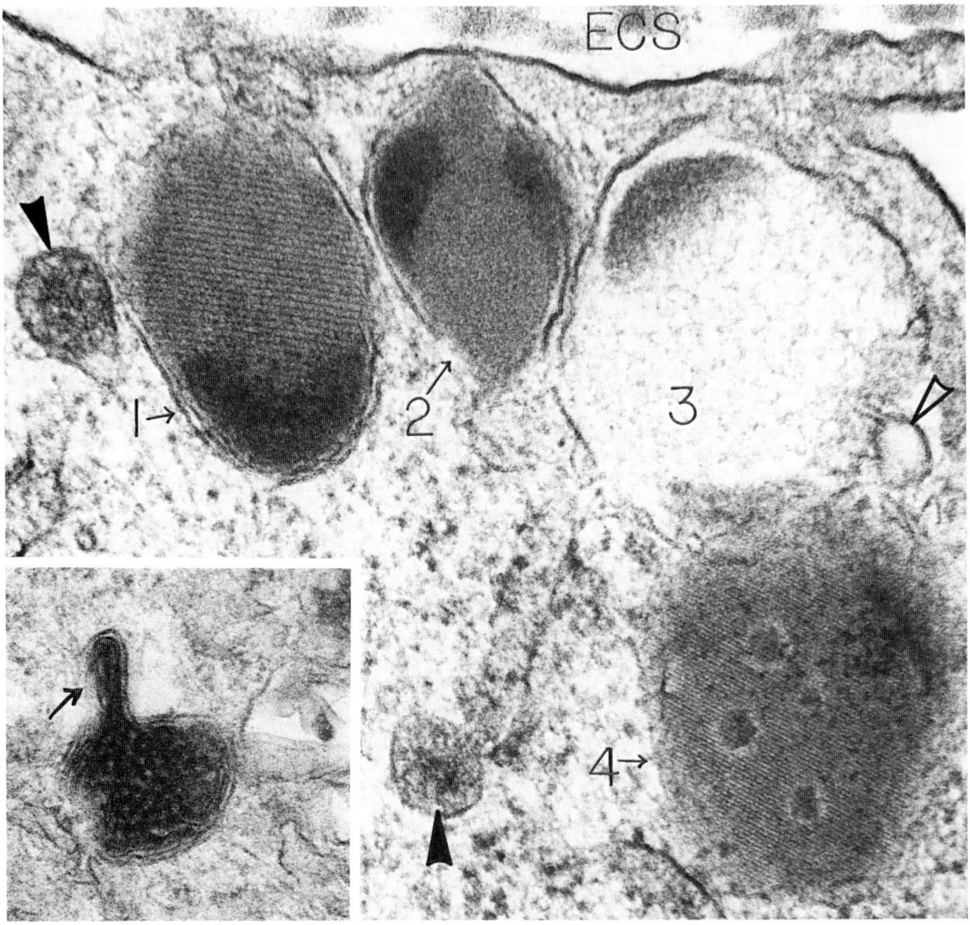

Figure 40 HSMCs in situ in skin biopsies of patients with bullous pemphigoid and fibrous histiocytoma (inset). The mast cell cytoplasm shows PMD. Granule 1 shows mixture of 8-nm parallel crystalline array and dense material; granule 2 shows finely granular material of several densities; granule 3 shows loss of nearly all contents; granule 4 shows 4-nm parallel crystalline array. Note four focal ring lesions in this granule. Cytoplasmic vesicles, either lucent (open arrowhead) or filled with dense granular material (closed arrowheads), are present. ECS = extracellular space. In the inset, a particle-filled vesicle (arrow) protrudes from a particle granule, reflecting vesicle budding as a mechanism for piecemeal granule losses. ×125,000; inset, ×73,500. (From Dvorak, A. M. and Kissell S, 1991, with permission.)

cells, we postulated that the empty granule containers are uniquely available for receiving new contents. Ultrastructural images documenting the accumulation of a wide variety of dense materials were then obtained in HSMCs present in wound healing (Dvorak AM and Kissell S, 1991) (Fig. 41). In contrast to PMD, where dense granule materials are focally altered and become widened, fragmented, and less dense (Fig. 40), the contents of granules in HSMCs in wound healing showed numerous irregular condensation foci of markedly dense new granule products within empty or partially empty granule containers (Dvorak AM and Kissell S, 1991) (Fig. 41). These new granule materials in HSMCs characteristically assumed numerous unique, intragranular dense patterns generally absent from unstimulated, normal HSMCs in vivo (Dvorak AM and Kissell S, 1991) and ex vivo (Dvorak AM et al., 1991c). Associated with this morphological evidence of recovery of HSMC granule contents in healing wounds was an exuberant proliferation of fibroblasts and angiogenesis. Recovering mast cells were encased in interstitial collagen adjacent to giant-sized, activated fibroblasts filled with expanded cisterns of membrane-bound ribosomes containing proteinaceous contents, interspersed with an angiogenesis response characteristic of granulation tissue (Dvorak AM and Kissel S, 1991).

Other investigators have described apparent mast cell recovery events during wound healing (Asboe-Hansen, 1971; Marckmann and Zachariae, 1964; Rasmussen, 1966; Wichmann, 1955). For example, mast cell numbers decreased in association with decreased histamine content of skin in early granulation tissue (Asboe-Hansen, 1971). Since most histamine in skin is associated with tissue mast cells (Riley and West, 1953), the parallel decrease in mast cell numbers and skin histamine content in early wound healing, with parallel increases in histamine and mast cell numbers in later wound healing (Asboe-Hansen, 1971; Marckmann and Zachariae, 1964; Rasmussen, 1966; Wichmann, 1955), suggests several possibilities. Recruitment of mast cell precursors to skin wounds could be responsible; division and growth of existing mast cells could increase mast cell numbers as well as skin histamine content; or mast cells could refill previously emptied granule containers. Our studies of HSMCs in wound healing, in the absence of mitosis, support the latter possibility—i.e., recovery of container contents. All three mechanisms, however, could act in concert to allow mast cell numbers and histamine levels to increase in healing wounds.

The presence of newly recruited, hypogranular mast cell precursors in in situ skin lesions is suggested by images of dense central granule nucleoids in mast cells that have reduced numbers of granules of smaller size than in normal mature cells and ultrastructural evidence of immaturity (Dvorak AM and Kissell S, 1991; Dvorak AM et al., 1976; Dvorak HF et al., 1974, 1976). Immature mast cells with evidence of granule immaturity exist in various cell-mediated immunological lesions of skin (Dvorak AM et al., 1976; Dvorak HF et al., 1974, 1976), chronic inflammatory disorders of gut (Dvorak AM, 1988c; Dvorak AM

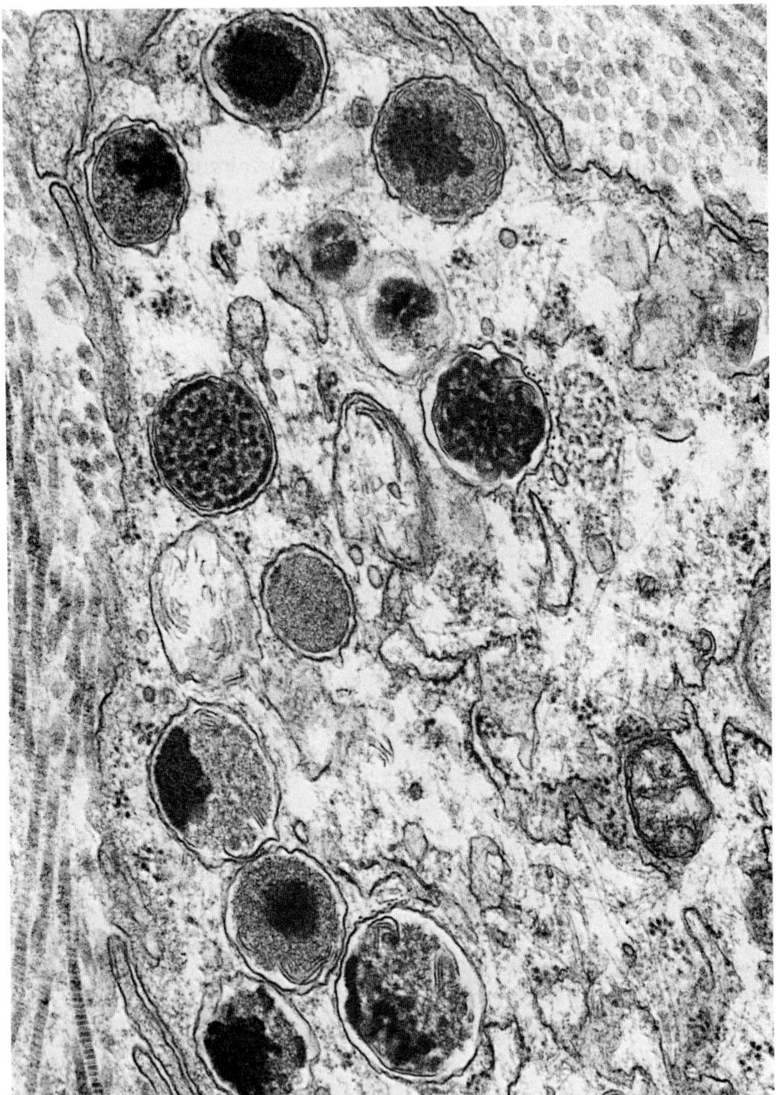

Figure 41 HSMC in situ in skin biopsy of dermal scar after excisions of melanoma and resection margins shows recovering granule matrix materials during wound healing. Note background of granule scrolls and finely granular material on which focal, homogeneously dense and very dense irregular threads or concentric, dense thick threads or dense particles are superimposed. The distribution of focal, homogeneously dense areas is either central or peripheral, in locations similar to those where piecemeal granule losses occur in releasing tissue mast cells (compare with PMD in Fig. 40). ×54,500. (From Dvorak, A. M. and Kissell S, 1991, with permission.)

et al., 1992a), neoplasms of lung (Peters et al., 1989, and Dvorak AM, unpublished data), as well as in newly developing mast cells cultured from human cord blood cells (Dvorak AM and Ishizaka T, 1992; Dvorak, AM, et al., 1992e; Furitsu et al., 1989). HLMCs recovering from AND in ex vivo experiments also reveal similar condensation of granule materials (Dvorak AM et al., 1988). Therefore, granule nucleoids are present in multiple circumstances, all of which are implicated in the production of human mast cell granule materials—i.e., in wound healing (Dvorak AM and Kissell S, 1991), in maturation of immature cells in multiple tissue locations of the body (Dvorak AM, unpublished data), in newly developing mast cells cultured from cord blood cell precursors (Dvorak AM and Ishizaka T, 1992; Dvorak, AM et al., 1992e; Furitsu et al., 1989), and in HLMCs ex vivo recovering from AND (Dvorak AM et al., 1986, 1987, 1988).

A number of electron microscopic studies of HSMCs in situ have appeared since our last literature review (up to 1987). (Dvorak AM, 1989c) Among these, several issues are addressed. For example, the apparent disappearance of mouse mast cells by light microscopic examination of graft-versus-host disease [viewed as a model for scleroderma (Claman et al., 1985] was investigated by electron microscopy (Claman et al., 1986). The missing mast cells that failed to stain with toluidine blue were visible in electron microscopic sections, leading the authors to dub them "phantom mast cells" (Claman et al., 1986), thus reestablishing the well-known fact that mast cells that cannot be visualized by light microscopy, for whatever reason, are readily identified with the electron microscope. "Phantom mast cells" (by this definition) are those that cannot be imaged by light microscopy but can be by electron microscopy. Investigation of the skin pathology associated with scleroderma revealed mat cell changes analogous to those reported in the mouse model of chronic graft-versus-host disease (Claman, 1989; Claman et al., 1986). In this instance, HSMCs were reported to be undergoing degranulation characterized by the "fusion of granules filled with pale, amorphous material" (Claman, 1989). These structures are, however, lipid bodies, not granules (Dvorak AM, 1991c; Dvorak AM et al., 1983b; Dvorak AM et al., 1992f; Galli et al., 1985; Weller et al., 1992). We have recently reviewed the varied ultrastructural images presented by lipid bodies in human mast cells as well as in numerous other mammalian cell types (Dvorak AM, 1991c; Galli et al., 1985). Lipid bodies are variably dense, nonmembrane-bound structures enmeshed in cytoskeletal filaments. The density of lipid bodies ranges from nearly electron-lucent to extremely dense (Figs. 2, 4, 6, 8, 15, 17–20, 23, 29B, 35). Some generalizations are possible among the observed densities of lipid bodies in different cell lineages when ultrastructural processing methods are kept constant. Dense lipid bodies generally are present in eosinophils (Weller and Dvorak AM, 1985; Weller et al., 1991a) and mast cells (Dvorak AM et al., 1983b, 1984, 1985b, 1986, 1987, 1988; Hammel et al., 1985); less dense lipid bodies are generally evident in neutrophils (Weller et al., 1989; Weller et al.,

1991b), macrophages (Dvorak AM et al., 1980a, 1983b), adipocytes (Galli et al., 1985), and fibroblasts (Dvorak AM, unpublished data). The observed density of these ubiquitous structures under standard processing conditions may reflect the ratio and type of phospholipids and neutral lipids present within them. Lipid bodies in most cell types that we regularly examine may also show variable areas of lucencies within them; numerous instances of fusion of lipid bodies are readily apparent in many mammalian cells (Dvorak AM, 1991c).

Thus, the "fused, swollen, pale granules" in clinically involved scleroderma skin (Fig. 2, in Claman, 1989) do not provide evidence for mast cell degranulation but do provide evidence for enhanced lipid body formation in a mast cell population (skin) that does not generally exhibit many lipid bodies in situ (Dvorak AM and Kissell S, 1991). The role of these arachidonic acid–containing structures (Dvorak AM, 1991c; Dvorak AM et al., 1983b, 1984, 1992f; Galli et al., 1985; Longworth et al., 1988; Weller and Dvorak AM, 1985; Weller et al., 1989, 1991a,b, 1992) in the pathobiology of mast cells and scleroderma shold be investigated further. Additionally, fibroblasts contained numerous pale lipid bodies in scleroderma (Figs. 3–5, in Claman, 1989). These cells should not be confused with "degranulating mast cells," wherever they exist (Table 3).

Light microscopic evaluation of human mast cells with specific antibodies for tryptase and chymase has provided interesting results regarding the distribution of mast cells containing these enzymes (Irani et al, 1989). Thus, while tryptase-containing mast cells predominate in lung alveoli and small intestinal mucosa, mast cells containing both enzymes are regularly present in skin, small intestinal submucosa, and tonsils (Irani et al., 1989). In particular, 99% of HSMCs were found to contain tryptase and chymase, suggesting considerable homogeneity in this population in adult skin (Irani et al., 1989). By ultrastructural analysis, HSMCs are also more homogeneous than are mast cells in other locations (Dvorak AM, 1989c; Dvorak AM and Kissell S, 1991); Dvorak AM et al., 1991c). Thus, we more regularly find crystal granule-containing cells in HSMC populations than in all other body locations (Dvorak AM and Kissell S, 1991; Dvorak AM et al., 1991c). Also of interest, immunomorphotyping of HSMCs from newborn foreskin tissue (a location with increased evidence of immature mast cells) shows cells that contain only chymase (Irani et al., 1989). These data suggest that during maturation of human mast cells (and perhaps in functional cycles of mature human mast cells), chymase appears first in immature mast cells (foreskin preparations); both enzymes are present in mature mast cells in locations that are less exposed to the repetitive release (and recovery) stimulated by environmental agents (skin and submucosa of the small intestine), and mast cells with tryptase alone predominate in locations where environmental exposures are extensive (lung, small intestine mucosa).

An attempt to subclassify human mast cells by immunogold localization of tryptase and chymase in ultrastructural preparations was made, but visualizing substructural granule patterns in the immunogold preparations was difficult (Craig and Schwartz, 1990; Craig et al., 1988, 1989). Until such substructural patterns are clearly and regularly visualized in immunogold preparations, classification of human mast cells based on these procedures remains uncertain. In general, the new studies (Craig et al., 1988, 1989) clearly show the granule location of chymase and tryptase in human mast cells; tryptase is more regularly associated with well-defined scrolls with lucent centers (and chymase is absent), perhaps because this pattern is more clearly visible than are other granule patterns in the immunogold preparations presented.

A recent ultrastructural evaluation of granule morphology in mast cells from multiple body sites (Weidner and Austen, 1990) confirmed the general ultrastructural evidence of remarkable diversity of human mast cells (reviewed in Dvorak AM, 1989c). The new study classified mast cells generally as "scroll-rich" or "scroll-poor," based on the presence or absence of well-defined scroll granules (Weidner and Austen, 1990). These studies (Weidner and Austen, 1990) confirmed the general presence of scroll-rich granules in human mast cells of lung or bowel mucosa origin and scroll-poor mast cells in skin, lymph nodes, breast, and bowel submucosa samples (reviewed in Dvorak AM, 1989c), as well as the frequent presence of mixed granules and cells with mixed granule populations of the scroll and crystal types (Dvorak AM, 1989c; Weidner and Austen, 1990). Scroll-poor mast cells, by definition, contained crystal granules, less well-defined scrolls, and amorphous granular material (Weidner and Austen, 1990). Such diversity of human mast cell granule architectural patterns makes immunogold subclassification of the enzyme contents of such granules difficult (Craig and Schwartz, 1990; Craig et al., 1988, 1989) until ultrastructural immunogold methods that are capable of imaging such patterns beneath the gold labels are done.

Because HSMCs in situ are infrequent in normal samples, many investigators have utilized the mast cell-rich dermal infiltrates of urticaria pigmentosa (UP) patients for ultrastructural studies (reviewed in Asboe-Hansen, 1971, and in Dvorak AM, 1989c). In general, some morphological atypicality [characterized by larger size, atypical, indented or bilobed nuclei, elongated narrow surface folds (Tharp et al., 1987a, 1988a,b) and increased numbers of scroll granules (Mirowski et al., 1990)] is recognized in mast cells of this origin, but the stimulated secretory biochemical analysis of this mast cell population, when isolated and examined ex vivo (Tharp et al., 1987a), does not differ from that of similarly prepared and examined HSMCs ex vivo (Lawrence et al., 1987; Lawrence et al., 1989; Tharp et al., 1987b). In certain cases, ultrastructural study of unstimulated UP skin biopsies has revealed typical intracytoplasmic degranulation channels with altered granule contents (Mirwoski et al., 1990) characteristic of AND (Dvorak AM, 1989c, 1991a).

HSMCs stimulated in situ by a variety of stimuli (including mechanical, antigen, or complement) have been studied by electron microscopy in biopsies of either normal or UP skin following such stimuli (Friedman and Kaliner, 1988; Kobayasi and Asboe-Hansen, 1969a; Moriyasu and Yamura, 1973; Swerlick et al., 1988; Yancey et al., 1985). In aggregate, these studies show that HSMCs express AND characterized by granule extrusion in these settings (Friedman and Kaliner, 1988; Kobayai and Asboe-Hansen, 1969a; Moriyasu and Yamura, 1973; Swerlick et al., 1988; Yancey et al., 1985). Thus, in HSMCs in situ, stimulated degranulation differs from the generalized formation of intracytoplasmic degranulation channels seen in stimulated HLMCs ex vivo (Caulfield et al., 1980; Dvorak AM et al., 1984, 1985b) and resembles that seen when HSMCs ex vivo are stimulated to degranulate (see next section; Dvorak AM et al., 1991c).

B. Ex Vivo

Functional studies of HSMCs using excised slices of skin have been available for some time (Greaves et al., 1972; Hermens et al., 1985; Tharp et al., 1983). More recently, efforts to improve on these studies have focused on the preparation of isolated skin cells from which variably pure mast cells of skin origin have been obtained (Benyon et al., 1986, 1987; Lawrence et al., 1987, 1989; Tharp et al., 1987b). These functional studies, in concert with similar studies using isolated mast cells of lung or gut origin, have revealed differences in eicosanoid production and in responsiveness to various secretory stimuli among mast cells of skin, lung, and gut origin (Lawrence et al., 1987; Tharp et al., 1987b).

Isolated HSMCs were prepared by enzymatic digestion of adult skin samples obtained from reduction mammoplasties and cultured overnight prior to electron microscopic studies (Dvorak AM et al., 1991c; Lawrence et al., 1987). Control, isolated HSMCs were well preserved and fully granulated (Fig. 42). Although all granule patterns reported for human mast cells were found, crystal granules were the most prevalant (Fig. 43), as is true for HSMCs in situ (Dvorak AM and Kissell S, 1991; Dvorak AM et al., 1991c). Moreover, single mast cells with individual crystal and scroll granules (Fig. 43), as well as mixed crystal-scroll granules, were evident. Lipid bodies (Fig. 43) occurred more frequently (Dvorak AM et al., 1991c) than in in situ HSMCs (Dvorak AM and Kissell S, 1991) but less frequently than in isolated mast cells of lung (Dvorak AM et al., 1983b), gut (Fox et al., 1985), synovial (Kopicky-Burd et al., 1988), or uterine (Massey et al., 1991) origin. The remainder of the ultrastructural features of isolated HSMCs was similar to their in situ counterparts (Dvorak AM and Kissell S, 1991). IgE-mediated AND of isolated HSMCs was accompanied by histamine release and characteristically showed extrusion of altered, membrane-free granules through multiple pores in the plasma membrane to the exterior of the cell (Fig. 44) (Dvorak AM et al., 1991c). Some cells also showed other morpho-

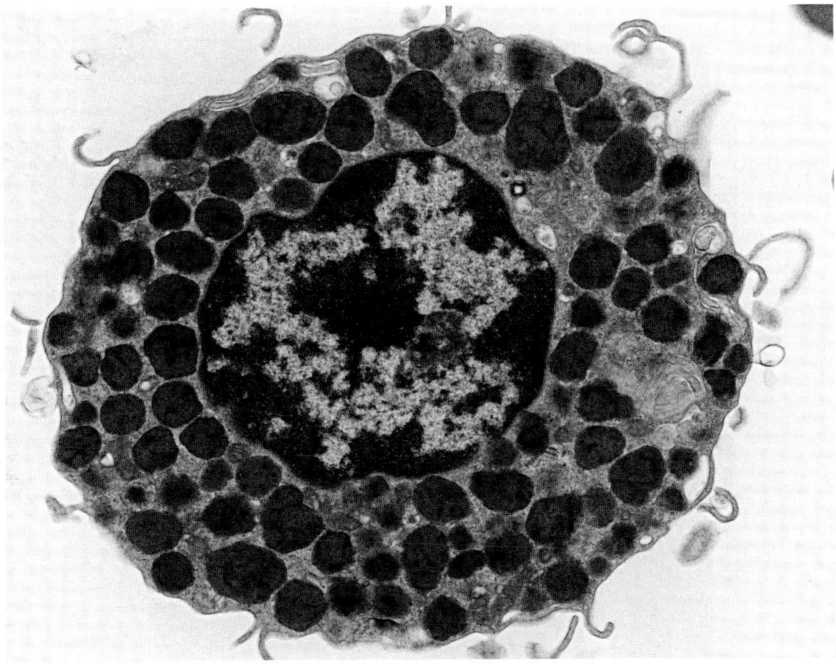

Figure 42 HSMC ex vivo shows well-preserved cell with full complement of dense granules. Lipid bodies are not present. ×11,000.

logical aspects of AND as expressed by isolated HLMCs (Dvorak AM et al., 1984, 1985b). These included granule swelling, fusion, alteration of matrix contents, degranulation channel formation, pore formation, and shedding of granules, membranes, and surface processes (Dvorak AM et al., 1991c).

The ultrastructural morphology of isolated HSMCs and their IgE-mediated degranulation (Dvorak AM et al., 1991c) shows some differences from similar studies of isolated HLMCs (Dvorak AM et al., 1983b, 1984, 1985b) and of HLMCs and HGMCs in biopsy samples (Dvorak AM, 1988c; Dvorak AM et al., 1992a,b; Peters et al., 1989). These differences include crystal granules as the predominant granule pattern, minor numbers of lipid bodies, and extrusion of granules during AND as characteristic for HSMCs (Dvorak AM et al., 1991c). By contrast, isolated HLMCs and HGMCs have more scroll granules and particle granules, respectively, and more lipid bodies (Dvorak AM et al., 1983b; Dvorak AM et al., 1984; Fox et al., 1985). In isolated HLMCs, AND is almost exclusively an intracellular fusion event characterized by the formation of complex degranulation channels within which altered granule matrix materials solubilize (Dvorak AM et al., 1984, 1985b). In addition to morphological

differences between mast cells of skin, lung, or gut origin, functional differences have been reported among mast cells of these organs (Lawrence et al., 1987, 1989). The ultrastructural morphology of isolated HSMCs (Dvorak AM et al., 1991c) is identical to that of skin mast cells in biopsy samples (Dvorak AM and Kissell S, 1991), thereby validating the usefulness of this new source of HSMCs for correlative functional and morphological studies.

Two recent ultrastructural studies of HSMCs ex vivo have reported degranulation responses to anti-IgE or substance P (Caulfield et al., 1990; Matis et al., 1990). In one study (Caulfield et al., 1990), HSMCs isolated from foreskins of patients 2–7 years of age were examined ex vivo. As in reports of others (reviewed in Dvorak AM, 1989c), this population of HSMCs was shown to contain primarily crystal granules. (Note: These authors equate three granule patterns with the generic term "crystal granules" as follows: scrolls, gratings, lattices. By this terminology, the lattice pattern ≈ to the longitudinal, regular parallel crystalline array of crystal granules; the grating pattern ≈ to the regular hexagonal array of the crystal pattern cut in cross-section; and the scroll pattern ≈ to scroll granules. Thus, some confusion may arise, since all scroll patterns are referred to as crystalline granules by these authors; scroll granules are thus not treated separately; and particle granules are not included at all.) The isolated HSMCs were exposed to either anti-IgE or substance P as secretagogues and subsequently examined by ultrastructure (Caulfield et al., 1990). These authors found that no ultrastructural differences existed in HSMCs between the morphology induced by these stimuli, despite numerous biochemical differences induced by these separate agents. In addition, and as in our study of isolated adult HSMCs (Dvorak AM et al., 1991c), they found both intracytoplasmic degranulation channel formation and granule extrusion to occur in stimulated HSMCs ex vivo (Caulfield et al., 1990). In another ultrastructural study of ex vivo HSMCs, organ cultures of skin slices from newborn foreskins were stimulated by substance P and examined by electron microscopy. In this system, extrusion of altered granule matrices to the cell's exterior was also illustrated (Matis et al., 1990).

VII. Human Uterine Mast Cells

A. Ex Vivo

Human uterine mast cells (HUMCs), prepared from hysterectomy specimens by mechanical and enzymatic dispersion, overnight culture, and separation on discontinuous Percoll gradients, were functionally and morphologically intact (Massey et al., 1991). Functional studies have shown that these isolated, purified HUMCs are unlike HSMCs but similar, with minor differences, to HLMCs as assayed in isolated preparations (Lawrence et al., 1987; Massey et al., 1991).

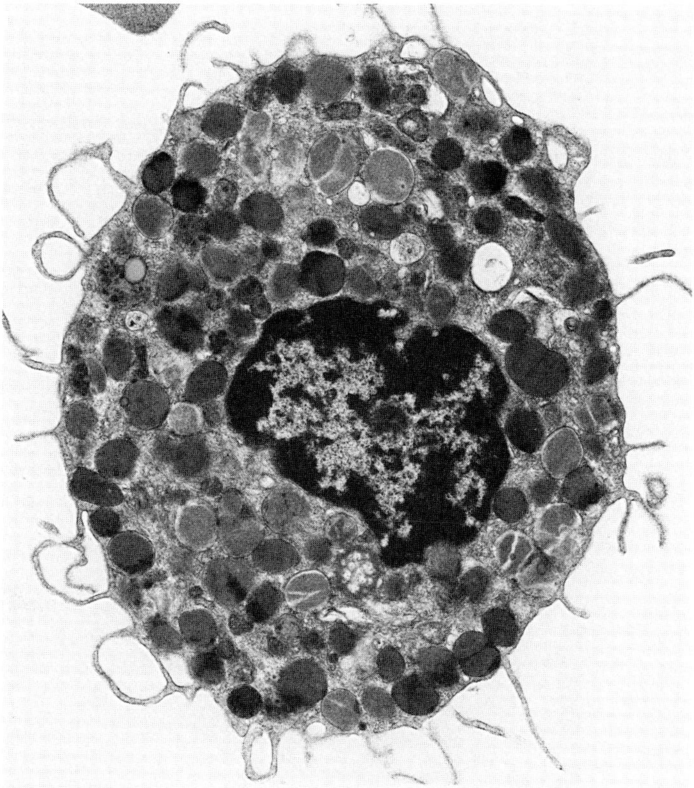

Figure 45 HUMC ex vivo is a mononuclear cell with narrow surface folds that is filled with dense granules. Several partially dense lipid bodies are seen. ×14,500.

The ultrastructural analysis of isolated HUMC preparations revealed large and small, well-preserved mast cells (Fig. 45) (Massey et al., 1991). Cell surfaces displayed narrow folds; nuclei were single-lobed, and many had large nucleoli and partly condensed chromatin; cytoplasmic contents were dominated by numerous large, membrane-bound granules and nonmembrane-bound lipid bodies. Additional cytoplasmic fetures included many cytoplasmic filaments, free ribosomes, and mitochondria. Cytoplasmic granules included several ultrastructural patterns (Figs. 46, 47). These included, in descending order of frequency, scrolls (Fig. 47) > crystals (Fig. 46) > homogeneously dense > combined scroll and crystals (Fig. 46) > reticular (thick irregular threads). Particle granules were conspicuously absent. Crystal granules displayed regular parallel arrays of several periodicities, as reported previously (Asboe-Hansen,

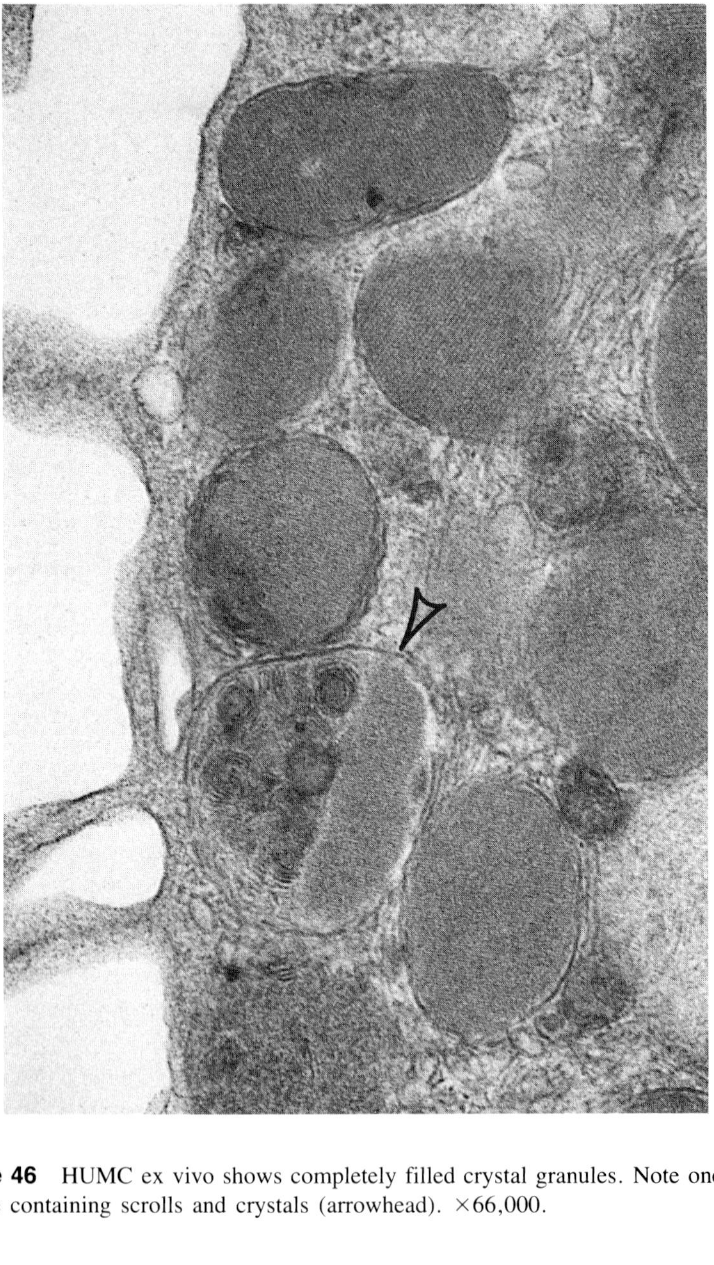

Figure 46 HUMC ex vivo shows completely filled crystal granules. Note one mixed granule containing scrolls and crystals (arrowhead). ×66,000.

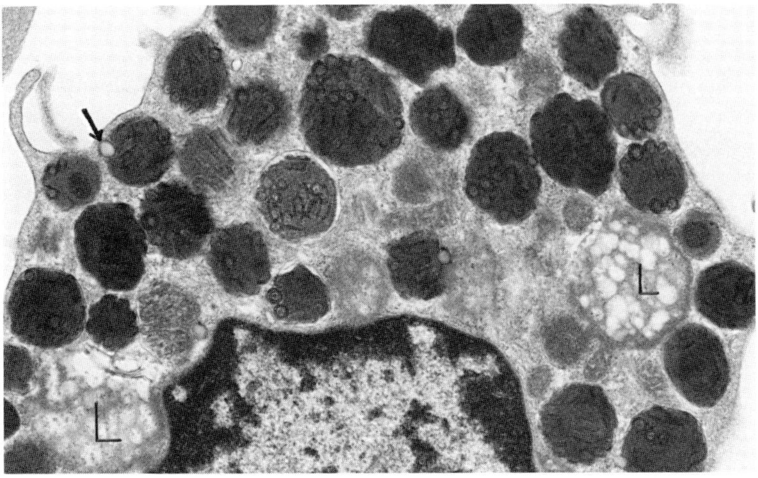

Figure 47 HUMC ex vivo shows scroll granules and two moderately dense lipid bodies (L) with numerous focal lucencies within them. One scroll granule also contains a similar focal, rounded, electron-lucent lipid structure (arrow). ×21,500.

1971; Dvorak AM, 1989c; Dvorak AM and Kissell S, 1991; Dvorak AM et al., 1991c); scroll granules either displayed lucent interiors or contained dense material in their centers, as reported (Dvorak AM, 1989c; Dvorak AM et al., 1984). Granules with dense central nucleoids surrounded by granule matrix, as in recovering or developing mast cell granules (Dvorak AM and Ishizaka T. 1992; Dvorak AM et al., 1992e; Dvorak AM and Kissell S, 1991), were present (Fig. 48). Somc enlarged granules resembled granule materials condensing and crystallizing in resolving degranulation channels (Dvorak AM et al., 1986). Several closed degranulation channels with less condensed, altered granule materials were present. Central canalicular structures, suggestive of antecedent (e.g., in vivo) resolution of degranulating cells (Dvorak AM et al., 1988), were also noted.

Nonmembrane-bound lipid bodies (Dvorak AM, 1989c, 1991b; Dvorak AM et al., 1983b, 1984) were very large, were encased in cytoplasmic filaments, and frequently displayed focal lucent areas (Figs. 48, 49). Many lucent areas consisted of small, round structures with punctate densities within them, similar to the changes in these generally dense structures that we noted in mast cells of gut origin (Fox et al., 1985).

Small mast cells with immature nuclei and diminished numbers of cytoplasmic granules were present (Fig. 49). These immature cells could reflect recovering mast cells after an antecedent degranulation event in the uterus in vivo (Dvorak AM et al., 1987) or maturation of newly recruited, immature mast cell

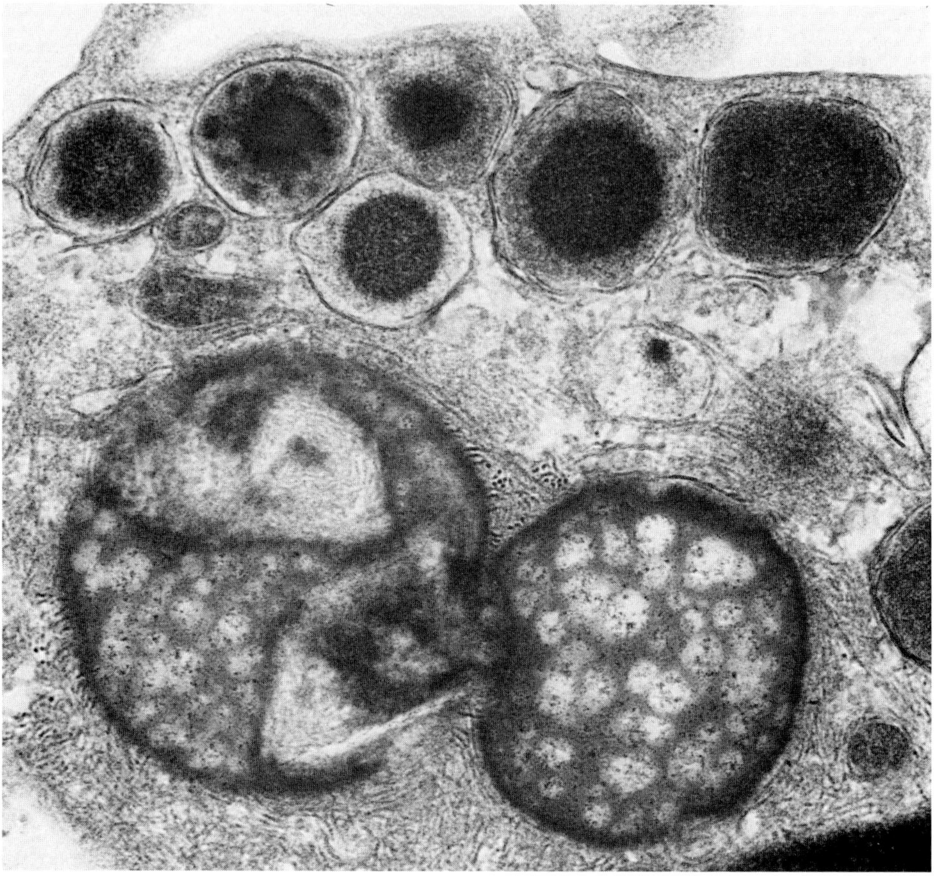

Figure 48 HUMC ex vivo shows two large lipid bodies enmeshed in intermediate filaments. Note focal particles within rounded lucent structures within the lipid bodies. The peripheral cytoplasm contains immature granules with condensing central nucleoids within them. ×52,000.

precursors into the uterus in vivo prior to surgery and subsequent isolation procedures.

VIII. Miscellaneous Human Mast Cells

A. In Situ

While biopsies of nearly all organ sites within which mast cells reside in humans have been examined by electron microscopy (Dvorak AM, unpublished data), several sites in addition to those already discussed are biopsied with more

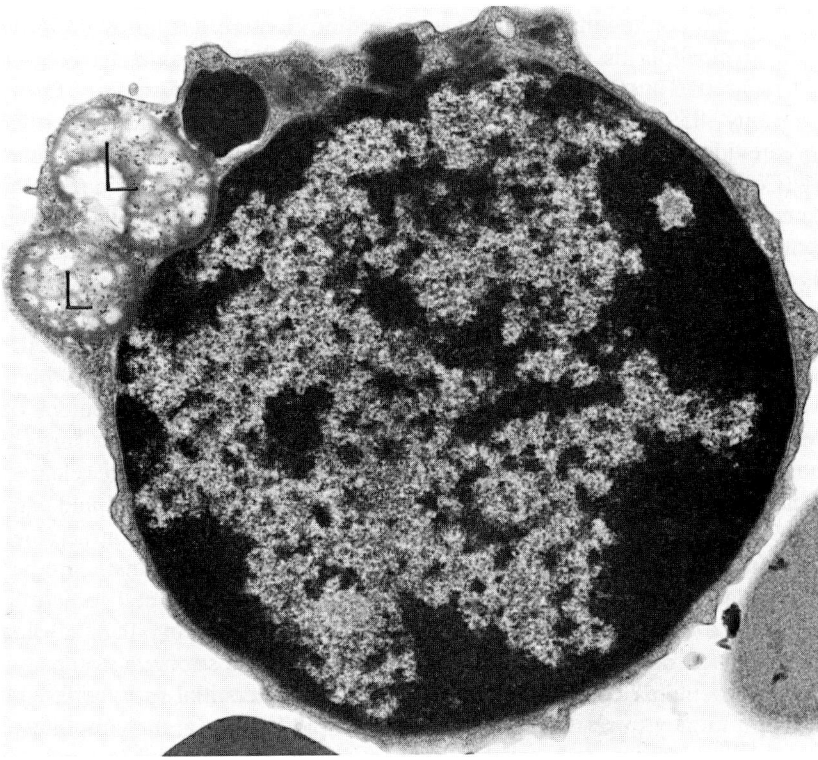

Figure 49 HUMC ex vivo is a small cell whose nucleus, with condensed chromatin, nearly fills the cell. Several dense granules and two large lipid bodies (L) are seen. ×16,000. (From Massey et al., 1991, with permission.)

frequency than others. These include kidney (Colvin et al., 1974; Dvorak AM and Monahan, 1985), breast (Dvorak HF et al., 1981; Weidner and Austen, 1990), and lymph nodes (Harris et al., 1982; Parmley et al., 1975; Weidner and Austen, 1990). We next discuss some ultrastructural observations regarding these sites.

Kidney

In a large study of kidney biopsies ($n = 42$), using giant 1μ, Epon-embedded, alkaline-Giemsa–stained sections, a striking and consistent increase in interstitial mast cells (HKMC) was found in several types of kidney diseases (Colvin et al., 1974). These diseases included chronic renal allograft rejection, analgesic nephropathy, chronic glomerulonephritis, chronic pyelonephritis, and malignant nephrosclerosis. Further, large numbers of mast cells were found within the

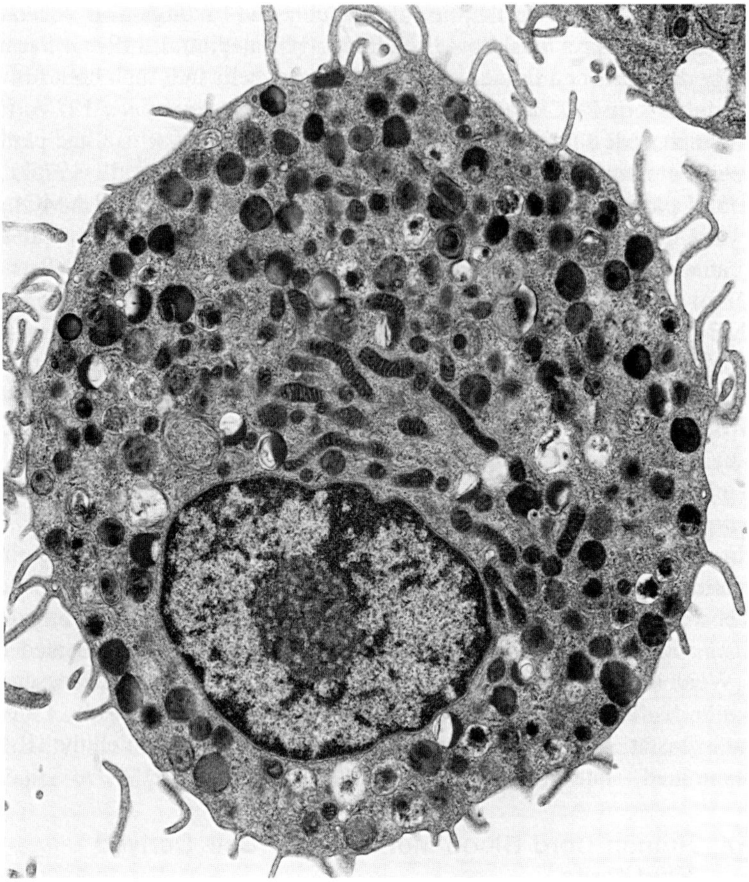

Figure 50 HCBMC in vitro. This nearly mature mast cell arose in human cord blood cells cocultured with 3T3 mouse skin fibroblasts. It has a monolobed nucleus with a large nucleolus, evenly distributed narrow surface folds, elongated mitochondria, free cytoplasmic ribosomes, and numerous small, membrane-bound dense granules. × 12,500.

Previously reported substructural granule patterns were present. The most conspicuous included regular crystalline arrays of several periodicities and orientations (Fig. 51), spirals and scrolls (Fig. 52), particles, and homogeneously dense areas. Many granules contained mixtures of these patterns. Most cultured HCBMCs expressed some granules with regular crystalline arrays (Fig. 51) like those most frequently present in HSMCs studied in situ (Dvorak AM and Kissell S, 1991) or ex vivo (Dvorak AM et al., 1991c). Scroll granules (Fig. 52),

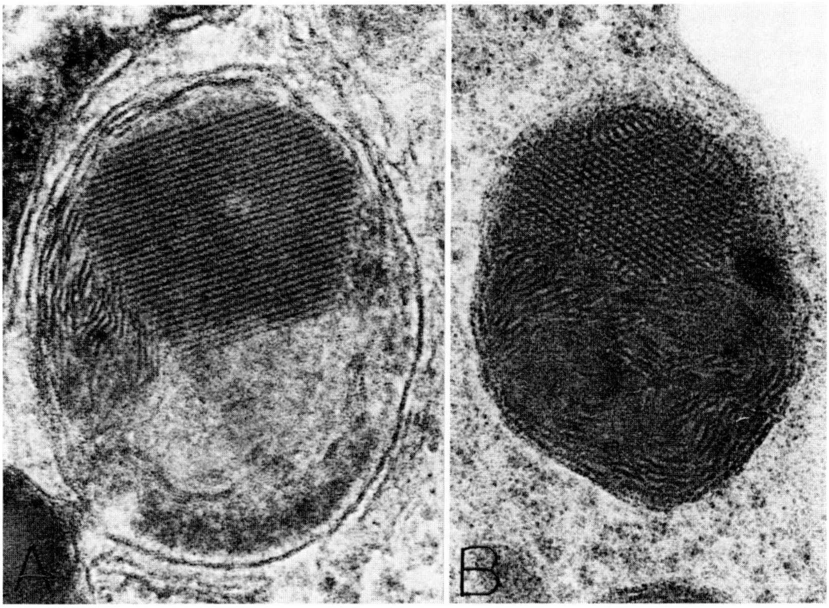

Figure 51 HCBMCs in vitro. High magnification images of crystals in mixed granules seen in (A) longitudinal and (B) cross-sections provide definitive proof that cells containing them are of the mast cell lineage. (A) ×97,000; (B) ×114,000.

typically found in HLMCs in situ (Peters et al., 1989) or ex vivo (Dvorak AM et al., 1984), were rare. Also, as in HSMCs, lipid bodies were rare (Dvorak AM, 1991a; Dvorak AM et al., 1991c; Furitsu et al., 1989). The mast cells that developed in these cultures were clearly different, by ultrastructural criteria, from mature basophils (Dvorak AM, 1988a; Dvorak AM et al., 1985a, 1989; Ishizaka et al., 1985), basophilic myelocytes (Dvorak AM, 1988a; Dvorak AM et al., 1985a, 1989), mature eosinophils (Dvorak AM et al., 1989, 1991a,b), and eosinophilic myelocytes (Dvorak AM, 1988a; Dvorak AM et al., 1985a, 1989, 1991a; Saito et al., 1988) arising in cultures of human cord blood cells containing various growth factors. Thus, culture conditions required for the development of human mast cells differ from those necessary for the development of basophils and support the morphological fact that basophils and mast cells are distinct and independent cellular lineages.

The sequential morphology of the development of HCBMC precursors is currently under investigation by electron microscopy (Dvorak AM and Ishizaka T, 1992; Dvorak AM et al., 1992e). Complete data are not yet available, but it is clear that immature mast cells (Fig. 53), as well as mature mast cells, are present

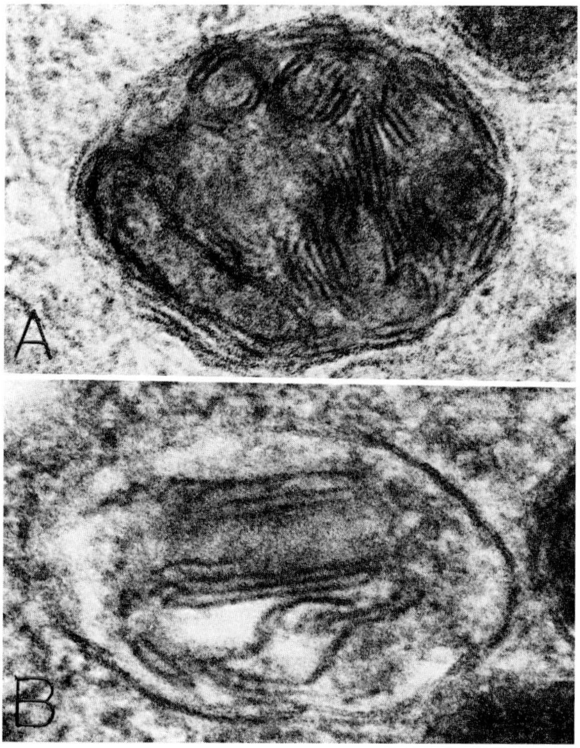

Figure 52 HCBMCs in vitro. High magnification images of scroll granules seen in (A) cross-section and (B) longitudinal views. (A) ×109,000; (B) ×158,000.

in 3-month-old cultures. Many of these cells are larger than mature cells, contain fewer and smaller granules, and display nuclear and cytoplasmic evidence of immature cells (Fig. 53). In particular, immature mast cells contained empty or partly full granules, often displaying dense central nucleoids superimposed on underlying granule materials (Fig. 54). This visual evidence of granule dense content condensation resembles, in part, granules in immature mast cells in situ, particularly in skin samples (Dvorak AM and Kissell S, 1991; Dvorak AM et al., 1976; Dvorak HF et al., 1976, 1979, 1980a,b) and granules recovering from PMD in wound healing (Dvorak AM and Kissell S, 1991).

X. Concluding Comments

The durability of morphological facts is assured and important to the understanding of cell biological events. Morphological facts do not change; it is our

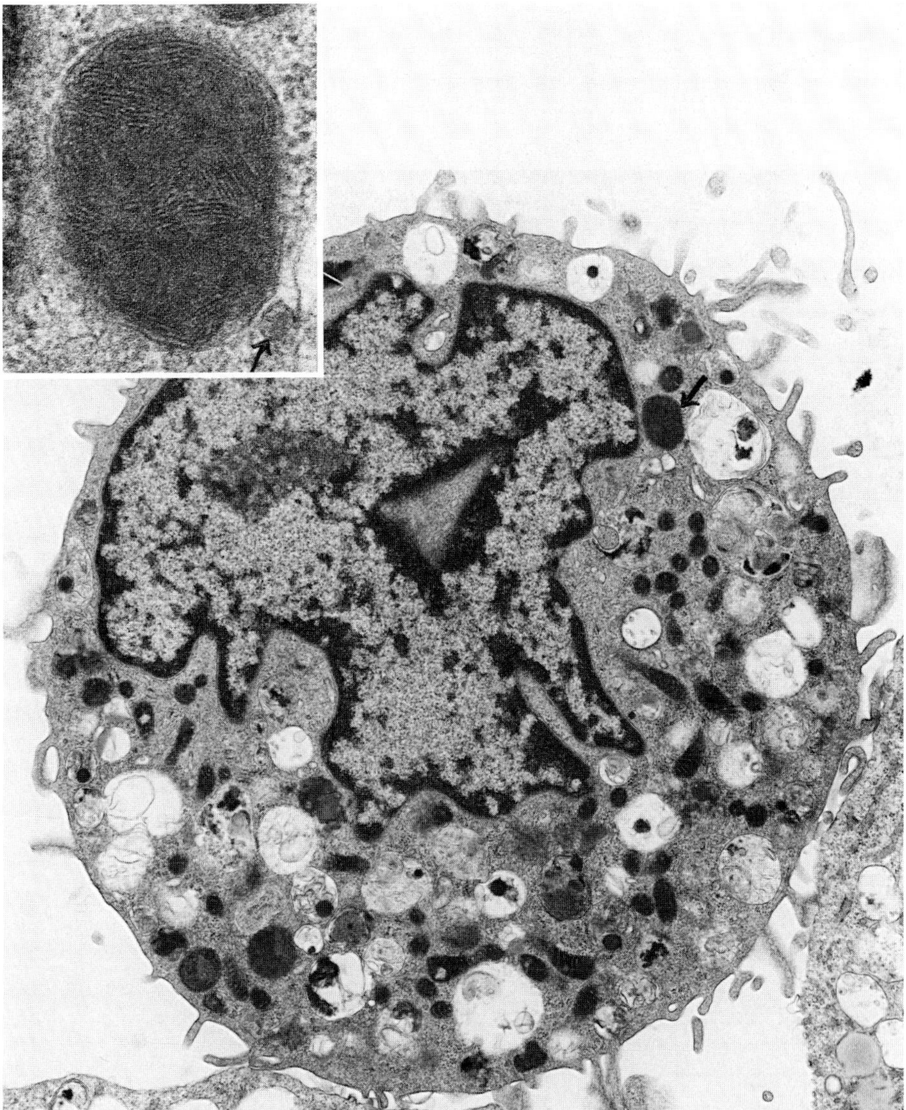

Figure 53 HCBMC in vitro. This immature mast cell arose in human cord blood cells cocultured with 3T3 cells and shows a large lobular nucleus with partially condensed chromatin and a large nucleolus. Narrow surface folds are short. The cytoplasm is filled with numerous large, partially filled granule containers among which smaller, mature granules with irregular crystalline arrays reside (arrow indicates mature granule, enlarged in the inset). Inset: Note small vesicle with dense material (arrow) adjacent to crystal granule. ×14,500; inset ×81,000.

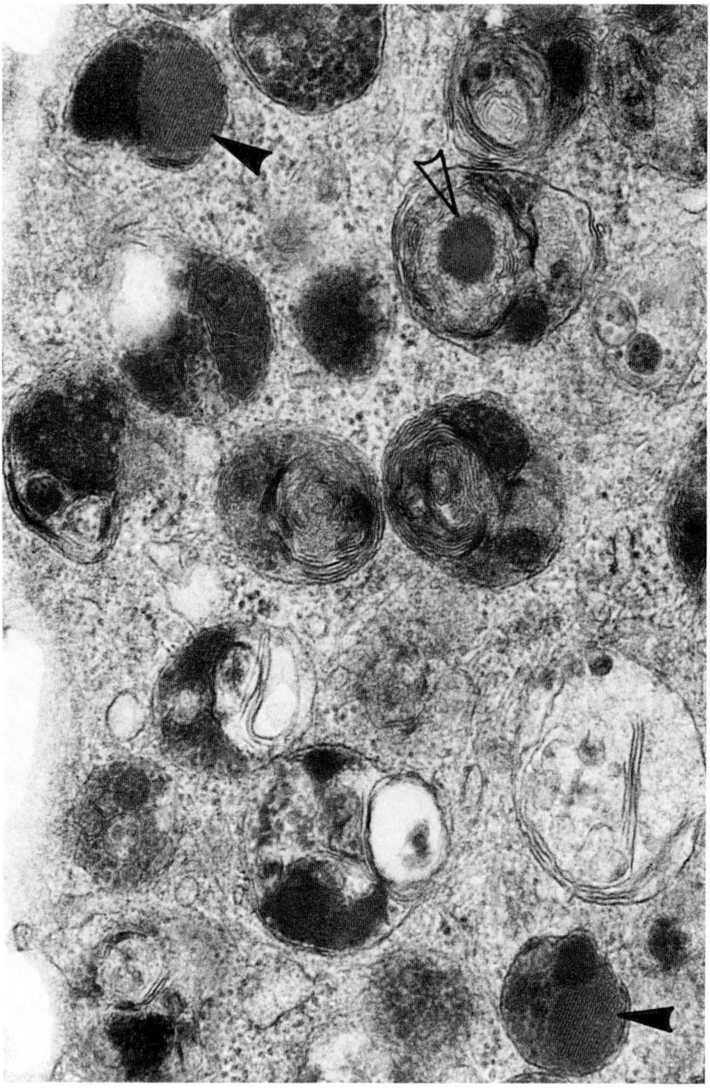

Figure 54 HCBMC in vitro. Another immature mast cell, developing in a coculture of human cord blood cells and 3T3 fibroblasts, shows marked heterogeneity of granule contents. Typical crystals within granules (closed arrowheads) definitively identify the mast cell lineage. Condensing central nucleoids of immature granules are seen (open arrowhead). A mixture of vesicles, lamellae, finely and coarsely granular, and homogeneously dense materials fill the immature granules of this immature mast cell. ×61,000.

interpretation of morphological facts that changes. We summarize in the tables the database (and results) on which the morphological facts that we present here were obtained. Table 1 lists the in situ, ex vivo, and in vitro sites, sources, and systems on which our ultrastructural observations of human mast cells are based; Table 2 lists human diseases from which we have obtained ultrastructural samples for study; Table 3 describes criteria for the identification of human mast cells and cells with which they have been confused; Table 4 lists the cellular sources and studies where we have shown incorporation of [^{3}H]arachidonic acid into lipid bodies; Table 5 gives the relative distribution of lipid bodies in various populations of human mast cells; Table 6 lists the circumstances in which we have identified degranulation processes (PMD/AND) in human mast cells; Table 7 summarizes morphological data obtained in ultrastructural analyses of the multiple sites, sources, and systems of human mast cells we have examined in situ, ex vivo, and in vitro. Much of these data have been published; a considerable amount of information has not been previously published, primarily because human mast cells were observed as side issues to larger targeted projects or to patient-care-related biopsies, and, in some instances, because the information gained was available in the publications of others as, for example, in HLNMCs (Parmley et al., 1975). This review has served, then, as a mechanism for us to assemble such morphological facts regarding human mast cells that we consider to be durable, albeit subject to changing interpretations by us and future investigators of mast cell biology. These facts follow:

1. Specific and unique granule architectural patterns allow identification of human mast cells, regardless of their origin.
2. Other morphological features (nucleus, lipid bodies, surface architecture, and the *absence* of features regularly present in other cells) support the lineage assignment of individual cells to that of human mast cells.
3. Lipid bodies are arachidonic acid–rich intracellular organelles, different from secretory granules, that are present in human mast cells but also are widespread in other mammalian cells; they may vary in incidence, size, density, and substructural details among human mast cell populations.
4. While all described ultrastructural granule patterns may be found in human mast cells of all organ sites, certain generalizations are true, as follows.
   a. HLMCs more generally have scroll granules.
   b. HGMCs more generally have scroll granules.
   c. HSMCs more generally have crystal granules.
   d. HSYMCs more generally have scroll granules.
   e. HUMCs more generally have scroll and crystal granules.

Table 7 Summary of Ultrastructural Studies of Human Mast Cells of Multiple Sites/Sources/Systems Examined In Situ, Ex Vivo, and In Vitro

Site/source/system	In situ	Ex vivo	In vitro	Lipid bodies	Granules predominant	Degranulation patterns
HLMC	+			+	Scroll	PMD
HLMC		+		+	Scroll	AND primarily characterized by cytoplasmic degranulation channels
HLMC			+	+	Scroll	DNK
HGMC	+			+	Scroll, particle	PMD, AND characterized by cytoplasmic degranulation channels and extrusion of granules
HGMC		+		+	Scroll, particle	DNK
HSYMC	+			+	Scroll	DNK
HSYMC		+		+	Scroll	DNK
HSMC	+			Rare	Crystal	PMD
HSMC		+		Increased over in situ but still rare	Crystal	AND primarily characterized by extrusion of granules
HUMC		+		+	Scroll, crystal	DNK
HCBMC			+	Rare	Crystal	DNK
HHMC	+			Rare	Scroll	AND characterized by cytoplasmic degranulation channels and extrusion of granules

HLMC = human lung mast cells; HGMC = human gastrointestinal mast cells; HSYMC = human synovial mast cells; HSMC = human skin mast cells; HUMC = human uterine mast cells; HCBMC = human cord blood-derived mast cells; HHMC = human heart mast cells; DNK = data not known; PMD = piecemeal degranulation; AND = anaphylactic degranulation.

   f. HHMCs more generally have scroll granules.
   g. HCBMCs more generally have crystal granules.
   h. HKMCs more generally have scroll granules (note small sample personally examined).
   i. HBMCs more generally have crystal and scroll granules.
   j. HLNMCs more generally have particle and crystal granules (Parmley et al., 1975).
   k. Particle granules are more generally found in intraepithelial human mast cells of gastrointestinal, respiratory, and kidney tubular origin.
   l. Particle granules are also present in HGMCs, HLMCs, HLNMCs; they are exceedingly rare in HSMCs and HCBMCs.
5. Human mast cells may contain granules primarily of one ultrastructural pattern; human mast cells may contain mixtures of individually patterned granules; individual granules within single human mast cells may display mixtures of known patterns.
6. Human mast cells with mixtures of scroll and crystal granules, although infrequent, are present in many tissue sites studied.
7. Human mast cells with mixtures of scroll and particle granules are more commonly identified in most sites and sources, except in HSMCs or HCBMCs.
8. Scroll granules (so-called discrete scrolls or empty scrolls) are associated with tryptase-positive human mast cells (MC_T) (Craig and Schwartz, 1990; Craig et al., 1988, 1989).
9. Crystal granules (so-called grating or lattice substructures, or compact, dense, nondiscrete scrolls) are associated with tryptase- and chymase-positive human mast cells (MC_{TC}), an immunogold ultrastructural finding (Craig and Schwartz, 1990; Craig et al., 1988, 1989) that needs direct, simultaneous demonstration of granule architectural patterns in immunogold preparations.
10. AND ultrastructural patterns differ in human mast cells of different sources; HLMCs ex vivo generally display intracytoplasmic fusion events, degranulation channel formation and alteration, and solubilization of granules within cytoplasmic degranulation channels; HSMCs ex vivo and in situ generally display granule extrusion events. Both patterns of AND have, however, been identified in human mast cells as follows: HLMCs ex vivo; HSMCs ex vivo; HGMCs in situ; HHMCs in situ.
11. HLMCs previously degranulated (AND) ex vivo recover by conservation and synthetic mechanisms.
12. In a closed system, wherein recruitment of nongranulated human mast cell precursors is impossible, and mitosis is absent, previously degranulated (AND) small HLMCs ex vivo that have shed all gran-

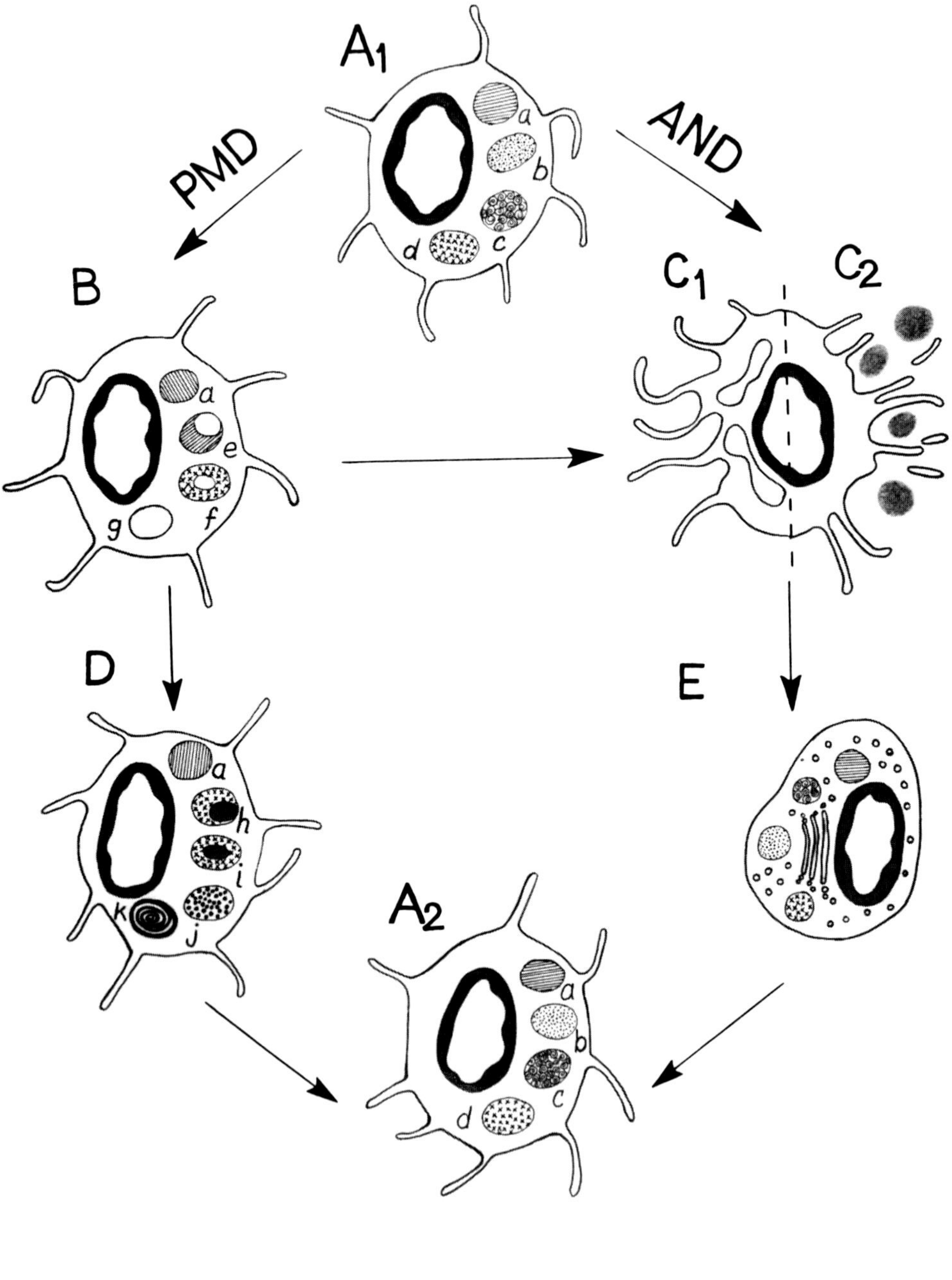
A1
PMD
AND
a
b
c
d
B
a
e
f
g
C1
C2
D
a
h
i
j
k
E
A2
a
b
c
d

ules and their containers undergo blast transformation and granule synthesis to reconstitute their cytoplasmic contents.

13. Nonfused human mast cell granules can increase in size by swelling and alteration of matrix contents and can reverse this process by condensation of matrix contents.
14. PMD of human mast cells in situ is widespread in human diseases involving multiple organ sites sampled for ultrastructural studies.
15. Two chronic inflammatory bowel diseases—ulcerative colitis and Crohn's disease—show extremely high degrees of PMD of HGMCs located in "so-called" uninvolved tissue sites—a morphological fact complemented by the demonstration of a high level of unprovoked histamine content in the uninvolved jejunal fluid of patients with inactive CD, a value that increases significantly during disease activity (Knutson et al., 1990).
16. PMD empties human mast cell granule containers, thereby setting the stage for refilling the previously emptied, conserved containers—a process identified in HSMCs in situ during wound healing.

A diagrammatic summary of the release and recovery responses of which human mast cells are capable is presented in Figure 55.

Figure 55 Schematic diagram summarizes release and recovery reactions of which human mast cells are capable. Mature mast cell (A_1) with full complement of granules displaying crystal (a), particle (b), scroll (c), and mixed (d) patterns. Given appropriate stimuli to produce AND (Dvorak, A. M. et al., 1984, 1985b, 1991c), mast cells develop intracytoplasmic channels that permeate the cytoplasm. Granule patterns are altered and solubilized within the intracytoplasmic channels (C_1). Degranulation pores open these channels to the exterior; individual membrane-free granules with swollen, altered matrices, free membranes, and cell processes are shed from actively degranulating cells (C_2). Recovery from fully expressed AND (Dvorak, A. M., 1989e) requires synthesis of new containers and granule contents (E). These actively synthesizing cells are filled with expanded Golgi structures, cytoplasmic vesicles, progranules, and newly forming granules (E) to produce a fully recovered mature mast cell with a full complement of granules (A_2). PMD of mast cells (B), identified in situ in numerous human diseases, for which specific stimuli are not yet known (Dvorak, A. M., 1992), is characterized by cells with unaltered granules (a), granules with focal losses of contents (e,f), and empty granule containers (g) (Dvorak, A. M. and Kissell S, 1991). Increasing the rate of vesicular transport of granule materials in PMD (B) could result in AND (C_1). Recovery from PMD, seen in mast cells in wound healing (D), shows increasing, complex focal (h,i), particulate (j), homogeneous, scroll- and threadlike (k) densities in empty or partly empty granule containers to produce a fully recovered mature mast cell with full complement of granules (A_2) displaying crystal (a), particle (b), scroll (c), and mixed (d) patterns (Dvorak, A. M. and Kissell S, 1991).

Acknowledgments

This work was supported by U.S.P.H.S. Grants CA 28834 and P30 AM 34854. We thank P. K. Gardner for word processing and editorial assistance. Technical assistance by P. Estrella, S. Kissell, L. Letourneau, R. Monahan-Earley, and E. Morgan is gratefully acknowledged. Discussions with and materials from Drs. H. F. Dvorak, S. J. Galli, T. Ishizaka, and L. M. Lichtenstein and numerous members of their laboratories have all made possible much of the work on which our reflections are based.

Discussion

Lichtenstein: Can you tell lung, skin, and uterus mast cells apart?
Dvorak: Yes. Skin mast cells usually contain crystal granules and few lipid bodies. Lung mast cells contain scroll granules, mixed granules, particle granules, and lipid bodies. Uterine mast cells contain scroll and crystalline granules and large numbers of large lipid bodies.
Kaliner: Friedman analyzed skin biopsies taken at various times after skin testing. He showed that the granule morphologies change progressively from a homogeneous pattern, to a crystalline pattern, to a solubilized granule. Don't you think that the various granule patterns you describe are stages in solubilization?
Dvorak: We have found no obligatory pattern of ultrastructural granule changes in kinetic studies of isolated human lung mast cells. In nonkinetic studies of isolated human skin mast cells and in spontaneously degranulating human heart and gut mast cells, no such pattern has been recognized.
Kennerly: Can you comment on the relevance of the fusion of vesicles emanating from the granule matrix to the membrane as has been suggested in rodent experiments?
Dvorak: This observation could reflect piecemeal degranulation.
Schwartz: When human mast cells are activated in vivo, is the degranulation process all or none? Does granule-to-granule fusion precede granule-membrane fusion?
Dvorak: Human lung mast cells and guinea pig basophils exhibit initial granule-granule fusion. Human skin mast cells and human basophils after IgE-mediated activation generally fuse single granules to the membrane.

References

Asboe-Hansen, G. (1971). *Mast Cells and the Skin*. International Academy of Pathology Monograph. Baltimore, Williams & Wilkins.

Barnett, M. L. (1975). Intrapithelial mast cells in gingival lichen planus: An ultrastructural study. *J. Invest. Dermatol.* 64:436–440.

Benyon, R. C., Church, M. K., Clegg, L. L., and Holgate, S. T. (1986). Dispersion and characterisation of mast cells from human skin. *Int. Arch. Allergy Appl. Immunol.* 79:332–334.

Benyon, R. C., Lowman, M. A., and Church, M. K. (1987). Human skin mast cells: Their dispersion, purification, and secretory characterization. *J. Immunol.* 138:861–867.

Bowyer, A. (1968). Observations on the granularity of mast cells in human skin. *Acta Dermatol. Venereol. (Stockh.)* 48:574–577.

Brown, L., Lanir, N., McDonagh, J., Czarnecki, K., Dvorak, A. M., and Dvorak, H. F. (1992). Fibroblast migration in fibrin gel matrices (submitted).

Burns, C. P., and Hoak, J. C. (1975). Freeze-etch studies of the granules of human mast cells and eosinophils. *J. Ultrastruct. Res.* 50:143–149.

Cable, W. J. L., Dvorak, A. M., Osage, J. E., and Kolodny, E. H. (1982). Fabry disease: Significance of ultrastructural localization of lipid inclusions in dermal nerves. *Neurology* 32:347–353.

Caulfield, J. P., Lewis, R. A., Hein, A., and Austen K. F. (1980). Secretion in dissociated human pulmonary mast cells. Evidence for solubilization of granule contents before discharge. *J. Cell Biol.* 85:299–312.

Caulfield, J. P., El-Lati, S., Thomas, G., and Church M. K. (1990). Dissociated human foreskin mast cells degranulate in response to anti-IgE and substance P. *Lab. Invest.* 63:502–510.

Ciano, P. S., Colvin, R. B., Dvorak, A. M., McDonagh, J., and Dvorak, H. F. (1986). Macrophage migration in fibrin gel matrices. *Lab. Invest.* 54:62–70.

Claman, H. N. (1989). Mast cell changes in a case of rapidly progressive scleroderma—Ultrastructural analysis. *J. Invest. Dermatol.* 92:290–295.

Claman, H. N., Jaffee, B. D., Huff, J. C., and Clark, R. A. F. (1985). Chronic graft-versus-host disease as a model for scleroderma. II. Mast cell depletion with deposition of immunoglobulins in the skin and fibrosis. *Cell Immunol.* 94:73–84.

Claman, H. N., Choi, K. L., Sujansky, W., and Vatter, A. E. (1986). Mast cell "disappearance" in chronic murine graft-vs-host disease (GVHD)—Ultrastructural demonstration of "phantom mast cells." *J. Immunol.* 137:2009–2013.

Colvin, R. B, Dvorak, A. M., and Dvorak, H. F. (1974). Mast cells in the cortical tubular epithelium and interstitium in human renal disease. *Hum. Pathol.* 5:315–326.

Cook, M. G., and Turnbull, G. J. (1975). A hypothesis for the pathogenesis of Crohn's disease based on an ultrastructural study. *Virchows Arch. Pathol. Anat. Histol.* 365:327–336.

Craig, S. S., and Schwartz, L. B. (1990). Human MC_{TC} type of mast cell granule: The uncommon occurrence of discrete scrolls associated with focal absence of chymase. *Lab. Invest.* 63:581–585.

Craig, S. S., Schechter, N. M., and Schwartz, L. B. (1988). Ultrastructural analysis of human T and TC mast cells identified by immunoelectron microscopy. *Lab. Invest.* 58:682–691.

Craig, S. S., and Schechter, N. M., Schwartz, L. B. (1989). Ultrastructural analysis of maturing human T and TC mast cells in situ. *Lab. Invest.* 60:147–157.

Dickersin, G. R., Lott, I. T., Kolodny, E. H., and Dvorak, A. M. (1980). A light and electron microscopic study of mannosidosis. *Hum. Pathol.* 11:245–256.

Dienstag, J. L., Rhodes, A. R., Bhan, A. K., Dvorak, A. M., Mihm, M. C., Jr., and

Wands, J. R. (1978). Urticaria associated with acute viral hepatitis type B. Studies of pathogenesis. *Ann. Intern. Med.* 88:34–40.

Dvorak, A. M. (1978). Biology and morphology of basophilic leukocytes. In *Immediate Hypersensitivity—Modern Concepts and Developments*. Edited by M. K. Bach. Immunology Series, Vol. 7. New York, Marcel Dekker, pp. 369–405.

Dvorak, A. M. (1979). Mast-cell hyperplasia and degranulation in Crohn's disease. In *The Mast Cell. Its Role in Health and Disease*. Edited by J. Pepys and A. M. Edwards. Kent, Pitman Medical Publishing Co, pp. 657–662.

Dvorak, A. M. (1986a). Mast-cell degranulation in human hearts. *N. Engl. J. Med.* 315:969–970.

Dvorak, A. M. (1986b). Morphologic expressions of maturation and function can affect the ability to identify mast cells and basophils in man, guinea pig, and mouse. In *Mast Cell Differentiation and Heterogeneity*. Edited by A. D. Befus, J. Bienenstock, and J. A. Denburg. New York, Raven Press, pp. 95–114.

Dvorak, A. M. (1987)—Procedural guide to specimen handling for the ultrastructural pathology service laboratory. *J. Electron. Microsc. Tech.* 6:255–301.

Dvorak, A. M. (1988a). Morphologic and immunologic characterization of human basophils, 1879 to 1985. *Riv. Immunol. Immunofarmacol.* 8:50–82.

Dvorak, A. M. (1988b). The fine structure of human basophils and mast cells. In *Mast Cells, Mediators and Disease*. Edited by S. T. Holgate. Immunology and Medicine Series. Dordrecht, The Netherlands, Kluwer Academic Publishers, pp. 29–97.

Dvorak, A. M. (1988c). Ultrastructural pathology of Crohn's disease. In *Inflammatory Bowel Diseases—Basic Research and Clinical Implications*. Edited by H. Goebell, B. M. Peskar, and M. Malchow. Lancaster, MTP Press, pp. 3–41.

Dvorak, A. M. (1988d). What is the evidence for damaged enteric autonomic nerves in Crohn's disease? In *Inflammatory Bowel Disease: Current Status and Future Approach*. Edited by R. P. MacDermott. Amsterdam, Elsevier, pp. 705–711.

Dvorak, A. M. (1989a). Axonal necrosis in Crohn's disease. In *Digestive Disease Pathology*, Vol. 2. Edited by S. Watanabe, M. Wolff, and S. C. Sommers. Philadelphia, Field and Wood, pp. 67–79.

Dvorak, A. M. (1989b). Gut autonomic nerve (GAN) tumors. In *Digestive Disease Pathology*, Vol. 2. Edited by S. Watanabe, M. Wolff, and S. C. Sommers. Philadelphia, Field and Wood, pp. 49–66.

Dvorak, A. M. (1989c). Human mast cells. In *Advances in Anatomy, Embryology, and Cell Biology*, Vol. 114. Berlin, Springer-Verlag, pp. 1–107.

Dvorak, A. M. (1989d). Metastatic intestinal adenocarcinomas identified by ultrastructural analysis of a site-specific organelle—The terminal web. In *Digestive Disease Pathology*, Vol. 2. Edited by S. Watanabe, M. Wolff, and S. C. Sommers. Philadelphia, Field and Wood, pp. 39–47.

Dvorak, A. M. (1989e). Recovery of human lung mast cells from anaphylactic degranulation utilizes a mixture of conservation and synthetic mechanisms. In *Mast Cell and Basophil Differentiation and Function in Health Disease*. Edited by S. J. Galli and K. F. Austen. New York, Raven Press, pp. 119–148.

Dvorak, A. M. (1989f). Ultrastructural monitoring of progress of Whipple's disease therapy. In *Digestive Disease Pathology*, Vol. 2. Edited by S. Watanabe, M. Wolff, and S. C. Sommers. Philadelphia, Field and Wood, pp. 81–90.

Dvorak, A. M. (1991b). Ultrastructure of human gastrointestinal system. Interactions among mast cells, eosinophils, nerves and muscle in human disease. In *Effects of Immune Cells and Inflammation on Smooth Muscle and Enteric Nerves*. Edited by W. J. Snape, Jr., and S. M. Collins. Boca Raton, FL, CRC Press. pp. 139–168.

Dvorak, A. M. (1991c). Biochemical contents of granules and lipid bodies—two distinctive organelles found in basophils and mast cells. In Basophil and Mast Cell Degranulation and Recovery. Vol. 4: Blood Cell Biochemistry series. Series Editor J. R. Harris, Vol Editor A. M. Dvorak. New York, Plenum.

Dvorak, A. M. (1992). Basophils and mast cells. Piecemeal degranulation in situ and ex vivo. A possible mechanism for cytokine-induced function in disease. In *Granulocyte Responses to Cytokines*. Edited by R. G. Coffey. New York, Marcel Dekker. pp. 169–271.

Dvorak, A. M. (1991a). *Basophil and Mast Cell Degranulation and Recovery*. Series editor J. R. Harris. Vol editor A. M. Dvorak. Blood Cell Biochemistry, Vol 4. London, Plenum. pp 1–415.

Dvorak, A. M., and Dickersin, G. R. (1979). Crohn's disease: Electron microscopic studies. In *Pathology Annual*—Part 2, Vol. 14. Edited by S. C. Sommers, and P. P. Rosen. New York, Appleton-Century-Crofts, pp. 259–306.

Dvorak, A. M., and Ishizaka, T. 1992. Ultrastructural identification of human mast cells arising in *in vitro* culture systems. In Progress in Allergy and Clinical Immunology. Vol. 2 Eds. Miyamoto, T., and Okuda, M. Göttingen, Hogrefe and Huber, pp. 75–84.

Dvorak, A. M., and Kissell, S. (1991). Granule changes of human skin mast cells characteristic of piecemeal degranulation and associated with recovery during wound healing in situ. *J. Leukocyte Biol.* 49:197–210.

Dvorak, A. M. and Monahan, R. A. (1982). Metastatic adenocarcinoma of unknown primary site. Diagnostic electron microscopy to determine the site of tumor origin. *Arch. Pathol. Lab. Med.* 106:21–24.

Dvorak, A. M. and Monahan, R. A. (1983). Crohn's disease—Mast cell quantitation using one micron plastic sections for light microscopic study. In *Pathology Annual*—Part I, Vol. 18. Edited by S. C. Sommers, and P. P. Rosen. New York, Appleton-Century-Crofts, pp. 181–190.

Dvorak, A. M., and Monahan, R. A. (1984a). Chronic abdominal pain, malaise, constipation and diarrhea in a forty year old woman: Crohn's disease. *Norelco Rep.* 31:18–44.

Dvorak, A. M., and Monahan, R. A. (1984b). Weight loss, fatigue, diarrhea, fever and lymphadenopathy in a forty eight year old male industrial engineer: Whipple's disease. *Norelco Rep.* 31:10–21.

Dvorak A. M., and Monahan, R. A. (1985). Abdominal pain, hepatomegaly and weight loss in a fifty four year old man: Renal cell carcinoma and adenoma. *Norelco Rep.* 32:61–66.

Dvorak, A. M., and Monahan-Earley, R. A. (1985). Rapidly progressive lung disease in a forty six year old woman with scleroderma: Bronchiolo-alveolar carcinoma. *Norelco Rep.* 32:22–28.

Dvorak, A. M., and Monahan-Earley R. A. (1986). *Diagnostic Ultrastructural Pathology*

(EM Pathology Monograph No. 1), Vol. 1. Mahwah, NJ, Electron Optics Publishing Group, pp. 1–98.

Dvorak, A. M., and Monahan-Earley, R. A. Diagnostic Ultrastructural Pathology I. A text-atlas of case studies illustrating the correlative clinical-ultrastructural pathologic approach to diagnosis. CRC Press, Boca Raton pp 1–512.

Dvorak, A. M., and Silen, W. (1985). Differentiation between Crohn's disease and other inflammatory conditions by electron microscopy. *Ann. Surg.* 201:53–63.

Dvorak, A. M., Mihm, M. C., Jr., and Dvorak, H. F. (1976). Morphology of delayed-type hypersensitivity reactions in man. II. Ultrastructural alterations affecting the microvasculature and the tissue and mast cells. *Lab. Invest.* 34:179–191.

Dvorak, A. M., Monahan, R. A., Osage, J. E., and Dickersin, G. R. (1978). Mast-cell degranulation in Crohn's disease. *Lancet* 1:498.

Dvorak, A. M., Roblin, R. O., Morgan, E. S., and Dvorak, H. F. (1979). Ultrastructure of the cell coat of untransformed and Simian virus 40-transformed fibroblasts. *J. Reticuloendothelial Soc.* 25:163–177.

Dvorak, A. M., Hammond, M. E., Morgan, E. S., and Dvorak, H. F. (1980a). Ultrastructural studies of macrophages: In vitro removal of cell coat with macrophage inhibition factor (MIF)-containing lymphocyte culture supernatants; chloroform extraction, phospholipase digestion, and autoradiographic studies. *J. Reticuloendothelial Soc.* 27:119–142.

Dvorak, A. M., Mihm, M. C., Jr., Osage, J. E., and Dvorak, H. F. (1980b). Melanoma. An ultrastructural study of the host inflammatory and vascular responses. *J. Invest. Dermatol.* 75:388–393.

Dvorak, A. M., Monahan, R. A., Osage, J. E., and Dickersin, G. R. (1980c). Crohn's disease: Transmission electron microscopic studies. II. Immunologic inflammatory response. Alterations of mast cells, basophils, eosinophils, and the microvasculature. *Hum. Pathol.* 11:606–619.

Dvorak, A. M., Osage, J. E., Monahan, R. A., and Dickersin, G. R. (1980d). Crohn's disease: Transmission electron microscopic studies. III. Target tissues. Proliferation of and injury to smooth muscle and the autonomic nervous system. *Hum. Pathol.* 11:620–634.

Dvorak, A. M., Cable, W. J. L., Osage, J. E., and Kolodny, E. H. (1981). Diagnostic electron microscopy. II. Fabry's disease: Use of biopsies from uninvolved skin. Acute and chronic changes involving the microvasculature and small unmyelinated nerves. In *Pathology Annual*—Part I, Vol. 16. Edited by S. C. Sommers, and, P. P. Rosen. New York, Appleton-Century-Crofts, pp. 139–158.

Dvorak, A. M., Mihm, M. C., Jr., Osage, J. E., Kwan, T. H., Austen, K. F., and Wintroub, B. U. (1982). Bullous pemphigoid, an ultrastructural study of the inflammatory response: Eosinophil, basophil and mast cell granule changes in multiple biopsies from one patient. *J. Invest. Dermatol.* 78:91–101.

Dvorak, A. M., Dvorak, H. F., and Galli, S. J. (1983a). Ultrastructural criteria for identification of mast cells and basophils in humans, guinea pigs, and mice. *Am. Rev. Respir. Dis.* 128(Suppl):S49–S52.

Dvorak, A. M., Dvorak, H. F., Peters, S. P., Schulman, E. S., MacGlashan, D. W., Jr., Pyne, K., Harvey, V. S., Galli, S. J., and Lichtenstein, L. M. (1983b). Lipid bodies: Cytoplasmic organelles important to arachidonate metabolism in macrophages and mast cells. *J. Immunol.* 131:2965–2976. [republished, *J. Immunol.* 132:1586–1597, 1984].

Dvorak, A. M., Galli, S. J., Schulman, E. S., Lichtenstein, L. M., and Dvorak, H. F. (1983c). Basophil and mast cell degranulation: Ultrastructural analysis of mechanisms of mediator release. *Fed. Proc.* 42:2510–2515.

Dvorak, A. M., Hammel, I., Schulman, E. S., Peters, S. P., MacGlashan, D. W., Jr., Schleimer, R. P., Newball, H. H., Pyne, K., Dvorak, H. F., Lichtenstein, L. M., and Galli, S. J. (1984). Differences in the behavior of cytoplasmic granules and lipid bodies during human lung mast cell degranulation. *J. Cell Biol.* 99:1678–1687.

Dvorak, A. M., Ishizaka, T., and Galli, S. J. (1985a). Ultrastructure of human basophils developing in vitro. Evidence for the acquisition of peroxidase by basophils and for different effects of human and murine growth factors on human basophil and eosinophil maturation. *Lab. Invest.* 53:57–71.

Dvorak, A. M., Schulman, E. S., Peters, S. P., MacGlashan, D. W., Jr., Newball, H. H., Schleimer, R. P., and Lichtenstein, L. M. (1985b). Immunoglobulin E–mediated degranulation of isolated human lung mast cells. *Lab. Invest.* 53:45–56.

Dvorak, A. M., Schleimer, R. P., Schulman, E. S., and Lichtenstein, L. M. (1986). Human mast cells use conservation and condensation mechanisms during recovery from degranulation. In vitro studies with mast cells purified from human lungs. *Lab. Invest.* 54:663–678.

Dvorak, A. M., Schleimer, R. P., and Lichtenstein, L. M. (1987). Morphologic mast cell cycles. *Cell Immunol.* 105:199–204.

Dvorak, A. M., Schleimer, R. P., and Lichtenstein, L. M. (1988). Human mast cells synthesize new granules during recovery from degranulation. In vitro studies with mast cells purified from human lungs. *Blood* 71:76–85.

Dvorak, A. M., Saito, H., Estrella, P., Kissell, S., Arai, N., and Ishizaka, T. (1989). Ultrastructure of eosinophils and basophils stimulated to develop in human cord blood mononuclear cell cultures containing recombinant human interleukin-5 or interleukin-3. *Lab. Invest.* 61:116–132.

Dvorak, A. M., Weller, P. F., Monahan-Earley, R. A., Letourneau, L., and Ackerman, S. J. (1990). Ultrastructural localization of Charcot-Leyden crystal protein (lysophospholipase) and peroxidase in macrophages, eosinophils and extracellular matrix of the skin in the hypereosinophillic syndrome. *Lab. Invest.* 62:590–607.

Dvorak, A. M., Ackerman, S. J., and Weller, P. F. (1991a). Subcellular morphology and biochemistry of eosinophils. In *Blood Cell Biochemistry: Megakaryocytes, Platelets, Macrophages and Eosinophils*, Vol. 2. Edited by J. R. Harris. London, Plenum, pp. 237–344.

Dvorak, A. M., Furitsu, T., Letourneau, L., Ishizaka, T., and Ackerman, S. J. (1991b). Mature eosinophils stimulated to develop in human cord blood mononuclear cell cultures supplemented with recombinant human interleukin-5. I. Piecemeal degranulation of specific granules and distribution of Charcot-Leyden crystal protein. *Am. J. Pathol.* 138:69–82.

Dvorak, A. M., Massey, W., Warner, J., Kissell, S., Kagey-Sobotka, A., and Lichtenstein, L. M. (1991c). IgE-mediated anaphylactic degranulation of isolated human skin mast cells. *Blood* 77:569–578.

Dvorak, A. M., Furitsu, T, Estrella, P, and Ishizaka, T. (1991d) Human lung-derived mature mast cells cultured alone or with mouse 3T3 fibroblasts maintain an ultrastructural phenotype different from that of human mast cells that develop from human cord blood cells cultured with 3T3 fibroblasts. AM. J. Pathol. 139:1309–1318.

Dvorak, A. M., McLeod, R. S., Onderdonk, A. B., Monahan-Earley, R. A., Cullen, J., Antonioli, D. A., Morgan, E., Blair, J. E., Estrella, P., Cisneros, R. L., Cohen, Z., and Silen, W. (1992a). Human gut mucosal mast cells. Ultrastructural observations and anatomic variation in mast cell-nerve associations in vivo. Int. Arch. Allergy Appl. Immunol. (in press).

Dvorak, A. M., McLeod, R. S., Onderdonk, A., Monahan-Earley, R. A., Cullen, J., Antonioli, D. A. Morgan, E., Blair, J. E., Estrella, P., Cisneros, R. L., Silen, W., Cohen, Z. (1992b). Ultrastructural evidence for piecemeal and anaphylactic degranulation of human gut mucosal mast cells in vivo (submitted).

Dvorak, A. M., Onderdonk, A. B., McLeod, R. S., Monahan-Early, R. A., Antonioli, D. A., Cullen J., Blair, J. E., Cisneros, R. L., Letourneau, L., Morgan, E., Silen, W., and Cohen, Z. (1992c). Exocytosis of granules from eosinophils in vivo. Ultrastructural observations in ulcerative colitis, Crohn's disease and familial polyposis syndrome patients with bacterial-infected continent ileal pouches (submitted).

Dvorak, A. M., Onderdonk, A. B., McLeod, R. S., Monahan-Earley, R. A., Cullen, J., Antonioli, D. A., Blair, J. E., Morgan, E., Cisneros, R. L., Estrella, P., Cohen, Z., and Silen, W. (1992d). Axonal necrosis of enteric autonomic nerves in continent ileal pouches. Possible implications for pathogenesis of Crohn's disease (submitted).

Dvorak, A. M., Furitsu, T., Kissell-Rainville, S., Ishizaka, T. (1992e) Ultrastructural identification of human mast cells resembling skin mast cells stimulated to develop in long-term human cord blood mononuclear cells co-cultured with 3T3 mouse skin fibroblasts. J. Leukocyte Biol. (in press)

Dvorak, A. M. , Schleimer, R. P., Dvorak, H. F., Lichtenstein, L. M., and Weller, P. F. (1992f) Human lung mast cell and alveolar macrophage cytoplasmic lypid bodies contain arachidonic acid and prostaglandin endoperoxide synthase (cyclooxygenase), the substrate and enzyme necessary for prostaglandin production. Int Arch Allergy Appl. Immunol. (in press)

Dvorak, H. F., and Dvorak, A. M. (1975). Basophilic leucocytes: Structure, function and role in disease. In *Clinics in Haematology*, Vol. 4: *Granulocyte and Monocyte Abnormalities*. Edited by M. A. Lichtman. London, Saunders, pp. 651–683.

Dvorak, H. F., Mihm, M. C., Jr., Dvorak, A. M., Johnson, R. A., Manseau, E. J., Morgan, E., and Colvin R. B. (1974). Morphology of delayed-type hypersensitivity reactions in man. I. Quantitative description of the inflammatory response. *Lab. Invest.* 31:111–130.

Dvorak, H. F., Mihm, M. C., Jr., and Dvorak, A. M. (1976). Morphology of delayed-type hypersensitivity reactions in man. *J. Invest. Dermatol.* 67:391–401.

Dvorak, H. F., Mihm, M. C., Jr., Dvorak, A. M., Barnes, B. A., Manseau, E. J., and Galli, S. J. (1979). Rejection of first-set skin allografts in man. The microvasculature is the critical target of the immune response. *J. Exp. Med.* 150:322–337.

Dvorak, H. F., Galli, S. J., and Dvorak, A. M. (1980a). Expression of cell-mediated hypersensitivity in vivo—Recent advances. In *International Review of Experimental Pathology*, Vol. 21. Edited by G. W. Richter, and M. A. Epstein. New York, Academic Press, pp. 119–194.

Dvorak, H. F., Mihm, M. C., Jr., Dvorak, A. M., Barnes, B. A., and Galli, S. J. (1980b). The microvasculature is the critical target of the immune response in vascularized skin allograft rejection. *J. Invest. Dermatol.* 74:280–284.

Dvorak, H. F., Dickersin, G. R., Dvorak, A. M., Manseau, E. J., and Pyne, K. (1981). Human breast carcinoma: Fibrin deposits and desmoplasia. Inflammatory cell type and distribution. Microvasculature and infarction. *J. Natl. Cancer Inst.* 67:335–345.

Dvorak, H. F., Galli, S. J., and Dvorak, A. M. (1986). Cellular and vascular manifestations of cell-mediated immunity. *Hum. Pathol.* 17:122–137.

Ehrlich, P. (1877). Beiträge zur Kenntnis der Anilinfärbungen und ihrer Verwendung in der mikroskopischen Technik. *Arch. Mikrosk. Anat.* 13:263–277.

Estensen, R. D. (1984). Eosinophilic myocarditis: a role for mast cells? *Arch. Pathol. Lab. Med.* 108:358–359.

Fedorko, M. E., and Hirsch, J. G. (1965). Crystalloid structure in granules of guinea pig basophils and human mast cells. *J. Cell Biol.* 26:973–976.

Fox, C. C., Dvorak, A. M., Peters, S. P., Kagey-Sobotka, A., and Lichtenstein, L. M. (1985). Isolation and characterization of human intestinal mucosal mast cells. *J. Immunol.* 135:483–491.

Friedman, M. M., and Kaliner, M. (1988). Ultrastructural changes in human skin mast cells during antigen-induced degranulation in vivo. *J. Allergy Clin. Immunol.* 82:998–1005.

Fujita, H., Asagami, C., Murozumi, S., Yamamoto, K., and Kinoshita, K. (1969). Electron microscopic studies of mast cells of human fetal skins. *J. Ultrastruct. Res.* 28:353–370.

Fujita, H., Asagami, C., Suetomi, Y., Araki, I., and Kinoshita, K. (1972). An ultrastructural study of mast granule formation in embryonic skin. *Acta Dermatol. Venereol.* (Stockh.) 52:249–256.

Furitsu, T., Saito, H., Dvorak, A. M., Schwartz, L. B., Irani, A-M. A., Burdick, J. F., Ishizaka, K., and Ishizaka, T. (1989). Development of human mast cells in vitro. *Proc. Natl. Acad. Sci. USA* 86:10039–10043.

Galli, S. J., Dvorak, A. M., and Dvorak, H. F. (1984). Basophils and mast cells: Morphologic insights into their biology, secretory patterns and function. In *Progress in Allergy. Mast Cell Activation and Mediator Release*, Vol. 34. Edited by K. Ishizaka. Basel, Karger, pp. 1–141.

Galli, S. J., Dvorak, A. M., Peters, S. P., Schulman, E. S., MacGlashan, D. W., Jr., Isomura, T., Pyne, K., Harvey, V. S., Hammel, I., Lichtenstein, L. M., and Dvorak, H. F. (1985). Lipid bodies—Widely distributed cytoplasmic structures that represent preferential nonmembrane repositories of exogenous [^{3}H]arachidonic acid incorporated by mast cells, macrophages, and other cell types. In *Prostaglandins, Leukotrienes, and Lipoxins. Biochemistry, Mechanism of Action, and Clinical Applications*. Edited by J. M. Bailey. New York, Plenum Press, pp. 221–239.

Galli, S. J., Dvorak, A. M., and Dvorak, H. F. (1990). Morphology, biochemistry, and function of basophils and mast cells. In *Hematology*, 4th ed. Edited by W. J. Williams, E., Beutler, A. J. Erslev, and M. A. Lichtman. New York, McGraw-Hill, pp. 840–845.

Ginsburg, R., Bristow, M. R., Kantrowitz, N., Baim, D. S., and Harrison, D. C. (1981). Histamine provocation of clinical coronary artery spasm: Implications concerning pathogenesis of variant angina pectoris. *Am. Heart J.* 102:819–822.

Glovsky, M. M., Dvorak, A. M., MacPhea, B., and Bastug, T. (1987). Basophil and skin mast cell histamine release, dermatographism and angioedema asociated with homozygous C7 complement deficiency. *J. Allergy Clin. Immunol.* 79:181 (abstract).

Greaves, M. W., Yamamoto, S., and Fairley, V. M. (1972). IgE-mediated hypersensitivity in human skin studied using a new in vitro method. *Immunology* 23:239–248.

Hammel, I., Dvorak, A. M., Peters, S. P., Schulman, E. S., Dvorak, H. F., Lichtenstein, L. M., and Galli, S. J. (1985). Differences in the volume distributions of human lung mast cell granules and lipid bodies: Evidence that the size of these organelles is regulated by distinct mechanisms. *J. Cell Biol.* 100:1488–1492.

Hammond, M. E., Roblin, R. O., Dvorak, A. M., Selvaggio, S. S., Black, P. H., and Dvorak, H. F. (1974). MIF-like activity in Simian virus 40-transformed 3T3 fibroblast cultures. *Science* 185:955–957.

Harris, N. L., Dvorak, A. M., Smith, J., and Dvorak, H. F. (1982). Fibrin deposits in Hodgkin's disease. *Am. J. Pathol.* 108:119–129.

Hashimoto, K., Gross, B. G., and Lever, W. F. (1966). An electron microscopic study of the degranulation of mast cell granules in urticaria pigmentosa. *J. Invest. Dermatol.* 46:139–149.

Haslam, P. L., Dewar, A., Butchers, P., Primett, Z. S., Newman-Taylor, A., and Turner-Warwick, M. (1987). Mast cells, atypical lymphocytes, and neutrophils in bronchoalveolar lavage in extrinsic allergic alveolitis. Comparison with other interstitial lung diseases. *Am. Rev. Respir. Dis.* 135:35–47.

Hermens, J. M., Ebertz, J. M., Hanifin, J. M., and Hirschman, C. A. (1985). Comparison of histamine release in human skin mast cells induced by morphine, fentanyl, and oxymorphone. *Anesthesiology* 62:124–127.

Hibbs, R. G., Burch, G. E., and Phillips, J. H. (1960). Electron-microscopic observations on the human mast cell. *Am. Heart J.* 60:121–127.

Irani, A-M. A., Bradford, T. R., Kepley, C. L., Schechter, N. M., and Schwartz, L. B. (1989). Detection of MC_T and MC_{TC} types of human mast cells by immunohistochemistry using new monoclonal anti-tryptase and anti-chymase antibodies. *J. Histochem. Cytochem.* 37:1509–1515.

Ishizaka, T., Dvoark, A. M., Conrad, D. H., Niebyl, J. R., Marquette, J. P., and Ishizaka, K. (1985). Morphologic and immunologic characterization of human basophils developed in cultures of cord blood mononuclear cells. *J. Immunol.* 134:532–540.

Kalsner, S., and Richards, R. (1984). Coronary arteries of cardiac patients are hyperreactive and contain stores of amines: A mechanism for coronary spasm. *Science* 223:1435–1437.

Kawanami, O., Ferrans, V. J., Fulmer, J. D., and Crystal, R. G. (1979). Ultrastructure of pulmonary mast cells in patients with fibrotic lung disorders. *Lab. Invest.* 40:717–734.

Knutson, L., Ahrenstedt, Ö, Odlind, B., and Hällgran, R. (1990). The jejunal secretion of histamine is increased in active Crohn's disease. *Gastroenterology* 98:849–854.

Kobayasi, T., and Asboe-Hansen, G. (1969a). Degranulation and regranulation of human mast cells. An electron microscopic study of the whealing reaction in urticaria pigmentosa. *Acta Dermatol. Venereol.* 49:369–381.

Kobayasi, T., and Asboe-Hansen, G. (1969b). Ultrastructure of mast-cell granules in squamous cell carcinoma. *Acta Dermatol. Venereol. (Stockh.)* 49:233–240.

Kopicky-Burd, J. A., Kagey-Sobotka, A., Peters, S. P., Dvorak, A. M., Lennox, D. W., Lichtenstein, L. M., and Wigley, F. M. (1988). Characterization of human synovial mast cells. *J. Rheumatol.* 15:1326–1333.

Lanir, N., Ciano, P. S., Van De Water, L., McDonagh, J., Dvorak, A. M., and Dvorak, H. F. (1988). Macrophage migration in fibrin gel matrices. II. Effects of clotting factor XIII, fibronectin, and glycosaminoglycan content on cell migration. *J. Immunol.* 140:2340–2349.

Lawrence, I. D., Warner, J. A., Cohan, V. L., Hubbard, W. C., Kagey-Sobotka, A., and Lichtenstein, L. M. (1987). Purification and characterization of human skin mast cells. Evidence for human mast cell heterogeneity. *J. Immunol.* 139:3062–3069.

Lawrence, I. D., Warner, J. A., Cohan, V. L., Lichtenstein, L. M., Kagey-Sobotka, A., Vavrek, R. J., Stewart, J. M., and Proud, D. (1989). Induction of histamine release from human skin mast cells by bradykinin analogs. *Biochem. Pharmacol.* 38:227–233.

Levi, R., Wolff, A., Robertson, D. A., and Graver, L. M. (1985). IgE-mediated hypersensitivity and ischemia as causes of endogenous cardiac histamine release. In *Advances in the Biosciences*. Vol. 51: *Frontiers in Histamine Research. A Tribute to Heinz Schild.* Edited by C. R. Ganellin and J-C. Schwartz. Oxford, Pergamon Press, pp. 305–308.

Levi-Schaffer, F., Austen, K. F., Caulfield, J. P., Hein, A., Gravellese, P. M., and Stevens, R. L. (1987). Coculture of human lung-derived mast cells with mouse 3T3 fibroblasts: Morphology and IgE-mediated release of histamine, prostaglandin D_2, and leukotrienes *J. Immunol.* 139:494–500.

Longworth, D. L., Monahan-Earley, R. A., Dvorak, A. M., and Weller, P. F. (1988). *Brugia malayi:* Arachidonic acid uptake into lipid bodies of adult parasites. *Exp. Parasitol.* 65:251–257.

Marckmann, A., and Zachariae, H. (1964). Histamine in full-thickness skin autografts of rat. *Proc. Soc. Exp. Biol. Med.* 117:705–708.

Massey, W. A., Guo, C-B., Dvorak, A. M., Hubbard, W. C., Bhagavan, B. S., Cohan, V. L., Warner, J. A., Kagey-Sobotka, A., and Lichtenstein, L. M. (1991). Human uterine mast cells. Isolation, purification, characterization, and ultrastructure pharmacology. J. Immunol. 147:1621–1627.

Matis, W. L., Lavker, R. M., and Murphy, G. E. (1990). Substance P induces the expression of an endothelial-leukocyte adhesion molecule by microvascular endothelium. *J. Invest. Dermatol.* 94:492–495.

McAuley, R. L., and Sommers, S. C. (1961). Mast cells in nonspecific ulcerative colitis. *Am. J. Dig. Dis.* 6:233–236.

Cytoplasmic lipid bodies of human eosinophils. Subcellular isolation and analysis of arachidonate incorporation. *Am. J. Pathol.* 138:141–148.

Weller, P. F., Ryeom. S. W., Picard, S. T., Ackerman, S. J., and Dvorak, A. M. (1991b). Cytoplasmic lipid bodies of neutrophils: Formation induced by *cis*-unsaturated fatty acids and mediated by protein kinase C. J. Cell Biol. 113:137–146.

Weller, P. F., Ryeom, S. W., and Dvorak, A. M. (1992). Lipid bodies: Structurally distinct, non-membranous intracellular sites of eicosanoid formation. In: Prostaglandins, Leukotrienes, Lipoxins and PAF. Edited by J. M. Bailey. New York, Plenum Press, pp 353–362.

Wichmann, B-E. (1955). The mast cell count during the process of wound healing. *Acta Pathol. Microbiol. Scand.* 108(Suppl):1–35.

Yancey, K. B., Hammer, C. H., Harvath, L., Renfer, L., Frank, M. M., and Lawley, T. J. (1985). Studies of human $C5_a$ as a mediator of inflammation in normal human skin. *J. Clin. Invest.* 75:486–495.

2

Structural Aspects of the High-Affinity Receptor for IgE

JUAN RIVERA

National Institute of Arthritis, Musculoskeletal, and Skin Diseases
National Institutes of Health
Bethesda, Maryland

I. Introduction

Mast cells, basophils, and their tumor analogs express on their surface membrane a glycoprotein that binds monomeric immunoglobulin E with high affinity. This receptor ($Fc_{\epsilon}RI$) is found exclusively on these cells and plays a central role in allergic diseases by mediating cellular secretion after exposure to allergen. The binding of monomeric IgE antibodies to the receptor on mast cells or basophils in itself does not lead to cellular activation. However, when cell bound IgE reacts with a multivalent antigen, such as pollen, the receptor is aggregated, leading to a plethora of biochemical and morphological changes that ultimately result in the degranulation of the cell and release of chemical mediators of the allergic response. Owing to its central role in transducing a specific signal from an extracellular to an intracellular environment, the receptor protein has been the focus of investigation as a potential target for therapeutic intervention.

In this chapter I focus on the current knowledge of the receptor's structure. I give less emphasis to the functional aspects of the receptor because this topic will be covered in detail in other chapters. However, I will consider how an understanding at a molecular level of the structure of the receptor may be used to study its function.

The studies presented in this chapter for the most part have utilized a histamine-releasing subline ($2H_3$+) of a neoplastic line of rat cells—the rat basophilic leukemia (RBL) cells (Eccleston et al., 1973; Barsumian et al., 1981). In general, the evidence derived from these studies, as far as the structure and functioning of the receptor are concerned, is applicable to the receptor on normal cells.

II. Structure of the Receptor

The receptor is a tetrameric protein comprised of three different polypeptides, as shown in Figure 1: a single α chain that contains the IgE binding site, a single β chain, and two γ chains that are covalently linked. This subunit structure for the receptor was defined by several means: (1) Incorporation of radioactive amino acids into cellular proteins results in a molar ratio of the subunits that is a small integral number (Metzger, 1983). (2) Other experiments showed that the α, β, and γ chains are coordinately synthesized and degraded and do not exchange in the plasma membrane independent of each other (Quarto et al., 1985). (3) The subunit structure of the receptor is tetrameric whether the receptor is isolated via IgE bound to the α chain or with monoclonal antibodies directed to the individual subunits. Therefore, the IgE does not induce the assembly of this subunit structure (Rivera et al., 1988). (4) Recent biosynthetic and transfection experiments confirmed the necessity of the three polypeptides for cell membrane expression of the rodent receptor (Blank et al., 1989; Rivera and Metzger, in preparation). It therefore seems reasonable to assume that the $\alpha\beta\gamma_2$ subunit structure is the unit receptor.

A. The α Chain

cDNAs corresponding to the rat, mouse, and human α chains have been cloned (Kinet et al., 1987; Kochan et al., 1988; Shimizu et al., 1988). The DNA sequence of the rat α shows 88% and 68% homology with the mouse and human α, respectively. By Northern blotting the major species of mRNA identified was 1.3 kb in rodents (Kinet et al., 1987) and 1.1 kb in humans (Thompson et al., 1990). These transcripts were found exclusively in cells of mast cell or basophil lineage.

The amino acid sequence for the α subunit is comprised of 245 residues. A hydropathicity plot of the α sequence suggests an N-terminal signal peptide and a single transmembrane domain. Cleavage of the leader peptide generates a 222-amino-acid protein with a predicted molecular weight of 27 kDa, whose extracellular N-terminal 181 residues contain two immunoglobulin-like domains (Kinet et al., 1987). The N-terminal segment contains seven potential sites for *N*-linked glycosylation. *O*-linked glycosylation is also suggested by previous studies (Kanellopoulos et al., 1980), but these sites remain to be identified. The heterogeniety in molecular weight (Kulczycki et al., 1976; Kanellopoulos et al., 1980; Hempstead et al., 1981) observed on SDS-PAGE for the mature α chain can potentially be explained by differences in glycosylation. That is, heterogeneity may result from differences in the number of sites utilized, which sites are utilized, and the type of carbohydrate added.

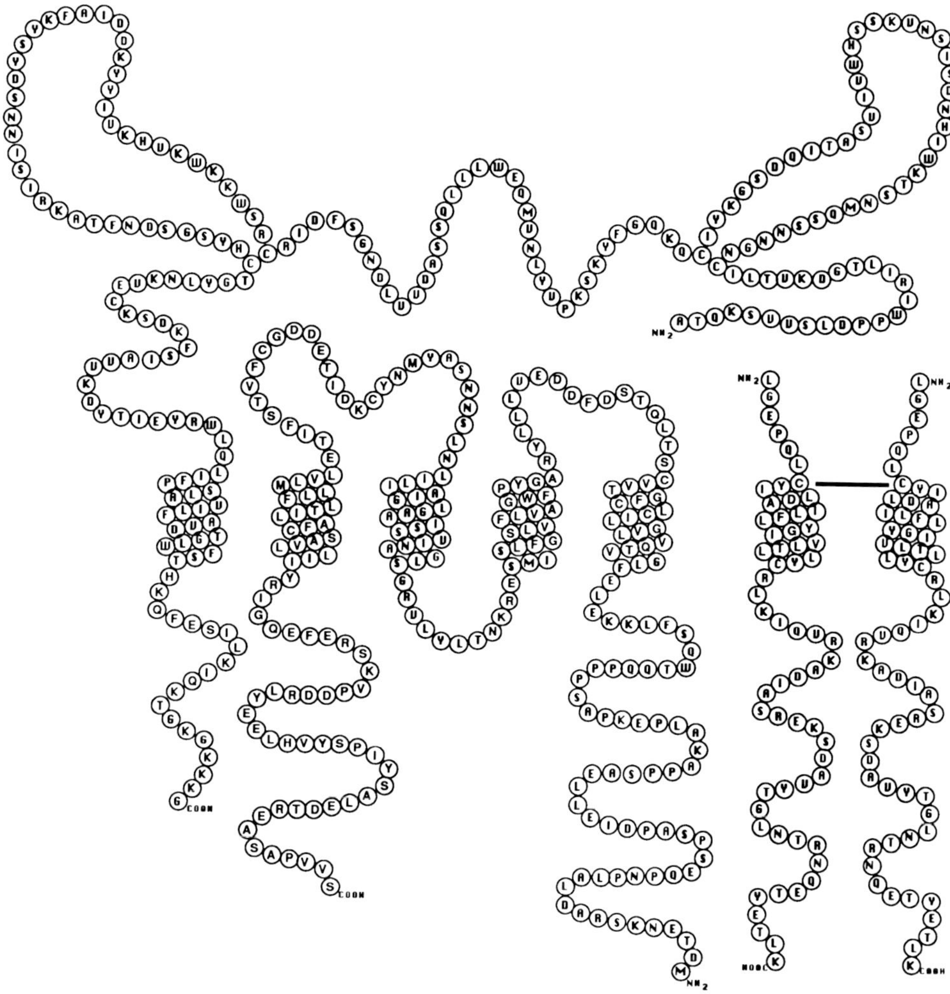

Figure 1 Model of the tetrameric receptor with high affinity for IgE. The amino acid sequence shown for each of the peptides is that of the fully processed cell surface expressed receptor. All the polypeptides are shown with the extracellular domains above the transmembrane alpha helices and the intracellular domains below. The α chain is shown on the left with a single transmembrane domain, an immunoglobulin-like extracellular domain, and a short intracellular tail. The β chain is depicted with four transmembrane domains with both the amino and carboxy termini intracellular. This topology predicts two extracellular and one intracellular loop. The disulfide-linked dimer of the γ chain is shown on the right as it is found in the native receptor.

B. The β Chain

The cDNAs of both rat and mouse β chains have been cloned (Kinet et al., 1988; Ra et al., 1989b). The homology of these sequences is 87%, with the homology evenly distributed between the untranslated and translated regions. In the RBL cells two major species of mRNA were observed by Northern blotting, a 1.75- and a 2.7-kb form. Which of these, if not both, is translated remains to be defined. In PT18 cells, a mouse mast cell line, both transcripts were also found to be present. However, in other cell lines tested, such as various macrophage lines, the transcripts were absent (Ra et al., 1989a).

The open reading frame of the rat sequence encodes a polypeptide of 243 amino acids with no apparent leader peptide. A hydropathicity plot of the predicted sequence suggests that the β chain crosses the plasma membrane four times (Kinet et al., 1988). The biochemical evidence for the predicted topology will be discussed later in this chapter.

The predicted molecular weight of the β chain from its cDNA is 26 kDa. Both in vitro and in vivo translation of the β chain lead to the production of a protein with an apparent molecular weight of 32 kDa in SDS-PAGE. However, in most in vivo isolates a second band at 28 kDa is also observed. The reason for the doublet of the β chain is not understood.

C. The γ Chain

The cDNA sequences for the mouse, rat, and human γ chains are now available (Ra et al., 1989b; Blank et al., 1989; Küster et al., 1990). The sequences are highly conserved, with 88% of the bases being conserved between rodent and human. In PT18 cells, RBL cells, and human basophils, only a single species of mRNA (0.85 kb) has been identified by Northern blots. In contrast to the α and β chains, the γ-chain mRNA has been identified in a variety of cell lines other than mast cells or basophils (Ra et al., 1989a). Recent studies establish the association of the γ chain with other receptors, previously referred to as FcγRIIa in the rodent (Ra et al., 1989a) and the human FcγRIII (Hibbs et al., 1989).

The amino acid sequence of the unprocessed γ chain contains 86 residues. A hydropathicity plot of the sequence predicts an N-terminal leader peptide of 18 amino acids in length. This is followed by five amino acids that comprise the extracellular domain and by a 21-amino-acid transmembrane segment and a 42-amino-acid cytoplasmic tail. The last six C-terminal amino acids of the γ chain are believed to be removed by a processing event that takes place before the γ chain is expressed on the plasma membrane (Blank et al., 1989). The fully processed γ chain is a polypeptide of 62 amino acids in length with a molecular mass of 7826 Da. Consistent with the biosynthetic studies, which revealed no incorporation of carbohydrate into the γ chain, no N-linked glycosylation sites are found in the γ-chain sequence.

In the plasma membrane the γ chain is found as a covalently crosslinked dimer in association with the α and β subunits (Perez-Montfort et al., 1983). The use of reducing agents, such as β-mercaptoethanol, leads to the monomer form of the γ chain. This observation suggest that dimerization of the γ chain in the native receptor results in the formation of a disulfide link.

III. Synthesis of the Receptor Subunits

A. The α Chain

Pulse-chase experiments aimed at identifying precursors of the α chain show that within 5 min of labeling, components reactive with IgE or with monoclonal antibodies directed to the α chain can be identified. The apparent molecular weights of these precursors in SDS-PAGE are 36, 38, and 40 kDa. Treatment of the precursors with endoglycosidase H (endo H), an enzyme that removes the N-linked high mannose sugars added early in the biosynthetic pathway (endoplasmic reticulum), generates a single band of 27 kDa, as predicted by the cDNA. However, precipitation with either IgE/anti-IgE or anti-α-chain antibodies, including one presumably directed at the intracellular aspect of the α chain, failed to identify the predicted species. The failure to identify in vivo a 27-kDa species of the α chain suggests that the unglycosylated form of the α chain is short-lived. A second IgE reactive component with an apparent molecular weight of 72 kDa was also precipitated with IgE/anti-IgE. This IgE-binding component was not susceptible to endo H and F and was resistant to sodium dodecyl sulfate and reducing agents. It is likely that this component is analogous to the aggregates of α chain observed upon tunicamycin treatment of cells transfected with truncated α chains (Blank et al., 1990). These aggregates appear to be degraded in the endoplasmic reticulum, as suggested by the time course of their disappearance and indirectly by the time course for maturation of the glycosylated α-chain precursors.

The ability to immunoprecipitate the glycosylated precursors of the α chain shows that the binding site for IgE on the α chain is formed during or shortly after the synthesis of the α chain. This suggests that extensive glycosylation is not a requirement for formation of the IgE binding site, in agreement with the studies of Hempstead et al. (1981).

The mature (55 kDa) α chain becomes evident 40–60 min after synthesis. This form is found on the cell surface membrane 120 min after synthesis. Treatment of the 55-kDa α chain with endo H did not result in any modification of the α chain. However, treatment with endo F generated a 27-kDa species, with about one-half the 55-kDa species remaining glycosylated. This suggests a difference in the complexity of the carbohydrate added to the α chains that may be responsible for the heterogeneity of the α chain.

in all cases dimers of the γ chain are found in association with the α chain or the $\alpha\beta$ complex. This suggests that the γ chains must interact with each other before they become associated with the other subunits to form the tetrameric structure. The assembly pathway detailed in the text is summarized in Figure 3.

The formation of a disulfide bond for dimerization of the γ chains is not a necessary requirement for interaction of the γ chains with each other or for their association with the α and β chains (Varin-Blank and Metzger, 1990).

The sequence of the γ reveals two cysteines that may be utilized to form the disulfide bridge. The issue of which of the cysteine residues is utlized in the disulfide bridge was recently addressed (Varin-Blank and Metzger, 1990). This

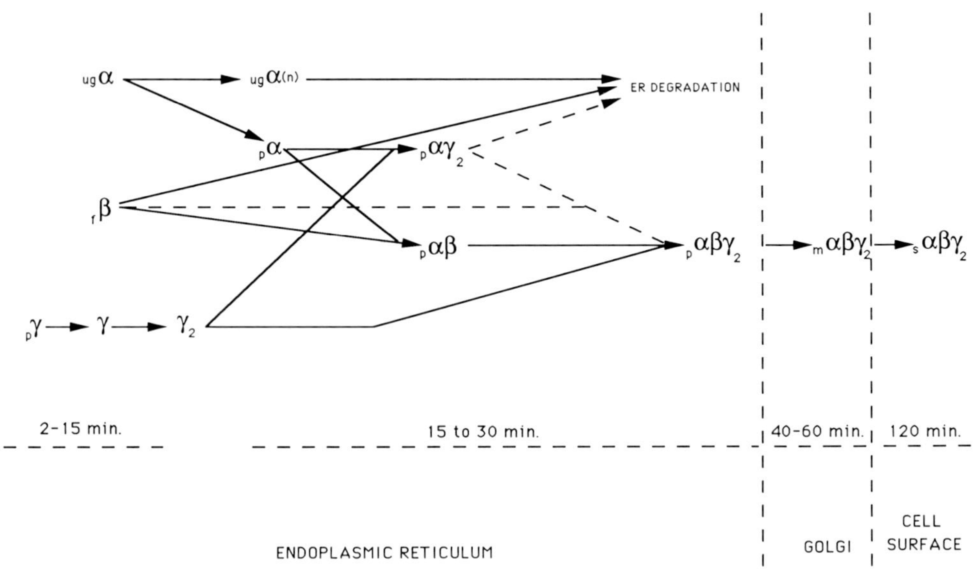

Figure 3 Model of the assembly pathway of the receptor. Synthesis of the receptor subunits is depicted on the left with assembly and maturation of the receptor depicted toward the right. Two major pathways are shown in the endoplasmic reticulum, leading to complete assembly of the receptor or degradation of unassembled subunits. Maturation (processing of *N*-linked sugars and the addition of *O*-linked sugars) of the assembled receptor is depicted to take place in the Golgi. Cell surface expression of the receptor was found to occur about 2 h after the synthesis of the constituent subunits. The solid lines represent pathways for which evidence is presented, and the dashed lines represent potential pathways for which evidence is unavailable. The subscripts represent the following: (1) u*g* denotes the unglycosylated α chain; (2) *p* denotes precursors to the mature form of the α and γ chains; (3) *f* denotes unassociated β chains, and (4) *m* and *s* denote the mature and surface expressed α chains.

study clearly shows that mutation of the cysteine 7–located N-terminal of the transmembrane segment, to a serine, results in the loss of the dimer form of the γ chain. In contrast, mutation of the cysteine 26–located C-terminal of the transmembrane segment does not result in the loss of dimers. Therefore, cysteine 7 must be responsible for the formation of the disulfide bridge since a mutation of this cysteine alone results in the loss of dimer formation. Interestingly, the mutation of the cysteine 7 to a serine that prevents covalent linkage of the γ chain had no effect on expression of the receptor, suggesting that such linkage is not required for the association of γ chains with α and β chains or for their cell surface expression.

V. Cell Surface Expression of the Receptor

Evidence of a completely assembled receptor as a prerequisite to cell surface expression is derived from studies on the assembly of the receptor and expression of the receptor in transfected COS cells (Blank et al., 1989; Rivera and Metzger, in preparation).

From pulse-chase studies the receptor is found to be assembled from its constituent subunits in the endoplasmic reticulum as detailed in the previous section. The presence of unassembled subunits or subunit complexes in cellular compartments other than the endoplasmic reticulum is not detected by use of monoclonal antibodies directed to the α and β chains. Isolation of the radiolabeled receptor via cell-bound IgE or with a monoclonal antibody directed to the α chain showed the presence of the assembled receptor on the cell surface within 90–120 min after synthesis. In all cases the molar ratio of incorporated radiolabeled amino acids was found to give a subunit structure of $\alpha\beta\gamma_2$.

The cell surface expression of the rodent receptor in transfected COS cells was possible only when the cDNAs for all three subunits were cotransfected (Blank et al., 1989). This result suggests that the complete assembly of the rodent receptor into its tetrameric structure is a prerequsite to the cell surface expression of this receptor. In contrast, the studies of Miller et al. (1989) show that the human α chain can be expressed in cells cotransfected with only the α and γ chains. Whether the structure of the human receptor for IgE is comprised of only α and γ subunits or the assembly pathway of the human receptor allows for expression of incompletely assembled receptors remains to be investigated.

VI. The Topology of the Receptor

The hydropathicity plots for each of the individual subunits provides a prediction of the extracellular and intracellular segments of each of the polypeptide sequences (Kinet, 1990). The α chain has an N-terminal hydrophilic sequence that forms the immunoglobulin-like domains. This segment also contains the IgE-binding site of the receptor and the putative N-linked glycosylation sites. Therefore, this segment is presumed to be on the extracellular aspect of the plasma membrane. More direct evidence comes from studies in which anti-peptide antibodies directed to a portion of the second immunoglobulin-like domain were shown to bind to intact RBL cells (Ra et al., 1988). Furthermore, recent evidence using mutated α chains, in which the predicted transmembrane and cytoplasmic sequence has been substituted or deleted, shows that these chimeric and truncated α chains contain the receptor-binding site for IgE that is predicted for the extracellular segment (Hakimi et al., 1990; Blank et al., 1990). The secretion of the human α chain from cells transfected with the truncated α chain also provides evidence for the predicted hydrophobic transmembrane segment since their is no stop-transfer of this truncated α chain. There is no direct proof that the segment following the transmembrane sequence is cytoplasmic, but it seems reasonable at this point to assume that this short hydrophilic segment is not incorporated in the cell membrane. Preliminary evidence from studies on the cell surface expression of mutated subunits indicate that the removal of the predicted cytoplasmic segment of the α chain had no effect on the cell surface expression of the receptor (Varin-Blank and Metzger, 1990), an unlikely finding if this segment was located in the membrane or was extracellular.

The topology of the β subunit has been more difficult to establish. Four possible transmembrane domains are predicted from the hydropathicity plots. Assuming that the β chain has four transmembrane domains, it follows that both the amino and carboxy termini are on the same side of the plasma membrane. That this is in fact the case is shown by two monoclonal antibodies that reacted with cell membranes but not intact cells (Rivera et al., 1988). The epitopes of these antibodies have been mapped; one was found to be reactive with an N-terminal peptide of 21 residues and the other to a C-terminal peptide of 113 residues (Kinet et al., 1988). Further evidence for the topology of the β chain shown in Figure 1 comes from studies on the expression of receptors containing mutant β chains (Varin-Blank and Metzger, 1990). These studies show that the only β-chain mutant that results in expression of the receptor contains the four transmembrane domains in the correct order with a deletion in the intracellular loop between the second and third domains (see Figure 4). This mutant expressed 38% of the wild-type receptor expression; all other permutations and deletions did not lead to cell surface expression of the receptor. The results provide strong evidence for the critical nature of the four presumptive transmembrane domains as the site of interaction with the other receptor subunits. This interaction presumably takes place in the plasma membrane; therefore, the deletion or exchange of any of these domains may impair the correct assembly of the receptor and be lethal to receptor expression.

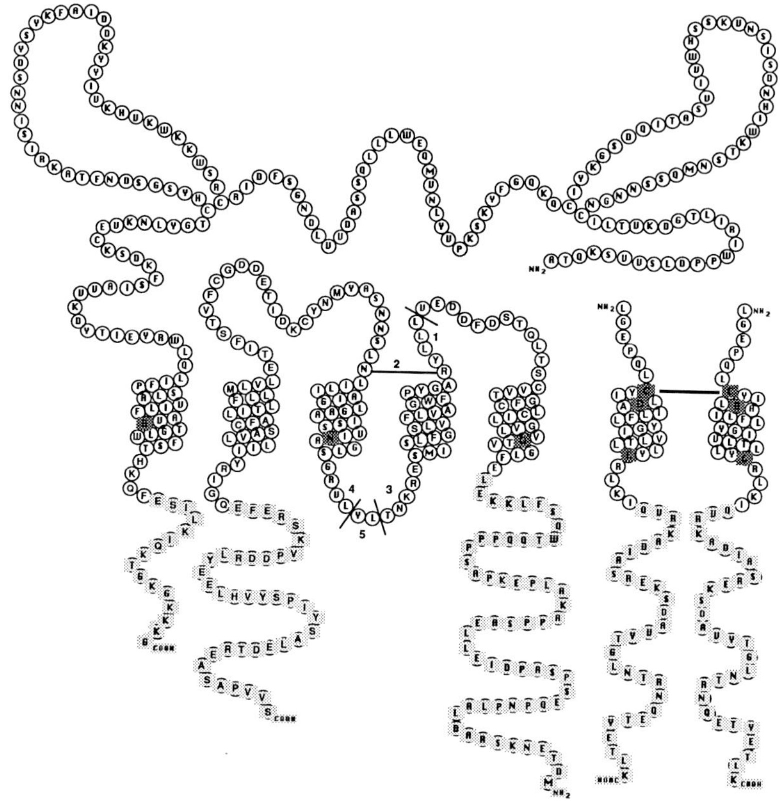

Figure 4 Mutant constructs of the high-affinity receptor for IgE. This figure depicts both deletional and site-specific mutations used for expression, immobilization, and internalization studies reviewed in the text. The light filled circles represent cytoplasmic tail deletions. For the β chain three tailless mutants were constructed, minus N_t, minus C_t, and minus $N_t + C_t$. The dark filled circles represent single mutations of the amino acid some of which are discussed in the text. The numbers shown on the β chain represent the following mutation: (1) mutant construct initiated at Leu^{94} and terminated at Thr^{123}, contains only the second transmembrane domain; (2) mutant construct that joins Arg^{97} to Asn^{151}, contains only transmembrane domains 1 and 4; (3) mutant construct that terminates β after Thr^{123}, contains only the first and second transmembrane domains; (4) mutant construct initiated at Leu^{126}, contains only the third and fourth transmembrane domains; and (5) a mutant in which constructs 3 and 4 were coexpressed leading to deletion of the intracellular loop structure.

Evidence for the topology of the γ chain as depicted in Figure 1 is derived from studies on the radiolabeling of the γ chain by various biochemical means. The γ chains can be iodinated on inverted vesicles but not on intact cells (Holowka and Baird, 1984). The γ chains were also found to be phosphorylated on threonine residues in vivo (Quarto and Metzger, 1986). Since both tyrosine and threonine residues are only found in the presumptive cytoplasmic tail, it is reasonable to assume that this segment is directed intracellularly. Moreover, antipeptide antibodies directed to the entire cytoplasmic tail of the γ chain react with soluble receptor but not with intact cells (J. Rivera, unpublished observation). By default, the short five-residue segment that precedes the transmembrane domain is assumed to be extracellular.

VII. Search for Receptor-Associated Molecules

One of the approaches in determining how the receptor transduces an extracellular signal to the intracellular environment is to define the molecules with which the receptor may interact to initiate the plethora of cellular changes observed. The recent isolation of the cDNAs for the receptor subunits now permits the study of functional characteristics of the genetically altered receptor. This in turn may lead to defining regions critical for receptor function and, ideally, epitopes for receptor-protein interactions. Several requirements must be met for the implementation of this strategy: first, the construction of the mutant cDNA and, more important, its expression on the cell surface; second, the availability of a suitable host cell that lacks the native receptor but that can respond to the aggregation of the transfected receptor by one of the available assays (Beaven et al., 1984).

Recently both these criteria have been met. The site-directed mutagenesis of the receptor subunits and the expression of different combinations of mutated receptor in transfected COS cells were recently reported (Varin-Blank and Metzger, 1990) (see Figure 4). These studies show that the removal of any single cytoplasmic domain of the receptor subunits has little effect on cell surface expression of the receptor. Moreover, the removal of all five cytoplasmic domains did not ablate cell surface expression, though it was reduced by sevenfold. This now permits the study of these mutants in a functionally suitable host. Loss of cell surface expression was observed when mutations were introduced in the transmembrane domains (Figure 4) of the receptor subunits (with most permutations done on the β subunit). In some cases minor changes produced major effects on expression. Clearly, this leads to greater difficulty in the study of the effects on receptor function by changes in the transmembrane region. Potentially more conservative changes may result in receptor expression. These studies, along with those on receptor subunit interaction and assembly

(Rivera and Metzger, in preparation) provide strong evidence for the critical role of the transmembrane domains in subunit interaction and assembly leading to the cell surface expression of the receptor.

Recently the well-known mastocytoma cell line P815, which lacks IgE receptors, was found to express some of the early signals of activation upon aggregation of transfected wild-type IgE receptors (Miller et al., 1990). The finding of the P815 cell line as a suitable host allows the study of the receptor mutants as these transfectants become available.

Other, more general characteristics of the unstimulated versus stimulated receptors can be studied in transient cultures of transfected cells such as COS cells. The interaction between the receptor and other cellular constituents such as cytoskeletal proteins has been described (Menon et al., 1986a) and correlated with secretion in mast cells. Both decreased translational mobility (Menon et al., 1986b) and internalization (Isersky et al., 1983) are initiated by the aggregation of the receptor. The effect of the deletion of the cytoplasmic domains of the receptor subunits on mobility and internalization has recently been studied (Mao et al., 1990). In general, these studies show that the interaction between the receptor and the cellular components involved in the immobilization and internalization of the receptor do not directly involve the cytoplasmic domains of the receptor. The only significant effect on the mobility of the receptor was observed in mutants containing a β chain with a truncated C-terminus. However, when the cytoplasmic domain of the α chain was substituted at the C-terminus of the β chain, the ability to immobilize the receptor by aggregation was restored. In contrast, while the β-chain C-terminal deletion caused a dramatic decrease in the rate of internalization, the substitution of the cytoplasmic domain of the α chain did not restore the ability of the receptor to internalize as efficiently. However, the fact that in the absence of the β chain the human α in the presence of only the rodent γ chain is internalized as efficiently as the wild-type receptor makes it unlikely that the C-terminus of the β chain contains a critically important epitope for receptor interaction with the endocytotic machinery. More likely, these effects are secondary, such as an effect on the receptor subunit conformation leading to loss of the ability to interact with other cellular proteins. Although it is clear that the cytoplasmic domain of many receptors that are internalized via coated pits is critical for this function (Davis et al., 1986: Iacopetta et al., 1988; Jing et al., 1990), this does not seem to be the case for the $Fc_{\epsilon}RI$. This finding is somewhat surprising since another member of the Fc-receptor family, namely the $Fc\gamma RII$, requires the cytoplasmic domain for efficient internalization (Miettinen et al., 1989).

The focus on the study of mutant receptors and the effects of these mutations on the function of the receptor is ideally suited for identifying critical regions of the receptor subunits that may serve as ligands to isolate other proteins involved in the signal transduction mechanism.

VIII. Concluding Remarks

As is evident from this chapter, in the last 3 years significant progress has been made in our understanding of receptor structure, topology, and requirements for expression. Unfortunately, less progress has been made in understanding the signal transduction mechanism of this receptor. In large part, the inability to identify and isolate active components from membrane vesicles or fragments precludes the reconstitution of receptor function in lipid vesicles or in other simple biological systems. The use of molecular genetics in the study of the receptor provides hope for the identification of other molecular components important to receptor function. Ideally, one or more of these components is specific to the function of the high-affinity receptor for IgE and would make a suitable target for therapeutic intervention.

Acknowledgments

A large part of the work reviewed in this chapter was done in the laboratory of Dr. Henry Metzger. I am indebted for his support and the critical reading of this manuscript.

Discussion

Ishizaka: Can you speculate on the role of the B chain in human FcϵRI?
Rivera: It may be required for expression in the rodent system, and a similar β-like chain may exist in the human but as of yet has not been isolated.
Lichtenstein: Please try to synthesize the intrachain events that initiate transduction—i.e., if the cytoplasmic part of the α chain is not necessary, where does the α chain "communicate"?
Rivera: Transmembrane regions are critical to the expression of the receptor. Mutants in this region versus the cytoplasmic domain seem to abolish the expression of the receptor, suggesting that this region is critical for subunit interaction.
Stevens: How does the high-affinity IgE receptor get to the plasma membrane? Have you looked at the normal and transfected cells at the EM level for specialized vesicles that carry this receptor but not various constituents of the secretory granule?
Rivera: We have no answer at present to this question.
Kennerly: Do any of the point mutations in any of the subunits abolish or diminish signal transduction?
Rivera: These mutants have not as of yet been characterized for signal transduction.

Kaplan: Is there variable glycosylation of the β subunit as a possible explanation why there are two persistent β bands on all your gels without interconversion or obvious proteolysis?
Rivera: There is no glycosylation of β subunit. Selective proteolysis has been considered as a cause of the double band, but this is speculative. As of yet there is no explanation.

References

Barsumian, E. L., Isersky, C., Petrino, M. G., and Siraganian, R. P. (1981). IgE-induced histamine release from rat basophilic leukemia cell lines: Isolation of releasing and nonreleasing clones. *Eur. J. Immunol* 11:317–323.

Beaven, M. A., Moore, J. P., Smith, G. A., Hesketh, T. R., and Metcalfe, J. C. (1984). The calcium signal and phosphatidylinositol breakdown in 2H3 cells. *J. Biol. Chem.* 259:7137–7142.

Blank, U., RA, C., Miller, L., Metzger, H., and Kinet, J-P. (1989). Complete structure and expression in transfected cells of high affinity IgE receptor. *Nature* 337:187–189.

Blank, U., Ra, C., and Kinet J-P. (1990). Characterization of truncated α chain products from human, rat and mouse high affinity receptor for immunoglobulin E. *J. Biol. Chem.* (in press).

Bonifacino, J. S., Suzuki, C. K., and Klausner, R. D. (1990). A peptide sequence confers retention and rapid degradation in the endoplasmic reticulum. *Science* 247:79–82.

Davis, C. G., Lehrman, M. A., Russell, D. W., Anderson, R. G., Brown, M. S., and Goldstein, J. L. (1986). The J.D. mutation in familial hypercholesterolemia: amino acid substitution in cytoplasmic domain impedes internalization of LDL receptors. *Cell* 45:15–24.

Eccleston, E., Leonard, B. J., Lowe, J. S., and Welford, H. J. (1973). Basophilic leukaemia in the albino rat and a demonstration of the basopoietin. *Nature New Biol.* 244:73–76.

Hakimi, J., Seals, C., Pettine, L. F., and Kochan, J. P. (1990). A chimaeric human $Fc_{\epsilon}RI$ alpha subunit that binds IgE. *FASEB J.* 4:A1047.

Hempstead, B. L., Parker, C. W., and Kulczycki, A., Jr. (1981). The cell surface receptor for immunoglobulin E. Effect of tunicamycin on molecular properties of receptor from rat basophilic leukemia cells. *J. Biol. Chem.* 256:10717–10723.

Hibbs, M. L., Selvaraj, P., Carpén, O., Springer, T. A., Küster, H., Jouvin, M-H. E., and Kinet, J-P. (1989). Mechanisms for regulating expression of membrane isoforms of FcgammaRIII (CD16). *Science* 246:1608–1611.

Holowka, D., and Baird, B. (1984). Lactoperoxidase-catalyzed iodination of the receptor for immunoglobulin E at the cytoplasmic side of the plasma membrane. *J. Biol. Chem.* 259:3720–3728.

Holowka, D., and Metzger, H. (1982). Further characterization of the beta-component of the receptor for immunoglobulin E. *Mol. Immunol* 19:219–227.

Iacopetta, B. J., Rothenberger, S., and Lukas, C. K. (1988). A role for the cytoplasmic domain in transferrin receptor sorting and coated pit formation during endocytosis. *Cell* 54:485–489.

Isersky, C., Rivera, J., Segal, D. M., and Triche, T. (1983). The fate of IgE bound to rat basophilic leukemia cells. II. Endocytosis of IgE oligomers and effect on receptor turnover. *J. Immunol.* 131:388–396.

Jing, S. Q., Spencer, T., Miller, K., Hopkins, C., and Trowbridge, I. S. (1990). Role of the human transferrin receptor cytoplasmic domain in endocytosis: Localization of a specific signal sequence for internalization. *J. Cell Biol.* 110:283–294.

Kanellopoulos, J. M., Liu, T. Y., Poy, G., and Metzger, H. (1980). Composition and subunit structure of the cell receptor for immunoglobulin E. *J. Biol. Chem.* 255:9060–9066.

Kinet, J-P. (1990). The high-affinity receptor for IgE. *Current Opinion Immunol.* 2:499–505.

Kinet, J-P., Metzger, H., Hakimi, J., and Kochan, J. (1987). A cDNA presumptively coding for the alpha subunit of the receptor with high affinity for immunoglobulin E. *Biochemistry* 26:4605–4610.

Kinet, J-P., Blank, U., Ra, C., Metzger, H., and Kochan, J. (1988). Isolation and characterization of cDNAs coding for the beta subunit of the high-affinity receptor for immunoglobulin E. *Proc. Natl. Acad. Sci. USA* 85:6483–6487.

Kinet, J-P., Metzger, H., Alber, G., Blank, U., Huppi, K., Jouvin, M-H. E., Küster, H., Miller, L., Ra, C., Rivera, J., and Varin-Blank, N. (1989). The high affinity receptor for immunoglobulin E: New developments. In *Progress in Immunology, VII*. Edited by F. Melchers, et al. Berlin, Springer-Verlag, pp. 716–723.

Klausner, R. D., and Sitia, R. (1990). Protein degradation in the endoplasmic reticulum. *Cell* 62:611–614.

Kochan, J., Pettine, L. F., Hakimi, J., Kishi, K., and Kinet, J-P. (1988). Isolation of the gene coding for the alpha subunit of the human high affinity IgE receptor. *Nucleic Acids Res.* 16:3584–3584.

Kulczycki, A., Jr., McNearney, T. A., and Parker, C. W. (1976). The rat basophilic leukemia cell receptor for IgE. I. Characterization as a glycoprotein. *J. Immunol.* 117:661–665.

Küster, H., Thompson, H., & Kinet, J-P. (1990). Characterization and expression of the gene for the human Fc receptor gamma subunit. Definition of a new gene family. *J. Biol. Chem.* 265:6448–6452.

Mao, S-Y., Varin-Blank, N., Edidin, M., and Metzger, H. (1990). Immobilization and internalization of mutated IgE receptors in transfected cells. *J. Biol. Chem.* (in press).

Menon, A. K., Holowka, D., Webb, W. W., and Baird, B. (1986a). Clustering, mobility, and triggering activity of small oligomers of immunoglobulin E on rat basophilic leukemia cells. *J. Cell Biol.* 102:534–540.

Menon, A. K., Holowka, D., Webb, W. W., and Baird, B. (1986b). Cross-linking of receptor-bound IgE to aggregates larger than dimers leads to rapid immobilization. *J. Cell Biol.* 102:541–550.

Metzger, H. (1983). The receptor on mast cells and related cells with high affinity for IgE. *Contemp. Top. Mol. Immunol.* 9:115–145.

Miettinen, H. M., Rose, J. K., and Mellman, I. (1989). Fc receptor isoforms exhibit distinct abilities for coated pit localization as a result of cytoplasmic domain heterogeneity. *Cell* 58:317–327.

Miller, L., Blank, U., Metzger, H., and Kinet, J-P. (1989). Expression of high-affinity binding of human immunoglobulin E by transfected cells. *Science* 244:334–337.

Miller, L., Alber, G., Varin-Blank, N., Ludowyke, R., and Metzger, H. (1990). Transmembrane signaling in P815 mastocytoma cells by transfected IgE receptors. *J. Biol. Chem.* 265:12444–12552.

Perez-Montfort, R., Kinet, J-P., and Metzger, H. (1983). A previously unrecognized subunit of the receptor for immunoglobulin E. *Biochemistry* 22:5722–5728.

Quarto, R., and Metzger, H. (1986). The receptor for immunoglobulin E: Examination for kinase activity and as a substrate for kinases. *Mol. Immunol.* 23:1215–1223.

Quarto, R., Kinet, J-P., and Metzger, H. (1985). Coordinate synthesis and degradation of the alpha-, beta-, and gamma-subunits of the receptor for immunoglobulin E. *Mol. Immunol.* 22:1045–1051.

Ra, C., Kochan, J., Hakimi, J., Danho, W., Metzger, H., and Kinet, J-P. (1988). The high affinity IgE receptor: Anti-peptide antibodies confirm isolated cDNA codes for alpha subunit. *FASEB J.* 2:A1248–A1248.

Ra, C., Jouvin, M-H. E., Blank, U., and Kinet, J-P. (1989a). A macrophage Fcg receptor and the mast cell receptor for IgE share an identical subunit. *Nature* 341:752–754.

Ra, C., Jouvin, M-H. E., and Kinet, J-P. (1989b). Complete structure of the mouse mast cell receptor for IgE (FcŒRI) and surface expression of chimeric receptors (rat-mouse-human) on transfected cells. *J. Biol. Chem.* 264:15323–15327.

Rivera, J., and Metzger, H. The high affinity receptor for IgE: Synthesis and assembly (in preparation).

Rivera, J., Kinet, J-P., Kim, J., Pucillo, C., and Metzger, H. (1988). Studies with a monoclonal antibody to the beta subunit of the receptor with high affinity for immunoglobulin E. *Mol. Immunol.* 25:647–661.

Shimizu, A., Tepler, I., Benfey, P. N., Berenstein, E. H., Siraganian, R. P., and Leder, P. (1988). Human and rat mast cell high-affinity immunoglobulin E receptors: Characterization of putative alpha-chain gene products. *Proc. Natl. Acad. Sci. USA* 85:1907–1911.

Thompson, H. L., Metcalfe, D. D., and Kinet, J-P. (1990). Early expression of high-affinity receptor for immunoglobulin E (FcŒRI) during differentiation of mouse mast cells and human basophils. *J. Clin. Invest.* 85:1227–1233.

Varin-Blank, N., and Metzger, H. (1990). Surface expression of mutated subunits of the high affinity mast cell receptor for IgE. *J. Biol. Chem.* 265:15685–15694.

Table 1 Mast Cell/Basophil Secretagogues

Hypoxia	
Drugs	Muscle relaxants Opioids Antibiotics Iodinated contrast media
Histamine-releasing factors	Neutrophils Eosinophils Lymphocytes Macrophages Platelets Endothelial cells Nasal washings
Calcium ionophone	A23187
Anaphylatoxins	C3a C4a C5a
Neurohormones	ATP Substance P Neurotensin
Physical stimuli	Heat Sunlight Cold Pressure
Cytokines	IL-1 IL-3 GM-CSF CTAP-3

cold, vibration, and pressure, also cause mast cell degranulation (Casale et al., 1986; Huston et al., 1986; Kaplan, 1983; Keahey et al., 1987; Soter et al., 1979); however, the mechanism is obscure. Finally, two areas of current research interest in mast cell secretagogues are the inflammatory cell-derived, histamine-releasing factors (HRF) and the neuropeptides. These topics are reviewed in depth below.

II. Inflammatory Cell-Derived, Histamine-Releasing Factors

The observation that late-phase allergic reactions are accompanied by recrudescence of histamine release in the absence of continued antigen stimulation (Durham et al., 1984; Naclerio et al., 1985) led to an intense search over the last 12 years for endogenously produced histamine-releasing factors. A number of the known cytokines, when examined, were found to have histamine-releasing activity. Included in this category are IL-1β (Submaranian et al., 1987), IL-3, and GM-CSF (Haak-Frendscho et al., 1988; MacDonald et al., 1989), which cause basophil histamine release at picomolar concentrations, and platelet factor 4 (Brindley et al., 1983) and IL-8 (White et al., 1989b), which cause basophil histamine release at less physiological micromolar concentrations. IL-2, IL-4, IL-5, IL-6, and G-CSF have no discernible basophil histamine-releasing activity (Alam et al., 1989). In addition, lymphocytes (Lett-Brown et al., 1979; Theuson et al., 1984), platelets (Orchard et al., 1986), monocytes (Schulman et al., 1988), alveolar macrophages (Schulman et al., 1985), neutrophils (White and Kaliner, 1987), and eosinophils (O'Donnell et al., 1983) have been shown to produce novel cytokines with histamine-releasing activity. Histamine-releasing activity has been observed in several human body fluids, including bronchoalveolar lavage fluid (Alam et al., 1990b; Broide et al., 1990), unstimulated nasal washings (MacDonald et al., 1987), and fluids bathing sites of cutaneous late-phase allergic reactions (Warner et al., 1986).

A. Characterization of the Production and Response to HRF

Most of what we know about these histamine-releasing factors (HRF) derives from studies employing nasal washings or HRF produced by neutrophils or mononuclear cells. Histamine-releasing activity for all these HRF has been detected using human basophils (Table 2). Thus far, only two studies have employed human mast cells in addition to basophils. Human lung mast cells responded to mononuclear cell-derived HRF, but were less sensitive than basophils (Schulman et al., 1985), and in another study, human cutaneous mast cells and basophils were equally responsive to the neutrophil-derived HRF (White et al., 1989a).

Atopics and nonatopics both produce and respond to neutrophil-derived HRF (White et al., 1987, 1989a). Whereas mononuclear cells of both atopics and nonatopics can be stimulated to produce HRF, only asthmatic subjects' mononuclear cells spontaneously produce HRF (Alam et al., 1984; Alam and Rozniecki, 1985). Likewise, both atopic and nonatopic basophils are capable of degranulating in response to mononuclear cell-derived HRF (Baeza et al., 1988). However, the basophils of atopic asthmatics are most sensitive, while the

Table 2 Inflammatory Cell-Derived Histamine-Releasing Factors

Source	Induces histamine release from	Characterization	IgE dependence	Identity
Lymphocytes	Human basophils	Anion exchange peak 1 eluting in the effluent	No	CTAP III
		Anion exchange peak 2 eluting with 0.5 M NaCl	Yes	Unidentified, Blocked N-terminus, 15–17 kDa
		Anion exchange peak 3 eluting before 1 M NaCl	No	Unidentified, Blocked N-terminus, 41 kDa
Platelets	Human basophils Human cutaneous MC	Anion exchange elute before 0.15 M NaCl	Yes	Unidentified
Alveolar macrophages	Human basophils	18 kDa	Yes	Unidentified
Neutrophils	Human basophils Human cutaneous MC RBL Rat and guinea pig cutaneous MC	2 kDa, 12 kDa, 25–40 kDa >200 kDa	No	Unidentified
Eosinophils	Human basophils	16 kDa	No	Major basic protein
Nasal washings	Human basophils	15–25 kDa	Yes	Unidentified
BAL	Human basophils	30–50 kDa	No	Unidentified

basophils of atopics and nonatopics have intermediate and low sensitivity, respectively, to mononuclear cell-derived HRF (Alam et al., 1990a). In contrast, while nasal HRF can be found in the nasal washings of all subjects, only basophils of atopic asthmatics respond to this product (MacDonald et al., 1987).

In an attempt to understand why basophils of atopic subjects, especially atopic asthmatics, are hyperresponsive to HRF, the relationship between HRF and IgE was studied. Desensitization of basophils to IgE-mediated degranulation rendered basophils unresponsive to nasal washings–derived HRF (MacDonald et al., 1987) as well as lung macrophage–derived HRF (Liu et al., 1986). Lactic acid treatment, which strips IgE from the basophil IgE receptor, also rendered the cells unresponsive to stimulation by both types of HRF. Responsiveness could be restored by passive sensitization with IgE-containing serum from atopic asthmatics responsive to HRF, but not by serum from normal controls. The data suggested that HRF stimulation of basophils was dependent on interaction of HRF with a subtype of IgE found only in certain atopic individuals, and this form of IgE was termed IgE(+).

Alam et al. (1990a) obtained similar results employing mononuclear cell–derived HRF in IgE-stripping experiments. Baeza et al. (1988), however, were unable to reproduce the cross-desensitization experiments using mononuclear cell–derived HRF. In addition, both nasal washings– and neutrophil-derived HRF caused equivalent amounts of histamine release from rat basophilic leukemia cells cultured in the absence of IgE and thus lacking surface bound IgE (White et al., 1988). Taken together, the data suggested that HRF was a heterogeneous mixture of factors, one or more of which might be IgE dependent.

B. Clinical Relevance of HRF

Only a few studies have addressed the clinical relevance of inflammatory cell–derived HRF. Alam et al. (1987) reported that the spontaneous production of HRF by cultured mononuclear cells of asthmatics was highly correlated with the subjects' bronchial reactivity to histamine. The correlation between spontaneous HRF production and hyperreactivity was found regardless of whether autologous or heterologous basophils were employed to assay HRF. Mononuclear cells of atopic asthmatics could be further stimulated by relevant antigen to produce more HRF. In a double-blinded, placebo-controlled trial, 2 years of grass immunotherapy significantly blunted antigen-stimulated HRF production (Kuna et al., 1989). Spontaneously produced HRF was decreased only in those patients who were clinically benefited, and the decrease correlated closely with the improvement in bronchial hyperreactivity to histamine. These results were confirmed and extended by Liao and Hsieh (1990), who further observed that basophil responsiveness to HRF is correlated with plasma histamine concentrations in new asthmatic patients and that responsiveness decreases after successful immunotherapy. The same authors also noted that successful immunotherapy results in a negative correlation between PHA-stimulated HRF production and airway hyperreactivity, while the same correlation is positive in poor immunotherapy responders. Taken together, the data suggest that HRF may contribute to asthma severity.

The relationship of HRF to atopic dermatitis with food allergy has also been studied (Sampson et al., 1989). Basophils of persons with atopic dermatitis and food allergy were found to have high rates of spontaneous histamine release compared with both normals and patients with atopic dermatitis without food allergy. Moreover, mononuclear cells of patients with atopic dermatitis and food allergy spontaneously produced an IgE-dependent HRF that caused histamine release only from basophils of other food allergic individuals. Strict dietary avoidance of the offending food reduced both the production of HRF and the rate of spontaneous basophil histamine release. Thus, HRF may account for the increased spontaneous histamine release seen in food allergic patients.

C. HRF Purification

Purification of the various HRFs has proven difficult (Table 2). As suggested by the IgE dependency studies, mononuclear cell–derived HRF consists of at least five factors (molecular weights of 11–12, 15–17, 25–27, 31–34, and over 80 kDa) identifiable by nondenaturing polyacrylamide gel electrophoresis (Baeza et al., 1989). About one-half of the activity in crude HRF could be bound by one of two IgE myelomas tested and migrated in three bands with apparent molecular weights of 14, 21 and 22 kDa. When crude HRF was fractionated by anion exchange chromatography, three peaks of HRF activity eluted with the effluent, at 0.5 M NaCl, and just before 1 M NaCl. The IgE binding factors eluted in the second fraction at 0.5 M NaCl. When the eluted material was subjected to SDS gel electrophoresis, it was found to contain a single 15–17-kDa peak of HRF activity. This fraction, which has a blocked N-terminus, is most likely the IgE-dependent factor previously described (MacDonald et al., 1987; Schulman et al., 1985). Histamine-releasing activity eluting from the anion exchange column just prior to 1 M NaCl (peak 3) consists predominantly of a 41-kDa HRF, also with a blocked N-terminus, with minor bands at 7, 11–12, 14–17, and 65–80 kDa. Material recovered in the effluent (peak 1) was the most heterogeneous, being composed predominately of an 11–12-kDa HRF, with additional activity at 15–18, 40–45, and 80–90 kDa. The 11–12 kDa fraction from peak 1 was purified into a wide band by acrylamide gel electrophoresis and electroelution. The upper and lower portions of the band were sequenced, and when the sequences were superimposed, the resultant sequence was identical to the first 36 amino acids of connective tissue activating peptide-III (Baeza et al., 1990). Recombinant CTAP-III, purified 11–12,000-Da HRF, the upper band (residues

1–21), and the lower band (residues 16–36) were all capable of inducing basophil histamine release. Thus, the only HRF thus far sequenced appears to be either CTAP-III or its breakdown products.

Neutrophil-derived HRF is also markedly heterogeneous. Fractionation of crude neutrophil HRF over a Sephadex G25 gel filtration column yields a consistent peak of HRF activity at 1400–2300 Da, with additional activity sometimes obtained in the void (>5000 Da) and/or the column (<1000 Da) volume (White et al., 1988). Fractionation over a Suparose 12 FPLC gel filtration column typically yields up to seven peaks of HRF activity. The most common consists of one to three peaks with molecular weights below 12 kDa, a peak at 25–45 kDa, and a peak with a molecular mass of greater than 200 kDa. Occasionally a peak at 12–18 kDa and a second peak above 200 kDa can be appreciated (White et al., 1991b). Attempts to isolate these peaks of HRF activity have been frustrated by rapid breakdown of the active material.

D. Manipulation of the Production and Activity of HRF

Little is known about the pharmacological manipulation of HRF. Sampson et al. (1989) reported that prolonged dietary avoidance markedly reduces the spontaneous generation of mononuclear cell–derived HRF in patients with atopic dermatitis and food allergies. Spontaneous production of monunuclear cell–derived HRF can also be reduced by specific antigen immunotherapy (Kuna et al., 1989). There are no published studies to date dealing with the pharmacological manipulation of the production and/or activity of mononuclear cell–derived HRF. The activity of neutrophil-derived HRF, however, can be inhibited in vitro by 10^{-7} to 10^{-5} M hydrocortisone (White et al., 1991a). Inhibition is first seen after 5–6 hr of preincubation with hydrocortisone and is maximal after 24 hr. In addition, inhibition was most marked in experiments utilizing the 1400–2300-Da HRF and minimal or absent when the >200-kDa HRF fractions were used. Manipulation of the production of neutrophil-derived HRF has also been studied. Nedocromil sodium, 10^{-7} to 10^{-4} M inhibits in vitro HRF production by isolated human neutrophils, but does not affect the activity of preformed neutrophil-derived HRF (White et al., 1991b).

Inasmuch as multiple HRFs might potentially be produced and released during inflammatory reactions, one might wonder why anaphylaxis does not often occur. One explanation might be that these factors are short-lived and only act locally at high concentrations. Alternatively, endogenous inhibitors of histamine release might be produced. Indeed, an 8-kDa factor produced by histamine-stimulated mononuclear cells has been described that specifically inhibits basophil histamine release induced by HRF, but not by other secretagogues such as allergen, anti-IgE, C5a, concanavalin A, or phorbol myristate acetate (Alam et al., 1888). This factor, termed HRIF, can also be recovered from bronchoalveolar lavage (BAL) fluid of normal subjects. A second, nonspecific inhibitor of basophil histamine release active against HRF, anti-IgE, concanavalin A, and *N*-formyl-methionine-leucyl-phenylalanine can also be identified in BAL fluid (Alam et al., 1990b). The identity of the nonspecific inhibitor is not known; however, the HRF-specific inhibitor is most likely IL-8 (Alam, 1990). Thus, endogenous factors exist that may be involved in the autoregulation of the activity of the various HRFs.

In summary, multiple HRFs are produced by inflammatory cells and these factors can be recovered from a variety of body fluids. The production of and response to these HRF correlate with disease severity both in asthma and in atopic dermatitis with food allergy. The production by inflammatory cells of an HRF-specific histamine release inhibitory factor suggests that mast cell/basophil activation during inflammation is under tight homeostatic control. Pharmacological manipulation of the production and activity of some of the HRFs can be achieved with nedocromil sodium and hydrocortisone, respectively, while production of others can be reduced by dietary allergen avoidance or by immunotherapy. It is likely that these HRF and HRIF contribute to the regulation of mast cell and basophil activity in allergic and other inflammatory disorders.

III. Neuropeptides and Mast Cells

Neuropeptides are a newly recognized group of neurotransmitters present both in the central nervous system and in peripheral nerves. In skin, the neuropeptides substance P, neurokinin A, somatostatin, neurotensin, and calcitonin gene-related peptide (CGRP) are found primarily in sensory nerves near epithelial surfaces, blood vessels, and glands (Cuello et al., 1978; Dalsgaard et al., 1983; Hartschuh et al., 1983; Landis and Fredieu, 1986). Neuropeptides cause vasodilation, vascular permeability, smooth muscle contraction, and activation of leukocytes and macrophages (Sertl et al., 1988; Payan and Goetzl, 1987; Hartung et al., 1986). Intradermal injection of substance P, neurokinin A, CGRP, somatostatin, vasoactive intestinal peptide, or neurotensin into human skin (Foreman and Jordan, 1983; Piotrowski and Foreman, 1986; Fuller et al., 1987) induces a wheal-and-flare response, and substance P has been released during acute inflammation in the rat skin (White and Helme, 1985; Helme et al., 1986; Yonehara et al., 1987).

To generate cutaneous inflammatory responses characterized by vasodilation and increased vascular permeability, intact sensory neurons in the injured area are required (Lewis, 1927). For example, vascular responses induced by the topical application of mustard oil, capsaicin, or xylene or by the intradermal injection of histamine require intact sensory innervation (Jancso et al., 1967; Bernstein et al., 1981). Electrical stimulation of peripheral nerves can mimic these reactions, leading to vasodilation and increased vascular permeability (Stricker, 1976; Jancso et al., 1968). These nerve-dependent vascular responses are referred to as neurogenic inflammation.

Cutaneous neurogenic inflammation involves the activation of sensory nerves with the release of vasoactive neuropeptides from sensory nerve endings (Lembeck and Holzer, 1979; Lembeck et al., 1982). Allergic skin reactions may also involve neurogenic components inasmuch as local application of capsaicin, a neurotoxin specific for sensory innervation, inhibits antigen-induced flare reactions and may also prevent heat- and cold-induced urticaria (Lundblad et al., 1987; Toth-Kasa et al., 1983).

Mast cells are found in close proximity to both myelinated and nonmyelinated nerve fibers (Wiesner-Menzeel et al., 1981; Newson et al., 1983) and may actually contact unmyelinated axons containing substance P and CGRP (Skofitsch et al., 1985; Stead et al., 1987). Thus, it is possible that neuropeptides interact with mast cells in producing local inflammation. Several neuropeptides, the best studied of which is substance P, have been shown to cause histamine release (Table 3) (Foreman and Jordan, 1983; Sertl and Kaliner, 1987; Sydbom, 1982; Shanahan et al., 1985; Ali et al., 1986; Barrett et al., 1986; Devillier et al., 1986; Lawrence et al., 1987; Ebertz et al., 1987; Foreman, 1987b; Church et al., 1989; Louis and Radermecker, 1990, 1991). Rat peritoneal mast cells release histamine in response to somatostatin, substance P, vasoactive intestinal peptide,

Table 3 Histamine-Releasing Activity of Sensory Neuropeptides

	Cell origin					
	Rat		Primates			
	Peritoneal	Mucosal (lung/ intestine)	Human skin	Human lung	Human basophil	Monkey (lung/ intestine)
Substance P	+	+	++	+	+	?
Neurokinin A	–	0	0	0	0	0
Somatostatin	++	-	0	0	0	0
Vasoactive intestinal peptide	++	-	0	0	0	-
Calcitonin gene-related peptide	+	0	0	0	0	0
Neurotensin	++	-	0	0	0	-

+, Activation of histamine release; -, no histamine-releasing activity; 0, unknown action; ?, uncertain histamine-releasing activity.

and neurotensin, whereas rat intestinal mast cells respond only to substance P (Ali et al., 1986). Whereas human skin and lung mast cells as well as human basophils respond to substance P, human skin mast cells are approximately 30-fold more sensitive than the latter cells. The threshold concentration of substance P required to activate basophil and lung mast cells is 100 μM, while human skin mast cells respond to 3–10 μM substance P (Louis and Radermecker, 1990, 1991). Thus, there is intraspecies heterogeneity of response of different mast cell populations of various neuropeptides. There is also heterogeneity of mast cell response to neuropeptides between species. Most mast cell populations in rats, mice, and hamsters respond to substance P, whereas guinea pig mast cells are completely resistant (Ali et al., 1986).

The mechanism whereby substance P induces mast cell/basophil degranulation is only partly defined. Substance P is an undecapeptide with a positively charged N-terminal (Arg-Pro-Lys-Pro) and a lipophilic C-terminal. Substance P–induced human skin degranulation occurs independent of the tachykinin receptors, NK-1, NK-2, and NK-3 (Church et al., 1989). Sequential removal of N-terminal amino acids leads to progressive loss of rat and human mast cell histamine-releasing activity, and experiments with synthetic peptides suggest that the positively charged N-terminus is essential, while a lipophilic C-terminus is also necessary, but the exact sequence is not critical (Church et al., 1989; Devillier et al., 1989). Furthermore, substance P–induced histamine release from rat peritoneal mast cells can be inhibited by pertussis toxin and by benzalkonium chloride (Bueb et al., 1990). Activation of phosphokinase C with 12-*0*-tetradecanoylphorbol-13-acetate (TPA), or inhibition of its breakdown with the diacylglycerol kinase inhibitor R 59022 or with the diacylglycerol lipase inhibitor RHC 80267, also inhibits substance P–induced histamine release from rat peritoneal mast cells (McLeod et al., 1990). These data suggest that activation by substance P is charge dependent and phosphokinase C sensitive, and that it occurs via activation of both a pertussis toxin–sensitive G protein and phospholipase C. Interestingly, substance P–induced degranulation of human lung mast cells, but not human skin mast cells or basophils, can be inhibited by the antiasthma drug nedocromil sodium (Louis and Radermecker, 1990).

Nanomolar concentrations of neuropeptides induce wheal-and-flare responses when injected into human skin (Hägermark et al., 1978). The substance P–induced flare, but not the wheal reaction, is closely correlated with the capacity of substance P to cause histamine release (Foreman and Jordan, 1983) and can be inhibited by antihistamines and mast cell depletion with compound 48/80 (Foreman and Jordan, 1983; Fuller et al., 1987; Jarizzo et al., 1983; Barnes et al., 1986). In contrast, neurokinin A and neurokinin B possess no histamine-releasing activity in vitro, but both can cause wheal-and-flare reactions in vivo (White and Helme, 1985; Devillier et al., 1986; Foreman, 1987a; Gamse et al., 1987). Thus, the mechanism whereby different neuropeptides cause vascular responses in the skin may vary and may not necessarily involve mast cell participation. The actions of the neuropeptides may be dependent on the concentration employed inasmuch as vascular permeability induced in rat skin by nanomolar concentrations of substance P and neurokinin A is not affected by antihistamines, whereas the response to micromolar concentrations can be inhibited partially with antihistamines (Andrews and Helme, 1987).

A convenient model to study whether sensory neuropeptides actually cause mast cell degranulation is antidromic electrical stimulation of cutaneous nerves. Electrical stimulation induces the release of substance P and other neuropeptides from sensory nerve endings in the skin, and the resultant cutaneous vascular responses can be prevented by pretreatment with capsaicin or substance P antagonists (White and Helme, 1985; Jancso et al., 1976; Lembeck and Holzer, 1979; Bernstein et al., 1981; Lundberg et al., 1985). The response elicited could reflect either the direct action of substance P on postcapillary venules or an indirect effect through substance P–induced mast cell degranulation. Stimulation of the auricular nerve in rats is reported to increase the proportion of degranulating mast cells and cause plasma protein extravasation that is partly inhibitable either by H_1 and H_2 antihistamines or by mast cell depletion with compound 48/80 (Lembeck and Holzer, 1979; Kiernan, 1972). Others, however, have been unable to confirm the latter results (Jancso et al., 1967; Kiernan, 1972; Gamse and Saria, 1987).

To investigate the role of mast cells in cutaneous neurogenic inflammation, the saphenous nerve of rats was electrically stimulated and vascular permeability within the area of the innervated nerve was measured (Kowalski and Kaliner, 1988; Kowalski et al., 1990). Electrical stimulation of the saphenous nerve produced extravasation of ^{125}I-labeled albumin into the skin within seconds, peaking 3–5 min later (Kowalski and Kaliner, 1988). Histologically, 86.5% of all mast cells in normal skin were found in the deep dermis, whereas the vessels leaking after electrical stimulation (visualized with the macromolecular tracer monastral blue B) were superficial. By electron microscopy, the vessels developing increased vascular permeability after electrical stimulation were identified as postcapillary venules (Kowalski et al., 1990). To assess the possible association of mast cell activation, the histamine content of the affected area of the skin was measured, and mast cell degranulation was sought histologically. Despite impressive plasma extravasation, no mast cell degranulation or decrease in skin histamine was observed through 15 min of electrical stimulation. However, by 30 min, a significant decrease in histamine content was produced, and the overall proportion of degranulating mast cells was increased by 35% above control. Measurement of plasma histamine showed that neurogenic inflammation was not accompanied by histamine release into the draining venous plasma (Kowalski and Kaliner, 1988).

To exclude the possibility that mast cell activation could occur without

(1987). Substance P-induced histamine release in human cutaneous mast cells. *J. Invest. Dermatol.* 88:366–371.

Erjavec, F., Lembeck, F., Florianc-Irman, T., Scofitch, G., Donner, J., Saria, A., and Holtzer, P. (1981). Release of histamine by substance P. *Naunyn-Schmiedeberg Arch. Pharmacol.* 317:67–70.

Foreman, J. C. (1987a). Neuropeptides and the pathogenesis of allergy. *Allergy* 42:1–11.

Foreman, J. C. (1987b). Substance P and calcitonin gene-related peptide: Effects on mast cells and in human skin. *Int. Arch. Allergy Appl. Immunol.* 82:366–371.

Foreman, J. C., and Jordan C. (1983). Histamine release and vascular changes induced by neuropeptides. *Agents Actions* 13:105–116.

Foreman, J. C., Mongar, J. L., and Gomperts, B. D. (1973). Calcium ionophores and movement of calcium ions following physiologic stimulus to a secretory process. *Nature* 245:249–251.

Fuller, R. W., Conradson, T. B., Dixon, C. M. S., Crossman, D. C., and Barnes, P. J. (1987). Sensory neuropeptide effects in human skin. *Br. J. Pharmacol.* 92:781–788.

Galli, S. J. (1987). New approaches for the analysis of mast cell maturation, heterogeneity, and function. *Fed. Proc.* 46:1906–1914.

Gamse, R., and Saria, A. (1987). Antidromic vasodilation in the rat hindpaw measured by laser Doppler flowmetry: Pharmacologic modulation. *J. Autonom. Nerv. Syst.* 19:105–111.

Gamse, T., Posch, M., Saria, A., and Jancso, G. (1987). Several mediators appear to interact in neurogenic inflammation. *Acta Physiol. Hungar.* 69:343–354.

Gorski, J. P., Hugli, T. E., and Muller, H. J. (1979). The third anaphylatoxin of the human complement system. *Proc. Natl. Acad. Sci. USA* 76:5299–5304.

Haak-Frendscho, M., Arai, N., Arai, K., Baeza, M. L., Finn, A., and Kaplan, A. P. (1988). Human recombinant granulocyte-macrophage colony-stimulating factor and interleukin 3 cause basophil histamine release. *J. Clin. Invest.* 82:17–20.

Haas, F., and Bergofsku, E. H. (1972). Role of the mast cell in the pulmonary pressor response to hypoxia. *J. Clin. Invest.* 51:3154–3162.

Hägermark, O., Hökfelt, T., and Pernow B. (1978). Flare and itch induced by substance P in human skin. *J. Invest. Dermatol.* 71.

Hartschuh, W., Weihe, E., and Reinecke, M. (1983). Peptidergic (neurotensin, VIP, substance P) nerve fibers in the skin. Immunohistochemical evidence of an involvement of neuropeptides in nociception, pruritus and inflammation. *Br. J. Dermatol.* 109(Suppl 25):14–17.

Hartung, H. P., Wolters, K., and Toyoka, K. V. (1986). Substance P binding properties and studies on cellular responses in guinea pig macrophages. *J. Immunol.* 136:3856–3863.

Helme, R., Koschorke, G. M., and Zimmerman, M. (1986). Immunoreactive substance P release from skin nerves in the rat by noxious thermal stimulation. *Neurosci. Lett.* 63:295–299.

Huston, D. P., Bressler, R. B., Kaliner, M., Sowell, L. K., and Baylor, M. W. (1986). Prevention of mast-cell degranulation by ketotifen in patients with physical urticarias. *Ann. Intern. Med.* 104:507–510.

Ishizaka, T., Chang, T. H., Taggart, M., and Ishizaka, K. (1972). Histamine release from rat mast cells by antibodies against rat basophilic leukemia cell membrane. *J. Immunol.* 108:339–345.

Jancso, N., Jancso-Gabor, A., and Szolcsanyi, J. (1967). Direct evidence for neurogenic inflammation and its prevention by denervation and by pretreatment with capsaicin. *Br. J. Pharmacol. Chemother.* 31:138–151.

Jancso, N., Jancso-Gabor, A., and Szolcsanyi, J. (1968). The role of sensory nerve endings in neurogenic inflammation induced in human skin and in the eye and paw of the rat. *Br. J. Pharmacol. Chemother.* 32:32–41.

Jarizzo, J., Coults, A., Eady, R., and Graves, M. (1983). Vascular responses of human skin to injection of substance P and mechanism of action. *Eur. J. Pharmacol.* 87:67–76.

Kaplan, A. P. (1983). Urticaria and angioedema. In *Allergy Principles and Practice.* Edited by E. Middleton, C. S. Reed, and E. S. Ellis. St Louis, Mosby, pp. 1341–1306.

Keahey, T. M., Indrisano, J., Lavker, R. M., and Kaliner, M. A. (1987). Delayed vibratory angioedema: Insights into pathophysiologic mechanisms. *J. Allergy Clin. Immunol.* 80:831–838.

Kiernan, J. A. (1972). The involvement of mast cells in vasodilation due to axon reflex in injured skin. *Q. J. Exp. Physiol.* 57:311–317.

Kitamura, Y., Go, S., and Hatanaka, K. (1978). Decrease of mast cell maturation, heterogeneity, and function. *Blood* 52:447–452.

Kowalski, M. L., and Kaliner, M. (1988). Neurogenic inflammation, vascular permeability and mast cells. *J. Immunol.* 140:1906–1914.

Kowalski, M. L., Sliwinska-Kowalski, M., and Kaliner, M. (1990). Neurogenic vascular permeability and mast cells. II. Further evidence indicating that mast cells are not involved in neurogenic inflammation. *J. Immunol.* 145:1214–1221.

Kuna, P., Alam, R., Kuzminska, B., and Rozniecki, J. (1989). The effect of preseasonal immunotherapy on the production of histamine-releasing factor (HRF) by mononuclear cells from patients with seasonal asthma: Results of a double-blind, placebo-controlled, randomized study. *J. Allergy Clin. Immunol.* 83:816–824.

Landis, S. C., and Fredieu, J. R. (1986). Coexistence of calcitonin gene-related peptide and vasoactive intestinal peptide in cholinergic sympathetic innervation of rat sweat glands. *Brain Res.* 377:177–179.

Lawrence, I. D., Warner, J. A., Cohan, V. L., Hubbart, W. C., Kagey-Sobotka, A., and Lichtenstein, L. M. (1987). *J. Immunol.* 139:3062–3069.

Lembeck, F., and Holzer, P. (1979). Substance P as neurogenic mediator of antidromic vasodilation and neurogenic plasma extravasation. *Naunyn-Schmiedeberg Arch. Pharmacol.* 310:175–183.

Lembeck, F., Donnerer, J., and Bartho, L. (1982). Inhibition of neurogenic vasodilation and plasma extravasation by substance P antagonists, somatostatin, and D-met^2, Pro^5-enkephalinamide. *Eur. J. Pharmacol.* 85:171–176.

Lett-Brown, M. A., Theuson, D. O., Plank D. E., Langford, M. P., and Grant, J. A. (1984). Histamine releasing activity. IV. Molecular heterogeneity of the activity from stimulated human thoracic duct lymphocytes. *Cell Immunol.* 87:434–444.

Lewis T. (1927). *The Blood Vessels of the Human Skin and Their Responses.* London, Shaw and Sons, p. 67.

Liao, T. N., and Hsieh, K. H. (1990). Altered production of histamine-releasing factor (HRF) activity and responsiveness to HRF after immunotherapy in children with asthma. *J. Allergy Clin. Immunol.* 86:894–901.

Louis, R. E., and Radermecker, M. F. (1990). Substance P-induced histamine release from human basophils, skin and lung fragments: effect of nedocromil sodium and theophylline. *Int. Arch. Allergy Appl. Immunol.* 92:329–333.

Louis, R. E., and Radermecker, M. F. (1991). Cutaneous and basophilic sensitivity to substance P and gastrin in non-atopic versus atopic subjects. *Allergy* 46: 30–34.

Lundberg, J. M., Saria, A., and Rosell, S. F. K. (1985). Substance P antagonist inhibits heat induced oedema in the rat skin. *Acta Physiol. Scand.* 120:145–146.

Lundblad, L., Lundberg, J. M., Anggard, A., and Zetterstrom, O. (1987). Capsaicin-sensitive nerves and the cutaneous allergy reaction in man. Possible involvement of sensory neuropeptides in the flare reaction. *Allergy* 42:20–31.

MacDonald, S. M., Lichtenstein, L. M., Proud, D., Plaut, M., Naclerio, R. M., MacGlashan D. W., and Kagey-Sobotka, A. (1987). Studies of IgE-dependent histamine releasing factors: Heterogeneity of IgE. *J. Immunol.* 139:506–512.

MacDonald, S. M., Schleimer, R. P., Kagey-Sobotka, A., Gillis, S., and Lichtenstein, L. M. (1989). Recombinant IL-3 induces histamine release from human basophils. *J. Immunol.* 142:3527–3532.

Margo, A. M. (1974). Involvement of IgE in con-A induced histamine release from human basophils in vitro. *Nature* 249:572–574.

McLeod, J., Hayes, N. A., and Foreman, J. C. (1990). Effect of 12-o-tetradecanoylphorbol-13-acetate (TPA) on substance P–induced histamine release from rat peritoneal mast cells. *Agents Actions* 30:140–142.

Metcalfe, D. D., Kaliner, M. A., and Donlon, M. A. (1981). The mast cell. *CRC Crit. Rev. Immunol.* 3:23–74.

Morrison, D. C., and Henson, P. M. (1978). Release of mediators from mast cells and basophils induced by different stimuli. In *Immediate Hypersensitivity-Modern Concepts and Development.* Edited by M. K. Bach. New York, Marcel Decker, pp. 431–502.

Naclerio, R. M., Proud, D., Togias, A. G., Adkinson, N. F., Meyers D. A., Kagey-Sobotka, A., Plaut, M., Norman P. S., and Lichtenstein L. M. (1985). Inflammatory mediators in late antigen-induced rhinitis. *N. Engl. J. Med.* 313:65–70.

Newson, B., Dahlström, A., Enerbäch, L., and Ahlman H. (1983). Suggesting evidence for a direct innervation of mucosal mast cells. An electron microscopic study. *Neuroscience* 10:565–570.

O'Donnell, M. C., Ackerman, S. J., Gleich, G. J., and Thomas, L. L. (1983). Activation of basophil and mast cell histamine release by eosinophil granule major basic protein. *J. Exp. Med.* 157:1981–1991.

Orchard, M. A., Kagey-Sobotka, A., Proud, D., and Lichtenstein, L. M. (1986). Basophil histamine release induced by a substance from stimulated human platelets. *J. Immunol.* 136:2240–2244.

Payan, K., and Goetzl, E. J. (1987). Substance p receptor–dependent responses of leukocytes in pulmonary inflammation. *Am. Rev. Respir. Dis.* 136:S39–S43.

Piotrowski, W., and Foreman, J. C. (1986). Some effects of calcitonin gene-related peptide in human skin and on histamine release. *Br. J. Dermatol.* 114:37–46.

Sampson, H. A., Broadbent, K. R., and Bernhisel-Broadbent, J. (1989). Spontaneous release of histamine from basophils and histamine releasing factor in patients with atopic dermatitis and food hypersensitivity.

Schulman, E. S., Liu, M. C., Proud, D., MacGlashan, D. W., Lichtenstein, L. M., and Plaut, M. (1985). Human lung macrophages induce hitamine release from basophils and mast cells. *Am. Rev. Respir. Dis.* 131:230–235.

Schulman, E. S., McGettigan, M. C., Post, T. J., Vigderman, R. J., and Shapiro. S. S. (1988). Human monocytes generate basophil histamine releasing activities. *J. Immunol.* 140:2369–2375.

Segal, D. M., Taurog, J. D., and Metzger, H. (1977). Dimeric immunoglobulin E. serves as a unit signal for mast cell degranulation. *Proc. Natl. Acad. Sci. USA* 74:2993–2998.

Sertl, K., and Kaliner, M. (1987). The influence of neurohormones and neuropeptides on mast cells. In *The Airways: Neural Control in Health and Disease*. Edited by M. A. Kaliner and P. Barnes. New York, Marcel Dekker, pp. 447–466.

Sertl, K., Wiederman, C., Kowalski, M. L., Hurtado, S., Plutchol, J., Linnoila, I., Pert, C. B., and Kaliner, M. A. (1988). The relationship between receptor distribution in rat lung and the capacity of substance P to stimulate vascular permeability. *Am. Rev. Respir. Dis.* 138:151–159.

Shanahan, F., Deneburg, J. A., Fox, J., Bienenstock, J., and Befus, D. (1985). Mast cell heterogeneity: Effects of neuroenteric peptides on histamine release. *J. Immunol.* 135:329–331.

Skoftisch, G., Savitt, J. M., and Jacobovitz, D. M. (1985). Suggestive evidence for a direct innervation of mucosal mast cells. An electron microscopic study. *Neuroscience* 10:565–570.

Soter, N. A., Wasserman, S., Pathak, M. A., Parish, J. A., and Austen K. F. (1979). Solar urticaria: Release of mediators into the circulation after experimental challenge. *J. Invest. Dermatol.* 72:282 (abstract).

Stead, R. H., Tomioka, M., Quinonez, G., Simon, G. T., Felten, S. Y., and Bienenstock, J. (1987). Intestinal mucosal mast cells in normal and nematode-infected rat intestines are in intimate contact with peptidergic nerves. *Proc. Natl. Acad. Sci. USA* 84:2975–2979.

Stricker, S. (1976). Untersuchung uber die Gefasswurzein des Ischiadicus. *Sitzung Kaiserlichen Akad. Wissenschaft. Wien* 3:173–185.

Sydbom, A. (1982). Histamine release from isolated rat mast cells by neurotensin and other peptides. *Agents Actions* 12:91–93.

Theuson, D. O., Speck, L. S., Lett-Brown, A., and Grant, J. A. (1979). Histamine-releasing activity (HRA). I. Production by mitogen or antigen stimulated human mononuclear cells. *J. Immunol.* 123:626–632.

Toth-Kasa, I., Jancso, G., Obal, F., and Husz, S. (1983). Involvement of sensory nerve endings in cold and heat urticaria. *J. Invest. Dermatol.* 80:34–36.

Warner, J. A., Pienkowski, M. M., Plaut, M., Norman, P. S., and Lichtenstein, L. M. (1986). Identification of histamine releasing factor(s) in the late phase of cutaneous IgE-mediated reactions. *J. Immunol.* 136:2583–2587.

White, D. M., and Helme, R. D. (1985). Release of substance P from peripheral nerve terminals following electrical stimulation of the sciatic nerve. *Brain Res.* 336:27–31.

White, M. V., and Kaliner, M. A. (1987). Neutrophils and mast cells. I. Human neutrophil-derived histamine releasing activity. *J. Immunol.* 139:1624–1630.

White, M. V., Kaplan, A. P., Haak-Frendscho, M., and Kaliner, M. (1988). Neutrophils and mast cells. Comparison of neutrophil derived histamine releasing activity with other histamine releasing factors. *J. Immunol.* 141:3537–3583.

White, M. V., Baer, H., Kuboto, Y., and Kaliner, M. (1989a). Neutrophils and mast cells: Characterization of cells responsive to neutrophil-derived histamine-releasing activity (HRA-N). *J. Allergy Clin. Immunol.* 84:773–780.

White, M. V., Yoshimura, T., Hook, W., Kaliner, M. A., and Leonard, E. J. (1989b). Neutrophil attractant/activation protein-1 (NAP-1) causes human basophil histamine release. *Immunol. Lett.* 22:151–54.

White, M. V., Igarashi, Y., Lundgren, J. D., Shelhamer, J., and Kaliner, M. (1991a). Hydrocortisone inhibits RBL mediator release induced by neutrophil derived histamine releasing activity (HRA-N) as well as by anti-IgE. *J. Immunol.* 147:667–673.

White, M. A., Phillips, R. L., and Kaliner, M. A. (1991b). Neutrophils and mast cells: Nedocromil sodium inhibits the generation of neutrophil-derived histamine-relasing activity (HRA-N). *J. Allergy Clin. Immunol.* 87:812–820.

Wiesner-Menzeel, L., Schultz, B., Vakilzadeh, G., and Czarnetzki, B. M. (1981). Electron microscopical evidence for a direct contact between nerve fibers and mast cells. *Acta Dermatovener.* 61:465–469.

Woodward, D. F., Owen, D. A. A., Pipkin, M. A., and Ledgard, S. E. (1985). Histamine involvement in the local and systemic microvascular effects produced by intradermal substance P. *Agents Actions* 17:126–130.

Yonehara, N., Shibutani, T., and Inoki, R. (1987). Contribution of substance P to heat-induced edema in rat paw. *J. Pharmacol. Exp. Ther.* 242:1071–1076.

4

Insights into Mast Cell Development and Function Derived from Analyses of Mice Carrying Mutations at *Beige, W*/c-*kit,* or *Sl*/*SCF* (c-*kit* Ligand) Loci

STEPHEN J. GALLI
EDWIN N. GEISSLER

Beth Israel Hospital
and Harvard Medical School
Boston, Massachusetts

BARRY K. WERSHIL

Massachusetts General Hospital
and Harvard Medical School
Boston, Massachusetts

JOHN R. GORDON

Western College of Veterinary Medicine
University of Saskatchewan
Saskatoon, Saskatchewan, Canada

MINDY TSAI

Beth Israel Hospital
Boston, Massachusetts

ILAN HAMMEL

Sackler School of Medicine
Tel-Aviv University
Tel-Aviv, Israel

I. Introduction

Mutant mice that express abnormalities in mast cell development or structure have represented an important and versatile resource for the investigation of many aspects of mast cell biology. And recently, the mast cell has proved to represent a valuable system for investigating the genes that are affected in the mutant animals. In this chapter, we will review some of the important aspects of mast cell biology that have been clarified by experiments performed in mutant beige *(bg)* mice or *W* or *Sl* mast cell–deficient mice. We will also review how studies with mast cells have helped to elucidate the nature and function of the products of the genes affected by these mutations.

II. Beige Mice

A. Value in Studies of Mast Cell Development and Function

The first mutation recognized to affect mast cell structure or development was the *bg* mutation, located on chromosome 13 of the domestic mouse (reviewed in

Silvers, 1979a). Mice homozygous for the beige mutation (e.g., C57BL/6-bg^J/bg^J beige mice) express defects similar to those of the human Chédiak-Higashi syndrome, a genetic disorder characterized by an autosomal dominant pattern of inheritance, pigment dilution, and impaired leukocyte-dependent host resistance to infection, and by the presence of very large cytoplasmic granules in melanocytes, granulocytes, and certain nonhematopoietic cells (reviewed in Silvers, 1979a; Hammel et al., 1987; Boxer, 1990). Besides humans and mice, similar syndromes have been reported in several other mammalian species (reviewed in Silvers, 1979a; Hammel et al., 1987; Boxer, 1990).

Chi and Lagunoff (1975) reported that the mast cells of beige mice contained extremely large cytoplasmic granules, which are readily recognized by either light microscopy or transmission electron microscopy (Fig. 1). Because of their giant granules, the mast cells derived from beige mice can be identified

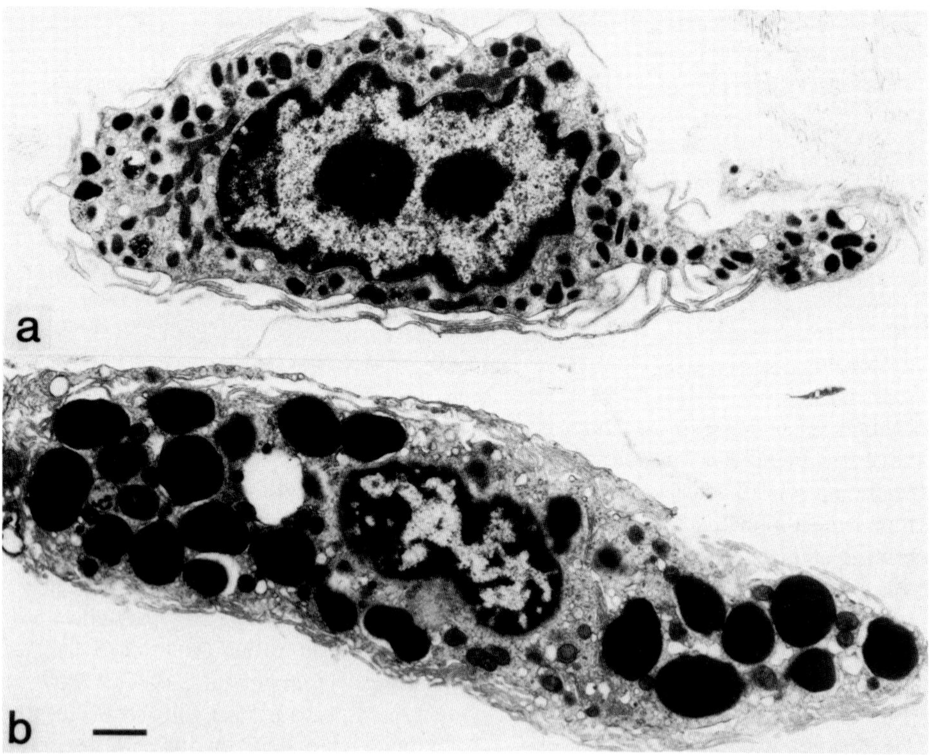

Figure 1 Dermal mast cells from the ear skin of a control (C57BL/6-bg^J/+ or +/+) mouse (a) or a beige (C57BL/6-bg^J/bg^J) mouse (b). The cytoplasmic granules of the beige mouse mast cell are much larger than those in the control cell. Bar, 1.0 μm. a and b, ×10,700. (From Hammel et al., 1987).

unequivocally even after their introduction into mice that have endogenous populations of normal mast cells (reviewed in Kitamura et al., 1985). Beige mice therefore represent excellent sources of bone marrow or mast cells for transplantation into genetically compatible recipients in experiments where identification of donor or recipient mast cells or granulocytes is desirable (reviewed in Kitamura et al., 1985). As described below, Kitamura and his associates have used this approach extensively to investigate the origin and development of mouse mast cells (Kitamura et al., 1985; Kanakura et al., 1987). In addition to the abnormalities affecting mast cells and granulocytes, beige mice have platelets that contain less than 1% of the normal level of serotonin, probably because they lack cytoplasmic dense bodies (Novak et al., 1984). By contrast, beige mouse mast cells are not deficient in serotonin (Weitzman et al., 1985). As a result, beige mice can be used in experiments evaluating the relative contribution of platelets, as opposed to mast cells, as a source of serotonin in inflammatory or immune responses (Galli and Hammel, 1984).

Recently, Nishimura et al. (1989) reported the discovery and characterization of a beige rat. This mutant exhibited giant cytoplasmic granules in mast cells and other cell types and had blood serotonin levels approximately one-tenth of those in the congenic normal rat. The beige rat may be of great value for certain mast cell studies that may be difficult to perform in mice.

B. Abnormalities in Unit Granule Formation and Pattern of Cytoplasmic Granule Enlargement in Beige Mouse Mast Cells

The product or products affected by mutations at the beige locus have not been identified (Justice et al., 1990). Nor is it clear whether all examples of the Chédiak-Higashi syndrome are due to mutations involving the same gene(s). Nevertheless, it has long been thought that the abnormal cytoplasmic granules that appear in cells affected by the mutations in the Chédiak-Higashi syndrome must reflect a profound defect in the generation or natural history of the affected granules (reviewed in Silvers, 1979a; Hammel et al., 1987; Boxer, 1990).

Two new findings that may shed light on the abnormalities of secretory granule formation in the Chédiak-Higashi syndrome were revealed by a detailed morphometric analysis of the ultrastructure of the cutaneous mast cells of C57BL/6-bg^J/bg^J mice and their normal littermates (Hammel et al., 1987). The "unit granule" volume of dermal mast cells in beige mice, i.e., the volume of the smallest size class of the mature cytoplasmic granules produced by this cell type, was ~18 times larger than that of the control mast cells. Hammel et al. (1991) showed that the volume of the unit granule can vary between the mast cells of different tissues in the same rats; e.g., the unit granule of volume of jejunal mucosal mast cells is ~5.5 × that of the mast cells in the ear pinna. However, the striking difference in the size of the unit granule volume of dermal mast cells in beige and control mice represents the first demonstration of a mutation that significantly alters the size of the unit granule in specific cell types. The magnitude of this effect of the beige mutation appears to vary according to cell lineage, in that the difference in the size of the unit granule in the pancreatic acinar cells of beige versus control mice (0.080 ± 0.03 versus 0.065 ± 0.003 μm^3, $p < 0.01$), while significant, was much less than that observed when dermal mast cell granules were compared (0.070 ± 0.002 versus 0.0038 ± 0.0003 μm^3, $p < 0.001$).

In addition to the marked enlargement of their unit granule volume, beige mouse mast cells exhibited a striking abnormality in the size distribution of their mature granules. Based on a study in the rat, Hammel et al. (1983) proposed that the mature cytoplasmic granules of mast cells and other cell types normally enlarge by a process of aggregation and fusion, but that only unit granules (i.e., mature granules of the smallest size class) could fuse with each other or with larger mature granules. Subsequently, Hammel et al. (1985) provided evidence that this "unit addition" pattern of cytoplasmic granule enlargement also occurred in human lung mast cells. This finding indicated that the process of aggregation and fusion of mature secretory granules is not restricted to the rat and may represent an important mechanism in the natural history of secretory granule enlargement in diverse species.

The unit addition pattern of secretory granule enlargement produces a distribution of granule sizes in which the most frequent granule size encountered in transmission electron micrographs, as judged by the volumes calculated from the actual cross-sectioned profile areas of these granules, is a multiple of the unit granule volume. In the case of the dermal mast cells of the normal littermates of beige mice, this most frequent granule size was 3 times the size of the unit granule (V_3 in Fig. 2a). By contrast, the size distribution of cytoplasmic granules in beige mouse mast cells conformed to the distribution that is predicted when granules of any size can aggregate and fuse randomly (Hammel and Lagunoff, 1982; Hammel et al., 1983), i.e., a granule size distribution in which the most frequently encountered size is that of the unit granule (V_1) and which includes many granules of very large size (Fig. 2b).

The molecular mechanisms that regulate the size of unit granules and determine the normal, unit addition pattern of secretory granule enlargement await clarification. Nevertheless, the abnormalities in beige mouse mast cell cytoplasmic granules revealed by the study of Hammel et al. (1987) suggest that the beige mutation profoundly affects the production and/or function of structure(s) necessary for unit granule formation in the Golgi region and for unit granule aggregation and fusion during granule enlargement outside the Golgi.

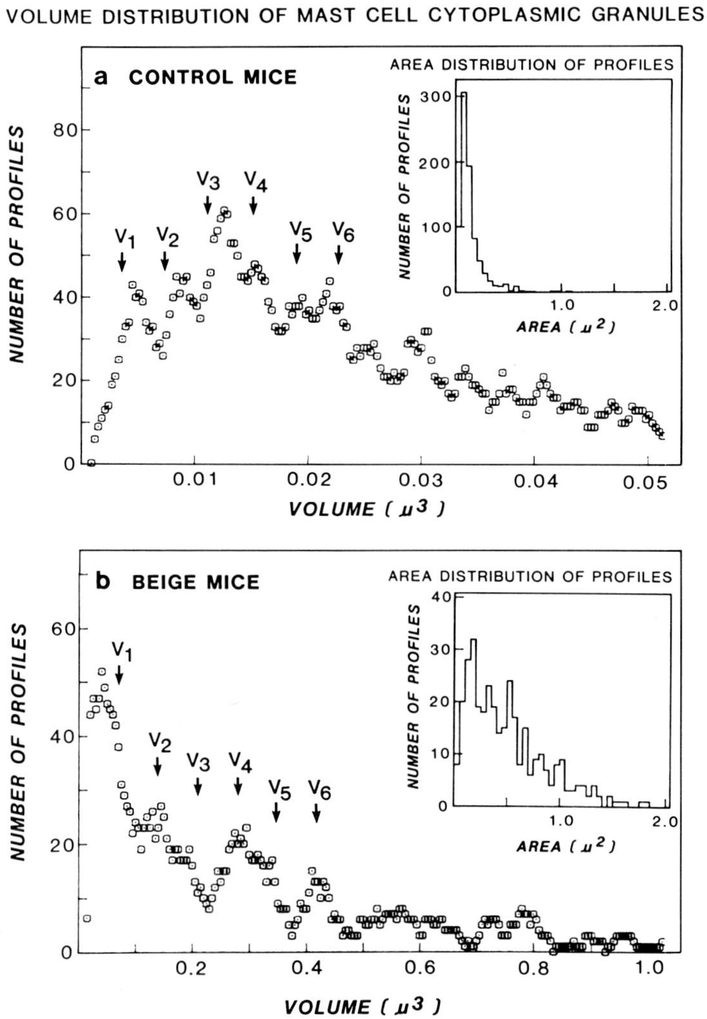

Figure 2 Moving bin histograms demonstrating periodic, multimodal distributions of control (a) or beige (b) mouse cutaneous mast cell granule equivalent volumes. The arrows (v_1, v_2, v_3, etc.) are placed at integral multiples of the mean intermodal distance, a value that defines the magnitude of the "unit volume." Insets show the distribution of the measured granule cross-sectioned (i.e., profile) areas. In (a), 826 granules (in 24 mast cells) were analyzed with a bin size of 0.0021 μm^3 moved every 0.0003 μm^3. In (b), 344 granules (in 28 mast cells) were analyzed with a bin size of 0.035 μm^3 moved every 0.005 μm^3. Note the difference in the volume ordinates in (a) and (b), reflecting the much larger size of mast cell granules in beige as opposed to normal mice. (From Hammel et al., 1987).

III. *W* or *Sl* Mutant Mast Cell–Deficient Mice

A. Introduction

The dominant white-spotting *(W)* locus on mouse chromosome 5, and the steel *(Sl)* locus on chromosome 10, had been studied by developmental biologists, hematologists, and geneticists for decades before it was clear that mutations at these loci influenced mast cell development. Indeed, mutations at *W* or *Sl* affect several important developmental programs, including gametogenesis, pigmentation, and hematopoiesis (Russell, 1979; Silvers, 1979b). Thus, most *W* or *Sl* mutations render the homozygous mutant animals sterile, devoid of coat pigmentation, and anemic (Russell, 1979; Silvers, 1979b). In 1978 and 1979, Kitamura et al. reported the important observations that mutations at *W* (Kitamura et al., 1978) or *Sl* (Kitamura and Go, 1979) also profoundly affect the development of mast cells. Subsequently, analyses of mice with mutations at *W* or *Sl* have provided many important insights into mast cell development, heterogeneity, and function (see below). Mast cell–deficient and congenic normal mice also have been used in efforts to determine the relative contribution of mast cells, as opposed to other sources, to the tissue content of such mediators as histamine (Yamatodani et al., 1982), serotonin (Inoue et al., 1985), heparin (Nakamura et al., 1981), and anticoagulantly active, heparin-like molecules associated with the microvasculature (Marcum et al., 1986).

W and *Sl* mutant mice, of course, also have been essential in efforts to identify and characterize both the products encoded at *W* and *Sl*, the tyrosine kinase growth factor receptor, c-*kit*, and a ligand for c-*kit*, respectively. We will discuss the structure and function of c-*kit* and its ligand in detail below, but first we will review some of the findings that originally suggested that the normal development of mouse mast cells reflected a receptor-ligand interaction between products encoded at *W* or *Sl*.

B. In Vivo Studies of Mast Cell Development in W/W^v and Sl/Sl^d Mice

The *W* or *Sl* mutant mice most commonly used in studies of mast cell development and function are $WBB6F_1$-W/W^v (W/W^v) or $WCB6F_1$-Sl/Sl^d (Sl/Sl^d) mice (reviewed in Galli and Kitamura, 1987; Kitamura et al., 1989). Mast cell deficiencies of variable magnitude are also expressed by mice with single or double doses of other mutant alleles at the *W* or *Sl* loci (Go et al., 1980; Geissler and Russell, 1983; Stevens and Loutit, 1982; Kohrogi et al., 1983; Galli and Kitamura, 1987). But except for W^n/W^n or *W/W* mice, which usually die in utero or within 2 weeks of birth, none of these mutants is as profoundly mast cell deficient as the W/W^v or Sl/Sl^d mice.

The genetic background and certain other important characteristics of W/W^v and Sl/Sl^d mice are depicted in Table 1. For the purposes of the present

Table 1 Characteristics of Genetically Mast Cell–Deficient WBB6F$_1$*W/W*^{v} or WCB6F$_1$-*Sl/Sl*^{d} Mice[a]

Characteristics	WBB6F$_1$-*W/W*^{v}	WCB6F$_1$-*Sl/Sl*^{d}
Genetic background[b]	WB/Re-*W*/+ × C57BL/6-*W*^{v}/+	WC/Re-*Sl*/+ × C57BL/6-*Sl*^{d}/+
Mutations	c-*kit* (Chromosome 5)	A ligand for c-*kit*[c] (Chromosome 10)
Site of defect resulting in mast cell deficiency	Stem cells/mast cell lineage itself	Tissue microenvironments required for mast cell development
Repair of mast cell deficiency with congenic +/+ bone marrow cells or mast cells	Yes	No
Repair of mast cell deficiency by injection of the c-*kit* ligand, SCF	No	Yes
Mast cells (% of +/+ level in adult, disease-free mice)	<1%[d]	<1%[d]
Mast cells develop in skin at sites of chronic idiopathic or PMA-induced dermatitis	Yes[e]	No[e]

[a]Both WBB6F$_1$-*W/W*^{v} and WCB6F$_1$-*Sl/Sl*^{d} mice also have a macrocytic anemia, lack hair pigmentation, and are sterile (Russell, 1979; Silvers, 1979b).
[b]The four possible genotypes of the F$_1$ mice (*W/W*^{v}, *W*/+, *W*^{v}/+, +/+, or *Sl/Sl*^{d}, *Sl*/+, *Sl*^{d}/+, +/+) can be distinguished according to coat color. The *W/W*^{v} and *Sl/Sl*^{d} mice are white with black eyes, the congenic +/+ mice are black, the various heterozygotes can be distinguished by the pattern of spotting.
[c]This c-*kit* ligand has been named: SCF (stem cell factor), KL (*k*it *l*igand), MGF (mast cell growth factor), and Steel factor (see text).
[d]The skin of adult *W/W*^{v} or *Sl/Sl*^{d} mice contains rare mast cells (~0.3% the number present in congenic +/+ mice). No mast cells at all have been observed in the following organs/sites: bone marrow, spleen, thymus, brain, heart, lung, kidney, urinary bladder, liver, stomach, ileum, cecum, mesentery, peritoneal cavity, hindlimb skeletal muscle, uterus.
[e]See Galli et al. (1987a) and Gordon and Galli (1990a).
Source: Modified from Galli, 1990.

discussion, it is important to emphasize that W/W^v and Sl/Sl^d mice are virtually devoid of mature, morphologically identifiable mast cells in all organs and anatomical sites examined (reviewed in Galli and Kitamura, 1987; Kitamura, 1989; Galli, 1990). Thus, as discussed in more detail in Kitamura (1989) and Galli (1990), W/W^v and Sl/Sl^d mice virtually lack both the "connective tissue–type mast cells" (CTMC) characteristic of the normal skin, peritoneal cavity, and gut muscularis propria, and the "mucosal mast cells" (MMC) characteristic of the mucosa of the gastrointestinal tissues.

Much of the early understanding of the nature of the defects caused by mutations at *W* or *Sl* was based on studies of transplantation of bone marrow among mutant and normal mice, and on attempts to reconstruct hematopoietic and stromal cells interactions in vitro (reviewed in Russell, 1979; Dexter and Moore, 1977). Such analyses indicated that the anemia and other hematological defect(s) in W/W^v mice reflected a problem intrinsic to the affected lineages, whereas the defect(s) in the Sl/Sl^d mice influenced the microenvironments necessary for the migration, proliferation, and/or survival of the affected lineages (Russell, 1979). For example, bone marrow transplantation of cells from the congenic normal +/+ mice cured the macrocytic anemia of W/W^v animals, but was without effect in Sl/Sl^d mice.

Kitamura et al. (1978) showed that transplantation of congenic +/+ bone marrow cells also repaired the mast cell deficiency of W/W^v mice. By contrast, the mast cell deficiency of Sl/Sl^d mice was refractory to bone marrow transplantation from the congenic +/+ mice. Moreover, transplantation of bone marrow from Sl/Sl^d mice repaired the mast cell deficiency of W/W^v animals (Kitamura and Go, 1979). These findings indicated that the mast cell deficiency of W/W^v mice, like their anemia, reflected a defect intrinsic to the mast cell lineage, whereas the mast cell deficiency of the Sl/Sl^d mouse reflected a problem in the microenvironments necessary for normal mast cell development. Beige mice were also used as donors of cells in several types of experiments designed to elucidate mast cell development (reviewed in Kitamura et al., 1985). The appearance in W/W^v recipients of mast cells with the giant cytoplasmic granules typical of beige mouse mast cells provided incontrovertible evidence that the newly appearing mast cells were of donor origin. This approach also demonstrated convincingly that mouse mast cells are derived from precursors that reside in the bone marrow and are similar to the cells that give rise to the spleen colony-forming cells (Kitamura et al., 1981). Additional studies by Kitamura and his associates employing the transfer of hematopoietic or lymphoid cells among beige, normal, and W/W^v mice have produced a detailed understanding of the embryonic development, normal differentiation, phenotypic heterogeneity, and proliferative potential of mouse mast cells (reviewed in Kitamura et al., 1985; Kitamura, 1989; Galli, 1990).

C. In Vitro Analyses of the Mechanism of Mast Cell Deficiency in W/W^v and Sl/Sl^d Mice

In order to study how particular cell-cell interactions are affected by mutations at defined loci, it is useful to be able to perform in vitro experiments employing the affected cell types. At first glance, one might expect that this approach would be impractical for analyzing the mast cell deficiency of mice with mutations at *W*, since adult animals with a double dose of mutations at this locus virtually lack the affected cell. Fortunately, however, cells in the mast cell lineage can in fact be generated in vitro from *W* mutant mice. In 1981, five groups reported that populations of cells with many features of mast cells could be generated by culturing normal mouse hematopoietic cells in media derived from mitogen-activated T cells, cloned Lyl+2– inducer T cells, or WEHI-3B tumor cells (Nabel et al., 1981; Nagao et al., 1981; Razin et al., 1981; Schrader, 1981; Tertian et al., 1981). While several different designations were proposed for these in vitro–derived cells, all of the currently available evidence supports our initial suggestion that they represent immature mast cells (Nabel et al., 1981; Galli et al., 1982; Galli, 1990). Subsequent work demonstrated that IL-3 was the factor critical for the growth of immature mast cells from mouse hematopoietic cells in vitro (Ihle et al., 1983). In this chapter, such cells will be designated IL-3-dependent, bone marrow-derived cultured mast cells (BMCMC).

Even though the tissues of W/W^v mice virtually lack mature mast cells, IL-3-dependent BMCMC can readily be generated from the bone marrow cells of W/W^v mice in numbers similar to those which can be produced from the bone marrow cells of the congenic normal mice (Yung and Moore, 1982; Suda et al., 1985; Nakano et al., 1985). However, both in vitro and in vivo studies revealed striking abnormalities in BMCMC of W/W^v origin. W/W^v BMCMC did not survive as long as populations of BMCMC of congenic +/+ origin when maintained in IL-3-containing media in vitro (Yung and Moore, 1982). And after adoptive transfer into the peritoneal cavity of W/W^v mice, W/W^v BMCMC virtually disappeared within 3 weeks of injection whereas +/+ BMCMC not only survived indefinitely, but also matured and acquired multiple phenotypic characteristics of normal peritoneal mast cells (Nakano et al., 1985). After subcutaneous or i.v. injection, BMCMC of $WBB6F_1$+/+ origin also survived and matured in the skin and other tissues of W/W^v mice (Nakano et al., 1985). By contrast, $WCB6F_1$-+/+ BMCMC failed to survive after injection into the skin of $WCB6F_1$-Sl/Sl^d animals (Gordon and Galli, 1990a).

The impaired ability of W/W^v BMCMC to survive in vitro or in vivo probably reflected abnormalities in the production and/or function of the *W* product in these cells. By contrast, the inability of normal BMCMC to survive in the tissues of Sl/Sl^d mice probably reflected abnormalities in the production and/or function of the *Sl* product in the dermal microenvironment of these mutants. To examine in detail the mechanisms by which abnormalities in *W* or *Sl* products influence mast cell development, Fujita and Kitamura and their associates (reviewed in Kitamura et al., 1989; Fujita et al., 1989) studied the interactions between BMCMC and 3T3 fibroblasts that had been generated from mutant mice of W/W^v or Sl/Sl^d genotype or from the congenic normal mice. This approach was based on observations of Ginsburg and his associates (reviewed in Ginsburg, 1963; Bland et al., 1982; Ginsburg et al., 1982; Davidson et al., 1986) indicating that feeder layers of mouse embryonic skin fibroblasts promoted the in vitro development and maturation of mouse mast cell populations, and the findings of Levi-Schaffer et al. (1986) demonstrating that coculture with 3T3 fibroblasts promoted the acquisition by BMCMC of multiple phenotypic characteristics of mature mast cells.

Fujita et al. (1988a,b) showed that when growth-arrested $WBB6F_1$-+/+ BMCMC were placed on monolayers of normal 3T3 cells (NIH/3T3 cells or 3T3 cells derived from $WBB6F_1$-+/+ or $WCB6F_1$-+/+ mice) in the absence of exogenous IL-3, the BMCMC were induced to make the transition from the G_1 to the S phase of the cell cycle and to proliferate and survive. By contrast, growth-arrested W/W^v BMCMC failed to transit G_1 and died when cocultured with normal 3T3 cells. $WCB6F_1$-+/+ or Sl/Sl^d BMCMC made the G_1 to S transition, proliferated, and survived on NIH/3T3 cells or $WCB6F_1$-+/+ 3T3 cells, but failed to do so on 3T3 cells derived from Sl/Sl^d embryos (Kitamura et al., 1989; Fujita et al., 1989). Finally, when membranes coated with 3T3 cells of $WCB6F_1$-+/+ origin were introduced into the peritoneal cavities of $WCB6F_1$-Sl/Sl^d mice, mast cells developed in association with the transplanted fibroblasts (Kitamura et al., 1989; Fujita et al., 1989).

The initial studies of Fujita and Kitamura (Kitamura et al., 1989; Fujita et al., 1989) indicated that contact between 3T3 cells and BMCMC was required for transmission of the critical signal between these cell types. However, Jarboe and Huff (1989) demonstrated that the proliferation of "mast cell–committed progenitors" (MCCP), and their maturation into cells with histochemical features of connective tissue–type mast cells (CTMC), was promoted by a soluble factor that was produced by embryonic fibroblasts derived from normal or W/W^v mice but not by fibroblasts of Sl/Sl^d mouse origin. Jarboe et al. (1989) provided evidence that the soluble factor did not represent any of a large panel of known cytokines and suggested that this factor might represent the *Sl* product and a ligand for the c-*kit* receptor. It is important to note that the MCCP that develop in the mesenteric lymph nodes of mice infected with the nematode *Nippostrongylus brasiliensis* lack cytoplasmic granules discernible by light microscopy and therefore probably represent an earlier stage of mast cell development than BMCMC. Another difference between BMCMC and MCCP is that BMCMC can be derived from W/W^v bone marrow cells cultured in the presence of IL-3, whereas the mesenteric lymph node cells of W/W^v mice infected with *N. brasiliensis* virtually lack MCCP. By contrast, Sl/Sl^d mice can generate apparently normal numbers of MCCP.

One explanation for the differences in the findings of Huff et al. (Jarboe and Huff, 1989; Jarboe et al., 1989) and Fujita and Kitamura et al. (Kitamura et al., 1989; Fujita et al., 1989) might be that MCCP can respond to a soluble fibroblast-derived factor whereas BMCMC cannot. Another explanation, which is in accord with the results of recent efforts to characterize fibroblast-derived factors with effects on mast cell development in mouse (Kitamura, personal communication) and human (Furitsu et al., 1989) systems, is that different fibroblast populations vary in their ability to produce soluble as opposed to cell-associated forms of the critical factor. Recently, Kitamura and his associates discovered a rat with a mutation in the c-*kit* tyrosine kinase domain (Kitamura, personal communication). Rats bearing two copies of the mutant *W* allele are profoundly mast cell–deficient, indicating that this animal may be useful for certain studies of mast cells or the c-*kit* receptor that may be difficult to perform in mice.

IV. Recognition that the *W* Locus Encodes c-*kit*

A. Identification of Allelism Between *W* and c-*kit*

Since the lineages affected by mutations at *W*, i.e., hematopoietic cells, melanocytes, and germ cells, are derived from all three embryonic germ layers, it was not initially clear how a mutation at a single locus might result in the pleiotropic effects observed in *W* mutant mice. One possibility was that *W* encoded a molecule whose expression is important to the development of each of the affected lineages during a critical stage of development. However, some *W* mutations result in severe defects in only one or two of the lineages that can be affected by mutations at this locus, demonstrating that some of the effects caused by *W* mutations can occur independently of one another. This observation raised the possibility that mutations at *W* influenced one or more of a group of closely linked genes, each of them affecting one of the lineages (Russell, 1979; Geissler et al., 1981).

The complexity of the developmental programs affected by *W* mutations, and the difficulty anticipated in obtaining large numbers of the affected cell types, suggested that a reverse genetics approach might be useful for identifying the gene product. Initially, several cloned DNA markers on mouse chromosome 5 were mapped to the *W* region to identify those which might be useful in a cloning strategy based on chromosome walking (Geissler et al., 1988a). One of the markers mapped in the *W* region was the c-*kit* protooncogene. The genetic proximity of c-*kit* and *W* was intriguing, since the presumed functional characteristics of c-*kit* were consistent with those predicted for the *W* gene product (Russell, 1979; Geissler et al., 1981).

The *kit* gene was first characterized as the viral oncogene (v-*kit*) of a feline sarcoma virus (HZ4-FeSV) (Besmer et al., 1986). cDNA cloning of the corresponding cellular sequences from both mouse and human tissues confirmed that v-*kit* arose by transduction and truncation of a cellular gene—the protooncogene c-*kit* (Yarden et al., 1987; Qiu et al., 1988). The murine c-*kit* gene was cloned from a mouse brain cDNA library (Qiu et al., 1988). The largest cDNA isolated encoded 5.1 of the full-length 5.5 kilobase pairs (kb) mRNA detected in the brain by Northern analysis. Nucleotide sequence analysis identified a 3-kb open reading frame extending from nucleotide 29 to 2954, followed by roughly 2 kb of untranslated sequence at the 3' end. The predicted amino acid sequence of c-*kit* displays extensive homology with the tyrosine protein kinase receptor superfamily, particularly with the transmembrane receptors for colony-stimulating factor-1 (CSF-1R or c-*fms*) and platelet-derived growth factor (PDGFR) (Yarden et al., 1987; Qiu et al., 1988). The 500-amino-acid (aa) extracellular domain of c-*kit* has homology with members of the immunoglobulin superfamily (Yarden et al., 1987). A 24-aa hydrophobic, putative transmembrane domain (residues 519–543) is followed by a 450-aa intracellular segment that contains the putative kinase region (residues 575–915). The kinase domain contains a possible ATP-binding site (residue 622), a putative autophosphorylation site (residue 821), and a poorly conserved, noncatalytic, hydrophilic stretch of 77 amino acids, the kinase insert domain, that divides the kinase domain in half (Yarden et al., 1987; Yarden and Ullrich, 1988).

The homology to CSF-1R suggested that the c-*kit* receptor might play a role in hematopoiesis, perhaps by promoting cell proliferation when stimulated by the c-*kit* ligand, which had not yet been identified. Presumably, as with other members of this receptor tyrosine kinase family, binding of the c-*kit* ligand to the external domain of the c-*kit* receptor would initiate a series of changes, including receptor dimerization and activation of the tyrosine kinase of the cytoplasmic domain. The activated kinase would then transmit a signal via phosphorylation of a critical substrate(s) associated with the plasma membrane, culminating in the endocytosis and degradation of the receptor.

In 1988, Chabot et al. reported data demonstrating that *W* and c-*kit* are closely linked on mouse chromosome 5. Geissler et al. (1988b) provided the first direct demonstration that *W* mutations influence the structure and expression of the gene encoding the c-*kit* receptor. These data included the finding that two spontaneous, phenotypically different *W* mutations were associated with distinct rearrangements of the c-*kit* locus. For one mutation, W^{44}, the site of the genetic rearrangement was shown to be confined to the c-*kit* structural gene, reducing the amount of c-*kit* message but apparently not altering its size. W^{44} most likely represents an insertion within an intervening sequence in the 5' end of the gene (Geissler et al., 1988b). Regardless of the precise mechanism that accounts for the altered expression of c-*kit* in the tissues of the W^{44}/W^{44} mouse, these results established that a genetic rearrangement confined to the c-*kit* structural gene is sufficient to produce a mutant *W* phenotype and, therefore, strongly supported the hypothesis that the c-*kit* protooncogene is allelic with the dominant-spotting *(W)* locus. Subsequently, additional spontaneous *W* mutations were shown to be associated with alterations in the c-*kit* structural gene, including several that comprise single base pair mutations in the region encoding the kinase domain (Bernstein et al., 1989; Nocka et al., 1990b; Reith et al., 1990; Tan et al., 1990).

The demonstration of allelism between *W* and c-*kit* represented a significant advance in efforts to understand the mechanism of *W* gene action. Moreover, mutations at *W* represented the first examples of germline mutations in a mammalian protooncogene. As a result, analysis of *W* gene action will also help to clarify the role of this protooncogene in normal mammalian development.

B. Expression of c-*kit* in Tissues of Normal and *W* Mutant Mice

Using an antibody prepared against the v-*kit* protein, a 145-kDa protein with autophosphorylating capacity was immunoprecipitated from the human A172 glioblastoma cell line (Yarden et al., 1987). Immunoprecipitations from cell types influenced by *W* mutations (e.g., mast cells and melanocytes) revealed the presence of several different isoforms, which are derived via posttranslational modifications of a single primary translation product (Nocka et al., 1989). At this time, there is no firm evidence for the existence of alternative splicing for the c-*kit* mRNA.

In the hematopoietic system, c-*kit* mRNA expression appears to be confined to those lineages which are influenced by *W* mutations (Andre et al., 1989; Nocka et al., 1989). c-*kit* is expressed in mast cells, and in early erythroid and myeloid cell lines, but not in myelomonocytic cell lines, in macrophage cell lines, or in T-cell–related cell lines (Andre et al., 1989; Nocka et al., 1989). On the other hand, autoradiographic studies with ^{125}I-labeled c-*kit* ligand indicate that the c-*kit* receptor is widely distributed among the bone marrow cells of adult mice, particularly on blasts, promyelocytes/myelocytes, promonocytes, monocytes, eosinophilic myelocytes, eosinophils, and some lymphocytes (Metcalf and Nicola, 1991). However, the number of receptors per cell varies extensively according to cell type, with blasts and some lymphocytes exhibiting the highest levels of labeling (Metcalf and Nicola, 1991). Evidence derived from studies of human basophils indicates that basophils lack detectable expression of the c-*kit* receptor (Valent et al., 1989; Lerner et al., 1991). Recently, Ogawa et al. (1991) provided evidence that depletion of adult mouse bone marrow of cells that express c-*kit* protein resulted in virtual elimination of hematopoietic progenitor cells responsive to IL-3, GM-CSF, or M-CSF, and also virtually eliminated CFU-S. c-*kit* mRNA is expressed in the embryonic and adult central nervous system of the rat, mouse, and cat (Yarden et al., 1987; Geissler et al., 1988b; Qiu et al., 1988). The significance of this intriguing finding is not yet clear, nor have gross abnormalities of central nervous system (CNS) structure of function been reported in *W* mutant mice.

Normal fetal liver cells express c-*kit* mRNA and protein, but the fetal livers of *W/W* embryos do not (Nocka et al., 1989). However, since brain and placental tissues of *W/W* embryos express detectable c-*kit* message, which is altered in size, the absence of c-*kit* mRNA in the *W/W* liver probably reflects the presence of reduced numbers of erythroid progenitors at this site (Nocka et al., 1989). The tissues of W/W^v mice express normal levels of c-*kit* mRNA, which is normal in size (Nocka et al., 1989). We and others have shown the BMCMCs from W/W^v mice also have undiminished levels of c-*kit* message and protein (Geissler et al., 1990; Nocka et al., 1989). Nevertheless, the c-*kit* protein expressed in W/W^v tissues retains little, if any, kinase activity owing to the effects of the *W* and W^v mutations on the structure of the gene product. Specifically, the W^v mutation results in an amino acid substitution in the kinase domain, which dramatically reduces the kinase activity, while *W* comprises a deletion of the transmembrane region of c-*kit*, which interferes with cell surface expression of the receptor (Nocka et al., 1990b).

C. The *Ws/Ws* Mast Cell–Deficient Rat

Recently, Kitamura and his associates have identified and characterized rats with mutations at the "white spotting" *(Ws)* locus (Niwa et al., 1991; Tsujimura et al., 1991). The *Ws* mutation is a deletion of 12 bases near the tyrosine kinase autophosphorylation site in the c-*kit* kinase (Tsujimura et al., 1991). Although newborn *Ws/Ws* rats are severely anemic, adult *Ws/Ws* rats exhibit a mild anemia but a profound mast cell deficiency (Niwa et al., 1991). Moreover, both male and female *Ws/Ws* rats are fertile. These features, the size of rats compared to mice, and the large number of studies that have already been performed with rat mast cells indicate that *Ws/Ws* rats may be extremely valuable resources for studies of mast cell development and function.

V. Recognition that *Sl* Encodes a Ligand for c-*kit*

A. Identification of Allelism Between *Sl* and the Gene for SCF, a c-*kit* Ligand

Identification of the c-*kit* receptor as the *W* gene product provided the conceptual framework and identified the biochemical and genetic reagents that assisted in the identification of the c-*kit* ligand. Consequently, three groups simultaneously reported the cloning and characterization of a novel growth factor that represented the product of the *Sl* locus and a ligand for the c-*kit* receptor (Williams et al., 1990; Copeland et al., 1990; Zsebo et al., 1990a,b; Martin et al., 1990; Huang et al., 1990; Anderson et al., 1990). Several names have been proposed for this c-*kit* ligand, including stem cell factor (SCF) (Zsebo et al., 1990b), kit ligand (KL) (Nocka et al., 1990a), mast cell growth factor (MGF) (Williams et al., 1990), and Steel factor (Witte, 1990). In this chapter, we will in most cases refer to this factor by the designations c-*kit* ligand or SCF.

Zsebo et al. (1990b) identified SCF as a growth factor for early hematopoietic progenitors based on its ability to promote colony formation in vitro by bone marrow cells derived from mice treated with 5-fluorouracil, characterized the aa sequence of the soluble SCF produced by Buffalo rat liver cells, showed that the factor had potent synergistic activities with other hematopoietic growth factors in semisolid cultures of mouse bone marrow cells, and demonstrated that SCF promoted the proliferation of Cl.MC/9, a cloned, IL-3-dependent immature mouse mast cell (Nabel et al., 1981). Martin et al. (1990) isolated and sequenced partial cDNA and genomic clones of rat SCF and partial and full-length cDNA and genomic clones of human SCF and demonstrated that truncated forms of the recombinant human protein could augment the in vitro proliferation of myeloid and lymphoid progenitors and could exhibit striking synergistic activities with several colony-stimulating factors, including EPO, IL-3, GM-CSF, and G-CSF.

Zsebo et al. (1990a) mapped the SCF gene to the Steel *(Sl)* locus on mouse chromosome 10 and showed that three mutations at the *Sl* locus, i.e., Sl^{12H}, *Sl*, and Sl^{d}, comprise deletions of some or all of the SCF coding sequences. Using stromal cell lines derived from homozygous lethal *Sl*/*Sl* embryos, Zsebo et al. (1990a) showed that the *Sl* mutation represents a deletion of all SCF coding sequences. Northern analyses of RNA from a stromal cell line derived from a Sl/Sl^{d} embryo and RNA isolated from the spleens of viable Sl/Sl^{d} mice showed that the Sl^{d} allele encodes an abundant, smaller-than-normal SCF transcript (Zsebo et al., 1990a). We also showed that the Sl^{d} mutation was associated with a novel SCF DNA restriction fragment length polymorphism. This finding suggested that the aberrant SCF transcript arose as a direct consequence of the Sl^{d} mutation, providing strong evidence that SCF is encoded at the *Sl* locus of the mouse (Zsebo et al., 1990a).

To demonstrate that SCF represented a ligand for c-*kit*, the cDNA for the entire murine c-*kit* (Qiu et al., 1988) was amplified from the SCF-responsive mast cell line Cl.MC/9 (Nabel et al., 1981) using PCR with primers designed from the published sequence. The ligand binding and transmembrane domains of human c-*kit*, encoded by amino acids 1–549 (Yarden et al., 1987), were cloned, the c-*kit* cDNAs were inserted into a mammalian expression vector, V19.8, and then transfected into COS-1 cells, and membrane fractions were prepared for binding assays using either rat or human ^{125}I-labeled SCF^{164}. There was no detectable specific binding of ^{125}I-SCF^{164} to membranes of COS-1 cells transfected with V19.8, alone. However, membranes of COS-1 cells expressing human recombinant c-*kit* ligand binding plus transmembrane domains did exhibit specific binding of ^{125}I-labeled hSCF^{164}. Similarly, membranes of COS-1 cells transfected with the full-length murine c-*kit* specifically bound rat ^{125}I-labeled SCF^{164}. Rat ^{125}I-labeled SCF^{164} bound similarly to both human and murine c-*kit*, while human ^{125}I-labeled SCF^{164} bound with lower avidity to murine c-*kit* than to human c-*kit*. These data are consistent with the pattern of SCF^{164} cross-reactivity between species, in that rat SCF^{164} induces proliferation of human bone marrow with a specific activity similar to that of human SCF^{164}, while human SCF^{164} induces proliferation of murine mast cells with a specific activity 800-fold less than that of the rat protein (Martin et al., 1990).

B. Demonstration that Recombinant Rat SCF Can Repair the Macrocytic Anemia and Mast Cell Deficiency of *Sl/Sl^d* Mice

The functional effects of recombinant forms of the c-*kit* ligand that were observed in vitro were consistent with the activities that might be predicted for a c-*kit* ligand. However, it was important to determine whether administration of recombinant c-*kit* ligand in vivo could influence the hematopoietic abnormalities expressed by *Sl* mutant mice. Zsebo et al. (1990a) demonstrated that treatment of *Sl/Sl^d* mice with pharmacological doses of recombinant rat SCF^{164} (rrSCF^{164}) resulted in a marked reduction of the severity of their macrocytic anemia. Moreover, the degree and the rate of resolution of the anemia were directly related to the dose of rrSCF^{164} administered. When rrSCF^{164} treatment was discontinued, the macrocytic anemia reappeared. In addition to increases in red cell numbers, rrSCF^{164}-treated *Sl/Sl^d* animals exhibited increases in multiple lineages of peripheral blood cells, with both leukocytosis and thrombocytosis. While the leukocytosis was primarily a result of increased neutrophils, lymphocytes and monocytes were also elevated.

We also showed that daily subcutaneous injection of rrSCF^{164} at 30 μg/kg for 3 weeks significantly increased the hematocrits of *Sl/Sl^d* mice and resulted in the appearance of large numbers of mast cells at the injection sites (Zsebo et al., 1990a). By contrast, treatment with vehicle alone did not significantly affect the hematocrit or the development of mast cells. The numbers of mast cells at sites of rrSCF^{164} injection in *Sl/Sl^d* mice actually exceeded the normal number of mast cells in the back skin of the congenic normal (+/+) mice (77.9 $\pm$ 16.9 versus 33.3 $\pm$ 3.6 per mm^2 of dermis; Galli et al., 1987a). The demonstration that administration of the recombinant c-*kit* ligand rrSCF^{164} repaired both the macrocytic anemia and the mast cell deficiency of *Sl/Sl^d* mice provided compelling evidence that the expression of these phenotypic abnormalities by *Sl/Sl^d* mice directly reflected the effects of these mutations on the c-*kit* ligand.

C. Structure and Tissue-Specific Expression of Alternative c-*kit* Ligands

The sequence of partial and full-length rat (Martin et al., 1990), mouse (Anderson et al., 1990; Huang et al., 1990; Zsebo et al., 1990a), and human (Martin et al., 1990) SCF cDNAs predicts a translation product that is a transmembrane protein comprising a 25-aa cleaved-signal peptide, a 189-aa extracellular ligand domain that includes a proteolytic cleavage site, a hydrophobic 21–23-aa membrane-spanning region, and a short (36–37 aa) intracellular domain. Northern analyses have shown that mouse 3T3 cells (Huang et al., 1990) and bone marrow–derived stromal cell lines (Anderson et al., 1990) express an abundant 6-kb SCF transcript as well as two smaller alternative transcripts, which are about 5 and 3 kb in size. While the significance of this finding is not yet clear, two forms of the SCF protein have been identified: a soluble factor comprising the first 164 or 165 aa of the extracellular domain and a transmembrane form comprising the full-length translation product (Zsebo et al., 1990b; Martin et al., 1990; Huang et al., 1990; Anderson et al., 1990; Flanagan et al., 1991).

Recently Flanagan et al. (1991) cloned and characterized two alternative SCF transcripts from the spleens of WCB6F$_1$ +/+ mice. The nucleotide sequence of one clone was identical to that of a previously reported mouse SCF cDNA (Anderson et al., 1990; Huang et al., 1990; Zsebo et al., 1990a). The second clone represented a novel splice variant that lacked an exon that encodes 27 amino acids in the juxtamembrane region of the extracellular domain. RNAse-protection studies indicated that the expression of these alternative SCF transcripts is regulated in a tissue-specific manner (Flanagan et al., 1991). Specifically, 3T3 cells and mouse brain and bone marrow tissues express both variants at about a 5 to 1 ratio, while in the spleen the alternative transcripts are present in nearly equimolar amounts. Furthermore, transfection of the longer cDNA clone into COS cells resulted in the appearance of equal amounts of both membrane-associated and soluble SCF proteins, 38 and 25 kDa, respectively. On the other hand, cells transfected with the shorter cDNA variant primarily expressed a 28-kDa cell-associated SCF and produced only trace amounts of a soluble 20-kDa protein (Flanagan et al., 1991). It is likely that the soluble form of SCF is derived from the larger cell-associated precursor by proteolysis in a fashion analogous to the processing of the secreted forms of CSF-1 and TGF-α from their membrane-associated precursors (Anderson et al., 1990; Huang et al., 1990; Martin et al., 1990; Zsebo et al., 1990a). The probable site of proteolytic cleavage in SCF is encoded by the exon that is missing from the shorter of the two SCF cDNAs described by Flanagan et al. (1991), a finding that probably explains the very low level of soluble SCF secreted by COS cells transfected with this cDNA variant.

Regardless of the mechanisms involved, these studies strongly suggest that tissue-specific regulation of alternative mRNA splicing could result in the differential expression of soluble as opposed to cell-associated forms of the SCF protein during development and cell differentiation. And such differential expression of forms of the SCF protein may importantly influence the expression of SCF-dependent effects in various tissues. In situ hybridization studies of developing mouse embryos identified expression of SCF mRNA not only in those tissues within which lineages affected by *Sl* mutations develop and/or migrate, but also within the central nervous system (Matsui et al., 1990). Taken together with work demonstrating c-*kit* mRNA in the developing mouse CNS (Orr-Urtegger et al., 1990), this finding suggests that c-*kit* and its ligand may have important effects in the development and/or function of the CNS and perhaps other organs and tissues not classically thought to be influenced by these products.

We have already noted that the predicted aa sequences of the receptors for SCF (c-*kit*) and CSF-1 (c-*fms*) revealed a strong structural homology that suggests an evolutionary relationship between the genes encoding these receptors (Yarden et al., 1987; Yarden and Ullrich, 1988). On the other hand, homologies between the ligands for these receptors were not readily apparent. Recently, however, Bazan (1991) reported that an evolutionary relationship between SCF and CSF-1 can be appreciated if one aligns their amino acid sequences by registering equivalent exons and regions with similar secondary structures. This comparison revealed a 16% identity of amino acids in the extracellular domains of these cytokines and identified similarities in the globular structure of the tertiary folds in their cytokine domains. Based on such findings, Bazan speculated that the interaction of SCF with the c-*kit* receptor may resemble the interactions of helical cytokines with the hematopoietic receptor superfamily.

VI. Activities of SCF in Mast Cell Development and Function

A. SCF Induces c-*kit*-Dependent Mouse Mast Cell Proliferation and Maturation In Vivo

Both direct and indirect lines of evidence indicate that either the soluble or the cell-associated forms of SCF can influence mast cell development and function. We already have noted that both W/W^v and Sl/Sl^d mice are profoundly deficient in mature mast cells in all organs and tissues, including those sites with predominant populations of connective tissue–type mast cells (CTMC) and those with large numbers of phenotypically distinct mucosal mast cells (MMC). Previous work indicated that IL-3 represented an important proliferative factor for mouse MMC in vivo (Abe and Nawa, 1988; Abe et al., 1988) and for immature mast cells (BMCMC) derived from the bone marrow cells of either normal (Ihle et al., 1983) or W/W^v mice (Yung and Moore, 1982; Suda et al., 1985; Nakano et al., 1985). Williams et al. (1990), Martin et al., (1990), Anderson et al. (1990), and

Zsebo et al. (1990b) showed that recombinant forms of the c-*kit* ligand induced proliferation of IL-3-dependent immature mouse mast cells in vitro, and Nocka et al. (1990a) showed that a natural form of the putative c-*kit* ligand purified from 3T3 cell-conditioned medium stimulated the proliferation of mouse peritoneal mast cells in vitro. Taken together, these findings indicated that, when administered in vitro, the c-*kit* ligand represented a proliferation factor for both immature mast cells and mature mast cells of the CTMC phenotype.

The study of Zsebo et al. (1990a) indicated that the subcutaneous injection of $rrSCF^{164}$, which encodes the processed soluble c-*kit* ligand secreted by Buffalo rat liver cells, permitted the development of mast cells in the dermis of Sl/Sl^d mice. Since the dermis of Sl/Sl^d mice ordinarily contains virtually no mast cells, the latter finding indicated that $rrSCF^{164}$ administered in vivo can induce the recruitment, proliferation, and/or maturation of mast cells in the skin. The dermis of the mouse normally contains predominantly mast cells of the CTMC phenotype (reviewed in Galli, 1990). However, the phenotype of the mast cells that appeared in the dermis of Sl/Sl^d mice injected with $rrSCF^{164}$ in the study of Zsebo et al. (1990a) was not reported. Nor was it determined whether SCF could influence mast cell development in normal mice.

We therefore examined the effects of $rrSCF^{164}$ on mast cell populations in normal mice and rats in vivo, using approaches that permitted the anatomical and phenotypic characterization of the responding cells as CTMC or MMC (Tsai et al., 1991a). As shown in Table 2, we found that daily subcutaneous injection of $rrSCF^{164}$ for 3 weeks induced a striking expansion of dermal mast cell populations in normal $WBB6F_1$-+/+ or $WCB6F_1$-+/+ mice, and in genetically mast cell–deficient $WCB6F_1$-Sl/Sl^d mice. In $WBB6F_1$-+/+ mice, mast cell numbers at sites injected with 100 or 30 μg of $rrSCF^{164}$/kg were 166× or 15× that in control sites injected with vehicle alone. In striking contrast to its effects on populations of dermal mast cells, $rrSCF^{164}$ had little or no effect on the hematocrit of normal mice of either genotype tested (Table 2).

The majority of the mast cells at $rrSCF^{164}$ injection sites, like dermal CTMC in the skin of untreated normal mice (Nakano et al., 1985; Galli et al., 1987a), exhibited cytoplasmic reactivity with the heparin-binding fluorescent dye berberine sulfate (Enërback, 1974), and many of them stained with safranin. Thus, injection of $rrSCF^{164}$ as the sole exogenous cytokine resulted in the development of dermal mast cells with characteristics of CTMC. Colocalization of immunohistochemical staining for bromodeoxyuridine (BrdU) incorporated into nuclear DNA and mast cell cytoplasmic granule staining with alcian blue (Arizono et al., 1990) indicated that morphologically identifiable mast cells were proliferating at sites of $rrSCF^{164}$ injection (Table 2). This finding indicated that the increased numbers of mast cells at sites of $rrSCF^{164}$ injection reflected at least in part the proliferation of differentiated dermal mast cells, not merely the recruitment, proliferation and/or maturation of mast cell precursors.

However, the skin of Sl/Sl^d mice ordinarily contains virtually no dermal

Table 2 c-*kit*-Dependent Stimulation of Proliferation of Mouse Dermal Mast Cells In Vivo by rrSCF^{164} [a]

Mouse genotype	rrSCF^{164} (μg/kg/day)	Hct (%) Before treatment	Hct (%) After treatment	Mast cells (no./mm^2 of dermis)	BrdU+ (% of mast cells)
WBB6F$_1$-+/+	100	48 ± 1.3	50 ± 0.7	4710 ± 1190[b]	16 ± 2.2[b]
WBB6F$_1$-+/+	30	50 ± 0.8	51 ± 0.3	454 ± 155[b]	13 ± 2.7[b]
WBB6F$_1$-+/+	0	51 ± 0.6	51 ± 0.5	31 ± 2	3.3 ± 1.2
WBB6F$_1$-*W/W^v*	100	39 ± 0.8	36 ± 3.4	0	—
WBB6F$_1$-*W/W^v*	30	40 ± 0.7	40 ± 2.5	0	—
WBB6F$_1$-*W/W^v*	0	40 ± 0.6	39 ± 0.2	0	—
WCB6F$_1$-+/+	30	46 ± 0.8	44 ± 2.7	122 ± 17[b]	36 ± 3.5[b]
WCB6F$_1$-+/+	0	47 ± 0.3	44 ± 0.4	29 ± 5	4.9 ± 0.7
WCB6F$_1$-*Sl/Sl^d*	30	30 ± 1.1	38 ± 1.7[b]	61 ± 24[b]	29 ± 5.7
WCB6F$_1$-*Sl/Sl^d*	0	30 ± 0.3	33 ± 0.6	0	—

[a]Mice were killed 24 hr after the last of 21 daily s.c. injections of rrSCF^{164} or vehicle for assessment of the number of mast cells/mm^2 of dermis at the injection site for quantification of the % of these mast cells which were proliferating, based on nuclear incorporation of bromeodeoyxuridine (BrdU). All results are expressed as mean ± SEM (n = 5–7).

[b]$p < 0.001$ versus value for mice treated with 0 μg/kg/day by Student's t-test (two-tailed).

Source: From Tsai et al., 1991a.

mast cells (Table 2 and Kitamura and Go, 1979). *Sl/Sl*^{d} mouse skin also ordinarily is virtually devoid of mast cell precursors (Hayashi et al., 1985). Thus, even though many differentiated mast cells were proliferating at rrSCF^{164} injection sites in *Sl/Sl*^{d} mice 3 weeks after initiation of treatment (Table 2), some of the effect of rrSCF^{164} in these mice must have reflected actions on the recruitment, survival, and/or induction of maturation of the mast cell precursors present in these animals (Kitamura and Go, 1979). An effect of rrSCF^{164} on mast cell maturation is also supported by the finding that many of the mast cells at rrSCF^{164} injection sites in *Sl/Sl*^{d} mice stained with berberine sulfate or safranin.

In contrast to the effects of rrSCF^{164} in *Sl/Sl*^{d} mice, injection of rrSCF^{164} into genetically mast cell–deficient WBB6F$_1$-*W/W*^{v} mice influenced neither the profound mast cell deficiency nor the anemia of these animals (Table 2). This result, together with work indicating that the *W* and *W*^{v} alleles encode c-*kit* products that express no *(W)* or markedly diminished *(W*^{v}*)* tyrosine kinase activity (Nocka et al., 1990b), indicates that the ability of rrSCF^{164} to induce the development of dermal CTMC in vivo requires that the rrSCF^{164} interacts with a functionally active c-*kit* receptor. The complete failure of even very high doses of rrSCF^{164} to induce cutaneous mast cell development in *W/W*^{v} mice is also noteworthy in light of reports that this mutant can develop mature dermal mast cells in association with a chronic idiopathic dermatitis (Galli et al., 1987a), in response to repeated epicutaneous applications of PMA (Gordon and Galli, 1990b), or as a result of treatment with IL-3 (Ody et al., 1990). The results of Tsai et al. (1991a) indicate that the appearance of mast cells in the skin of *W/W*^{v} mice in these settings probably does not reflect increased local production of endogenous c-*kit* ligand, but instead may be due to other effects such as the activation of either alternative signaling mechanisms or processes distal to the interaction between c-*kit* and its ligand.

B. In the Rat, SCF Induces the Development In Vivo of Mast Cells with Phenotypic Characteristics of CTMC or MMC

Even though s.c. administration of rrSCF^{164} increased the Hct of *Sl/Sl*^{d} mice (Table 2), indicating a response of SCF-sensitive cells at a location distal from the SCF injection site, the effects of rrSCF^{164} on mast cell populations were most striking in the vicinity of the s.c. injection sites. For example, no mast cells appeared in the skin contralateral to rrSCF^{164} injection sites in *Sl/Sl*^{d} mice or in the gastric tissues of these animals. To assess the systemic effects of rrSCF^{164} on mast cell development and phenotype, we turned to the rat. Huntley et al. (1990) reported highly sensitive and specific ELISA methods for quantifying tissue content of mast cell–specific proteases associated with CTMC and MMC (RMCP I and RMCP II, respectively) in this species. In collaboration with George F. J. Newlands and Hugh R. P. Miller, we quantified levels of RMCP I and RMCP II in the tissues of rrSCF^{164}-treated and control rats, in addition to determining mast cell numbers in these tissues (Tsai et al., 1991a).

We found that daily intravenous administration of rrSCF^{164} to rats at a dose of 25 μg/kg/day for 14 days increased mast cell numbers systemically and also produced striking increases in levels of both types of rat mast cell–associated proteases (Table 3). In the skin, lung, and liver, rrSCF^{164} treatment resulted in marked increases in numbers of mast cells and in tissue content of the CTMC-associated protease, RMCP I, but no significant changes in levels of the MMC-associated protease, RMCP II. In the spleen, rrSCF^{164} treatment resulted in striking expansion of mast cell populations, as well as marked increases in levels of both RMCP I and RMCP II. However, the total amount of RMCP II in the spleens of rrSCF^{164}-treated animals was much less than the corresponding amounts of RMCP I. Similar results were obtained when the bone marrow and peritoneal cells of rrSCF^{164}-treated or control rats were examined (Tsai et al., 1991a). rrSCF^{164} treatment significantly expanded populations of mast cells in the mucosa, submucosa, and muscularis propria of the glandular stomach, and in the mucosa and submucosa of the ileum (Table 3). MMC predominate in the mucosa of these organs, whereas CTMC predominate in the submucosa and muscularis propria (Enërback, 1986; Miller et al., 1989; Huntley et al., 1990). rrSCF^{164} treatment increased the content of both RMCP II (p = 0.018 by the two-tailed Student's t-test) and RMCP I (p = 0.045 by the one-tailed Student's t-test) in the glandular stomach and also significantly increased the content of both proteases in the ileum (Table 3). Moreover, when the protease content of the mast cells present in the skin or ileal mucosa of rrSCF^{164}-treated rats was examined by immunohistochemistry, the pattern of staining was similar to that observed in the control rats (Tsai et al., 1991a). Thus, according to the anatomical distribution and the protease phenotype of the expanded populations of mast cells that appeared in rrSCF^{164}-treated rats, i.v. administration of rrSCF^{164} to rats markedly expanded populations of CTMC and also significantly increased levels of gastrointestinal MMC.

The findings of Tsai et al. (1991a), taken together with the observation that W/W^v and Sl/Sl^d mice virtually lack both CTMC and MMC (Crowle and Reed, 1984; Nakano et al., 1985; Kitamura et al., 1989), indicate that interactions between c-*kit* and its ligand importantly influence the normal development of both CTMC and MMC. On the other hand, the effect of i.v. treatment with rrSCF^{164} on CTMC populations in the rat appeared to be greater than the effect on MMC populations. Whether this finding reflected differences in the bioavailability of rrSCF^{164} in various anatomical locations after i.v. administration, or other factors, was not determined.

In addition to demonstrating that SCF can induce mast cell hyperplasia in adult rats, the study of Tsai et al. (1991a) also raises the possibility that the mast cell proliferation associated with certain immunological or pathological re-

Table 3 Systemic Effects of rrSCF^{164} on Mast Cell Populations and Tissue Mast Cell Protease Content in the Rat[a]

Tissue	rrSCF^{164} (μg/kg/day)	Mast cells (no./mm^2 of tissue)	RMCP I (μg/g of tissue)	RMCP II (μg/g of tissue)
Skin	25	87 ± 7***	69 ± 7***	ND[b]
	0	26 ± 3	27 ± 3	ND
Lung	25	48 ± 6***	13 ± 1.2***	10 ± 1.6
	0	7 ± 0.4	3.8 ± 0.8	11 ± 1.2
Liver	25	62 ± 10***	35 ± 8**	1.2 ± 0.3
	0	3.6 ± 0.4	0.4 ± 0.06	0.8 ± 0.1
Spleen	25	204 ± 40***	92 ± 24**	14.2 ± 5.0*
	0	0.07 ± 0.02***	0.7 ± 0.08	0.10 ± 0.004
Glandular Stomach				
Mucosa	25	50 ± 9**		
Submucosa	25	144 ± 36*	5.9 ± 1.2	19 ± 1.3*
Muscularis propria	25	32 ± 5**		
Mucosa	0	12 ± 3		
Submucosa	0	45 ± 8	3.3 ± 0.4	13 ± 1.7
Muscularis propria	0	12 ± 2		
Ileum				
Mucosa	25	80 ± 14*		
Submucosa	25	146 ± 51*	1.4 ± 0.5*	508 ± 83*
Muscularis propria	25	ND		
Mucosa	0	38 ± 12**		
Submucosa	0	19 ± 4*	0.2 ± 0.1	272 ± 5
Muscularis propria	0	ND		

[a]Rats were killed ~24 hr after the last injection of 14 daily i.v. injections of rrSCF^{164} or vehicle for assessment of mast cell numbers and measurement of content of rat mast cell–associated proteases I and II (RMCP I and RMCP II) in various tissues. All results are expressed as mean ± SEM (n = 5–8).
* ** *** = $p < 0.05$, 0.01, or 0.001 versus value for rats treated with 0 μg/kg/day by Student's t = test (two-tailed).
[b]ND, not detected.
Source: From Tsai et al., 1991a.

sponses may reflect, in part, excessive local or even systemic production of forms of the c-*kit* ligand. Thus, the administration of exogenous SCF not only produced significant expansions of populations of CTMC and MMC in sites ordinarily containing large numbers of mast cells, such as the skin and stomach, but also resulted in the appearance of many mast cells at sites that typically contain very few mast cells, such as the liver, spleen, and bone marrow. Because of the structure of their microvasculature, the liver, spleen, and bone marrow represent examples of anatomical sites that would develop particularly high interstitial concentrations of SCF after intravenous administration of the cytokine. Indeed, the permeability characteristics of the microvasculature of various organs may represent a very important factor governing the patterns of changes in mast cell populations observed in subjects treated systemically with SCF.

C. SCF Induces Mouse Mast Cell Proliferation, Maturation, and Heparin Synthesis In Vitro

Our in vivo studies indicated that administration of $rrSCF^{164}$ as the only exogenous cytokine induced the proliferation and maturation of CTMC in the mouse and greatly expanded populations of CTMC in the rat. To assess in more detail the effects of $rrSCF^{164}$ on mast cell proliferation and maturation, we analyzed mast cell populations exposed to $rrSCF^{164}$ in vitro (Tsai et al., 1991b). We first demonstrated that $rrSCF^{164}$, like a candidate c-*kit* ligand purified from BALB/3T3 fibroblast conditioned medium (Nocka et al., 1990a), can induce proliferation of mature as well as immature, IL-3-dependent mast cells (Fig. 3). $rrSCF^{164}$ induced proliferation of the IL-3-dependent cloned mast cell line PT-18 (Fig. 3a), IL-3-dependent BMCMC from either BALB/c mice (Fig. 3b) or $WBB6F_1$-+/+ mice (Fig. 3c), and purified mouse PMC, which comprise an IL-3-independent population of mature CTMC mast cells (reviewed in Galli, 1990) (Fig. 3d). BMCMC derived from $WBB6F_1$-W/W^v mice exhibited a very weak proliferative response to $rrSCF^{164}$, which was statistically significant (p = 0.014 versus cells maintained without $rrSCF^{164}$ by two-tailed Student's t-test) only at a concentration of $rrSCF^{164}$ of 500 ng/ml (Fig. 3d). This result is consistent with previous work indicating that the W and W^v alleles encode c-*kit* products that express no (W) or markedly diminished (W^v) tyrosine kinase activity (Nocka et al., 1990b) and indicates that the effects of $rrSCF^{164}$ on mast cell proliferation in vitro require the interaction of the cytokine with a functional *c-kit* receptor.

We found that the cells in Figure 3 that responded to the proliferative effects of $rrSCF^{164}$ were morphologically identifiable mast cells rather than less mature precursors. Ninety percent ($WBB6F_1$-+/+ BMCMC, PMC) to 100% (PT-18) of the cells tested were mast cells according to staining with neutral red. And >98% of the cells proliferating in response to $rrSCF^{164}$ were identified as

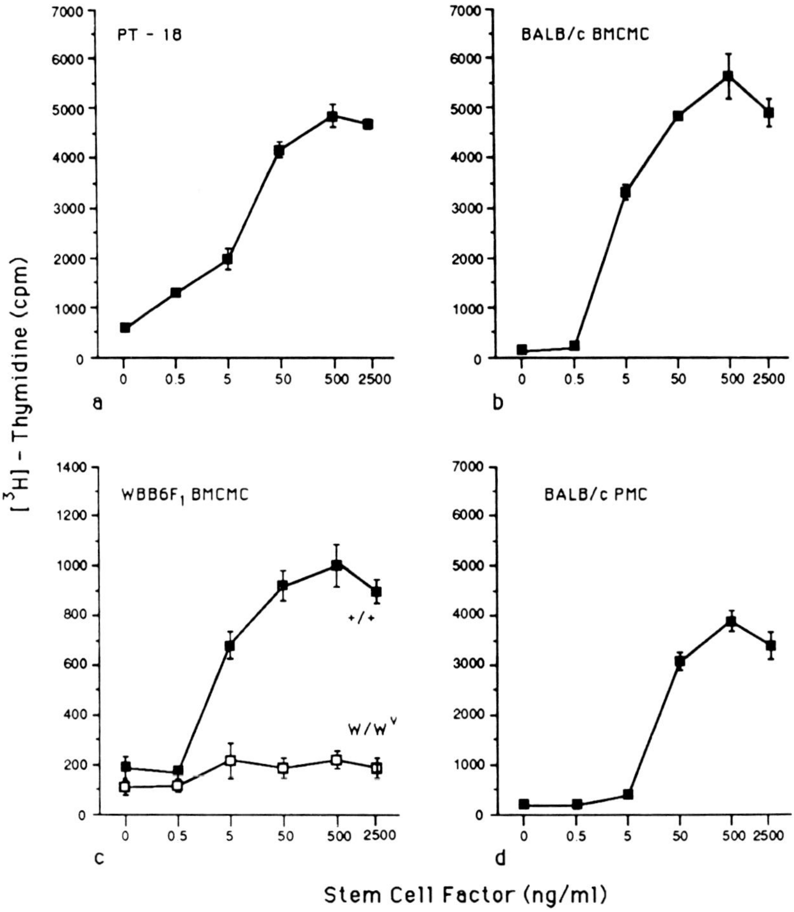

Figure 3 The c-*kit* ligand, rrSCF^{164}, induces c-*kit*-dependent proliferation of both IL-3-dependent immature mouse mast cells and mature, IL-3-independent mouse mast cells. (a) The cloned, IL-3-dependent PT-18 mast cell line. (b) Four-week-old primary populations of IL-3-dependent BMCMC from BALB/c mice. (c) Four-week-old populations of BMCMC derived from WBB6F$_1$-*W/W^v* mice or the congenic normal (+/+) mice. (d) Purified peritoneal mast cells (PMC) from retired breeder BALB/c mice. Data shown are mean ± SEM (n = 3–5/point) of ^{3}H-thymidine, expressed as cpm, incorporated over a period of 4 hr. Four-hour incorporation of ^{3}H-thymidine observed after incubating cells in IL-3-containing conditioned medium instead of in rrSCF^{164} was 11384 ± 420 cpm for PT18 cells, 3234 ± 214 cpm for BALB/c BMCMC, 6656 ± 441 cpm for WBB6F$_1$-+/+ BMCMC, 10065 ± 899 cpm for WBB6F$_1$-*W/W^v* BMCMC, and 222 ± 30 cpm (Not significantly different than the value for PMC incubated without growth factors: 193 ± 29 cpm) for PMC. (From Tsai et al., 1991b).

mast cells by colocalization of immunohistochemical staining for bromodeoxyuridine incorporated into nuclear DNA and mast cell cytoplasmic granule staining with alcian blue (Arizono et al., 1987).

Both dermal mast cells and PMC are regarded as T-cell-independent CTMC populations that do not proliferate in response to IL-3 alone (reviewed in Galli, 1990; Tsuji et al., 1990a,b). As shown in the legend of Figure 3, we confirmed that purified PMC did not proliferate in response to IL-3-containing medium, whereas all of the IL-3-dependent populations, including BMCMC derived from $WBB6F_1$-W/W^v mice, gave the expected proliferative response. IL-3-dependent BMCMC and PMC are representative of immature and mature stages of mast cell development (reviewed in Galli, 1990). Thus, $rrSCF^{164}$ can stimulate proliferation of the mast cell lineage at a later period of its development than can IL-3.

We also found that $rrSCF^{164}$ could promote mast cell maturation (Table 4). In accord with previous work (Galli et al., 1982; Nakano et al., 1985; Levi-Schaffer et al., 1986; Kanakura et al., 1988), we found that BMCMC maintained under our usual conditions in IL-3-containing medium had a very low histamine content and were consistently negative for cytoplasmic staining with either berberine sulfate or safranin. By contrast, freshly isolated PMC exhibited strong cytoplasmic staining for berberine sulfate or safranin. We found that when BMCMC were maintained in $rrSCF^{164}$ (50 ng/ml) for 4 weeks, many of the cells acquired reactivity for berberine sulfate or safranin. Moreover, BMCMC maintained in $rrSCF^{164}$ had a histamine content that was ~30 times that of BMCMC maintained in IL-3-containing medium.

To confirm that the acquisition of reactivity with berberine sulfate by BMCMC maintained in $rrSCF^{164}$ reflected an increased ability of these populations to synthesize heparin, we collaborated with Helen Thompson and Dean D. Metcalfe to analyze biochemically the [^{35}S] proteoglycans synthesized by BMCMC maintained in the presence or absence of $rrSCF^{164}$. In accord with previous work (Razin et al., 1982; Galli et al., 1982; Sredni et al., 1983; Levi-Schaffer et al., 1986; Otsu et al., 1987; Kanakura et al., 1988), we found that BMCMC maintained in IL-3-containing medium incorporated [^{35}S] sulfate predominantly into chondroitin sulfates. Indeed, these [^{35}S] macromolecules were susceptible to complete degradation by treatment with chondroitin ABC lyase and thus contained no detectable [^{35}S] heparin. By contrast, BMCMC maintained 4–6 weeks in $rrSCF^{164}$ (50 ng/ml) incorporated a substantial amount of [^{35}S] sulfate into heparin, as judged by degradation of the [^{35}S]-labeled macromolecules by treatment with either heparinase or nitrous acid. Thus, 41–70% (mean ± SD = 51 ± 13%, n = 4) of the [^{35}S] proteoglycans synthesized by BMCMC maintained 4–6 weeks in $rrSCF^{164}$ were susceptible to degradation by treatment with heparinase, and 45–55% (mean ± SD = 50 ± 4%, n = 4) of the [^{35}S] proteoglycans were susceptible to degradation by nitrous

Table 4 Histochemical Characteristics and Histamine Content of Various Populations of Mouse Mast Cells

Mast cells[a]	Alcian blue/safranin (%)[b]			Berberine sulfate (%)[b]				Histamine[c] (pg/cell)
	AB+/S–	AB+>S+	S+>AB+	–	±	+	++	
BMCMC (CM-4 wk)	100	0	0	100	0	0	0	0.08 ± 0.02
BMCMC (CM-8 wk)	100	0	0	100	0	0	0	0.08 ± 0.04
BMCMC (CM-4 wk/SCF-4 wk)	33 ± 3	47 ± 3	20 ± 2	44 ± 16	16 ± 2	40 ± 15	0	2.23 ± 0.39
PMC (SCF-2 wk)	0	5 ± 1	95 ± 1	6 ± 1	23 ± 7	69 ± 2	2 ± 1	2.53 ± 0.23
PMC (freshly isolated)	0	0	100	0	0	0	100	20.9 ± 2.7

[a]Bone marrow–derived cultured mast cells (BMCMC) were maintained in IL-3-containing conditioned medium (CM) for 4 or 8 weeks or were maintained in CM for 4 weeks and then transferred to medium lacking IL-3 but containing rrSCF^{164} (50 ng/ml) for an additional 4 weeks. Peritoneal mast cells (PMC) were used immediately after purification or after 2 weeks in medium containing rrSCF^{164} (50 ng/ml). Medium containing rrSCF^{164} was replaced 2–3 × per week.

[b]Staining of mast cells in cytocentrifuge preparations for alcian blue(AB)/safranin(S) or berberine sulfate; at least 100 cells were examined in each preparation. AB+/S– = all granules AB+, no granules S+; AB+>S+ = more AB+ than S+ granules; S+>AB+ = more S+ than AB+ granules. Berberine sulfate: – = no berberine sulfate positive granules. ± = occasional weakly positive granules; + = many positive granules; ++ = many intensely positive granules. Data shown are mean ± SEM (n = 3–8/point).

[c]Histamine content was determined by a fluorometric method. Data shown are mean ± SEM (n = 3–8/point).

Source: From Tsai et al., 1991b.

acid. The [^{35}S]-labeled macromolecules were identified as proteoglycans by their susceptibility to degradation by NaOH into molecules of smaller molecular weight (Kanakura et al., 1988).

rrSCF^{164} also induced phenotypic changes in PMC. Nocka et al. (1990a) reported that a candidate c-*kit* ligand purified from conditioned medium of BALB/3T3 fibroblasts stimulated the proliferation of PMC in vitro and that the cytoplasmic granules of these cells stained with berberine sulfate. We also found that many PMC maintained in vitro with rrSCF^{164} retained reactivity with berberine sulfate (Table 4). However, our results indicate that some PMC maintained in rrSCF^{164} had no detectable cytoplasmic staining with berberine sulfate or exhibited diminished reactivity with safranin (Table 4). In addition, PMC maintained in rrSCF^{164} had a histamine content very similar to that of BMCMC maintained in rrSCF^{164} but only ~12% that of freshly isolated PMC (Table 4).

Our findings demonstrated that rrSCF^{164} not only can promote the proliferation of either immature or mature mast cells, but also can induce changes in the phenotype of these populations. BMCMC maintained in rrSCF^{164} both proliferated and became more mature. This finding indicates that SCF can induce immature, IL-3-dependent mast cells to acquire phenotypic characteristics of CTMC, including the ability to synthesize substantial amounts of heparin. This observation also identifies an in vitro system in which the administration of SCF as the sole exogenous cytokine can influence both the proliferation and the maturation of a cellular lineage expressing c-*kit*. Mature, IL-3-independent PMC also proliferated in response to rrSCF^{164}. But in this case, the cells maintained in rrSCF^{164} had a substantially lower histamine content and, as a population, exhibited less mature histochemical characteristics than the mast cells initially placed in culture. However, PMC maintained in rrSCF^{164} had a much higher histamine content and more mature histochemical staining characteristics than did PMC propagated in medium containing IL-3 and IL-4 (Kanakura et al., 1988).

Even though rrSCF^{164} promoted BMCMC maturation and permitted PMC to retain phenotypic features that were more mature than those of PMC grown in IL-3 and IL-4, the characteristics of BMCMC or PMC maintained in rrSCF^{164} differed from those of freshly purified PMC. This finding may indicate that the soluble form of SCF used in our experiments (Martin et al., 1990) influences mast cell maturation differently than the membrane-associated form of SCF (Flanagan and Leder, 1990; Anderson et al., 1990; Flanagan et al., 1991), which may be encountered by mast cells in vivo. However, both the histochemical staining characteristics and the histamine or heparin content of BMCMC maintained in soluble rrSCF^{164} were quite similar to those reported for BMCMC cocultured with skin-derived 3T3 fibroblasts (Levi-Schaffer et al., 1986), a system that favors contact between mast cells and membrane-associated c-*kit* ligand. For example, when BMCMC that became adherent to 3T3 fibroblasts during coculture for 14 days were analyzed, 39 ± 7% of the cells' [^{35}S] proteoglycans were susceptible to degradation by nitrous acid treatment (Levi-Schaffer et al., 1986). In our study, the corresponding value for BMCMC maintained for 4–6 weeks in $rrSCF^{164}$ was 50 ± 4%. Thus, according to multiple criteria including heparin synthesis, exposure to soluble $rrSCF^{164}$ can reproduce mast cell maturation-inducing effects of coculture of BMCMC with 3T3 cells.

Nevertheless, BMCMC cultured with $rrSCF^{164}$ did not acquire, nor did PMC cultured with $rrSCF^{164}$ retain, a phenotype fully identical to that of resident PMC. As additional phenotypic characteristics of BMCMC or PMC maintained with or without SCF are examined, we expect that additional differences may be detected. Such differences may indicate that SCF is not sufficient to induce full maturation of mast cells with the CTMC phenotype. Nerve growth factor (NGF) can induce the in vivo hyperplasia of both CTMC (Aloe and Levi-Montalcini, 1977; Marshall et al., 1990) and MMC (Marshall et al., 1990) in neonatal, but not in adult rats. Matsuda et al. (1991) recently reported that NGF, when administered together with IL-3, promoted the maturation of BMCMC, as assessed by the mast cells' histamine content, ultrastructure, and berberine sulfate reactivity. Moreover, production of soluble NGF by Swiss albino 3T3 fibroblasts was enhanced when the fibroblasts were cocultured with BMCMC and IL-3, and addition of a monoclonal antibody against NGF to the coculture system containing BMCMC, IL-3, and 3T3 cells interfered with the acquisition of berberine sulfate reactivity by the BMCMC. When taken together with observations indicating that BMCMC fail to survive when cocultured with 3T3 cells derived from Sl/Sl^d mice (Kitamura et al., 1989; Fujita et al., 1989), the findings of Matsuda et al. (1991) raise the possibility that, under certain circumstances, optimal maturation of BMCMC in vitro may require both SCF and NGF.

The observation that BMCMC or PMC maintained in $rrSCF^{164}$ differ in phenotype from freshly isolated PMC also may reflect, at least in part, the active proliferation of mast cell populations maintained in SCF. PMC proliferating in vitro in response to IL-3 and IL-4 contained much less histamine and exhibited less mature histochemical characteristics than freshly isolated PMC (Nakahata et al., 1986; Hamaguchi et al., 1987; Kanakura et al., 1988). And we found that the expanded population of dermal mast cells at sites of s.c. injection of $rrSCF^{164}$ in $WCB6F_1$-+/+ mice exhibited more variable intensity of cytoplasmic staining with berberine sulfate or safranin than did the nonproliferating dermal mast cell populations in control mice (Tsai et al., 1991b). In addition, the effects of $rrSCF^{164}$ on the numbers of mast cells in various tissues of rats treated with the cytokine for 3 weeks were more striking than the corresponding effects on the mast cell–associated protease content of these tissues (Tsai et al., 1991a). Taken together, all these findings support the hypothesis that populations of proliferating CTMC contain mast cells exhibiting phenotypic characteristics that are different, and may be considered more immature, than those of the resting populations (reviewed in Galli, 1990).

The mechanisms by which SCF influences mast cell proliferation and maturation remain to be fully elucidated. Our experiments with BMCMC derived from $WBB6F_1$-*W/W^v* mice (Tsai et al., 1991b), and similar work reported by others (Nocka et al., 1990a), indicates that the effects of SCF on mast cell proliferation in vitro require that the c-*kit* ligand interacts with a functionally competent c-*kit* receptor. The failure of $rrSCF^{164}$ to induce mast cell development in the skin of $WBB6F_1$-*W/W^v* mice indicates that the ability of SCF to affect the development of dermal mast cells in vivo also requires a functionally active c-*kit* receptor. However, the subsequent events leading to mast cell proliferation and/or maturation are not fully understood. By itself, SCF has relatively modest effects on the proliferation of hematopoietic or lymphoid cells in vitro, but it acts in potent synergy with other cytokines to influence the development of specific erythroid, myeloid, or lymphoid lineages (Zsebo et al., 1990a,b; Martin et al., 1990; Anderson et al., 1990). We have found that $rrSCF^{164}$ can activate certain mouse mast cell populations to release their mediators (Galli et al., 1991b). Preliminary data indicate that the concentrations of $rrSCF^{164}$ required to observe these effects in vitro are at least an order of magnitude higher than those required to induce proliferation of the same mast cell populations (Galli et al., 1991b). But c-*kit* receptor-dependent activation of dermal mast cells in vivo is observed at doses of $rrSCF^{164}$ identical to or even lower than those we used to induce proliferation of these populations (Wershil et al., 1992).

Activation of mast cell populations generated in vitro, either via the $Fc_\epsilon RI$ or by other mechanisms, induces these cells to develop increased levels of mRNA for a variety of cytokines and/or to secrete the products (Young et al., 1987; Plaut et al., 1989; Wodnar-Filipowicz et al., 1989; Burd et al., 1989; Gordon and Galli, 1990a). Some of these cytokines, e.g., IL-3 and IL-4, can promote or augment mast cell proliferation (reviewed in Plaut et al., 1989; Wodnar-Filipowicz et al., 1989; Burd et al., 1989; Gordon et al., 1990); others, e.g., GM-CSF (Bressler et al., 1989) and IFN-γ (Takagi et al., 1990) have activities that can suppress mast cell proliferation. In light of these findings, it will be of interest to determine whether one of the actions of SCF is to induce mast cells to generate other cytokines with autocrine effects on mast cell proliferation and/or maturation. Recently, Razin et al. (1991) reported evidence that contact with 3T3 fibroblasts induces mouse PMC or BMCMC to develop increased levels of IL-3 mRNA. And Matsuda et al. (1991) suggested that BMCMC stimulated with IL-3 may induce increased production of NGF by 3T3 cells. Finally, Marshall et al. (1990) have provided evidence that the ability of NGF to induce mast cell hyperplasia in neonatal rats may, in part, reflect the release by NGF-activated mast cells of factors with autocrine effects on mast cell proliferation.

These findings support previous lines of evidence indicating that an intricate pattern of bidirectional communication exists between mast cells and fibroblasts (reviewed in Kitamura, 1989; Stevens and Austen, 1989; Galli, 1990) and suggest that certain interesting aspects of these "conversations" are mediated by growth factors that may have complex autocrine and/or paracrine effects on mast cell development. IgE may also participate in these interactions, since activation of BMCMC via the $Fc_{\epsilon}RI$ promotes the generation of cytokines with autocrine effects on mast cell development (reviewed in Gordon et al., 1990) and diminishes levels of c-*kit* mRNA (Geissler et al., 1990). $Fc_{\epsilon}RI$-dependent stimulation may also enhance the generation of mast cell-committed progenitors (Ashman et al., 1991).

We feel that considerable additional work will be required to explain fully the specific interactions between SCF and other factors that may contribute to the regulation of mast cell proliferation or maturation under different circumstances in vitro or in vivo. In light of the evidence indicating that soluble forms of SCF have potent synergistic effects with several other cytokines in regulating hematopoietic cell development and lineage commitment in vitro, it will be important to investigate whether some of the effects of SCF on mast cell development reflect interactions between SCF and other growth factors that have positive or negative effects on mast cell proliferation and/or maturation. Indeed, we already have found that the addition of SCF markedly augments the generation of BMCMC from bone marrow cells maintained in IL-3-containing medium (Frankel, Galli, et al., unpublished data).

It will also be of interest to search for differences in the responsiveness of mast cells to soluble, as opposed to cell-associated, forms of the c-*kit* ligand. Flanagan et al. (1991) reported that cultured medium conditioned by COS cells expressing either of the wild-type mouse variant SCF cDNAs could stimulate the proliferation of mouse mast cells, and that the relative ability of the culture supernatants to stimulate mast cell proliferation was proportional to the relative concentration of soluble SCF. However, the wild-type, membrane-associated form of SCF promoted mast cell adherence as well as stimulated mast cell proliferation. By contrast, BMCMC did not adhere to transfected COS cells expressing the form of SCF encoded by the Sl^d allele. Flanagan et al. (1991) showed that the Sl^d cDNA comprises an insertion/deletion within the SCF gene that removes 242 bp at the 3' end of the coding sequence. The truncated Sl^d transcript encodes almost all of the extracellular domain of SCF but is lacking the coding sequence for both the transmembrane and intracellular domains of the wild-type protein. Expression of the Sl^d cDNA in transfected COS cells results in the secretion of a soluble product capable of stimulating mast cell proliferation but fails to result in the appearance of the membrane-associated form of SCF (Flanagan et al., 1991).

In light of these findings and our observations that local injection of $rrSCF^{164}$ can induce the appearance of mature mast cells in the skin of Sl/Sl^d

mice (Tsai et al., 1991a), it will be of interest to reexamine the mechanism responsible for the severe mast cell deficiency exhibited by Sl/Sl^d mice. One possibility is that Sl/Sl^d stromal cells in vivo, unlike COS cells transfected with Sl^d cDNA, fail to produce a soluble, biologically active form of the Sl product. Another possibility is that the amounts of soluble c-*kit* ligand produced by Sl/Sl^d stromal cells in vivo are insufficient to induce mast cell development. But whatever the explanation for the lack of mast cell development in Sl/Sl^d mice, the work of Flanagan et al. (1991), supports other lines of evidence (reviewed in Russell, 1979; Kitamura et al., 1989) indicating that, in many circumstances, biologically significant effects of the *Sl* product are mediated through membrane-associated forms of the molecule. Moreover, it is possible that SCF regulates certain aspects of mast cell adherence, migration, or development in concert with other molecules in the interstitium or associated with cell surfaces. Mast cells can interact with stromal cell products other than SCF, such as laminin (Thompson et al., 1989). In addition, Morrison-Graham and Weston (1989) have reported that the skin of Sl/Sl^d embryos produces an extracellular matrix that differs from that of the congenic normal embryos in its ability to enhance melanocyte differentiation in vitro and in its ultrastructural characteristics. This finding raises the possibility that SCF can influence the organization or characteristics of other components of the interstitium.

D. SCF Induces Mast Cell Activation and c-*kit*-Dependent Signal Transduction

It will be important to define in detail the signal transduction pathways activated by interactions between the c-*kit* receptor and SCF. We have found that SCF can activate certain mouse mast cell populations for mediator release, particularly when administered intradermally (Galli et al., 1991b; Wershil et al., 1992). Dermal mast cell activation by $rrSCF^{164}$ in vivo is c-*kit*-dependent and occurs at doses of cytokine as low as 140 fmole/site (Wershil et al., 1992). Thus, on a molar basis, $rrSCF^{164}$ is at least 10-fold more potent as an activator of dermal mast cells than is substance P (Yano et al., 1989). On the other hand, activation of mast cells for mediator release by SCF in vitro requires very high concentrations of the cytokine (usually 500 ng/ml or more) (Galli et al., 1991b), and the extent to which the biochemical changes associated with such activation resemble those observed after IgE-dependent mast cell activation (reviewed in Ishizaka, 1988) has not been reported.

However, two groups have investigated the patterns of signal transduction mediated by activation of c-*kit* receptor tyrosine kinase. Rottapel et al. (1991) recently reported that the c-*kit* ligand induced the c-*kit* receptor of BMCMC to autophosphorylate on tyrosine and to bind phosphatidylinositol 3'-kinase (P13K) and phospholipase C-γ1(PLC-γ1) and provided evidence that tyrosine phosphorylation of the c-*kit* receptor promoted complex formation with P13K.

This study showed that the c-*kit* receptor is distinct from CSF-1R by virtue of its ability to bind to PLC-γ1 and is different from the PDGFR in that it apparently cannot bind to the Ras GTPase-activating protein. Rottapel et al. (1991) therefore proposed that the distinct affinities of these receptors for their cytoplasmic ligands, together with variation in their pattern of tissue-specific expression, may determine their specific biological effects. Furthermore, they suggested that the variable effects of distinct *W* mutations on different cell lineages might be controlled by the availability of individual substrates within the different lineages.

Lev et al. (1991) investigated the signal transduction mediated by a chimeric receptor kinase composed of the extracellular ligand-binding domain of the epidermal growth factor (EGF) receptor and the transmembrane and cytoplasmic domains of c-*kit*. They demonstrated that upon binding EGF, the ligand-receptor complex underwent endocytosis and degradation and showed that the activated c-*kit* kinase strongly associated with P13K and an 85-kDa phosphoprotein and coupled to modified PLC-γ1 and the Raf1 protein kinase, but did not significantly change levels of inositol phosphate. Based on the differences between the signaling that was observed after ligand binding to this chimeric receptor and that induced via the receptors for CSF-1 or PDGF, Lev et al. (1991) proposed that each receptor in this family is coupled to a specific combination of signal transducers, which determines a receptor-specific program of gene expression.

One of the elements involved in both c-*kit*-dependent and CSF-1-dependent signal transduction may be encoded at the *mi* locus on mouse chromosome 6 (Silvers, 1979c). Mutant mice of the *mi/mi* genotype are osteopetrotic owing to a monocyte/macrophage defect and are also mast cell-deficient (Stevens and Loutit, 1982; Stechschulte et al., 1987), probably owing to an inability of the mast cell lineage to respond to the proliferative and perhaps other effects of the c-*kit* ligand (Ebi et al., 1990). Dubreuil et al., (1991) showed that transfection of the CSR-1R (c-*fms*) gene rendered mast cells derived from *W* mutant mice, but not mast cells derived from *mi/mi* mice, able to proliferate in response to coculture with fibroblasts. These findings suggested that binding of ligand to either the c-*kit* or the c-*fms* receptor activates similar or overlapping signal transduction pathways, and that the *mi* locus may encode an element common on these pathways.

Figure 4 summarizes the structure of the c-*kit* receptor and SCF and presents current understanding of the role of c-*kit* receptor/SCF interactions in regulating mast cell development.

VII. Chromosomal Location of c-*kit* and *SCF* in Humans

As illustrated by the *W*/c-*kit* and *Sl/SCF* loci, the genetic colocalization of cloned genes and mutations causing genetic disease may comprise preliminary evidence

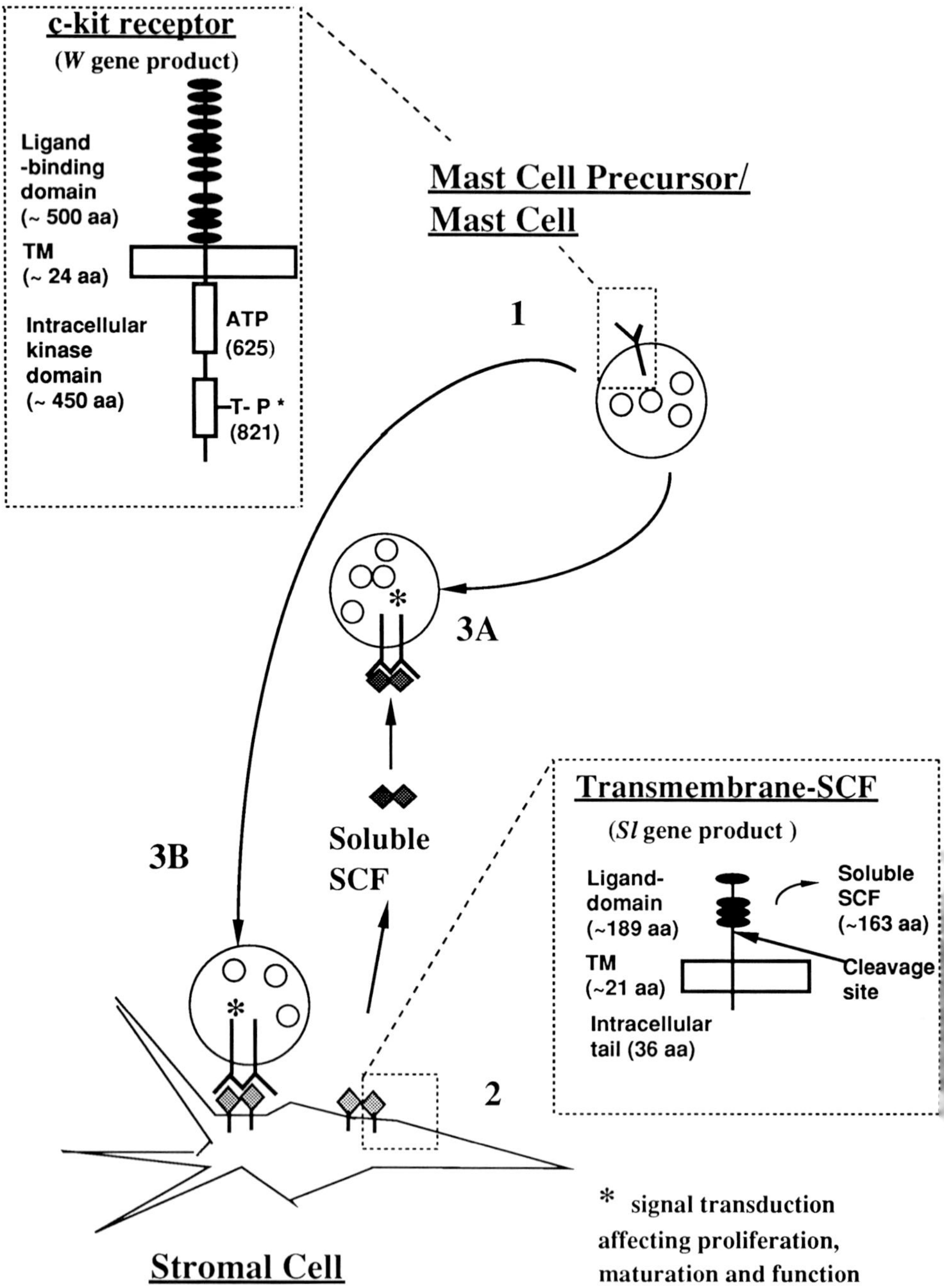
c-kit receptor
(W gene product)
Ligand -binding domain (~ 500 aa)
TM (~ 24 aa)
Intracellular kinase domain (~ 450 aa)
ATP (625)
T- P * (821)
Mast Cell Precursor/ Mast Cell
1
3A
3B
Soluble SCF
Transmembrane-SCF
(Sl gene product)
Ligand-domain (~189 aa)
TM (~21 aa)
Intracellular tail (36 aa)
Soluble SCF (~163 aa)
Cleavage site
2
Stromal Cell
* signal transduction affecting proliferation, maturation and function

for their allelism. Of course, rigorous genetic and biochemical proof of their allelism would elucidate the molecular basis for the pathology. In the human genome, the c-*kit* locus maps in the centromeric regions of chromosome 4 between 4q11 and 4q21, an area that has well-defined genetic homology to the *W* region of mouse chromosome 5 (Yarden et al., 1987). At present, a locus producing an autosomal dominant piebaldism is the only human genetic disorder which maps in this region and whose phenotypic effects resemble in part those which rise from mutant *W* gene action. The first evidence for a genetic locus controlling this trait was the description of a mentally retarded child with integumental pigmentary changes by Funderburk and Crandall (1974). Cytogenetic analysis of the circulating lymphocytes of this patient revealed a translocation and interstitial deletion of the proximal long arm of chromosome 4. Subsequently, Lacassie et al. (1977) reported an independent case of dominant piebaldism and mild mental retardation in a child with a deletion of 4q11–4q21 as its only chromosome abnormality.

Recent reports that c-*kit* is expressed in the developing and adult mammalian brain (Orr-Urtegger et al., 1990) are intriguing in this context and suggest that the mental retardation exhibited by these individuals could also reflect

---

Figure 4 c-*kit* receptor/c-*kit* receptor ligand (SCF) interactions in mast cell development. (1) Precursors of mast cells and cells in the mast cell lineage express the c-*kit* receptor on their surface. The box shows a diagram of the structure of the mouse c-*kit* receptor, including the transmembrane (TM) portion, an ATP binding site, and the tyrosine autophosphorylation (T-P*) site. Black ovals indicate approximate position of cysteine residues in the extracellular domain. The 21-aa signal peptide of the newly synthesized product is not shown. (2) A stromal cell (e.g., a fibroblast) expresses transmembrane-SCF. The box shows a diagram of the structure of the transmembrane-SCF, including the cleavage site for generation of soluble SCF and the approximate position of cysteine residues (black ovals) in the extracellular domain. The 25-aa signal peptide of the newly synthesized product is not shown. Much of the soluble SCF forms noncovalently linked dimers. At least three alternatively spliced forms of transmembrane-SCF have been described (see text), the longest of which is diagrammed. (3) Interaction of the mast cell precursor or mast cell with the soluble (A) or transmembrane (B) SCF induces signal transduction in the mast cell precursor/mast cell and also c-*kit* receptor dimerization and internalization of the receptor-ligand complex. The c-*kit* receptor/SCF interaction has been shown to favor recruitment/survival of mast cell precursors, to induce proliferation of both immature and mature mast cells in the mast cell lineage, to promote the maturation of immature mast cells, and, in certain circumstances, to induce mast cell mediator release. Based on the phenotypic abnormalities expressed by *W* or *Sl* mutant mice, the c-*kit* receptor/SCF interaction is also likely to influence the migration of mast cell precursors and mast cells. SCF may influence mast cell migration, proliferation, maturation, and function directly or in association with other soluble or cell-associated factors. It is possible that interactions between transmembrane-SCF and the c-*kit* receptor can induce signal transduction in the cell expressing the transmembrane-SCF.

altered c-*kit* expression in the developing CNS. The hematological parameters of these individuals were not reported. Therefore, the extent to which the piebald syndrome resembles the *W* mutant phenotype is not known. The availability of molecular probes for the c-*kit* product may facilitate the colocalization of c-*kit* with other human genetic disorders, such as the Diamond-Blackfan syndrome (Diamond et al., 1961; Brody, 1982), whose phenotypic effects resemble those of *W* mutations.

The *Sl*/*SCF* locus on mouse chromosome 10 maps in the vicinity of genes that have been localized to the long arm of human chromosome 12 (reviewed in Geissler et al., 1991). We recently reported the use of somatic cell hybrid lines to localize the human *SCF* locus to the long arm of chromosome 12, between 12q14.3 and 12qter (Geissler et al., 1991). In addition to localizing the *Sl* homolog in humans, these data provide further evidence for the conservation of synteny between the long arm of human chromosome 12 and the distal end of mouse chromosome 10 (reviewed in Geissler et al., 1991).

The localization of *SCF* to the long arm of human chromosome 12 supports other evidence that abnormalities in the c-*kit* signaling pathway might be involved in malignancies of hematopoietic cells or other instances of neoplastic transformation. Briefly, this evidence is as follows: both the truncated viral c-*kit* oncogene (Besmer et al., 1986) and the closely related tyrosine kinase receptor protooncogene c-*fms* (CSF-1R) (Rohrschneider et al., 1989) have transforming potential; both W^x/W^v and Sl/Sl^d mice express a much higher incidence of lymphocytic leukemia than their congenic normal littermates (reviewed in Russell, 1979); c-*kit* mRNA is expressed in the blast cells of patients with acute myeloblastic leukemia (AML) but not in blasts from patients with acute lymphoblastic leukemia (ALL) or in myeloid blasts derived from normal marrow (Wang et al., 1989), and analysis of the expression of c-*kit* protein on the cell surface confirmed these findings (Lerner et al., 1991). Recent reports have demonstrated the expression of c-*kit* transcripts in human small lung cell cancer tumor samples and tumor-derived cell lines (Seikido et al., 1991) and in human testicular germ cell tumors (Strohmeyer et al., 1991).

The significance of the expression of c-*kit* in AML blasts and other neoplasms and the role of *W*/c-*kit* and *Sl*/*SCF* mutations in leukemogenesis are not yet clear. However, these observations are consistent with the hypothesis that aberrant expression of the c-*kit* signaling pathway may be involved in the development of neoplasias in both mouse and human. Evidence supporting this hypothesis recently has been reported by Rottapel et al. (1991), who found that c-*kit* is constitutively phosphorylated in the absence of c-*kit* ligand in the mouse mastocytoma cell line P 815.

A role for aberrant *SCF* expression in neoplastic development has not yet been demonstrated. However, the localization of *SCF* to human chromosome 12 is intriguing in the context of previous reports of aneuploidy and translocations of chromosome 12 in patients with several forms of malignant or premalignant hematopoietic abnormalities or with tumors originating within nonhematopoietic tissues that are likely to express c-*kit* or *SCF*, including malignant gliomas, testicular tumors, and uterine leiomyomas (reviewed in Geissler et al., 1991). It is possible that aberrant expression of *SCF* subsequent to a chromosome rearrangement involving the *SCF* locus may participate in the etiology of some of these tumors. On the other hand, it is possible that other genes or chromosome 12 may be involved in the development and/or expansion of some of these tumors. Thus, without direct investigation of these neoplasms, the role of *W*/c-*kit* and/or *Sl/SCF* in their pathogenesis remains uncertain.

VIII. Analysis of Mast Cell Function Using W/W^v and Sl/Sl^d Mice: A Versatile and Powerful General Approach for Identifying and Quantifying the Roles of Mast Cells in Biological Responses

There is no dearth of clues about the possible roles of mast cells in biological responses. Mast cells represent rich sources of histamine, heparin, proteases, and many other biologically active mediators (reviewed in Metcalfe et al., 1981; Schwartz and Austen, 1984; Galli, 1987; Galli and Lichtenstein, 1988). Mast cells also express surface receptors for immunoglobulins of the IgE class, which, when occupied by intact IgE, prime the cells to release stored and newly generated mediators in response to encounters with specific antigens (reviewed in Ishizaka, 1988; Metzger et al., 1989). The remarkable variety of mediators potentially derived from mast cells, and the recognition that mast cells can release these mediators in response to stimulation by many different signals in addition to IgE and specific antigen (e.g., anaphylatoxins, certain neuropeptides, basic compounds derived from leukocytes, and components of insect venoms), has encouraged speculation that mast cells may play important roles in diverse immunological, pathological, and physiological processes (reviewed in Metcalfe et al., 1981; Schwartz and Austen, 1984; Galli et al., 1984; Galli, 1987).

Unfortunately, proof of the importance of mast cells in specific immunological or pathological responses has been difficult to obtain. There are several reasons why this is so (reviewed in Galli, 1987, 1990). Many "mast cell–associated" mediators are also produced by other cell types. As a result, even convincing evidence that one of these mediators has a critical role in a particular biological response is not, by itself, sufficient evidence that the mast cell is important in that response. Pharmacological experiments employing antagonists of individual mast cell–associated mediators, or inhibitors of mast cell activation, can provide important information about the role of these mediators, and/or the effects of these drugs, in the process under study. However, such experiments may not necessarily elucidate the role of the mast cell itself. Indeed, the extent to which efforts at pharmacological inhibition of mast cell activation can clarify the role of the mast cell depends on the strength of the evidence documenting that the effects of the drugs used are selective for the mast cell.

Analysis of mast cell function in vivo is further complicated by the fact that mast cell activation usually results in the elaboration of multiple mediators, which may have diverse, and sometimes even opposing, biological effects. The *net* biological consequences of the combined activities of all of these mediators may be difficult to predict. Finally, it is now widely accepted that individual mast cell populations can express significant variation in multiple aspects of phenotype, including morphology, mediator content, and response to drugs and secretagogues; such evidence of "mast cell heterogeneity" suggests that phenotypically distinct mast cells may have different roles in health and disease (reviewed in Enërback, 1986; Galli, 1990).

A useful approach for identifying and quantifying the roles of mast cells in biological responses in vivo is to search for differences in the expression of biological responses in anatomical sites that differ only in that one site contains mast cells and the other does not (Galli, 1987; Galli and Kitamura, 1987). Our general approach for evaluating the roles of mast cells in biological responses is shown in Table 5.

Briefly, if W/W^v and Sl/Sl^d mice express a particular biological response differently than do the congenic normal (+/+) mice, this may reflect the virtual absence of mature mast cells in the mutants or some other effect of their *W* or *Sl* mutations. If the response of W/W^v mice is normalized after bone marrow transplantation from the congenic +/+ mice, this finding indicates that the mast

Table 5 General Scheme for Investigating Mouse Mast Cell Function In Vivo

1. Search for quantitative differences in the expression of biological responses in genetically mast cell–deficient WBB6F$_1$-W/W^v and WCB6F$_1$-Sl/Sl^d mice and the congenic normal (+/+) mice.
2. Compare the responses in W/W^v mice and W/W^v mice that have received bone marrow transplantation from congenic +/+ mice.
   Note: This determines whether the response abnormally expressed in W/W^v mice has a *bone marrow–dependent component.*
3. Analyze the response in W/W^v mice selectively reconstituted with mast cells.
   Note: This determines whether the response abnormally expressed in W/W^v mice has a mast cell–dependent component.
4. Define the mechanism(s) by which mast cells contribute to the response.

Source: Modified from Galli, 1990.

cell and/or some other bone marrow–dependent lineage accounted for the abnormality in the response. To discriminate between contributions of the mast cell as opposed to other bone marrow–derived elements, one then should attempt to analyze W/W^v mice selectively repaired of their mast cell deficiency by the injection of cultured, growth factor–dependent mast cells (i.e., BMCMC) derived from congenic +/+ mouse bone marrow cells (Nakano et al., 1985; Galli and Kitamura, 1987; Galli et al., 1989a,b; Wershil et al., 1989). Such adoptively transferred mast cell populations gradually acquire multiple phenotypic characteristics of the native mast cell populations present in the same anatomical sites in normal mice (reviewed in Galli, 1990).

In theory, W/W^v mice systemically repaired of their mast cell deficiency by i.v. administration of BMCMC of congenic +/+ origin can be used to investigate the contribution of mast cells to biological responses elicited in virtually any organ or anatomical site. In practice, there are a number of difficulties with this approach. These include the number of BMCMC that must be transferred to achieve levels of mast cells in the recipients' tissues that approximate those in the congenic +/+ mice, the fact that the distribution of the adoptively transferred mast cell populations within specific organs may differ from that observed in normal mice, and the observations of Nakano et al. (1989a) indicating that a very small number of hematopoietic stem cells with extensive proliferative potential (as few as one) can result in repair of the anemia of W/W^v mice. Moreover, the progeny of these adoptively transferred stem cells can also differentiate into myeloid cells (macrophages, neutrophils, megakaryocytes, and mast cells) and lymphoid cells (Nakano et al., 1989b).

The +/+ BMCMC populations used for repair of the mast cell deficiency of W/W^v mice ordinarily contain no detectable CFU-S, nor does the i.v. injection of W/W^v mice with up to 1.0×10^6 +/+ BMCMC correct the anemia of the recipients (Nakano et al., 1985). However, the studies of Nakano et al. (1989a,b) suggest that even a few stem cells with extensive proliferative potential present in a population of +/+ BMCMC adoptively transferred into W/W^v recipients might result in repair of the recipients' anemia and the production of myeloid and lymphoid cells of donor origin; i.e., under these circumstances, the repair of the recipients' mast cell deficiency would not be selective. In fact, the i.v. transfer of large numbers (e.g., $\geq 1.0 \times 10^7$) of +/+ BMCMC into W/W^v mice sometimes results in correction of the recipients' anemia, as well as repair of their mast cell deficiency (Wershil, Yano, and Galli, unpublished data). By contrast, when the +/+ BMCMC are injected intradermally, one routinely obtains selective local reconstitution of dermal mast cell populations, without such systemic effects as the correction of the W/W^v recipients' anemia or the appearance of mast cells in distant anatomical sites (Nakano et al., 1985; Galli and Kitamura, 1987; Galli et al., 1989a). An additional advantage of W/W^v mice selectively repaired of their mast cell deficiency by local intradermal transplanta-

et al., 1981; Schwartz and Austen, 1984; Ishizaka, 1988; Galli and Lichtenstein, 1988). However, a variety of other cell types may also contribute to the pathogenesis of IgE-dependent reactions. These cells include basophils, which express $Fc_{\epsilon}RI$ and can elaborate many mediators with effects similar to those of the mast cell (reviewed in Metcalfe et al., 1981; Schwartz and Austen, 1984; Ishizaka, 1988; Galli and Lichtenstein, 1988), and monocytes, macrophages, platelets, and perhaps eosinophils, which can interact with IgE or complexes of IgE via $Fc_{\epsilon}RII$/CD23 or by other mechanisms (reviewed in Kikutani et al., 1989; Capron et al., 1989; Galli et al., 1989a). Genetically mast cell–deficient, congenic normal, and mast cell–reconstituted, mast cell–deficient mice provide a means to discriminate between the roles of mature mast cells, as opposed to other potential effectors, in IgE-dependent responses.

Perhaps the simplest experimental model of an IgE-dependent immediate hypersensitivity response is passive cutaneous anaphylaxis (PCA): IgE of known antigenic specificity is injected directly into the skin of an immunologically naïve recipient, specific antigen is administered systemically (generally intravenously) at some suitable later interval, and then the intensity of the ensuing reaction is assessed. At least three groups demonstrated that mast cell–deficient mice were unable to express IgE-dependent PCA responses (Thomas and Schrader, 1983; Askenase et al., 1983; Inagaki et al., 1986). To prove that this inability to express PCA reflected the mutants' mast cell deficiency, rather than another phenotypic abnormality of the mice, we investigated whether long-term selective local repair of the dermal mast cell deficiency of W/W^v mice rendered the animals competent to express IgE-dependent PCA (Wershil et al., 1987).

Using the approach outlined in Table 5, we found that essentially all of the tissue swelling, augmented vascular permeability, and deposition of crosslinked ^{125}I-fibrin associated with PCA reactions was mast cell–dependent (Wershil et al., 1987). More recently, we found that the early phase of tissue swelling that occurred at sites of PCA reactions in normal or mast cell–reconstituted mice was followed by an influx of granulocytes, composed predominantly of neutrophils, which reached maximal levels 6–12 hr after antigen challenge (Wershil et al., 1991a). Moreover, even though tissue swelling at these sites diminished progressively from 2 to 24 hr after antigen challenge, swelling at the reaction sites remained significantly greater than that at control sites for at least 24 hr. Analyses of mast cell–reconstituted W/W^v mice indicated that both the persistent tissue swelling (Fig. 5) and the neutrophil influx (Fig. 6) observed 6 hr after antigen challenge were essentially entirely mast cell–dependent.

In many allergic patients, intradermal challenge with specific antigen or anti-IgE induces an immediate wheal-and-flare reaction, which is followed, 4–8 hr later by a period of persistent swelling and leukocyte infiltration termed the late-phase cutaneous reaction (reviewed in Galli and Lichtenstein, 1988;

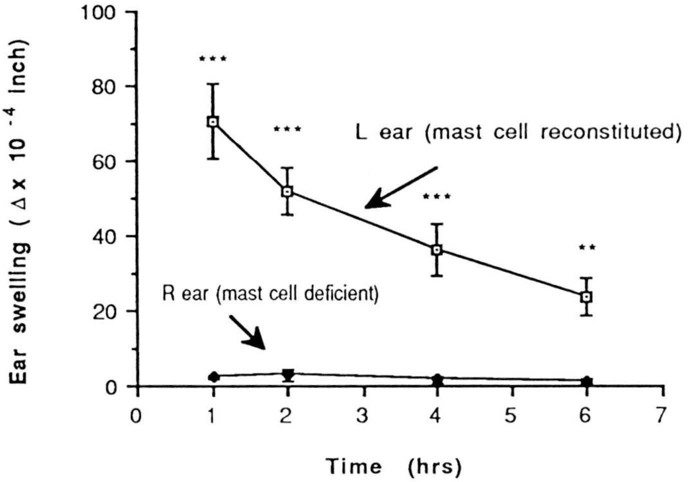

Figure 5 The ear swelling associated with IgE-dependent cutaneous reactions in the mouse is mast cell-dependent. Ear swelling responses were determined in both mast cell–reconstituted (left, L) and mast cell–deficient (right, R) ears of WBB6F$_1$-*W*/W^v mice that had been injected > 10 weeks before the experiment with WBB6F$_1$-+/+ BMCMC. Both ears were injected with IgE anti-DNP antibodies, and 1 day later, the mice were challenged with DNP$_{30\text{-}40}$-HSA i.v. Data represent mean ± SEM (n = 4/point). Significant differences between values for L and R ears are shown as $^{**}p < 0.02$, $^{***}p < 0.001$. (From Wershil et al., 1991a).

Lemanske and Kaliner, 1988). Late-phase reactions (LPRs) were initially studied in detail in the skin. However, it is now clear that late consequences of IgE-dependent reactions, notably including infiltration of the reaction sites with blood-borne leukocytes, also occur in the respiratory tract and other anatomical locations. Indeed, it has been argued compellingly that many of the clinically significant consequences of IgE-dependent reactions, in both the respiratory tract and the skin, reflect the actions of the leukocytes recruited to these sites during the LPRs, rather than the direct effects of the mediators released by mast cells and other cells at early intervals after antigen challenge (reviewed in Galli and Lichtenstein, 1988; Lemanske and Kaliner, 1988). Several lines of evidence derived from both clinical and animal studies suggested that the leukocyte infiltration associated with LPRs occurs as a result of mast cell degranulation. On the other hand, several other potential effector cells, including basophils, lymphocytes, monocytes, platelets, and perhaps eosinophils, also represent potential sources of proinflammatory mediators in IgE-dependent responses.

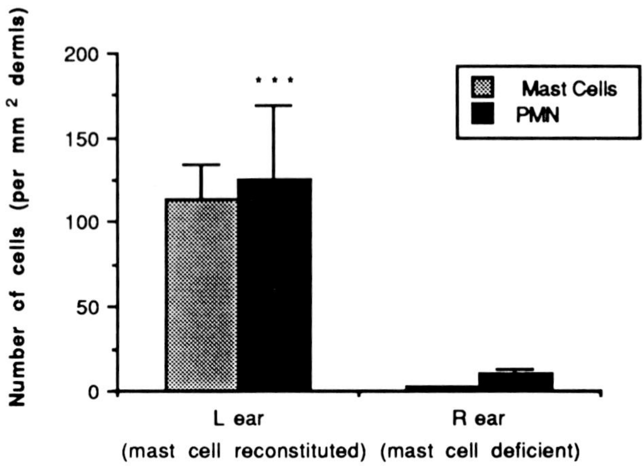

Figure 6 The neutrophil infiltration associated with IgE-dependent cutaneous reactions in the mouse is mast cell–dependent. The total numbers of mast cells and neutrophils were measured in the mast cell–reconstituted left (L) and mast cell–deficient right (R) ears of WBB6F$_1$-*W*/*W*^{v} mice that > 10 weeks earlier underwent local reconstitution of the left ear with WBB6F$_1$-+/+ BMCMC. Data are from the same mice shown in Figure 5, in which IgE had been injected into both ears 1 day before antigen challenge (mean ± SEM). (From Wershil et al., 1991a).

B. Role of TNF-α in IgE- and Mast Cell–Dependent Leukocyte Infiltration

The study of Wershil et al. (1991a) indicates that, in the mouse, the tissue swelling and leukocyte infiltration associated with cutaneous LPRs are indeed mast cell–dependent. This model system also provided an opportunity to investigate potential mechanisms by which mast cells might recruit leukocytes to LPRs. As reviewed in detail in Wershil et al. (1991a), the influx of leukocytes into sites of mast cell degranulation might reflect the actions of several mast cell–derived mediators, including products of arachidonic acid oxidation, chemotactic peptides or proteins, and/or several different cytokines. Burd et al. (1989) and Gordon and Galli (1990a) showed that upon activation via the Fc$_\epsilon$RI, IL-3-dependent or -independent cloned mouse mast cells developed increased levels of mRNA for at least six cytokines with demonstrated or potential ability to elicit leukocyte infiltration: TNF-α, IL-1α, MIP-1α, MIP-1β, TCA3, and JE. IgE-dependent activation of cloned mouse mast cells also resulted in the release of bioactivity for TNF-α (Gordon and Galli, 1990a) and IL-1 (Burd et al., 1989).

However, studies of cytokine production by the populations of mature mouse mast cells that participate in expressions of biological responses in vivo have been very limited. Indeed, the only detailed studies of cytokine production by mature mouse mast cells have focused on TNF-α. Young et al. (1987) demonstrated that mouse peritoneal mast cells contained a cytolytic activity with immunological and functional similarities to TNF-α. Gordon and Galli (1990a) demonstrated that the TNF-α-like cytolytic activity of mouse mast cells represented a product of the TNF-α gene, and that freshly isolated mouse peritoneal mast cells constitutively contained, on a per cell basis, approximately twice as much TNF-α bioactivity as do mouse peritoneal macrophages stimulated with LPS. Moreover, Gordon and Galli (1991) demonstrated that IgE-dependent activation of both in vitro–derived mast cells and freshly isolated peritoneal mast cells resulted in the rapid release of preformed stores of TNF-α followed by the synthesis and sustained release of large quantities of newly formed TNF-α.

TNF-α can be produced by many cell types besides the mast cell, including monocytes/macrophages, T cells, B cells, and neutrophils (reviewed in Beutler and Cerami, 1989; Gordon and Galli, 1990a; Gordon et al., 1990). However, in mouse skin, challenge with IgE and specific antigen results in much higher levels of TNF-α mRNA when mast cells are present than when these cells are absent. Gordon and Galli (1991) injected an anti-DNP mouse monoclonal IgE into the skin of normal mice, W/W^v mice, and mast cell–reconstituted, genetically mast cell–deficient W/W^v mice. The next day, $DNP_{30-40}HSA$ was injected intravenously and 45 min later, the reaction sites were harvested for Northern analysis. This study demonstrated that challenge with specific antigen induced substantially higher levels of TNF-α mRNA at skin sites containing mast cells than at identically challenged sites in mast cell–deficient W/W^v mice that were devoid of mast cells (Fig. 7).

Taken together, the in vitro and in vivo studies of Gordon and Galli (1991) indicate that mast cells probably represent a biologically significant source of TNF-α during IgE-dependent responses and define a mechanism whereby stimulation of mast cells via the $Fc_\epsilon RI$ can account for both the rapid release of preformed stores of the cytokine and the sustained release of newly synthesized product. We have proposed that these experiments also identify TNF-α as the first of a newly recognized class of mast cell–associated mediators (Gordon and Galli, 1991). Mast cell–associated mediators classically are divided into the preformed mediators, which are stored in the cells' cytoplasmic granules and are released upon exocytosis, and the newly synthesized mediators, which are not stored but are produced and secreted only after appropriate stimulation of the cells (Metcalfe et al., 1981; Schwartz and Austen, 1984; Galli and Lichtenstein, 1988). However, mast cells activated via the $Fc_\epsilon RI$ release TNF-α with a prolonged kinetics that reflects the contributions of both preformed and newly synthesized pools of product (Gordon and Galli, 1991).

Given the many potential mechanisms by which mast cells might influence leukocyte infiltration in LPRs, we were interested in determining the extent to

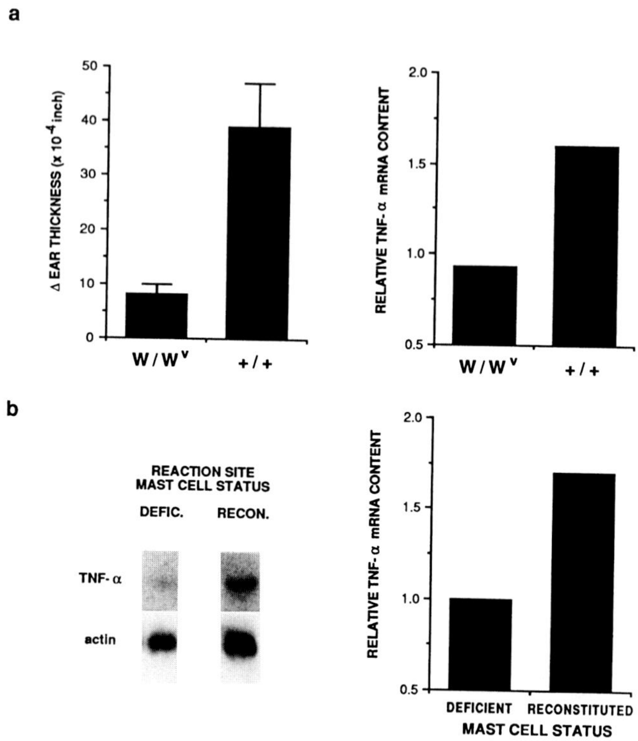

Figure 7 TNF-α mRNA induction following specific immunological challenge of IgE-sensitized skin in mice is mast cell–dependent. (a) Left panel, IgE-dependent dermal inflammatory responses in IgE-sensitized skin of genetically mast cell–deficient WBB6F$_1$-*W/W^v* (*W/W^v*) mice or the congenic normal WBB6F$_1$-+/+ (+/+) mice, as measured by ear swelling 30 min following intravenous antigen challenge. Right panel, relative TNF-α mRNA levels 45 min after antigen challenge in biopsies of cutaneous reaction sites obtained from the *W/W^v* and +/+ mice shown in the left panel, as determined by laser densitometric scanning of Northern blot autoradiographs. The levels of actin mRNA in the biopsies were used as internal standards to control for RNA loading on the Northern blots (see Gordon and Galli, 1991). (b) Mast cell reconstitution of one ear of *W/W^v* mice repairs the defect in IgE-dependent TNF-α mRNA in the mast cell–reconstituted ears, but not in the contralateral, mast cell–deficient ears. Left panel, Northern blot analysis of the TNF-α and actin mRNA levels within reaction sites in mast cell–deficient (Defic.) ears and the contralateral mast cell–reconstituted (Recon.) ears of *W/W^v* mice (~5 μg of olig-dT-selected mRNA/lane). Right panel, graphic presentation of relative TNF-α mRNA levels in the mast cell-deficient and mast cell–reconstituted reaction sites, as determined by laser densitometric analysis of the Northern blot in the left panel. As in (a), the relative TNF-α mRNA content was corrected for variation in mRNA loading, by reference to the actin signals. (From Gordon and Galli, 1991.)

which TNF-α might contribute to this aspect of the reaction. We therefore tested the ability of a polyclonal rabbit anti-TNF-α antiserum to interfere with the development of inflammation at sites of IgE-dependent cutaneous mast cell activation (Wershil et al., 1991a). The rabbit antibody used in this study had been raised against recombinant mouse TNF-α and was able to inhibit completely the cytotoxicity of either recombinant mouse TNF-α or mast cell–derived TNF-α against L929 cells in vitro (Gordon and Galli, 1990a). In addition, this antibody was able to inhibit by ~84% the neutrophil infiltration induced by the intradermal injection of recombinant mouse TNF-α into the skin of normal mice (Wershil et al., 1991a). When compared to the effect of similar dilutions of normal rabbit serum, the rabbit anti-TNF-α was able to diminish by 47 ± 7% the neutrophil infiltration measured 6 hr after elicitation of IgE-dependent cutaneous mast cell activation in the skin of normal mice (Fig. 8).

Notably, our anti-TNF-α antiserum was more effective at diminishing the leukocyte infiltration elicited by recombinant mouse TNF-α than that observed after mast cell activation (Wershil et al., 1991a). One possible explanation for this difference is that the intradermally injected recombinant mouse TNF-α was more accessible to the antiserum than was endogenous TNF-α of mast cell

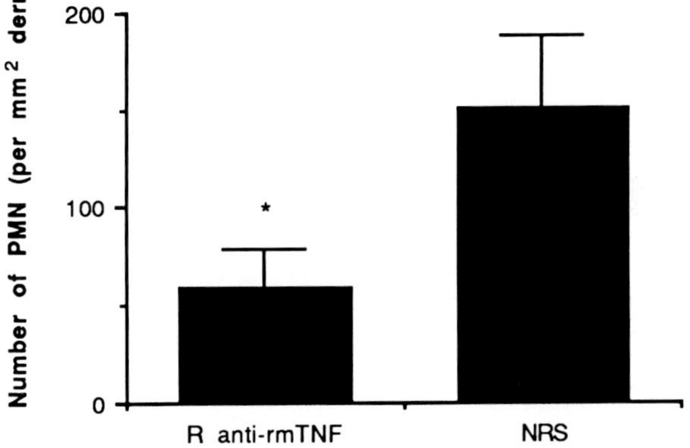

Figure 8 Inhibition of the neutrophil infiltration associated with IgE-dependent reactions by a rabbit anti-recombinant mouse TNF-α antiserum (R anti-rm TNF). Both ears of C57BL/6 mice were injected with IgE anti-DNP antibodies. The next day the left ears were injected with 20 μl of a 1 : 100 dilution of R anti-rm TNF antiserum and the right ears were injected with 20 μl of a 1 : 100 dilution of normal rabbit serum (NRS) in the same vehicle. The mice were immediately challenged with $DNP_{30\text{-}40}$-HSA i.v. and sacrificed 6 hr later for measurement of neutrophil infiltration. Data represent mean ± SEM ($n = 8$). Significant differences between the left and right ears are shown as $*p < 0.05$. (From Wershil et al., 1991a).

origin. In mouse mast cells generated in vitro, a significant fraction of the TNF-α bioactivity is associated with the cells' cytoplasmic granules (Young et al., 1987). If the same is true for dermal mast cells, the physical association of TNF-α with other components of the mast cell granule may have limited the antiserum's access to the cytokine. Moreover, the recombinant mouse TNF-α was given as a single injection, whereas mast cells activated via the $Fc_{\epsilon}RI$ in vitro release TNF-α over a prolonged period after stimulation (Gordon and Galli, 1991).

Our findings thus support the hypothesis that TNF-α contributes to the mast cell–dependent leukocyte infiltration associated with cutaneous LPRs. This result is not surprising, in light of many studies demonstrating that TNF-α can promote leukocyte infiltration by effects on both vascular endothelial cells and leukocytes (reviewed in Pober, 1987; Bevilacqua et al., 1987; Beutler and Cerami, 1989). Moreover, using an organ culture system, Klein et al. (1989) demonstrated that IgE-dependent activation of human foreskin mast cells resulted in the expression of a TNF-α–inducible leukocyte adherence molecule (ELAM-1) on adjacent vascular endothelial cells. Klein et al. (1989) also demonstrated that antibodies to TNF-α inhibited the development of augmented expression of ELAM-1 in tissue fragments challenged with agents to induce mast cell activation. Although the cellular source of the TNF-α responsible for the augmented ELAM-1 expression observed in this model system was not initially identified, recent work by this group has demonstrated the presence of both immunoreactive TNF-α and TNF-α mRNA in human skin mast cells (Walsh et al., 1991). These findings support the possibility that mast cell–derived TNF-α may contribute to the leukocyte infiltration observed in IgE-dependent cutaneous LPRs in humans.

Recent data raise the possibility that mast cell–derived TNF-α may also contribute to LPRs expressed in human lung. We have provided preliminary evidence that purified human lung mast cells can release TNF-α upon stimulation via the $Fc_{\epsilon}RI$ (Gordon et al., 1991). And Wegner et al. (1990) showed in a primate model of asthma that a monoclonal antibody to intercellular adhesion molecule (ICAM-1), a leukocyte adherence structure whose expression on the surface of vascular endothelial cells can be augmented by IL-1, TNF-α, or IFN-γ, attenuated both airway eosinophilia and airway hyperresponsiveness.

On the other hand, it is unlikely that TNF-α is the sole mediator by which mast cells influence leukocyte recruitment. Indeed, several mast cell products, acting alone or perhaps in concert with mediators from other cells that are recruited to these reactions, may contribute to the leukocyte infiltration that follows IgE-dependent mast cell activation. This possibility represents another explanation for the inability of our anti-TNF-α antibody to block completely the leukocyte infiltration at sites of IgE-dependent skin reactions (Wershil et al., 1991a). This possibility is also supported by the work of Leung et al. (1991), who analyzed the augmented expression of ELAM-1 by vascular endothelial cells at sites of intradermal antigen challenge of the skin in vivo, or in skin organ cultures challenged with allergen in vitro. The in vivo studies demonstrated that augmented ELAM-1 expression occurred concomitantly with the appearance of leukocyte infiltrates 3–4 hr after intradermal challenge in all atopic patients tested but in only one of four apparently normal controls. However, inhibition of the allergen-induced augmented ELAM-1 expression that was observed in the organ culture system required simultaneous treatment with antisera to both TNF-α and IL-1.

C. Mast Cell–Leukocyte Cytokine Cascades in IgE-Dependent and Other Inflammatory Responses

While the evidence indicating that mast cells represent a significant source of many multifunctional cytokines is steadily increasing (reviewed in Gordon et al., 1990; Galli et al., 1991a), it would be misleading to discuss mast cell cytokine production without emphasizing that the mast cell represents just one among many potential sources of these biologically active compounds. In certain IgE-dependent responses, including some of those elicited in the skin, mast cells may represent the most significant initial source of multifunctional cytokines. But as these reactions evolve, additional sources of cytokines may be activated and/or recruited. For example, the neutrophils that are recruited to certain mast cell–dependent responses may represent a source of additional TNF-α (reviewed in Galli et al., 1991a). By contrast, other leukocytes recruited to sites of mast cell activation may represent sources of cytokines not produced in significant quantities by the mast cell itself.

We recently reported that hamster and human eosinophils represent a source of TGF-α mRNA and product, whereas the mat cells in these sites were negative for TGF-α (Elovic et al., 1990; Wong et al., 1990). TGF-α has a number of biological actions, such as the promotion of epithelial cell proliferation, which might contribute to some of the pathological changes associated with chronic allergic reactions. For example, eosinophil-derived TGF-α may contribute to the bronchial epithelial proliferation observed in patients with allergic asthma and to the epidermal proliferation that can develop at sites of chronic atopic dermatitis (reviewed in Wong et al., 1990; Galli et al., 1991a). Eosinophils probably can produce a number of cytokines in addition to TGF-α. Recently, we found that the eosinophils of patients with blood eosinophilia due to the idiopathic hypereosinophilic syndrome, Job's syndrome, or drug-related hypersensitivity express both TGF-β_1 mRNA and immunoreactive TGF-β_1 product (Wong et al., 1991). TGF-β_1 is a multifunctional cytokine with potent effects on the extracellular matrix, suggesting that eosinophil-derived TGF-β_1 may importantly contribute to the interstitial fibrosis observed in many settings associated with eosinophil infiltration of tissues, including the subbasement membrane fibrosis characteristics of allergic asthma (reviewed in Wong et al., 1991).

It is likely that mast cell-derived cytokines, and cytokines derived from neutrophils, eosinophils, and other recruited leukocytes, participate importantly in a wide range of biological responses beyond those associated with IgE. Indeed, we feel that the pathogenesis of IgE-dependent reactions and many other mast cell–associated responses may be importantly influenced by a complex sequence of events that we have termed a mast cell–leukocyte cytokine cascade (Gordon et al., 1990; Galli et al., 1991a). According to this hypothesis, certain critical features of the reactions are initiated by mast cell–derived cytokines whereas later aspects of the reaction are critically regulated by cytokine activities derived from leukocytes recruited to the reaction site. The studies outlined briefly above indicate that mast cell–deficient and congenic normal mice, and W/W^v mice locally repaired of their dermal mast cell deficiency, represent excellent model systems in which to investigate the roles of mast cell–leukocyte cytokine cascades in the initiation, progression, and perhaps resolution of IgE-dependent responses and other biological reactions elicited in the skin. In theory, similar approaches can be taken to investigate mast cell function, and mast cell–leukocyte cytokine cascades, in other anatomical sites as well. For example, Qureshi and Jakschik (1988) injected +/+ BMCMC i.p. to investigate the role of mast cells in intraperitoneal inflammation, and Wershil et al. (1991b) reported that local reconstitution of gastric mast cell populations in W/W^v mice can be achieved by the direct injection of +/+ BMCMC into the stomach wall.

D. Role of Mast Cells in IgE-Dependent Resistance to the Feeding of Ticks and in Reactions to Substance P

All the available evidence indicates that the expression of IgE-dependent passive cutaneous anaphylaxis or IgE-dependent cutaneous LPRs in the mouse depends entirely on the presence of dermal mast cells. The mast cells' role in these reactions can thus be characterized as "essential," in that no detectable reactions occur in the absence of this cell type. Mast cell–reconstituted W/W^v mice also have been used to analyze several other biological responses. Only a few of these may represent additional examples of responses in which the role of the mast cell is essential. Thus, IgE-dependent resistance to the cutaneous feeding of larval *Haemaphysalis longicornis* ticks requires the presence of dermal mast cells (Matsuda et al., 1987, 1990), as does the leukocyte infiltration observed when substance P is injected either into subcutaneous air chambers (Matsuda et al., 1989) or directly into the skin (Yano et al., 1989). Recruitment of granulocytes at sites of substance P administration requires relatively high doses of the compound, whereas much smaller quantities elicit augmented vascular permeability, tissue swelling, and deposition of cross-linked ^{125}I-fibrin (Yano et al., 1989); all these consequences of intradermal administration of substance P also appear to require the presence of a population of dermal mast cells (Matsuda et al., 1989; Yano et al., 1989).

The studies of the role of mast cells in resistance to the feeding of *H. longicornis* ticks and in inflammatory responses to substance P can be used to make two different, but equally important, points concerning experiments conducted with mast cell–reconstituted *W/W^v* mice. The first is that this approach represents a powerful and versatile way to ask specific questions concerning mast cell function in vivo. The second is that one should be cautious about using the results of these experiments to draw overly broad conclusions about mast cell biology. For example, the studies of immune resistance to the feeding of *H. longicornis* ticks represent the strongest evidence yet available that the mast cell can be critical to the expression of an IgE-dependent host response that confers actual benefit to the host. But this finding does not prove that mast cells are important in all forms of host immunity to parasite infection. Indeed, many studies of the responses of normal, mast cell–deficient, and bone marrow– or mast cell–reconstituted *W/W^v* mice infected with various internal parasites have not yet produced a clear picture of the role of the mast cell in the responses (reviewed in Reed, 1989; Wershil et al., 1989). There is no question that some of these reactions are associated with striking mast cell hyperplasia at sites of infection in the gut, and that in some of the responses, extensive mast cell activation occurs in association with expulsion of the parasites. Yet, for some parasites, there is little or no impairment of host resistance in the mast cell–deficient animals; for other parasites, host resistance is abnormal in the *W/W^v* animals, but it is not clear that this is due to the mast cell deficiency of the mutants.

Even in the case of resistance to ectoparasites, such as ticks, the importance of the mast cell as an effector of host resistance may vary according to the species of parasite. For example, *W/W^v* mice exhibit resistance to the feeding of larval *Dermacentor variabilis* ticks that may be only slightly impaired compared to that observed in the congenic normal (+/+) mice (den Hollander and Allen, 1985; Steeves and Allen, 1990). *W/W^v* mice have basophils (Jacoby et al., 1984), and many basophils are detected at cutaneous feeding sites of *D. variabilis* larvae in both *W/W^v* and +/+ mice (Steeves and Allen, 1990). Basophils represent an alternative effector cell that can participate in IgE-dependent responses in mice. Moreover, basophils appear to be required for the expression of immune resistance to the cutaneous finding of *Amblyomma americanum* larval ticks in the guinea pig (Brown et al., 1982). In mice, it is possible that immune resistance to the feeding of certain species of ticks reflects an essential contribution by cutaneous mast cells, whereas, for other species of ticks, the basophil plays a more important role.

In the case of substance P, the importance of the mast cells' contribution may depend on the route of administration of the agonist. When substance P was administered intradermally, we found that virtually all the effects of substance P on tissue swelling, vascular permeability, and granulocyte infiltration were mast cell–dependent (Yano et al., 1989). For example, injection of as little as 2 pmol of substance P into +/+ mice caused significant cutaneous swelling, whereas injection of up to 2500× larger doses (5 nmol) of substance P into the skin of genetically mast cell–deficient W/W^v or Sl/Sl^d mice produced effects not significantly different than those observed after injection of vehicle alone. These findings support the hypothesis that release of endogenous substance P can induce mast cell activation and mast cell–dependent inflammation, at least under some circumstances (reviewed in Yano et al., 1989).

However, our experiments did not directly evaluate the effects of the release of endogenous substance P on the mast cell. Nor do our findings rule out the possibility that other effects of substance P can be mediated independently of the mast cell. Indeed, evidence has already been reported that indicates that certain of the effects of substance P on the vasculature are mast cell–independent. For example, Kowalski and Kaliner (1988) showed that electrical stimulation can induce an apparently mast cell–independent augmentation of vascular permeability in the rat, which is detected within a few minutes after stimulation. The procedure we employed in our studies was not well suited for identifying neuropeptide-dependent changes induced within a few minutes of challenge, since the intradermal injection of 20 μl of fluid itself causes an increase in ear thickness during this interval. Kowalski et al. (1990) later showed that W/W^v and +/+ mice exhibit indistinguishable alterations in vascular permeability in response to intravenous substance P. Recently, we have confirmed that, at certain doses, substance P administered intravenously induces alterations of vacular permeability and deposition of cross-linked ^{125}I-fibrin that are not significantly different in normal and mast cell–deficient mice (Takeishi, Wershil, and Galli, unpublished data). These latter observations are compatible with the finding that the vasodilatory effects of intra-arterial substance P in human skin, unlike the effects introduced by intradermal administration of the peptide, are not inhibited by antihistamines (reviewed in Yano et al., 1989).

Taken together, these studies indicate that the extent to which the vascular effects of substance P are mast cell–dependent may be critically influenced by the route of administration of the peptide. Thus, intravenous or intra-arterial administration favors direct interactions with vascular endothelial cells, whereas intradermal injection facilitates interactions with interstitial elements such as mast cells. Further, it should be appreciated that the reactions induced by substance P, and other neuropeptides that can activate mast cells, are likely to be under complex regulatory control in vivo. The effects observed in particular organs or tissues will depend on such factors as the concentration of the endogenous neuropeptide that might be achieved in the immediate vicinity of its release, the proximity of mast cells to sites of neuropeptide release, the sensitivity of that particular mast cell population to direct or indirect activation by neuropeptide-dependent mechanisms, and the local distribution and activity of enzymes capable of degrading the neuropeptides. Many, perhaps all, of these factors exhibit considerable species and anatomical variation (reviewed in Yano et al., 1989).

Nevertheless, the findings of Yano et al. (1989) indicate that virtually all of substance P's ability to elicit cutaneous swelling and leukocyte infiltration on intradermal injection into mouse skin is mast cell–dependent. This result, taken together with evidence indicating that human cutaneous mast cells are particularly sensitive to stimulation by substance P (reviewed in Yano et al., 1989), suggests that the wheal component of the response to intradermal injection of substance P in human skin might reflect in part mast cell–dependent effects of the peptide, not solely the direct actions of substance P on the vasculature.

X. The Use of Mast Cell–Reconstituted *W/W^v* Mice to Evaluate the Contribution of Mast Cells to Reactions Which Can Be Detectably Expressed in Mast Cell–Deficient Mice

The group of biological responses in which mast cells make an important but nonessential contribution is probably much larger than the set of reactions in which the role of the mast cell is essential. For example, a variety of inflammatory responses can be elicited in the tissues of mast cell–deficient mice, but the intensity of these responses, and/or the rates of their development, may be significantly augmented when mast cells are present. In reactions such as these, the mature mast cell represents an important effector cell, yet cannot be considered essential for the development of the reaction. In other biological responses, studies with mast cell–deficient and mast cell–reconstituted W/W^v mice detected no significant mast cell–dependent contribution at all. Table 6 summarizes the results of several studies in which mast cell–reconstituted mice were used to evaluate the specific roles of mast cells in individual biological responses.

While each study listed in Table 6 addressed a number of interesting aspects of mast cell function, a few points established by this work merit emphasis. First, it may be difficult to use data derived from in vitro studies to predict the results of direct tests of mast cell function in vivo. In the case of the acute inflammation induced by the epicutaneous application of phorbol 12-myristate 13-acetate (PMA), we found that the magnitude of the tissue swelling and leukocyte infiltration associated with the reactions in normal or mast cell-

Table 6 Roles of Mast Cells in Biological Responses, as Determined by Studies with Mast Cell–Deficient and Congenic Normal Mice and W/W^v Mice Locally Repaired of Their Mast Cell Deficiency by Injection of +/+ BMCMC

Biological response	Anatomical site	Findings
I. Mast cells essential for the response		
IgE-dependent inflammation	Skin	Mast cells required for both early and late phases of tissue swelling, ^{125}I-fibrin deposition, and leukocyte infiltration (Wershil et al., 1987; Wershil et al., 1991a)
IgE-dependent resistance to the feeding of larval *Haemaphysalis longicornis* ticks	Skin	Mast cells required for expression of resistance to feeding of larval ticks (Matsuda et al., 1987, 1990)
IgE-dependent inflammation	Stomach	Mast cells required for ^{125}I-fibrin deposition and leukocyte infiltration (Wershil et al., 1991b)
Substance P–induced inflammation	Skin	Mast cells required for tissue swelling, ^{125}I-fibrin deposition, and leukocyte infiltration induced by i.e. injection substance P into skin (Yano et al., 1989). and for eosinophil infiltration induced by injection of substance P into subcutaneous air chambers (Matsuda et al., 1989), but not for increased vascular permeability induced by i.v. administration of substance P (Kowalski et al., 1990; Takeishi, Wershil, and Galli, unpublished data)

II. Mast cells augment aspects of the response		
Inflammation induced by epicutaneous phorbol 12-myristate 13-acetate	Skin	Mast cells increase the tissue swelling and leukocye infiltration associated with the response (Wershil et al., 1988)
Inflammation induced by thioglycollate	Peritoneal cavity	Mast cells increase the rate of development and the duration of leukocyte infiltration, but do not affect the peak levels of leukocytes in the exudate (Qureshi and Jakschik, 1988)
Inflammation induced by immune complexes	Peritoneal cavity	Mast cells increase the rate of development and magnitude of leukocyte infiltration (Ramos et al., 1990)
Angiogenesis associated with growth of B16-BL6 melanoma	Skin	Mast cells increase rate, but not magnitude, of blood vessel growth, as judged by quantification of blood vessels in ears transilluminated at various intervals after local injection of tumor cells (Starkey et al., 1988).
III. Mast cells do not detectably contribute to the response		
T-cell–dependent contact sensitivity	Skin	Mast cells do not detectably affect the tissue swelling, ^{125}I-fibrin deposition, or leukocyte infiltration associated with the response (Mekori et al., 1987, and see text).

References

Abe, T., and Nawa, Y. (1988). Worm explusion and mucosal mast cell response induced by repetitive IL3 administration in *Strongyloides ratti* infected nude mice. *Immunology*, 63:181–185.

Abe, T., Ochiai, H., Mimamishima, Y., and Nawa, Y. (1988). Induction of intestinal mastocytosis in nude mice by repeated injection of interleukin-3. *Int. Arch. Allergy Appl. Immunol.* 86:356–358.

Alizadeh, H., and Murrell, K. D. (1984). The intestinal mast cell response to *Trichinella spiralis* infection in mast cell-deficient W/W^v mice. *J. Parasitol.* 70:767–773.

Aloe, J., and Levi-Montalcini, R. (1977). Mast cells increase in tissue of neonatal rats injected with the nerve growth factor. *Brain Res.* 133:358–366.

Anderson, D. M., Lyman, S. D., Baird, A., Wignall, J. M., Eisenman, J., Rauch, C., March, C. J., Boswell, H. S., Gimpel, S. D., Cosman, D., and Williams, D. E. (1990). Molecular cloning of mast cell growth factor, a hematopoietin that is active in both membrane bound and soluble forms. *Cell* 63:235–243.

Andre, C., d'Auriol, L., Lacombe, C., Gisselbrecht, S., and Galibert, F. (1989). *c-kit* mRNA expression in human and murine hematopoietic cell lines. *Oncogene* 4:1047–1048.

Arizono, N., Koreto, O., Nakao, S., Iwai, Y., Kushima, R., and Takeoka, O. (1987). Phenotypic changes in mast cells proliferating in the rat lung following infection with *Nippostrongylus brasiliensis*. *Virchows Arch. B* 154:1–7.

Arizono, N., Shiota, Y., Yamada, M., Matsumoto, Y., Yoshikawa, H., Matsuda, S., and Tegoshi, T. (1990). Bromodeoxyuridine labeling studies on the proliferation of intestinal mucosal mast cells in normal and athymic rats. *APMIS* 98:369–376.

Ashman, R. I., Jarboe, D. L., Conrad, D. H., and Huff, T. F. (1991). The mast cell committed progenitor—In vitro generation of committed progenitors from bone marrow. *J. Immunol.* 146:211–216.

Askenase, P. W., Van Loveren, H., Kraueter-Kops, S., Yacov, Y., Meade, R., Theoharides, T. C., Nordlung, J. J., Scovern, H., Gershon, M. D., and Ptak, W. (1983). Defective elicitation of delayed-type hypersensitivity in W/W^v and Sl/Sl^d mast cell–deficient mice. *J. Immunol.* 131:2687–2894.

Bazan, F. (1991). Genetic and structural homology of stem cell factor and macrophage colony-stimulating factor. *Cell* 65:9–10.

Bernstein, A., Chabot, B., Dubreuil, P., Reith, A., Nocka, K., Majumder, S., Ray, P., and Besmer, P. (1989). The mouse *W*/c-*kit* locus. *CIBA Found. Symp.* 148:158–172.

Besmer, P., Murphy, J. E., George, P. C., Qiu, F., Bergold, P. J., Lederman, L., Snyder, H. W., Jr., Brodeur, D., Zuckerman, E. E., and Hardy, W. D. (1986). A new acute transforming feline retrovirus and relationship of its oncogene *v-kit* with the proetin kinase gene family. *Nature* 320:415–421.

Beutler, B., and Cerami, A. (1989). The biology of cachectin/TNF - α primary mediator of the host response. *Annu. Rev. Immunol.* 7:625–655.

Bevilacqua, M. P., Wheeler, M. E., Pober, J. S., Fiers, W., Mendrick, D. L., Cotran, R. S., and Gimbrone, M. A., Jr. (1987). Endothelial-dependent mechanisms of leukocyte adhesion: regulation by interleukin 1 and tumor necrosis factor. In *Leukocyte Emigration and Its Sequellae*. Edited by H. Z. Movat. New York, S. Karger, pp. 79–93.

Bland, C. E., Ginsburg, H., Silbert, J. E., and Metcalfe, D. D. (1982). Mouse heparin proteoglycan. Synthesis by mast cell-fibroblast monolayers during lymphocyte-dependent mast cell proliferation. *J. Biol. Chem.* 257:8661–8666.

Boxer, L. A. (1990). Qualitative abnormalities of neutrophils. In *Hematology*, 4th ed. Edited by W. J. Williams, E. Beutler, A. J. Erslev, and M. A. Lichtman. New York, McGraw-Hill, pp. 821–839.

Bressler, R. B., Thompson, H. L., Keffer, J. M., and Metcalfe, D. (1989). Inhibition of the growth of IL-3-dependent mast cells from murine bone marrow by recombinant granulocyte-macrophage colony-stimulating factor. *J. Immunol.* 143:135–139.

Brody, J. (1982). Diamond-Blackfan syndrome in a father and son. *Aust. Pediatr. J.* 18:128–129.

Brown, S. J., Galli, S. J., Gleich, G. J., and Askenase, P. W. (1982). Ablation of immunity to *Amblyomma americanum* by anti-basophil serum: cooperation between basophils and eosinophils in expression of immunity to ectoparasites (ticks) in guinea pigs. *J. Immunol.* 129:790–796.

Burd, P. R., Rogers, H. W., Gordon, J. R., Martin, C. A., Jayaraman, S., Wilson, S. D., Dvorak, A. M., Galli, S. J., and Dorf, M. E. (1989). Interleukin 3-dependent and -independent mast cells stimulated with IgE and antigen express multiple cytokines. *J. Exp. Med.* 170:245–257.

Capron, A., Capron, M., Grangette, C., and Dessaint, J. P. (1989). IgE and inflammatory cells. In *IgE, Mast Cells and the Allergic Response. Ciba Foundation Symposium No. 147*. Edited by D. Chadwick, D. Evered, and J. Whelan. Chichester, UK, Wiley, pp. 153–170.

Chabot, B., Stephenson, D. A., Chapman, V. M., Besmer, P., and Bernstein, A. (1988). The protooncogene c-kit encoding a transmembrane tyrosine kinase receptor maps to the mouse *W* locus. *Nature* 335:88–89.

Chi, E. Y., and Lagunoff, D. (1975). Abnormal mast cell granules in the beige (Chediak-Higashi syndrome) mouse. *J. Histochem. Cytochem.* 23:117–122.

Copeland, N. G., Gilbert, D. J., Cho, B. C., Donovan, P. J., Jenkins, N. A., Cosman, D., Anderson, D., Lyman, S. D., and Williams, D. E. (1990). Mast cell growth gactor maps near the steel locus on mouse chromosome 10 and is deleted in a number of steel alleles. *Cell* 63:175–183.

Crowle, P. K., and Reed, N. D. (1984) Bone marrow origin of mucosal mast cells. *Int. Arch. Allergy Appl. Immunol.* 73:242–247.

Davidson, S., Kinarty, A., Coleman, R., Reshef, A., and Ginsburg, H. (1986). Fibroblasts are required for mast cell granule synthesis. In *Mast Cell Differentiation and Heterogeneity*. Edited by A. D. Befus, J., Bienenstock, and J. A. Denburg. New York, Raven Press, pp. 115–124.

den Hollander, N., and Allen, J. R. (1985). *Dermacentor variabilis*: Resistance to ticks acquired by mast cell-deficient and other strains of mice. *Exp. Parasitol.* 59:169–179.

Dexter, T. M., and Moore, M. A. S. (1977). In vitro duplication of and "cure" of haemopoietic defects in genetically anemic mice. *Nature* 269:412–414.

Diamond, L. K., Allen, D. M., and Magill, F. B. (1961). Congenital (erythroid) hypoplastic anemia. *Am. J. Dis. Child.* 102:403–415.

Dubreuil, P., Forrester, L., Rottapel, R., Reedijk, M., Fujita, J., and Bernstein, A. (1991). The c-*fms* gene complements the mitogenic defect in mast cells derived from mutant *W*, but not *mi* (*microphthalmia*), mice. *Proc. Natl. Acad. Sci. USA* 88:2341–2345.

Ebi, Y., Kasugai, T., Seino, Y., Onoue, H., and Kanemoto, T., Kitamura, Y. (1990). Mechanism of mast cell deficiency in mutant mice of mi/mi genotype—An analysis by co-culture of mast cells and fibroblasts. *Blood* 75:1247–1251.

Elovic, A., Galli, S. J., Weller, P. F., Chang, A. L. C., Chiang, T., Chou, M. Y., Donoff, R. B., Gallagher, G. T., Matossian, K., McBride, J., Tsai, M., Todd, R., and Wong, D. T. W. (1990). Production of transforming growth factor-alpha by hamster eosinophils. *Am. J. Pathol.* 137:1425–1434.

Enerbäck, L. (1974). Berberine sulphate binding to mast cell polyanions: A cytofluorometric method for the quantitation of herparin. *Histochemistry*. 42:301–313.

Enerbäck, L. (1986). Mast cell heterogeneity: The evolution of the concept of a specific mucosal mast cell. In *Mast Cell Differentiation and Heterogeneity*. Edited by A. D. Befus, J. Bienenstock, and J. A. Denburg. New York, Raven Press, pp. 1–26.

Flanagan, J. G., and Leder, P. (1990). The c-*kit* ligand: A cell surface molecule altered in steel mutant fibroblasts. *Cell* 63:185–194.

Flanagan, J. G., Chan, D. C., and Leder, P. (1991). Transmembrane form of the *kit* ligand growth factor is determined by alternative splicing and is missing in the Sl^d mutant. *Cell* 64:1025–1035.

Frankel, S. K., Tsai, M., Gordon, J. R., Iemura, A., Zsebo, K. M., Geissler, E. N., and Galli, S. J. Effects of combinations of the rat c-*kit* ligand, stem cell factor, and other growth factors on the development and characteristics of bone marrow–derived or peritoneal mast cell-derived cultured mouse mast cells in vitro. (in preparation).

Fujita, J., Nakayama, H., Onoue, H., Ebi, Y., Kanakura, Y., Kuriu, A., and Kitamura, Y. (1988a). Failure of W/W^v mouse-derived cultured mast cells to enter S phase upon contact with NIH/3T3 fibroblasts. *Blood* 72:463–468.

Fujita, J., Nakayama, H., Onoue, H., Kanakura, Y., Nakano, T., Asai, H., Takeda, S., Honjo, T., and Kitamura, Y. (1988b). Fibroblast-dependent growth of mouse mast cells in vitro: Duplication of mast cell depletion in mutant mice of W/W^v genotype. *J. Cell. Physiol.* 134:78–84.

Fujita, J., Onoue, H., Ebi, Y., Nakayama, H., and Kanakura, Y. (1989). In vitro duplication and in vivo cure of mast-cell deficiency of Sl/Sl^d mutant mice by cloned 3T3 fibroblasts. *Proc. Natl. Acad. Sci. USA* 86:2888–2891.

Funderbuck, S. J., and Crandall, B. F. (1974). Dominant piebald trait in a retarded child with a reciprocal translocation and a small intercalary deletion. *Hum. Genet.* 26:715–722.

Furitsu, T., Saito, H., Dvorak, A. M., Schwartz, L. B., Irani, A. M., Burdick, J. F., Ishizaka, K., and Ishizaka, T. (1989). Development of human mast cells in vitro. *Proc. Natl. Acad. Sci, USA* 86:10039–10043.

Galli, S. J. (1987). New approaches for the analysis of mast cell maturation, heterogeneity, and function. *Fed. Proc.* 46:1906–1914.

Galli, S. J. (1990). New insights into "the riddle of the mast cells": Microenvironmental regulation of mast cell development and phenotypic heterogeneity. *Lab. Invest.* 62:5–33.

Galli, S. J., and Dvorak, A. M. (1984). What do mast cells have to do with delayed hypersensitivity? *Lab. Invest.* 50:365–368 (editorial).

Galli, S. J., and Hammel, I. (1984). Unequivocal delayed hypersensitivity in mast cell–deficient and beige mice. *Science* 226:710–713.

Galli, S. J., and Kitamura, Y. (1987). Animal model of human disease. Genetically mast cell-deficient W/W^v and Sl/Sl^d mice: Their value for the analysis of the roles of mast cells in biological responses in vivo. *Am. J. Pathol.* 127:191–198.

Galli, S. J., and Lichtenstein, L. M. (1988). Biology of mast cells and basophils. In *Allergy: Principles and Practice,* 3rd ed. Edited by E. Middleton, Jr., C. E. Reed, E. F. Ellis, N. F. Adkinson Jr., and J. W. Yuninger. St. Louis, Mosby, pp. 106–134.

Galli, S. J., Dvorak, A. M., Marcum, J. A., Ishizaka, T., Nabel, G., Der Simonian, H., Pyne, K., Goldin, J. M., Rosenberg, R. D., Cantor, H., and Dvorak, H. F. (1982). Mast cell clones: A model for the analysis of cellular maturation. *J. Cell Biol.* 95:435–444.

Galli, S. J., Dvorak, A. M., and Dvorak, H. F. (1984). Basophils and mast cells: Morphologic insights into their biology, secretory patterns and function. *Prog. Allergy* 34:1–141.

Galli, S. J., Arizono, N., Murakami, T., Dvorak, A. M., and Fox, J. G. (1987a). Development of large numbers of mast cells at sites of idiopathic chronic dermatitis in genetically mast cell-deficient $WBB6F_1$-W/W^v mice. *Blood* 69:1661–1666.

Galli, S. J., Wershil, B. K., Bose, R., Walker, P. A., and Szabo, S. (1987b). Ethanol-induced acute gastric injury in mast cell-deficient and congenic normal mice. Evidence that mast cells can augment the area of damage. *Am. J. Pathol.* 128:131–140.

Galli, S. J., Wershil, B. K., Gordon, J. R., and Martin, T. R. (1989a). Mast cells: Immunologically specific effectors and potential sources of multiple cytokines during IgE-dependent responses. In *IgE, Mast Cells and the Allergic Response. Ciba Foundation Symposium No. 147.* Edited by D. Chadwick, D. Evered, and J. Whelan. Chichester, UK, Wiley, pp. 53–73.

Galli, S. J., Wershil, B. K., Yano, H., Arizono, N., Gordon, J. R., and Murakami, T. (1989b). Analysis of the roles of phenotypically distinct mast cell populations in non-immunological responses. In *Mast Cell and Basophil Differentiation and Function in Health and Disease.* Edited by S. J. Galli, and K. F. Austen. New York, Raven Press, pp. 255–273.

Galli, S. J., Gordon, J. R., and Wershil, B. K. (1991a). Cytokine production by mast cells and basophils. *Curr. Opinion Immunol.* 3:865–873.

Galli, S. J., Tsai, M. T., Langley, K. E., Zsebo, K. M., and Geissler, E. N. (1991b). Stem cell factor (SCF), a ligand for *c-kit,* induces mediator release from some populations of mouse mast cells. *FASEB J.* 5:A1092 (abstract).

Geissler, E. N., and Russell, E. S. (1983). Analysis of hematopoietic effects of new dominant spotting (*W*) mutants of the mouse. II. Effects on mast cell development. *Exp. Hematol.* 11:461–466.

Geissler, E. N., McFarland, E. D., and Russell, E. S. (1981). Analysis of pleiotropism at the dominant white-spotting (*W*) locus of the house mouse. *Genetics* 97:337–361.

Geissler, E. N., Cheng, S. V., Gusella, J. F., Housman, D. E. (1988a). Genetic analysis of the dominant white spotting (*W*) region of mouse chromosome 5: Identification of cloned DNA markers near *W*. *Proc. Natl. Acad. Sci. USA* 85:9635–9639.

Geissler, E. N., Ryan, M. A., and Housman, D. E. (1988b). The dominant-white spotting (*W*) mutations of the mouse encodes the c-*kit* protooncogene. *Cell* 55:185–192.

Geissler, E., Gordon, J. R., Tsai, M., and Galli, S. J. (1990). Activation of mast cells down-regulates mRNA for c-*kit* tyrosine kinase receptor. *FASEB J.* 4:A1704 (abstract).

Geissler, E., Liao, M., Brook, J., Martin, F., Zsebo, K., Housman, D., and Galli, S. (1991). Stem cell factor (SCF), a novel hematopoietic growth factor and a ligand for the c-*kit* tyrosine kinase receptor, maps on human chromosome 12 between 12q14.3 and 12qter. *Som. Cell Mol. Gen.* 17:207–214.

Ginsburg, H. (1963). The in vitro differentiation and culture of normal mast cells from mouse thymus. *Am. NY Acad. Sci.* 103:20–39.

Ginsburg, H., Ben-Shahar, D., and Ben-David, E. (1982). Mast cell growth on fibroblast monolayers. Two-cell entities. *Immunology* 45:371–380.

Go, S., Kitamura, Y., and Nishimura, M. (1980). Effect of *W* and W^v alleles on production of tissue mast cells in mice. *J. Hered.* 71:41–44.

Gordon, J. R., and Galli, S. J. (1990a). Mast cells as a source of both preformed and immunologically inducible TNF-α/cachectin. *Nature* 346:274–276.

Gordon, J. R., and Galli, S. J. (1990b). Phorbol 12-myristate 13-acetate-induced development of functionally active mast cells in W/W^v but not Sl/Sl^d genetically mast cell–deficient mice. *Blood* 75:1637–1645.

Gordon, J. R., and Galli, S. J. (1991). Release of both preformed and newly synthesized tumor necrosis factor α (TNF-α)/cachectin by mouse mast cells stimulated by the $Fc_\epsilon RI$. A mechanism for the sustained action of mast cell-derived TNF-α during IgE-dependent biological responses. *J. Exp. Med.* 174:103–107.

Gordon, J. R., Burd, P. R., and Galli, S. J. (1990). Mast cells as a source of multifunctional cytokines. *Immunol. Today* 11:458–464.

Gordon, J. R., Post, T., Schulman, E. S., and Galli, S. J. (1991). Characterization of mouse mast cell TNF-α induction in vitro and in vivo, and demonstration that purified human lung mast cells contain TNF-α. *FASEB J.* 5:A1009 (abstract).

Ha, T.-Y., and Reed, N. D. (1987). Systemic anaphylaxis in mast cell-deficient mice of W/W^v and Sl/Sl^d genotypes. *Exp. Cell. Biol.* 55:63–68.

Ha, T.-Y., Reed, N. D., and Crowle, P. K. (1986). Immune response potential of mast cell-deficient W/W^v mice. *Int. Arch. Allergy Appl. Immunol.* 80:85–94.

Hamaguchi, Y., Kanakura, Y., Fujita, J., Takeda, S.-I., Nakano, T., Tarui, S., Honjo, T., and Kitamura, Y. (1987). Interleukin 4 as an essential factor for in vitro clonal growth of murine connective tissue-type mast cells. *J. Exp. Med.* 165:268–273.

Hammel, I., and Lagunoff, D. (1982). Morphometric analysis of secretory granule formation. *J. Cell Biol.* 95:404a (abstract).

Hammel, I., Lagunoff, D., Bauza, M., and Chi, E. (1983). Periodic, multi-modal distribution of granule volumes in mast cells. *Cell. Tissue Res.* 228:51–59.

Hammel, I., Dvorak, A. M., Peters, S. P., Schulman, E. S., Dvorak, H. F., Lichtenstein, L. M., and Galli, S. J. (1985). Differences in the volume distributions of human lung mast cell granules and lipid bodies: evidence that the size of these organelles is regulated by distinct mechanisms. *J. Cell Biol.* 100:821–839.

Hammel, I., Dvorak, A. M., and Galli, S. J. (1987). Defective cytoplasmic granule formation. I. Abnormalities affecting tissue mast cells and pancreatic acinar cells of beige mice. *Lab. Invest.* 56:321–328.

Hammel, I., Arizono, N., and Galli, S. J. (1991). Mast cells in rat dermis and jejunal lamina propria show a five-fold difference in unit granule volume. *Cell Tissue Res.* 265:329–334.

Hayashi, C., Sonoda, T., Nakano, T., Nakayama, H., and Kitamura, Y. (1985). Mast-cell precursors in the skin of mouse embryos and their deficiency in embryos of *Sl/Sl^d* genotype. *Dev. Biol.* 109:234–241.

Huang, E., Nocka, K., Beier, D. R., Chu, T-Y., Buck, J., Lahm, H-W., Wellner, D., Leder, P., and Besmer, P. (1990). The hematopoietic growth factor KL is encoded at the *Sl* locus and is the ligand of the *c-kit* receptor, the gene product of the *W* locus. *Cell* 63:225–233.

Huntley, J. F., Mackellar, A., Newlands, G. F. J., Irvine, J., and Miller, H. R. (1990). Mapping of the rat mast cell granule proteinaes RMCP I and II by enzyme-linked immunosorbent assay and paired immunofluorescence. *APMIS* 98:933–944.

Ihle, J. N., Keller, J., Oroszlan, S., Henderson, L. E., Copeland, R. D., Fitch, F., Prystowsky, M. B., Goldwasser, E., Schrader, J. W., Palaszynski, E., Dy, M., and Lebel, B. (1983). Biological properties of homogeneous interleukin 3. I. Demonstration of WEHI-3 growth-factor activity, mast cell growth-factor activity, P cell-stimulating factor activity and histamine-producing factor activity. *J. Immunol.* 131:282–287.

Inagaki, N., Goto, S., Nagai, H., and Koda, A. (1986). Homologous passive cutaneous anaphylaxis in various strains of mice. *Int. Arch. Allergy Appl. Immunol.* 81:58–62.

Inoue, F., Hasegawa, H., Nishimura, M., Yanagisawa, M., and Ichiyama, A. (1985). Distribution of 5-hydroxytryptamine (5HT) in tissue of a mutant mouse deficient in mast cell (*W/W^v*). Demonstration of the contribution of mast cells to the 5HT content in various organs. *Agents Actions* 16:295–301.

Ishizaka, T. (1988). Mechanisms of IgE-mediated hypersensitivity. In *Allergy: Principles and Practice,* 3rd ed. Edited by E. Middleton, Jr., C. E. Reed, E. F. Ellis, N. F. Adkinson, Jr., and J. W. Yuninger. St. Louis, Mosby, pp. 71–93.

Jacoby, W., Cammarata, P. V., Findlay, S., and Pincus, S. (1984). Anaphylaxis in mast cell-deficient mice. *J. Invest. Dermatol.* 83:302–304.

Jarboe, D. L., and Huff, T. F. (1989). The mast cell-committed progenitor. II. *W/W^v* mice do not make mast cell-committed progenitors and *Sl/Sl^d* fibroblasts do not support development of normal mast cell-committed progenitors. *J. Immunol.* 7:2418–2423.

Jarboe, D. L., Marshall, J. S., Randolph, T. R., Kukolja, A., and Huff, T. F. (1989). The mast cell-committed progenitor. I. Description of a cell capable of IL-3-independent proliferation and differentiation without contact fibroblasts. *J. Immunol.* 142:2405–2417.

Justice, M. J., Silan, C. M., Ceci, J. D., Buchberg, A. M., Copeland, N. G., and Jenkins, N. A. (1990). A molecular genetic linkage map of mouse chromosome 13 anchored by the beige (*bg*) and satin (*sa*) loci. *Genomics* 6:341–351.

Kanakura, Y., Sonoda, S., Nakano, T., Fujita, J., Kuriu, A., Asai, H., and Kitamura, Y. (1987). Formation of mast-cell colonies in methylcellulose by mouse skin cells and development of mucosal-like mast cells from the cloned cells in the gastric mucosa of W/W^v mice. *Am. J. Pathol.* 129:168–176.

Kanakura, Y., Thompson, H., Nakano, T., Yamamura, T-i., Asai, H., Kitamura, Y., Metcalfe, D. D., and Galli, S. J. (1988). Multiple bidirectional alterations of phenotype and changes in proliferative potential during the in vitro and in vivo passage of clonal mast cell populations derived from mouse peritoneal mast cells. *Blood* 72:877–885.

Kikutani, H., Yokota, A., Uchibayashi, N., Yukawa, K., Tanaka, T., Sugiyama, K., Barsumian, E. L., Suemura, M., and Kishimoto, T. (1989). Structure and function of Fc_ϵ receptor II (Fc_ϵRII/CD23): A point of contact between the effector phase of allergy and B cell differentiation. In *IgE, Mast Cells and the Allergic Response. Ciba Foundation Symposium No. 147.* Edited by D. Chadwick, D. Evered, and J. Whelan. Chichester, UK, Wiley, pp. 23–35.

Kitamura, Y. (1989). Heterogeneity of mast cells and phenotypic changes between subpopulations. *Annu. Rev. Immunol.* 7:59–76.

Kitamura, Y., and Go, S. (1979). Decreased production of mast cells in Sl/Sl^d mice. *Blood* 53:492–497.

Kitamura, Y., Go, S., and Hatanaka, S. (1978). Decrease of mast cells in W/W^v mice and their increase by bone marrow transplantation. *Blood* 52:447–452.

Kitamura, Y., Yokoyama, M., Matsuda, H., Ohno, T., and Mori, K. J. (1981). Spleen colony-forming cell as common precursor for tissue mast cells and granulocytes. *Nature* 291:159–160.

Kitamura, Y., Sonoda, T., Nakano, T., Hayashi, C., and Asai, H. (1985). Differentiation processes of connective tissue mast cells in living mice. *Int. Arch. Allergy Appl. Immunol.* 77:144–150.

Kitamura, Y., Nakayama, H., and Fujita, J. (1989). Mechanism of mast cell deficiency in mutant mice of W/W^v and Sl/Sl^d genotype. In *Mast Cell and Basophil Differentiation and Function in Health and Disease.* Edited by S. J. Galli and K. F. Austen. New York, Raven Press, pp. 15–25.

Klein, L. M., Lavker, R. M., Matis, W. L., and Murphy, G. F. (1989). Degranulation of human mast cells induces an endothelial antigen central to leukocyte adhesion. *Proc. Natl. Acad. Sci. USA* 86:8972–8976.

Kohrogi, T., Yokoyama, M., Taguchi, T., Kitamura, Y., and Tutikawa, K. (1983). Effect of Sl^t mutant allele on production of tissue mast cells in mice. *J. Hered.* 74:375–377.

Kowalski, M. L., and Kaliner, M. A. (1988). Neurogenic inflammation, vascular permeability, and mast cells. *J. Immunol.* 140:3905–3911.

Kowalski, M. L., Sliwinska-Kowalska, M., and Kaliner, M. A. (1990). Neurogenic inflammation, vascular permeability, and mast cells. II. Additional evidence indicating that mast cells are not involved in neurogenic inflammation. *J. Immunol.* 145:1214–1221.

Lacassie, Y., Thurmon, T. F., Tracy, M. C., and Pelias, M. Z. (1977). Piebald trait in a retarded child with an interstitial deletion of chromosome 4. *Am. J. Hum. Genet.* 29:641–642.

Lemanske, R. F., Jr., and Kaliner, M. A. (1988). Late phase allergic reactions. In *Allergy: Principles and Practice,* 3rd ed. Edited by E. Middleton Jr., C. E. Reed, E. F. Ellis, N. F. Adkinson, Jr., and J. W. Yuninger. St. Louis, Mosby, pp. 224–246.

Lerner, N. B., Nocka, K. H., Cole, S. R., Qiu, F. H., Strife, A., Ashman, L. A., and Besmer, P. (1991). Monoclonal antibody YB8.B5 identifies the human *c-kit* protein product. *Blood* 1876–1883.

Leung, D. Y. M., Pober, J. S., and Cotran, R. S. (1991). Expression of endothelial-leukocyte adhesion molecule-1 in elicited late phase allergic reactions. *J. Clin. Invest.* 87:1805–1809.

Lev, S., Givol, D., and Yarden, Y. (1991). A specific combination of substrates is involved in signal transduction by the *kit*-encoded receptor. *EMBO J.* 10:647–654.

Levi-Schaffer, F., Austen, K. F., Gravallese, P. M., and Stevens, R. L. (1986). Coculture of interleukin 3-dependent mouse mast cells with fibroblasts results in a phenotypic change of the mast cells. *Proc. Natl. Acad. Sci. USA* 83: 6485–6488.

Marcum, J. A., McKenney, J. B., Galli, S. J., Jackman, R. W., and Rosenberg, R. D. (1986). Anticoagulantly active heparinlike molecules from mast cell-deficient mice. *Am. J. Physiol.* 250:H879–H888.

Marshall, J. S., Stead, R. H., McSharry, C., Nielsen, L., and Bienenstock, J. (1990). The role of mast cell degranulation products in mast cells hyperplasia. I. Mechanism of action of nerve growth factor. *J. Immunol.* 144:1886–1892.

Martin, F. H., Suggs, S. V., Langley, K. E., Lu, H. S., Ting, J., Okino, K. H., Morris, C. F., McNiece, I. K., Jacobsen, F. W., Mendiaz, E. A., Birkett, N. C., Smith, K. A., Johnson, M. J., Parker, V. P., Flores, J. C., Patel, A. C., Fisher, E. F., Erjavec, H. O., Herrera, C. J., Wypych, J., Sachdev, R. K., Pope, J. A., Leslie, I., Wen, D., Lin, C-H., Cupples, R. L., and Zsebo, K. M. (1990). Primary structure and functional expression of rat and human stem cell factor DNAs. *Cell* 63:203–211.

Martin, T. R., Galli, S. J., Katona, I. M., and Drazen, J. M. (1989). Role of mast cells in anaphylaxis. Evidence for the importance of mast cells in the pulmonary alterations and death induced by anti-IgE in mice. *J. Clin. Invest.* 83:1375–1383.

Matsuda, H., Nakano, T., Kiso, Y., and Kitamura, Y. (1987). Normalization of anti-tick response of mast cell-deficient W/W^v mice by intracutaneous injection of cultured mast cells. *J. Parasitol.* 73:155–160.

Matsuda, H., Kawakita, K., Kiso, Y., Nakano, T., and Kitamura, Y. (1989). Substance P induces granulocyte infiltration through degranulation of mast cells. *J. Immunol.* 142:927–931.

Matsuda, H., Watanabe, N., Kiso, Y., Hirota, S., Ushio, H., Kannan, Y., Azuma, M., Koyama, H., and Kitamura, Y. (1990) Necessity of IgE antibodies and mast cells for manifestation of resistance against larval *Haemaphysalis longicornis* ticks in mice. *J. Immunol.* 144:259–262.

Matsuda, H., Kannan, Y., Ushio, H., Kiso, Y., Kanemoto, T., Suzuki, H., and Kitamura, Y. (1991). Nerve growth factor induces development of connective tissue–type mast cells in vitro from murine bone marrow cells. *J. Exp. Med.* 174:7–14.

Matsui, Y., Zsebo, K. M., and Hogan, B. L. M. (1990) Embryonic expression of a haematopoietic growth factor encoded by the *Sl* locus and the ligand for *c-kit*. *Nature* 347:667–669.

Mekori, Y. A., and Galli, S. J. (1985). Undiminished immunological tolerance to contact sensitivity in mast cell-deficient W/W^v and Sl/Sl^d mice. *J. Immunol.* 135:879–885.

Mekori, Y. A., and Galli, S. J. (1990). [^{125}I] Fibrin deposition occurs at both early and late intervals of IgE-dependent and contact sensitivity reactions elicited in mouse skin. Mast cell-dependent augmentation of fibrin deposition at early intervals in combined IgE-dependent and contact sensitivity reactions. *J. Immunol.* 145:3719–3727.

Mekori, Y. A., Weitzman, G. L., and Galli, S. J. (1985). Reevaluation of reserpine-induced suppression of contact sensitivity. Evidence that reserpine interferes with T lymphocyte function independently of an effect on mast cells. *J. Exp. Med.* 162:1935–1953.

Mekori, Y. A., Dvorak, H. F., and Galli, S. J. (1986). ^{125}I-Fibrin deposition in contact sensitivity reactions in the mouse. Sensitivity of the assay for quantitating reactions after active or passive sensitization. *J. Immunol.* 136:2018–2025.

Mekori, Y. A., Chang, J. C. C., Wershil, B. K., and Galli, S. J. (1987). Studies of the role of mast cells in contact sensitivity responses. Passive transfer of the reaction into mast cell-deficient mice locally reconstituted with cultured mast cells: Effect of reserpine on transfer of the reaction with DNP-specific cloned T cells. *Cell. Immunol.* 109:39–52.

Metcalf, D., and Nicola, N. A. (1991). Direct proliferative actions of stem cell factor on murine bone marrow cells in vitro: Effects of combination with colony-stimulating factors. *Proc. Natl. Acad. Sci. USA* 88:6239–6243.

Metcalfe, D. D., Kaliner, M., and Donlon, M. A. (1981). The mast cell. *CRC Crit. Rev. Immunol.* 2:23–74.

Metzger, H., Kinet, J-P., Blank, U., Miller, L., and Ra, C. (1989). The receptor with high affinity for IgE. In *IgE, Mast Cells and the Allergic Response. Ciba Foundation Symposium No. 147.* Edited by D. Chadwick, D. Evered, and J. Whelan. Chichester, UK, Wiley, pp. 93–113.

Miller, H. R. P., Huntley, J. F., Newlands, G. F. J., Mackellar, S., Irvine, J., Haig, D. M., MacDonald, A., Lammas, A. D., Wakelin, D., and Woodbury, R. G. (1989). Mast cell granule proteases in mouse and rat: a guide to mast cell heterogeneity and activation in the gastrointestinal tract. In *Mast Cell and Basophil Differentiation and Function in Health and Disease.* Edited by S. J. Galli, and K. F. Austen. New York, Raven Press, pp. 81–91.

Morrison-Graham, K., and Weston, J. (1989). Mouse mutants provide new insights into the role of extracellular matrix in cell migration and differentiation. *Trends Genet.* 5:116–121.

Nabel, G., Galli, S. J., Dvorak, A. M., Dvorak, H. F., and Cantor, H. (1981). Inducer T lymphocytes synthesize a factor that stimulates proliferation of cloned mast cells. *Nature* 291:332–334.

Nagao, K., Yokoro, K., and Aaronson, S. A. (1981). Continuous lines of basophil/mast cells derived from normal mouse bone marrow. *Science* 212:333–335.

Nakahata, T., Kobayashi, T., Ishiguro, A., Tsuji, K., Naganuma, K., Ando, O., Yagi, Y., Tadokoro, K., and Akabane, T. (1986). Extensive proliferation of mature connective-tissue type mast cells in vitro. *Nature* 324:65–67.

Nakamura, N., Kojima, J., Okamoto, S., and Kitamura, Y. (1981). Absence of heparin in glycosaminoglycan fractions isolated from the skin of genetically mast cell–depleted W/W^v mice. *Biochem. Int.* 3:449–456.

Nakano, T., Sonoda, T., Hayashi, C., Yamatodani, A., Kanayama, Y., Yamamura, T., Asai, H., Yonezawa, Y., Kitamura, Y., and Galli, S. J. (1985). Fate of bone marrow–derived cultured mast cells after intracutaneous, intraperitoneal and intravenous transfer into genetically mast cell–deficient W/W^v mice. Evidence that cultured mast cells can give rise to both connective tissue-type and mucosal mast cells. *J. Exp. Med.* 162:1025–1043.

Nakano, T., Waki, N., Asai, H., and Kitamura, Y. (1989a). Effect of 5-fluorouracil on "primitive" hematopoietic stem cells that reconstitute whole erythropoiesis of genetically anemic W/W^v mice. *Blood* 73:425–430.

Nakano, T., Waki, N., Asai, H., and Kitamura, Y. (1989b). Lymphoid differentiation of the hematopoietic stem cell that reconstitutes total erythropoiesis of a genetically anemic W/W^v mouse. *Blood* 73:1175–1179.

Nishimura, M., Inoue, M., Nakano, T., Nishikawa, T., Miyamoto, M., Kobayashi, T., and Kitamura, Y. (1989). Beige rat: A new animal model of Chediak-Higashi syndrome. *Blood* 74:270–273.

Niwa, Y., Kasugai, T., Ohno, K., Morimoto, M., Yamazaki, M., Dohmae, K., Nishimune, Y., Kondo, K., and Kitamura, Y. (1991). Anemia and mast cell depletion in mutant rats that are homozygous at "white-spotting (*Ws*)" locus. *Blood* 78:1936–1941.

Nocka, K., Majumder, S., Chabot, B., Ray, P., Cervonne, M., Bernstein, A., and Besmer, P. (1989) Expression of the c-*kit* protooncogene in known cellular targets of *W* mutations in normal and *W* mutant mice: evidence for an impaired c-*kit* kinase in mutant mice. *Genes Dev.* 3:816–826.

Nocka, K., Buck, J., Levi, E., and Besmer, P. (1990a). Candidate ligand for the *c-kit* transmembrane kinase receptor: KL, a fibroblast derived growth factor stimulates mast cells and erythroid progenitors. *EMBO J.* 10:3287–3294.

Nocka, K., Tan, J., Chiu, E., Chu, T. Y., Ray, P., Traktman, P., and Besmer, P. (1990b). Molecular bases of dominant negative and loss of function mutations at the murine c-*kit*/white spotting locus: W^{37}, W^v, W^{41} and *W*. *EMBO J.* 9:1805–1813.

Novak, E. K., Hui, S-W., and Swank, R. T. (1984). Platelet storage pool deficiency in mouse pigment mutations associated with seven distinct genetic loci. *Blood* 63:536–544.

Ody, C., Kindler, V., and Vassalli, P. (1990). Interleukin 3 perfusion in W/W^v mice allows the development of macroscopic hematopoietic spleen colonies and restores cutaneous mast cell number. *J. Exp. Med.* 172:403–6.

Ogawa, M., Matsuzaki, Y., Nishikawa, S., Hayashi, S.-I., Kunisada, T., Sudo, T., Kina, T., Nakauchi, H., and Nishikawa, S. I. (1991). Expression and function of c-*kit* in hemopoietic progenitor cells. *J. Exp. Med.* 174:63–71.

Orr-Urtegger, A., Avivi, A., Zimmer, Y., Givol, D., Yarden, Y., and Lonai, P. (1990). Developmental expression of c-*kit,* a protooncogene encoded by the *W* locus. *Development* 109:911–923.

Otsu, K., Nakano, T., Kanakura, Y., Asai, H., Katz, H. R., Austen, K. F., Stevens, R. L., Galli, S. J., and Kitamura, Y. (1987). Phenotypic changes of bone marrow–derived mast cells after intraperitoneal transfer into W/W^v mice that are genetically deficient in mast cells. *J. Exp. Med.* 165:615–627.

Perdue, M. H., Masson, S., Wershil, B. K., and Galli, S. J. (1991). The role of mast cells in ion transport abnormalities associated with intestinal anaphylaxis. Correction of the diminished secretory response in genetically mast cell–deficient W/W^v mice by bone marrow transplantation. *J. Clin. Invest.* 87:687–693.

Plaut, M., Pierce, J. H., Watson, C. J., Hanley-Hyde, J., Nordan, R. P., and Paul, W. E. (1989). Mast cell lines produce lymphokines in response to cross-linkage of FceRI or to calcium ionophores. *Nature* 339:64–67.

Pober, J. S. (1987). Effects of tumour necrosis factor and related cytokines on vascular endothelial cells. *CIBA Found. Symp.* 131:170–184.

Qiu, F., Ray, P., Brown, K., Barker, P. E., Jhanwar, S., Ruddle, F. H., and Besmer, P., (1988). Primary structure of c-*kit*: Relationship with the CSF-1/PDGF receptor kinase family-oncogenic activation of v-*kit* involves deletion of extracellular domain and C-terminus. *EMBO J.* 7:1003–1011.

Qureshi, R., and Jakschik, B. A. (1988). The role of mast cells in thioglycollate-induced inflammation. *J. Immunol.* 141:2090–2096.

Ramos, B. F., Qureshi, R., Olsen, K. M., and Jakschik, B. A. (1990). The importance of mast cells for the neutrophil influx in immune complex-induced peritonitis in mice. *J. Immunol.* 145:1868–1873.

Razin, E., Cordon-Cardo, C., and Good, R. A. (1981). Growth of a pure population of mouse mast cells in vitro with conditioned medium derived from concanavalin A–stimulated splenocytes. *Proc. Natl. Acad. Sci. USA* 28:2559–2561.

Razin, E., Stevens, R. L., Akiyama, F., Schmid, K., and Austen, K. F. (1982). Culture from mouse bone marrow of a subclass of mast cells possessing a distinct chondroitin sulfate proteoglycan with glycoaminoglycans rich in *N*-acetylgalactosamine-4,6-disulfate. *J. Biol. Chem.* 257:7229–7236.

Razin, E., Leslie, K. B., and Schrader, J. W. (1991). Connective tissue mast cells in contact with fibroblasts express IL-3 mRNA. Analysis of single cells by polymerase chain reaction. *J. Immunol.* 146:981–987.

Reed, N. R. (1989). Function and regulation of mast cells in parasitic infections. In *Mast Cell and Basophil Differentiation and Function in Health and Disease*. Edited by S. J. Galli, and K. F. Austen. New York, Raven Press, pp. 205–215.

Reith, A., Rottapel, R., Giddens, E., Brady, C., Forrester, L., and Bernstein, A. (1990). W mutant mice with mild or severe developmental defects contain distinct point mutations in the kinase domain of the c-kit transmembrane receptor. *Genes Dev.* 4:390–400.

Rohrschneider, L. R., Rothwell, V. M., and Nicola, N. A. (1989). Transformation of murine fibroblasts by a retrovirus encoding the murine *c-fms* protooncogene. *Oncogene* 4:1015–1022.

Rottapel, R., Reedijk, M., Williams, D. E., Lyman, S. D., Anderson, D. M., Pawson, T., and Bernstein, A. (1991) The *Steel/W* transduction pathway: *kit* autophosphorylation and its association with a unique subset of cytoplasmic signaling proteins is induced by the Steel factor. *Mol. Cell. Biol.* 11:3043–3051.

Russell, E. S. (1979). Hereditary anemias of the mouse: a review for geneticists. *Adv. Genet.* 20:357–459.

Schrader, J. W. (1981). The in vitro production and cloning of the P cell, a bone marrow–derived null cell that expresses H-2 and Ia-antigens, has mast cell–like granules, and is regulated by a factor released by activated T cells. *J. Immunol.* 131:452–458.

Schwartz, L. B., and Austen, K. F. (1984). Structure and function of the chemical mediators of mast cells. *Prog. Allergy* 34:271–321.

Seder, R. A., Paul, W. E., Dvorak, A. M., Sharkis, S. J., Kagey-Sobotka, A., Niv, Y., Finkelman, F. D., Barbieri, S. A., Galli, S. J., and Plaut, M. (1991). Mouse splenic and bone marrow cell populations that express high-affinity Fc_{ϵ} receptors and produce interluekin 4 are highly enriched in basophils. *Proc. Natl. Acad. Sci. USA* 88:2835–2839.

Seikido, Y., Obata, Y., Ueda, R., Hida, T., Suyama, M., Shimokata, K., Ariyoshi, Y., and Takahashi, T. (1991). Preferential expression of c-kit protooncogene transcripts in small cell lung cancer. *Cancer Res.* 51:2416–2419.

Silvers, W. K., (1979a). Beige, silver, greying with age and other determinants. In *The Coat Color of Mice. A Model for Mammalian Gene Action and Interaction.* New York, Springer-Verlag, pp. 125–146.

Silvers, W. K. (1979b). Dominant spotting, patch and rump-white; steel, flexed tail, splotch and varitint-waddler. In *The Coat Color of Mice. A Model for Mammalian Gene Action and Interaction.* New York, Springer-Verlag, pp. 206–241.

Silvers, W. K. (1979c). Microphthalmia and other considerations. In *The Coat Color of Mice. A Model for Mammalian Gene Action and Interaction.* New York, Springer-Verlag, pp. 268–291.

Sredni, B., Friedman, M. M., Bland, C. E., and Metcalfe, D. D. (1983). Ultrastructural, biochemical, and functional characteristics of histamine-containing cells cloned from mouse bone marrow: tentative identification as mucosal mast cells. *J. Immunol.* 131:915–922.

Starkey, J. R., Crowle, P. K., and Taubenberger, S. (1988). Mast-cell-deficient W/W^v mice exhibit a decreased rate of tumor angiogenesis. *Int. J. Cancer* 15: 48–52.

Stechschulte, D. J., Sharma, R., Dileepan, K. N., Simpson, K. M., Aggarwal, N., Clancy, J., Jr., and Jilka, R. (1987). Effects of the *mi* allele on mast cells, basophils, natural killer cells and osteoclasts in C57Bl/6J mice. *J. Cell. Physiol.* 132:565–570.

Steeves, E. B., and Allen, J. R. (1990). Basophils in skin reactions of mast cell-deficient mice infested with *Dermacentor variabilis*. *Int. J. Parasitol.* 20:655–667.

Stevens, J., and Loutit, J. F. (1982). Mast cells in spotted mutant mice. (*W Ph mi*). *Proc. R. Soc. (Lond.)* 215:405–409.

Stevens, R. L., and Austen, K. F. (1989). Recent advances in the cellular and molecular biology of mast cells. *Immunol. Today* 10:381–386.

Strohmeyer, T., Peter, S., Hartmann, M., Munemitsu, S., Ackermann, R., Ullrich, A., and Slamon, D. J. (1991). Expression of the *hst-1* and *c-kit* protooncogenes in human testicular germ cell tumors. *Cancer Res.* 51:1811–1816.

Suda, T., Suda, J., Spicer, S. S., and Ogawa, M. (1985). Proliferation and differentiation in culture of mast cell progenitors derived from mast cell progenitors derived from mast cell-deficient mice of genotype *W/W^v*. *J. Cell. Physiol.* 122:187–192.

Takagi, M., Koike, K., and Nakahata, T. (1990). Antiproliferative effect of IFN-gamma on proliferation of mouse connective-tissue type mast cells. *J. Immunol.* 145:1880–1884.

Takeishi, T., Martin, T. R., Katona, I. M., Finkelman, F. D., and Galli, S. J. (1991). Differences in the expression of the cardiopulmonary alterations associated with anti-IgE-induced or active anaphylaxis in mast cell–deficient and normal mice. Mast cells are not required for the cardiopulmonary changes associated with certain fatal anaphylactic responses. *J. Clin. Invest.* 88:598–608.

Tan, J. C., Nocka, K., Ray, P., Traktman, P., and Besmer, P. (1990). The dominant W^{42} spotting phenotype results from a missense mutation in the c-*kit* receptor kinase. *Science* 247:209–212.

Tertian, G., Yung, Y. P., Guy-Grand, D., and Moore, M. A. S. (1978). Long term in vitro culture of murine mast cells. I. Description of a growth-factor dependent culture technique. *J. Immunol.* 127:788–794.

Thomas, W. R., and Schrader, J. W. (1983). Delayed hypersensitivity in mast cell–deficient mice. *J. Immunol.* 130:2565–2567.

Thompson, H. L., Burbelo, P. D., Yamada, Y., Kleinman, H. K., and Metcalfe, D. D. (1989). Mast cells chemotax to laminin with enhancement factor after IgE-mediated activation. *J. Immunol.* 143:4188–4192.

Tsai, M., Shih, L., Newlands, G. F. J., Takeishi, T., Langley, K. E., Zsebo, K. M., P, M. H. R., Geissler, E. N., and Galli, S. J. (1991a). The rat c-*kit* ligand, stem cell factor, induces the development of connective tissue-type and mucosal mast cells in vivo. Analysis by anatomical distribution, histochemistry and protease phenotype. *J. Exp. Med.* 174:125–131.

Tsai, M., Takeishi, T., Thompson, H., Langley, K. E., Zsebo, K. M., Metcalfe, D. D., Geissler, E. N., and Galli, S. J. (1991b). Induction of mast cell proliferation, maturation and heparin synthesis by the rat c-*kit* ligand, stem cell factor. *Proc. Natl. Acad. Sci. USA* 88:6382–6386.

Tsuji, K., Nakahata, T., Takagi, M., Kobayashi, T., Ishiguro, A., Kikuchi, T., Naganuma, K., Koike, K., Miyajima, A., Arai, K., and Akabane, T. (1990a). Synergistic action of phorbol ester and IL-3 in the induction of "connective" tissue–type mast cell proliferation *J. Immunol.* 144:678–684.

Tsuji, K., Nakahata, T., Takagi, M., Kobayashi, T., Ishiguro, A., Kikuchi, T., Naganuma, K., Koike, K., Miyajima, A., Arai, K., and Akabane, T. (1990b). Effects of interleukin-3 and interleukin-4 on the development of connective tissue–type mast cells: interleukin-3 supports their survival and interleukin-4 triggers and supports their proliferation synergistically with interleukin-3. *Blood* 75:421–427.

Tsujimura, T., Hirota, S., Nomura, S., Niwa, Y., Yamazaki, M., Tono, T., Morii, E.,

Kim, H.-M., Kondo, K., Nishimune, Y., and Kitamura, Y. (1991). Characterization of *Ws* mutant allele of rats: A 12 base deletion in tyrosine kinase domain of c-*kit* gene. *Blood* 78:1942–1946.

Valent, P., Ashman, L. K., Hinterberger, W., Eckersberger, E., Majdic, O., Lechner, K., and Bettelheim, P. (1989). Mast cell typing: demonstration of a distinct hematopoietic cell type and evidence for immunophenotypic relationship to mononuclear phagocytes. *Blood* 73:1778–1785.

Walsh, L. J., Trinchieri, G., Waldorf, H. A., Whitaker, D., and Murphy, G. F. (1991). Human dermal mast cells contain and release tumor necrosis factor α which induces endothelial leukocyte adhesion molecule-1. *Proc. Natl. Acad. Sci. USA* 88:4220–4224.

Wang, C., Curtis, J. E., Geissler, E. N., McCulloch, E. A., and Minden, M. (1989). The expression of the protooncogene c-*kit* in blast cells of acute myeloblastic leukemia. *Leukemia* 3:699–702.

Wegner, C. D., Gundel, R. H., Reilly, P., Haynes, N., Letts, L. G., and Rothlein, R. (1990). Intracellular adhesion molecule-1 (ICAM-1) in the pathogenesis of asthma. *Science* 247:456–459.

Weitzman, G., Galli, S. J., Dvorak, A. M., and Hammel, I. (1985). Cloned mouse mast cells and normal mouse peritoneal mast cells. Determination of serotonin content and ability to synthesize serotonin in vitro. *Int. Arch. Allergy Appl. Immunol.* 77:189–191.

Wershil, B., Mekori, Y. A., and Galli, S. J. (1989). The contribution of mast cells to immunological responses with IgE- and/or T cell-mediated components. In *Mast Cell and Basophil Differentiation and Function in Health and Disease*. Edited by S. J. Galli and K. F. Austen. New York, Raven Press, pp. 229–246.

Wershil, B. K., Mekori, Y. A., Murakami, T., and Galli, S. J. (1987). ^{125}I-Fibrin deposition in IgE-dependent immediate hypersensitivity reactions in mouse skin. Demonstration of the role of mast cells using genetically mast cell–deficient mice locally reconstituted with cultured mast cells. *J. Immunol.* 139:2605–2614.

Wershil, B. K., Murakami, T., and Galli, S. J. (1988). Mast cell-dependent amplification of an immunologically nonspecific inflammatory response. Mast cells are required for the full expression of cutaneous acute inflammation induced by phorbol 12-myristate 13-acetate. *J. Immunol.* 140:2356–2360.

Wershil, B. K., Wang, Z., Gordon, J. R., and Galli, S. J. (1991a). Recruitment of neutrophils during IgE-dependent cutaneous late phase responses in the mouse is mast cell dependent: partial inhibition of the reaction with antiserum against tumor necrosis factor-alpha. *J. Clin. Invest.* 87:446–453.

Wershil, B. K., Wang, Z-S., and Galli, S. J. (1991b). Evidence of mast cell–dependent neutrophil infiltration during IgE-dependent gastric inflammation in the mouse: does this represent a gastric late phase reaction (LPR)? *Gastroenterology* 100:A625 (abstract).

Wershil, B. K., Tsai, M., Geissler, E. N., Zsebo, K. M., and Galli, S. J. (1992). The rat *c-kit* ligand, stem cell factor, induces c-*kit* receptor-dependent mouse mast cell activation in vivo. Evidence that signaling through the c-*kit* receptor can induce expression of cellular function. J. Exp. Med. 175:245–255.

Williams, D. E., Eisenman, J., Baird, A., Rauch, C., Ness, K. V., March, C. J., Park,

L. S., Martin, U., Mochizuki, D., Boswell, H. S., Burgess, G. S., and Lyman, S. D. (1990). Identification of a ligand for the c-*kit* proto-oncogene. *Cell* 63:167–174.

Witte, U. N. (1990). Steel locus defines new multipotent growth factor. *Cell* 63:5–6.

Wodnar-Filipowicz, A., Heusser, C. H., and Moroni, C. (1989). Production of the haemopoietic growth factors GM-CSF and interleukin-3 by mast cells in response to IgE receptor–mediated activation. *Nature* 339:150–152.

Wong, D. T. W., Weller, P. F., Galli, S. J., Elovic, A., Rand, T. H., Gallagher, G. T., Chiang, T., Chou, M. Y., Matossian, K., McBride, J., and Todd, R. (1990). Human eosinophils express transforming growth factor-alpha *J. Exp. Med.* 172:673–681.

Wong, D. T. W., Elovic, A., Matossian, K., Nagura, N., McBride, J., Chou, M. Y., Gordon, J. R., Rand, T. H., Galli, S. J., and Weller, P. F. (1991). Eosinophils from patients with blood eosinophils express transforming growth factor β1. *Blood* 78:2702–2707.

Yamatodani, A., Maeyama, K., Watanabe, T., Wada, H., and Kitamura, Y. (1982). Tissue distribution of histamine in a mutant mouse deficient in mast cells. Clear evidence for the presence of non-mast-cell histamine. *Biochem. Pharmacol.* 31:305–309.

Yano, H., Wershil, B. K., Arizono, N., and Galli, S. J. (1989). Substance P–induced augmentation of cutaneous vascular permeability and granulocyte infiltration in mice is mast cell dependent. *J. Clin. Invest.* 84:1276–1286.

Yarden, Y., and Ullrich, A. (1988). Growth factor receptor tyrosine kinases. *Annu. Rev. Biochem.* 57:443–478.

Yarden, Y., Kuang, W-J., Yang-Feng, T., Coussens, L., Munemitsu, S., Dull, T. J., Chen, E., Schlessinger, J., Francke, U., and Ullrich, A. (1987). Human proto-oncogene c-*kit*: A new cell surface receptor tyrosine kinase for an unidentified ligand. *EMBO J.* 6:3341–3351.

Young, J. D-E., Liu, C., Butler, G., Cohn, Z. A., and Galli, S. J. (1987). Identification, purification, and characterization of a mast cell-associated cytolytic factor related to tumor necrosis factor. *Proc. Natl. Acad. Sci. USA* 84:9175–9179.

Yung, Y-P., and Moore, M. A. S. (1982). Long-term in vitro culture of murine mast cells. III. Discrimination of mast cell growth-factor and granulocyte CSF. *J. Immunol.* 129:1256–1261.

Zsebo, K. M., Williams, D. A., Geissler, E. N., Broudy, V. C., Martin, F. H., Atkins, H. L., Hsu, R-Y., Birkett, N. C., Okino, K. H., Murdock, D. C., Jacobsen, F. W., Langley, K. E., Smith, K. A., Takeichi, T., Cattanach, B. M., Galli, S. J., and Suggs, S. V. (1990a). Stem cell factor (SCF) is encoded at the *Sl* locus of the mouse and is the ligand for the c-*kit* tyrosine kinase receptor. *Cell* 63:213–224.

Zsebo, K. M., Wypych, J., McNiece, I. K., Lu, H. S., Smith, K. A., Karkare, S. B., Sachdev, R. K., Yuschenkoff, V. N., Birkett, N. C., Williams, L. R., Satyagal, V. N., Tung, W., Bosselman, R. A., Mendiaz, E. A., and Langley, K. E. (1990b). Identification, purification, and biological characterization of hematopoietic stem cell factor from buffalo rat liver-conditioned medium *Cell* 63:195–201.

5

The Origin and Development of Murine and Human Mast Cells

ARNOLD S. KIRSHENBAUM

Johns Hopkins University Hospital, Baltimore
Homewood Hospital, Baltimore
and National Institute of Allergy and Infectious Diseases
National Institutes of Health
Bethesda, Maryland

MENACHEM ROTTEM and DEAN D. METCALFE

National Institute of Allergy and Infectious Diseases
National Institutes of Health
Bethesda, Maryland

JULIE P. GOFF

Georgetown University Medical Center
Rockville, Maryland

I. Introduction

Murine and human mast cells originate in vivo from pluripotent cells that can be found in highest number in the bone marrow. In vitro studies using mouse bone marrow have shown that the addition of IL-3 to bone marrow cultures gives rise to pure cultures of mast cells from Thy 1+ progenitor cells. IL-4 is synergistic with IL-3 in promoting murine mast cell growth and development but does not support mast cell growth alone, while GM-CSF can be shown to inhibit mast cell proliferation. Early mouse bone marrow–derived mast cells possess high-affinity IgE receptors, although the cells may lack the characteristic granular morphology of mature mast cells. Rodent bone marrow–derived mast cells resemble mucosal mast cells histochemically, but acquire the phenotypic properties of connective tisssue mast cells when cocultured with 3T3 fibroblasts. In humans, mast cells originate from CD34+ pluripotent progenitor cells. Mast cell proliferation requires recombinant human (rh)IL-3 and can be enhanced when CD34+ cells are cultured in the presence of rhIL-3 and stem cell factor (rhSCF). rhSCF appears to mature cultured human mast cells, giving rise to characteristic ultrastructural

Moore, 1984). By 14 days, a homogeneous culture of mast cells is observed. These mast cells have granules containing chondroitin sulfate E proteoglycans. After 1 week of culture in IL-3, one-third of mouse bone marrow cells have been reported to have IgE receptors (Prystowsky et al., 1984; Razin et al., 1984), and by 3 weeks all cells are positive (Prystowsky et al., 1984).

Buoyant density and velocity sedimentation studies indicate that mast cell precursors are low-density cells (Yung and Moore, 1984). Flow cytometric analysis of surface marker expression in cultures of mouse bone marrow cells stimulated with IL-3 has substantiated the presence of subpopulations of Thy 1.2+ cells, which appear transiently and possess IgE receptors, CR3 receptors, or neither of these receptors (Bender et al., 1988). The data suggested that Thy 1.2+ precursor cells give rise to granulocytes and mast cells. Committed mast cell progenitors, however, harvested from the mesenteric lymph nodes of mice infected with *Nippostrongylus braziliensis* appear to lack Thy 1.2 positivity (Jarboe et al., 1989). Further evidence for this differentiation scheme was provided from Coulter volume and perpendicular light scatter distributions, which showed an increase in volume and perpendicular light scatter as Thy 1.2+ cells differentiated into mast cells and a decrease in volume and perpendicular light scatter as Thy 1.2+ cells differentiated into granulocytes (Bender et al., 1988).

Murine mast cells derived from bone marrow cultures supplemented with IL-3 express transcripts for $Fc_{\epsilon}RI$ subunits and possess high-affinity surface IgE receptors by 1 week in culture. The cells bearing IgE receptors often contained few, if any, granules and could not be identified histochemically using traditional staining procedures (Fig. 1) (Rottem et al., 1992). The expression of transcripts and the number of receptor-positive cells continued to increase over 3 weeks in culture. Similarly, a progressively larger number of cells became granulated, resembling mature murine mast cells (Fig. 1). Cellular histamine content rose concurrently. The majority of IgE receptor–bearing cells could be grown in liquid suspension cultures for 1 week, removed, and subsequently shown to be committed mast cell progenitors, giving rise to mast cell colony-forming units (CFUs) in agarose (Rottem et al., 1992). The early appearance of IgE receptors during mast cell differentiation may be important for these cells to respond to IgE-mediated stimuli before granulation. Non-B, non-T cells of splenic origin produce IL-4 when cultured with IL-3 in response to crosslinking of $Fc_{\epsilon}RI$ receptors, and it has been suggested that these cells are early mast cells or basophils (Ben-Sasson et al., 1990). In addition, single bone marrow–derived and connective tissue mast cells, when cocultured with mouse 3T3 fibroblasts, were shown to synthesize detectable amounts of IL-3 mRNA, as determined by polymerase chain reaction (Razin et al., 1991). Thus, one can speculate that rodent mast cells might, under certain microenvironmental conditions, produce

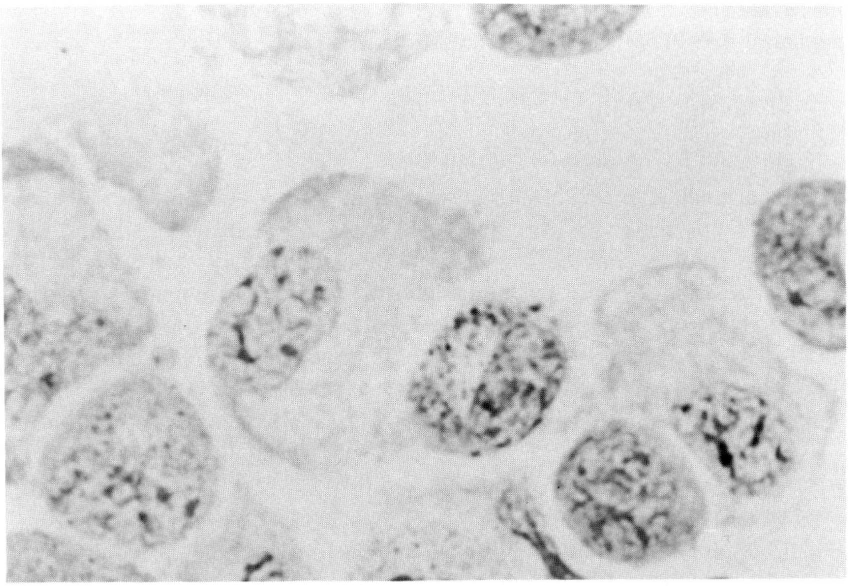

a

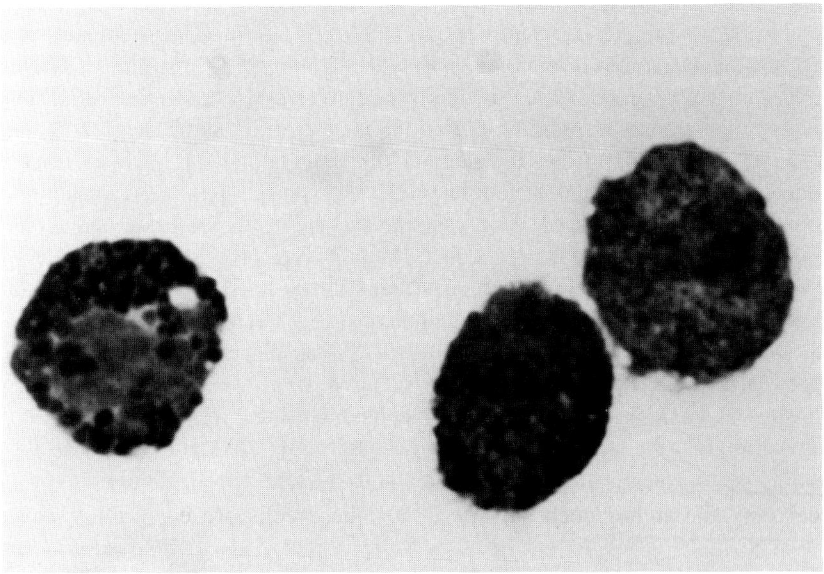

b

Figure 1 Early stage in murine mast cell diffentiation. (a) bone marrow cells grown in IL-3-supplemented medium for 5 days and positively sorted on the basis of IgE receptors; (b) cells from the same culture grown for an additional 14 days in agarose.

mRNA and bioactivity for the mast cell growth factors IL-3 and IL-4, autostimulating the growth and proliferation of mast cell precursor cells.

III. Origin of Human Mast Cells

A. Stem Cell Origin of Human Mast Cells

Human mast cells have been difficult to culture from blood or bone marrow in sufficient number for studying mast cell growth and differentiation. Liquid suspension cultures provide a simple, reproducible system for studying cell growth characteristics. Unlike the rodent model, however, human peripheral or cord blood or bone marrow mononuclear cells separated by density sedimentation and grown in liquid suspension cultures give rise to cultures rich in basophils rather than mast cells (Tadokoro et al., 1983; Ishizaka et al., 1985; Otsuka et al., 1986). Similarly, single-lineage and mixed CFUs containing basophils but not mast cells were observed when mononuclear cells were cultured in methylcellulose in the presence of rhIL-3 (Leary et al., 1987, 1988). Human mast cell CFUs have been grown in agar, although CFUs were too few in number for adequate growth and characterization studies (McCarthy et al., 1986).

Small numbers of mast cells have recently been cultured and studied using a technique whereby human bone marrow–derived mononuclear cells are suspended over agar (Kirshenbaum et al., 1989b) or agarose (Kirshenbaum et al., 1989c), the structure of which resembles that of chondroitin sulfates (Kennedy, 1979), in the presence of rhIL-3 (interphase cultures). These mast cells, identified by histochemical staining techniques, peaked in number by 2–3 weeks (1–5%), had high-affinity IgE receptors (Kirshenbaum et al., 1989a), and contained the human mast cell neutral protease tryptase, within cytoplasmic granules. Mast cells cultured over agarose surfaces did not have characteristic granule ultrastructural patterns seen in human lung or skin mast cells.

Having shown that human mast cells could arise under specific culture conditions from bone marrow mononuclear cells, it remained to be determined whether mast cells arise from committed T-cell, B-cell, eosinophil, or macrophage progenitor cells, or a mast cell progenitor cell directly derived from pluripotent CD34+ human progenitor cells. Previous reports were conflicting, suggesting that human skin, colon, and spleen mast cells did not possess T-cell, B-cell, or monocyte markers (Rimmer and Horton, 1987) although they may possess surface membrane antigens associated with a late stage of monocyte/macrophage but not basophil differentiation (Valent et al., 1989). Using immune adherence (panning) and complement lysis to remove committed T-cell (CD2), B-cell (CD19 and 20), eosinophil, or macrophage (CD14) precursors from human bone marrow, bone marrow–derived mononuclear cells continued to give rise to mast cells. Mast cells were effectively removed, however, when CD34+ pluripotent progenitor cells were depleted from bone marrow cells. CD34+

cells, highly enriched (>99% CD34+) using immunomagnetic selection, were then cultured in the presence of rhIL-3 over agarose surfaces. Mast cells again were observed in small numbers (Kirshenbaum et al., 1991). Mast cell granules contained homogenous dense material but no scroll, lattice, or reticular patterns seen in mature skin or lung mast cells. Human mast cells, therefore, were shown to originate from pluripotent CD34+ human progenitor cells and appeared to require additional conditions in vitro for the development of mast cell granule ultrastructure.

B. CD34+ Cell/3T3 Fibroblast Cocultures and the Effect of rhSCF

Mouse 3T3 fibroblasts permit human mast cell differentiation in vitro from human cord blood mononuclear cells (Furitsu et al., 1989). To confirm that mast cells are derived from CD34+ cells, CD34+ cells were cocultured with 3T3 fibroblasts in the presence of rhIL-3. Over 6 weeks, adherent CD34+ cells gave rise to cultures containing oval or spindle-shaped metachromatically staining cells with numerous cytoplasmic extensions (Fig. 2) (Kirshenbaum et al., 1991). Using simultaneous immunogold labeling, these cells were shown to have IgE

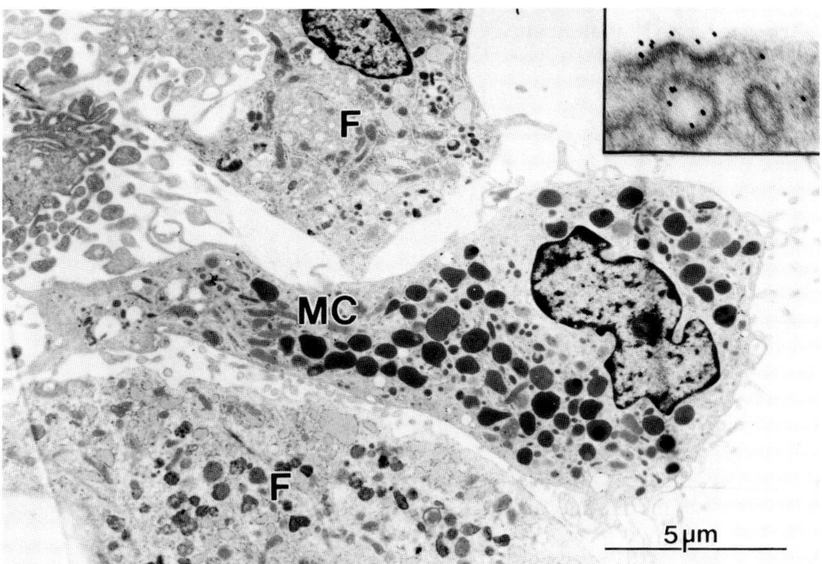

Figure 2 Human mast cells derived from CD34+ positive human bone marrow cells cocultured for 6 weeks with 3T3 fibroblasts. Mast cell surface stains positive for IgE receptors (inset). F = fibroblast; MC = mast cell. (From Kirshenbaum et al., 1991, by permission.)

IV. Conclusions

Mast cells originate from pluripotential progenitor cells in murine and human bone marrow, but their exact relation to other cell lineages is still unclear. Acquisition of IgE receptors appears to occur early in the development of murine mast cells, before cells exhibit the morphological characteristics of mature cells. Immature murine and human mast cell progenitors are presumed to migrate to specific tissue sites where cells mature under the influence of microenvironmental factors to exhibit tissue-specific phenotypes.

Discussion

Denburg: Have you studied cytokine receptors (such as for IL-3) on the surface of mast cell precursors?

Metcalfe: IL-3 receptors have been shown to be low in number to absent on mature human mast cells, but not on human basophils.

Bienenstock: In your coculture systems with 3T3 fibroblasts do you always include IgE, and is it critical to results?

Metcalfe: IgE does not appear to be essential in our human basophil/mast cell cultures.

Kennedy: Do protein synthesis inhibitors affect adhesion to laminin in $Fc_{\epsilon}RI$-stimulated mast cells?

Metcalfe: No. New protein synthesis is not required for a bone marrow–derived mast cell to bind to laminin.

Hohman: Is it possible that activated mast cells detach from laminin because the cells secrete an enzyme that degrades either laminin or the receptor?

Metcalfe: It appears that detachment can occur in the absence of granule release.

Platts-Mills: Where is laminin expressed? Is it primarily a component of nerve sheaths?

Metcalfe: No. laminin is found in a number of structures, including basement membrane.

Platts-Mills: Mast cells must survive in skin for at least 12 weeks since PK sites can be detected for that long; so presumably something is keeping them stable.

Metcalfe: There are undoubtedly additional binding proteins that alone or in combination and with specific factors may achieve mast cell stasis.

Rivera: Do mast cells attach to laminin when the receptor is aggregated in the absence of Ca^{2+}

Metcalfe: Mast cell attachment to laminin is a Ca-dependent process.

References

Anderson, D. M., Lyman, S. D., Baird, A., Wignall, J. M., Eisenman, J., Rauch, C., March, C. J., Boswell, H. S., Gimpel, S. D., Cosman, D., and Williams, D. E.

(1990). Molecular cloning of mast cell growth factor, a hematopoietin that is active in both membrane bound and soluble forms. *Cell* 63:235–243.

Ashman, R. I., Jarboe, D. L., Conrad, D. H., and Huff, T. F. (1991). The mast cell committed progenitor. In vitro generation of committed progenitors from bone marrow. *J. Immunol.* 146:211–216.

Bender, J. G., Van Epps, D. E., and Stewart, C. C. (1988). Characterization of granulocytes and mast cells in cultures of mouse bone marrow stimulated with IL-3. *J. Cell Physiol.* 135:71–78.

Ben-Sasson, S. Z., Le Gros, G., Conrad, D. H., and Finkelman, F. D. (1990). Cross-linking Fc receptors stimulate splenic non-B, non-T cells to secrete interleukin 4 and other lymphokines. *Proc. Natl. Acad. Sci. USA* 87:1421–1425.

Bressler, R. B., Thompson, H. L., Keffer, J. M., and Metcalfe, D. D. (1989). Inhibition of the growth of IL-3 dependent mast cells from murine bone marrow by recombinant granulocyte macrophage colony stimulating factor. *J. Immunol.* 143:135–139.

Burnet, F. M. (1977). The probable relationship of some or all mast cells to the T-cell system. *Cell. Immunol.* 30:358–360.

Copeland, N. G., Gilbert, D. J., Cho, B. C., Donovan, P. J., Jenkins, N. A., Cosman, D., Anderson, D., Lyman, S. D., and Williams, D. E. (1990). Mast cell growth factor maps near the steel locus on mouse chromosome 10 and is deleted in a number of steel alleles. *Cell* 63:175–183.

Czarnetzki, B. M., Sterry, W., Bazin, H., and Kapveram, K. J. (1982). Evidence that tissue mast cells derived from mononuclear phagocytes. *Int. Arch. Allergy Appl. Immunol.* 67:44–48.

Ehrlich, P. (1878) Beirtrage zur Theorie und Praxis dee Histologischen Farbung. Ph.D. thesis. Leipzig University.

Flanagan, J. G., and Leder, P. (1990). The *kit* ligand: A cell surface molecule altered in steel mutant fibroblasts. *Cell* 63:185–194.

Fung, M. C., Hapel, A. J., Ymer, S., Cohem, D. R., Johnson, R. M., Campbell, H. D., and Young I. G. (1984). Molecular cloning of cDNA for murine interleukin-3. *Nature (Lond.)* 307:233–237.

Furitsu, T., Saito, H., Dvorak, A. M., Schwartz, L. B., Irani, A-M. A., Burdick, J. F., Ishizaka, K., and Ishizaka, T. (1989). Development of human mast cells in vitro. *Proc. Natl. Acad. Sci. USA* 86:10039–10043.

Hamaguchi, Y., Kanakura, Y., Fujita, J., Takeda, S-I., Nakano, T., Tarui, S., Honjo, T., and Kitamura, Y. (1987). Interleukin 4 as an essential factor for in vitro clonal growth of murine connective tissue type mast cells. *J. Exp. Med.* 165: 268–273.

Huang, E., Nocka, K., Beier, D. R., Chu, T-Y., Buck, J., Lahm, H-W., Wellner, D., Leder, P., and Besmer, P. (1990). The hematopoietic growth factor KL is encoded by the *Sl* locus and is the ligand of the c-*kit* receptor, the gene product of the W locus. *Cell* 63:225–233.

Ihle, J. N., Keller, J., Orsozlan, S., Henderson, L. E., Copeland, T. D., Fitch, F., Prystowsky, M. B., Goldwasser, E., Schrader, J. W., Palaszynski, E., Dy, M., and Lebel, B. (1983). Biological properties of homogeneous interleukin 3. I. Demonstration of WEHI-3 growth factor activity, mast cell growth factor activity, P cell stimulating factor activity and histamine producing factor activity. *J. Immunol.* 131:282–287.

Ishizaka, T., Dvorak, A. M., Conrad, D. H., Niebyl, J. R., Marquetti, J. P., and Ishizaka, K. (1985). Morphologic and immunologic characterization of human basophils developed in cultures of cord blood mononuclear cells. *J. Immunol.* 134:532–540.

Jarboe, D. L., Marshall, J. S., Randolph, T. R., Kukolja, A., and Huff, T. F. (1989). The mast cell-committed progenitor. I. Description of a cell capable of IL-3-independent proliferation and differentiation without contact with fibroblasts. *J. Immunol.* 142:2405–2417.

Kennedy, J. F. (1979). Proteoglycans—Biological and chemical aspects in human life. In *Studies of Organic Chemistry*. Section 2. New York, Elsevier, p. 167.

Kirshenbaum, A. S., Dreskin, S. C., and Metcalfe, D. D. (1989a). A staphylococcal protein A rosetting assay for the demonstration of high affinity IgE receptors on rIL-3-dependent human basophil-like cells grown in mixed cultures. *J. Immunol.* 123:55–62.

Kirshenbaum, A. S., Goff, J. P., Dreskin, S. A., Irani, A-M., Schwartz, L. B. and Metcalfe, D. D. (1989b). Interleukin 3–dependent growth of basophil-like and mast-like cells from human bone marrow. *J. Immunol.* 142:2424–2429.

Kirshenbaum, A. S., Goff, J. P., and Metcalfe, D. D. (1989c). Human macrophages cultured on agar but not agarose resemble mast cells. *Immunology* 68: 120–125.

Kirshenbaum, A. S., Kessler, S. W., Goff, J. P., and Metcalfe, D. D. (1991). Demonstration of the origin of human mast cells from CD34+ bone marrow progenitor cells. *J. Immunol.* 146:1410–1415.

Kirshenbaum, A. S., Goff, J. P., Kessler, S. W., Mican, J. M., Zsebo, K., and Metcalfe, D. D. (1992). Effect of IL-3 and stem cell factor on the appearance of human basophils and mast cells from CD 34^+ pluripotent progenitor cells. *J. Immunol.* 148:772–777.

Kitamura Y., and Go, S. (1979). Decreased production of mast cells in Sl/Sl^d anemic mice. *Blood* 53:492–497.

Kitamura, Y., Go, S., and Hatanaka, S. (1978). Decrease of mast cells in W/W^v mice and their increase by bone marrow transplantation. *Blood* 52:447–452.

Kitamura, Y., Yokohama, M., Matsuda, H., Ohno, T., and Mori, K. J. (1981). Spleen colony-forming cell as common precursor for tissue mast cells and granulocytes. *Nature* (*Lond.*) 291:159–160.

Lanotte, M., Arock, M., Lacaze, N., and Guy-Grand, D. (1986). Murine basophil-mast differentiation: Toward optimal conditions of selective growth and maturation of basophil-mast or allied cells. *J. Cell Physiol.* 129:199–226.

Leary, A. G., Yang, Y-C., Clark, S. C., Gasson, J. C., Golde, D. W., and Ogawa, M. (1987). Recombinant gibbon interleukin-3 supports formation of human multilineage colonies and blast cells colonies in culture: comparison with recombinant with recombinant granulocyte-macrophage colony stimulating factor. *Blood* 87: 1343–1348.

Leary, A. G., Ikebuchi, K., Hirai, Y., Wong, G. G., Yang, Y-C., Clark, S. C., and Ogawa, M. (1988). Synergism between interleukin-6 and interleukin-3 in supporting proliferation of human hematopoietic stem cells: Comparison with interleukin-1a. *Blood.* 71:1759–1763.

Lee, F., Yokota, T., Otsuka, T., Meyerson, P., Villaret, D., Coffman, R., Mosmann, T., Rennick, D., Roehm, N., Smith, C., Zlotnik, A., and Arai, K-I. (1986). Isolation and characterization of a mouse interleukin cDNA clone that expresses B cell stimulatory fator 1 activities and T cell and mast cell stimulating activities. *Proc. Natl. Acad. Sci. USA* 83:2061–2065.

Martin, F. H., Suggs, S. V., Langley, K. E., Lu, H. S., Ting, J., Okino, K. H., Morris, C. F., McNiece, I. K., Jacobsen, F. W., Mendiaz, E. A., Birkett, N. C., Smith, K. A., Johnson, M. J., Parker, V. P., Flores, J. C., Patel, A. C., Fisher, E. F., Erjavec, H. O., Herrera, C. J., Wypych, J., Sachdev, R. K., Pope, J. A., Leslie, I., Wen, D., Lin, C-H., Cupples, R. L., and Zsebo, K. M. (1990). Primary structure and functional expression of rat and human stem cell factor DNAs. *Cell* 63:203–211.

McCarthy, J. H., Mandel, T. E., Garsa, O. M., and Metcalf, D. (1986). The presence of mast cells in agar cultures. *Exp. Hematol.* 8:562–567.

Metcalf, D. (1986). The molecular biology and functions of the granulocyte macrophage colony stimulating factors. *Blood* 67:257–267.

Nabel, G., Galli, S. J., Dvorak, A. M., Dvorak, H. F., and Cantor, H. (1981). Inducer T lymphocytes synthesize a factor that stimulates proliferation of cloned mast cells. *Nature* (*Lond.*) 291:332–334.

Nagao, K., Yokoro, K., and Aaronson, S. A. (1981). Continuous lines of basophil/mast cells derived from normal mouse bone marrow. *Science* 212:333–335.

Nakahata, T., Kobayashi, T., Ishiguro, A., Tsuji, K., Naganuma, K., Ando, O, Yagi, Y., Tadokoro, K., and Akabane, T. (1986). Extensive proliferation of mature connective tissue type mast cells in vitro. *Nature* (*Lond.*) 324:65–67.

Nakano, T., Kanakura, Y., Nakahata, T., Matsuda, H. and Kitamura, Y. (1987). Genetically mast cell deficient W/W^v mice as a tool for studies of differentiation and function of mast cells. *Fed. Proc.* 46:1920–1923.

Otsuka, H., Dolovich, J., Befus, A. D., Telizyn, S., Bienenstock, J., and Denburg, J. A. (1986). Basophilic cell progenitors, nasal metachromatic cells, and peripheral blood basophils in ragweed allergic patients. *J. Allergy Clin. Immunol.* 78:365–371.

Prystowsky, M. B., Otten, G., Naujokas, M. F., Vardiman, J., Ihle, J. N., Goldwasser, E., and Fitch, F. W., (1984). Multiple hematopoietic lineages are found after stimulation of mouse bone marrow precursor cells with interleukin 3. *Am. J. Pathol.* 117:171–179.

Razin, E., Cordon-Cardo, C., and Good, R. A. (1981). Growth of a pure population of mouse mast cells in vitro with conditioned medium derived from concanavalin A–stimulated splenocytes. *Proc. Natl. Acad. Sci. USA* 28:2559–2561.

Razin, E., Ihle, J. N., Seldin, D., Mencia-Huerta, J-M., Katz, H. R., Leblanc, P. A., Hein, A., Caulfield, J. P., Austen, K. F., and Stevens, R. L. (1984). Interleukin 3: A differentiation and growth factor for the mouse mast cell that contains chondroitin sulfate E proteoglycan. *J. Immunol.* 132:1479–1486.

Razin, E., Leslie, K. B., and Schrader, J. W. (1991). Connective tissue mast cells in contact with fibroblasts express IL-3 mRNA. Analysis of single cells by polymerase chain reaction. *J. Immunol.* 146:981–987.

Rennick, D., Lee, F. D., Yokota, T., Arai, K-I., Cantor, H., and Nabel, G. J. (1985). A cloned MCGF cDNA encodes a multilineage hematopoietic growth factor: Multiple activities of interleukin 3. *J. Immunol.* 134:910–914.

Rimmer, E. F., and Horton, M. A. (1987). Origin of human mast cell studied by dual immunofluorescence. *Clin. Exp. Immunol.* 68:712–718.

Rottem, M., Barbieri, S., and Kinet, J.-P., and Metcalfe, D. D. (1992). Kinetics of the appearance of $Fc_{\epsilon}RI$-bearing cells in interleukin-3-dependent mouse bone marrow cultures: correlation with histamine content and mast cell maturation. *Blood.* 79:972–980.

Schrader, J. W. (1981). The in vitro production and cloning of the P cell, a bone marrow derived null cell that expressed H-2 and Ia antigens, has mast cell-like granules, and is regulated by a factor released by activated T cells. *J. Immunol.* 126:452–458.

Sonoda, T., Ohno, T., and Kitamura, Y. (1982). Concentration of mast-cell progenitors in bone marrow, spleen, and blood of mice determined by limiting dilution analysis. *J. Cell Physiol.* 112:136–140.

Sonoda, T., Kitamura, Y., Haku, Y., Hara, H., and Mori, K. J. (1983). Mast cell precursors in various hematopoietic colonies of mice produced in vivo and in vitro. *Br. J. Hematol.* 53:611–620.

Sredni, B., Friedman, M. M., Bland, C. D., and Metcalfe, D. D. (1983). Ultrastructural, biochemical, and functional characteristics of histamine-containing cells cloned from mouse bone marrow: Tentative identification as mucosal mast cell. *J. Immunol.* 131:915–922.

Tadokoro, K., Stadler, B. M., and de Weck, A. L. (1983). Factor dependent in vitro growth of normal bone marrow derived basophil-like cells. *J. Exp. Med.* 158:857–871.

Tan, J. C., Nocka, K., Ray, P., Traktman, P., and Besmer, P. (1990). The dominant *W42 spotting* phenotype results from a missense mutation in the c-*kit* receptor kinase. *Science* 247:209–212.

Tertian, G., Yung, Y. P., Guy-Grand, D., and Moore, M. A. S. (1981). Long term in vitro culture of murine mast cells. I. Description of a growth factor dependent culture technique. *J. Immunol.* 127:788–794.

Thompson, H., Metcalfe, D. D., and Kinet, J. P. (1990). Early expression of high-affinity receptor for immunoglobulin E (FceRI) during differentiation of mouse mast cells and human basophils. *J. Clin. Invest.* 85:1227–1233.

Valent, P., Ashman, L. K., Hinterberger, W., Eckersberger, F., Majdic, O., Lechner, K., and Bettelheim, P. (1989). Mast cell typing: Demonstration of a distinct hematopoietic cell type and evidence of immunophenotypic relationship to mononuclear phagocytes, *Blood* 73:1778–1785.

Yokota, T., Lee, F., Rennick, D., Hall, L., Arai, N., Mosmann, T., Nabel, T., Cantor, H., and Arai, K. (1984). Isolation and characterization of mouse cDNA clone that expresses mast cell growth factor activity in monkey cells. *Proc. Natl. Acad. Sci. USA* 81:1070–1074.

Yung, Y. P., and Moore, M. A. S. (1984). Mast cell growth factor: Its role in mast cell differentiation, proliferation, and maturation. In *Contemporary Topics in Molecular Immunology*. Vol. 10. Edited by F. P. Inman and S. Gillis. New York, Plenum Press, pp. 147–179.

Zsebo, K. M., Wypych, J., McNiece, I. K., Lu, H. S., Smith, K. A., Karkare, S. B., Sachdev, R. K., Yuschenkoff, V. N., Birkett, N. C., Williams, L. R., Satyagal,

V. N., Weifong, T., Bosselman, R. A., Mendiaz, E. A., and Langley, K. E. (1990a). Identification, purification, and biological characterization of hematopoietic stem cell factor from buffalo rat liver-conditioned medium. *Cell* 63:195–201.

Zsebo, K. M., Williams, D. A., Geissler, E. N., Broudy, V. C., Martin, F. H., Atkins, H. L., Hsu, R-Y., Birkett, N. C., Okino, K. H., Murdock, D. C., Jacobsen, F. W., Langley, K. E., Smith, K. A., Takeishi, T., Cattanach, B. M., Galli, S. J., and Suggs, S. V. (1990b). Stem cell factor is encoded at the *Sl* locus of the mouse and is the ligand for c-*kit* tyrosine kinase receptor. *Cell* 63:213–224.

Zucker-Franklin, D., Grusky, G., Hirayama, N., and Schnipper, E. (1981). The presence of mast cell precursors in rat peripheral blood. *Blood* 58:544–551.

6

Heterogeneity of Human Mast Cells

LAWRENCE B. SCHWARTZ

Medical College of Virginia
Richmond, Virginia

I. Introduction

The presence of more than one type of mast cell in humans is a critical concept relevant to the role of mast cells in health and disease. Variations in fixation properties provided the first experimental evidence suggesting the existence of different types of human mast cells (Strobel et al., 1981), somewhat similar to the situation described in rodents (Enerback, 1966). Accordingly, intestinal mucosal mast cells (MMC) displayed metachromatic staining after fixation in Carnoy's solution, but not when fixed in neutral buffered formalin. In contrast, connective tissue mast cells (CTMC) found in the intestinal submucosa retained their metachromatic staining properties regardless of the fixative used. However, Craig et al. (1986) found that, in humans, the number of mast cells visualized by toluidine blue staining decreases both in the intestinal mucosa and submucosa when aldehyde fixatives are used instead of Carnoy's fluid. Furthermore, these fixation-dependent methods are limited by the inability to recognize different types of mast cells in a single section. Thus, these apparent differences did not provide precise criteria for identification of different types of mast cells in humans. In this review, mast cell heterogeneity will refer to differences between mast cells relating to function, maturity, lineage, and both qualitative and quantitative compositional features. Mast cell type will refer to the two mast cell subsets defined below on the basis of protease composition, which are thought to reflect developmental pathways.

Evidence for the unambiguous presence of two types of human mast cells was based on finding distinct protease patterns in mast cells in different tissues (Irani et al., 1986; Schechter et al., 1990). MC_{TC} cells contain tryptase, chymase, a cathepsin G–like protease, and carboxypeptidase; MC_T cells contain only tryptase (Table 1). Immunohistochemical techniques distinguish between these two types of mast cells in the same tissue section, thus allowing for an accurate quantitation of their respective numbers at various organ sites as well as in the dispersed cell preparations used for biochemical or functional studies. The characteristic tissue distribution of each mast cell type defines the target organ and consequently the physiological response to release of mediators and suggests that both types are mature cells with distinct roles. Functional studies of mast cells dispersed from different tissues suggest further heterogeneity. Although all mast cells respond to IgE-mediated and A23187 signals, basic peptides, substance P, and complement anaphylatoxins activate skin, but not lung or colonic mucosa-derived mast cells (Lawrence et al., 1987; Tharp et al., 1987; Benyon et al., 1987; Church et al., 1982). Disodium cromoglycate and nedocromil modestly inhibit histamine release from mast cells recovered by bronchoalveolar lavage, but show minimal, if any, inhibition of degranulation of mast cells in preparations of dispersed human lung, intestinal mucosa, and skin (Flint et al., 1985; Church and Hiroi, 1987; Befus et al., 1987; Pearce et al., 1974) or in vivo in skin (Ting et al., 1983). Comparison of the results obtained by these various studies is somewhat complicated by the lack of standardization of the experimental methods used to disperse and purify mast cells from human tissues and variations from tissue to tissue in accessory cell populations that copurify

Table 1 Selected Characteristics of Human MC_T and MC_{TC} Cells

Characteristic	MC_T	MC_{TC}
Neutral protease	Tryptase	Tryptase Chymase Cathepsin G Carboxypeptidase
Granule ultrastructure	Discrete scrolls	Gratings/Lattices
T-lymphocyte dependence	+	–
Activation by complement anaphylatoxin	–	+
Inhibition of histamine release by cromolyn	+	–

with mast cells. Whether the functional differences appreciated in mast cells derived from different human tissues reflect lineage-related differences or simply the local effects of the tissue microenvironment needs to be resolved. The following review will summarize information on these mast cell neutral proteases, the distribution of the two types of human mast cells in different tissues, and studies relating to the lineage of MC_T and MC_{TC} cells.

II. The Neutral Proteases of Human Mast Cells

A. Tryptase

Tryptase is a serine endoprotease with specificity for trypsin-like substrates (Schwartz et al., 1981) and serves as a specific marker for human mast cells relative to other cell types (Castells et al., 1987; Schwartz, 1985; Irani et al., 1989a). With electron microscopic techniques, positive staining for tryptase occurs in immature mast cells at a time when granule formation first begins (Craig et al., 1989). Preliminary evidence in mast cells developed in vitro from human fetal livers indicates that tryptase appears in granules prior to their acquisition of metachromatic staining properties. Thus, tryptase may serve as a marker for immature forms of mast cells, as they first become granulated. Threefold greater amounts of tryptase were found in mast cells derived from adult foreskin (35 $\mu g/10^6$ mast cells; 99% MC_{TC} cells) than in those from adult lung (12 $\mu g/10^6$ mast cells; 93% MC_T cells) (Schwartz et al., 1987a) by ELISA (Wenzel et al., 1986), a quantitative but not qualitative difference between mast cells from these two tissues.

Active tryptase is a tetramer that is stabilized by its ionic association with heparin proteoglycan and appears to be stored in and released from mast cells as a complex with proteoglycan (Alter et al., 1987; Schwartz and Bradford, 1986; Schwartz et al., 1990). When free in physiological buffer or plasma, tryptase inactivation proceeds rapidly and is associated with conversion of the tetrameric form to that of a monomer. No active site inhibitor of tryptase has been found in human tissues and fluids (Alter et al., 1990), suggesting that the association of tryptase with heparin is the primary means of regulating its enzymatic activity in vivo. Two major cDNA variants of tryptase, called α- and β-tryptase, and four variants of β-tryptase have been detected (Vanderslice et al., 1990; Miller et al., 1989, 1990). Both major cDNA species are represented in the normal haploid human genome on chromosome 16. Whether isoenzymes of tryptase exist, each containing different ratios of the cDNA products, is not known.

The biological role of tryptase is unsolved. Of potential interest are the generation of C3a from C3 (Schwartz et al., 1983), destruction of the clotting activity of fibrinogen (Schwartz et al., 1985), activation of prostromelysin (which in turn activates procollagenase) (Gruber et al., 1989), and enhancement of pulmonary smooth muscle contractility to histamine (Sekizawa et al., 1989). The prolonged retention in tissues of tryptase as a complex with heparin and perhaps other proteases after its release from mast cells suggests that an effect on the local tissue microenvironment or on recruited plasma proteins is likely.

Because of its selective concentration in secretory granules of human mast cells, tryptase levels in complex biological fluids such as serum serve as an indicator of mast cell activation. This permits the precise diagnosis of allergic reactions in both antemortem (Schwartz et al., 1987b, 1989) and postmortem samples (Yunginger et al., 1991). Mast cell activation also has been implicated in aspirin-induced immediate hypersensitivity reactions, high serum levels being found after anaphylaxis and after upper respiratory reactions associated with intestinal involvement (Bosso et al., 1989). In addition, analysis of tryptase levels in skin chamber fluids during cutaneous allergic reactions indicates that mast cell degranulation occurs in the early phase, but not in the late phase, of the allergic response (Shalit et al., 1988, 1990; Schwartz et al., 1987a). Further, basophils rather than mast cells appear to be the cell source of the elevated levels of histamine found during the late-phase cutaneous response. Similar results have been found in bronchoalveolar lavage fluid (BALF) after endobronchial allergen challenge of sensitive subjects (Sedgwick et al., 1990). In addition, elevated levels of tryptase in BALF taken from atopic asthmatics at baseline suggest ongoing mast cell activation occurs as a component of the chronic inflammatory state (Wenzel et al., 1988). Interestingly, tryptase levels are not elevated after exercise-induced bronchospasm, suggesting mast cells do not participate in this response (Broide et al., 1990). The elevated levels of tryptase in nasal lavage fluid and in tears, respectively, are the best pieces of evidence for mast cell activation in the nasal allergic response (Castells and Schwartz, 1988) and in ocular diseases, including allergic, vernal, and giant papillary cell conjunctivitis. Thus, measurements of tryptase in various biological fluids provide an objective means to assess mast cell involvement.

B. Chymase

Chymase is a serine endoprotease with specificity for chymotrypsin-like substrates (Schechter et al., 1986) and has been selectively localized to human mast cells of the MC_{TC} type by light (Irani et al., 1989a) and electron (Craig and Schwartz, 1990; Craig et al., 1988) microscopy. Levels of chymase as determined by radioimmunoassay were undetectable in extracts of lung mast cells, even though 7% were of the MC_{TC} type, and averaged 4.5 $\mu g/10^6$ mast cells in extracts of adult foreskin mast cells (99% MC_{TC} cells) (Schwartz et al., 1987b). Chymase-like enzymatic activity in mast cells from adult foreskin was 25-fold higher than in mast cells from lung. The source of the low level of chymase-like activity attributed to lung mast cells may be MC_{TC} cells, which comprise 7% of the lung mast cells. No evidence now exists for a chymase in MC_T cells or for additional human chymase enzymes in MC_{TC} cells (other than the cathepsin G–like protease described below).

Chymase is a monomer, optimally active at neutral pH. Like tryptase, chymase binds tightly to heparin, but unlike tryptase, is not stabilized by this interaction. Chymase is inhibited by many of the proteins that inhibit serine proteases, such as lima bean and soybean trypsin inhibitors and chymostatin. In plasma, α_1-antichymotrypsin, α_1-proteinase inhibitor, and α_2-macroglobulin are the major inhibitors of chymase; however, even these inhibitors are inefficient, serving as better substrates than inhibitors (Schechter et al., 1989). Thus, chymase, like tryptase, is resistant to inhibition by the protease inhibitors present in plasma. The biological activity of chymase, like that of tryptase, is unsolved. Of potential interest are the in vitro observations that chymase converts angiotensin I to II approximately fourfold more efficiently than angiotensin-converting enzyme (Wintroub et al., 1984), inactivates bradykinin (Reilly et al., 1982), and attacks the lamina lucida of the basement membrane at the dermal-epidermal junction of human skin (Briggaman et al., 1984).

C. Cathepsin G

Cathepsin G is a neutral protease found in neutrophils and monocytes. The presence of a cathepsin G–like protein in MC_{TC} cells has been demonstrated by immunohistochemistry using a polyclonal goat anti–cathepsin G antibody (Schechter et al., 1990). The staining of MC_{TC} cells could be blocked by preincubation of the antiserum with purified cathepsin G but not with chymase, indicating lack of cross-reactivity of the antibody with the proteinases. Double-labeling techniques using monoclonal murine antichymase antibody and the polyclonal goat anti–cathepsin G antibody showed a one to one correlation between chymase-containing and cathepsin G–containing mast cells, indicating the presence of cathepsin G in MC_{TC} but not MC_T cells. Western blot analysis of extracts of dispersed cutaneous mast cells showed a stained band at 30,000 Da. This comigrated with chymase and a minor species of cathepsin G present in neutrophils. The major form of cathepsin G migrates at 28,000 Da. Analysis of the catalytic chymotryptic activity in extracts of cutaneous mast cells revealed approximately 30% to be inhibited by aprotinin and anti–cathepsin G antibody, both of which inhibit cathepsin G and not chymase. These results indicate that substantial levels of this cathepsin G–like protease are present in MC_{TC} cells and extend the compositional differences between MC_{TC} and MC_T types of human mast cells.

D. Elastase

Elastase is a neutral protease which, like cathepsin G, is found in neutrophils, monocytes, and macrophages (Campbell et al., 1989). Immunohistochemistry with a polyclonal rabbit antielastase antibody failed to stain mast cells in human skin, lung, and small intestine, demonstrating the absence of elastase in MC_T as well as in MC_{TC} cells (Schechter et al., 1990).

E. Carboxypeptidase

Mast cell carboxypeptidase activity originally was identified in rodent mast cells (Everitt and Neurath, 1980; Schwartz et al., 1982). Later, a human carboxypeptidase was detected and localized to secretory granules in human mast cells dispersed from skin and lung by the IgE-mediated release of an activity that cleaves the carboxyterminal His^9-Leu^{10} bond of angiotensin I and behaves like a zinc metalloexopeptidase (Goldstein et al., 1987). Human mast cell carboxypeptidase is a monomeric enzyme with a M_r of 34,500 Da by SDS-PAGE electrophoresis (Goldstein et al., 1989). Based on the cDNA-derived amino acid sequence of the catalytic portion of the enzyme, the human enzyme is 86% identical to mouse mast cell carboxypeptidase A and has a calculated M_r of 36,100 Da and a net positive charge of 16 (Reynolds et al., 1989). Overall, the human enzyme is more homologous to human pancreatic carboxypeptidase B than A. However, the composition of the catalytic site is more homologous to human pancreatic carboxypeptidase A, as are its substrate specificities. Human mast cell carboxypeptidase removes carboxyterminal Phe and Leu residues, but does not recognize carboxyterminal Arg or Lys residues. However, unlike bovine pancreatic carboxypeptidase A, the human mast cell enzyme does not cleave des-Arg^9 bradykinin or substance P. The human enzyme has been called either human mast cell carboxypeptidase A or simply human mast cell carboxypeptidase (HMC-CP).

Two monoclonal murine antibodies were prepared against human mast cell carboxypeptidase purified from human skin. Western blots performed with CP_1 identified the 35,000-Da band of protein corresponding to mast cell carboxypeptidase (unpublished data). The monoclonal anti-HMC-CP antibodies selectively stained the MC_{TC} type of human mast cell. MC_T cells were not stained. Mast cells dispersed from neonatal foreskin, adult facial skin, and adult foreskin contain 0.5, 5, and 16 pg of carboxypeptidase per mast cell, respectively, as estimated by the enzymatic activity in mast cell extracts and the specific activity of the purified enzyme (Goldstein et al., 1989). Such levels presumably reflect the percentage and maturity of the MC_{TC} cells in each preparation. These findings extend the biochemical differences between MC_T and MC_{TC} types of human mast cells to include compositional differences in carboxypeptidase content as well as in the content of chymase.

F. Summary

The simultaneous, selective, and abundant presence of tryptase, chymase, carboxypeptidase, and a cathepsin G–like proteinase in the MC_{TC} type of human mast cell (Table 2) suggests a specialized function for this type of mast cell, requiring the collaborative actions of chymase, HMC-CP, and a cathepsin G–like proteinase. Such concerted activity has not yet been demonstrated with the human mast cell proteases. In the rat system, chymase I and the carboxypeptidase A isolated from the secretory granules of rat peritoneal mast cells sequentially degrade apolipoprotein B (Kokkonen et al., 1986). This facilitates uptake of low-density lipoprotein particles by macrophages, which then have the appearance of foam cells (Kokkonen and Kovanen, 1989). Because MC_{TC} cells in humans are the predominant mast cell type in periarteriolar and perivenular tissues (Irani et al., 1986), a concerted effect of released mast cell proteases on lipoprotein uptake by human macrophages similar to that observed in the rat may have a bearing on atherogenesis.

III. The Tissue Distribution and Morphology of MC_T and MC_{TC} Mast Cells

In 1986 two types of human mast cells were recognized by immunohistochemical techniques that were referred to as MC_T (containing tryptase alone) and MC_{TC} (containing tryptase and chymase) (Irani et al., 1986). The clear distinction between MC_T and MC_{TC} cells allows for an accurate analysis of their distribution at various organ sites. In most tissues examined, a mixture of MC_T and MC_{TC} cells is seen, the relative distribution of which varies markedly with the anatomical site. Therefore, MC_T and MC_{TC} cells cannot be distinguished from one another based on their location alone. In histologically normal tissues, MC_T cells are the predominant type of mast cells seen in the alveolar septa of the lung and in the small intestinal mucosa, while MC_{TC} cells predominate in the skin and in the small intestinal submucosa (Table 3). These observations have been confirmed histochemically with synthetic substrates selective for chymotryptic and tryptic protease activities (Osman et al., 1989). Therefore, in terms of tissue

Table 2 Neutral Proteases in Human MC_T and MC_{TC} Cells

	Content (pg/cell)	
Protease	MC_T	MC_{TC}
Tryptase	10	35
Chymase	ND	4.5
Carboxypeptidase	ND	10
Cathepsin G	ND	+
Elastase	ND	ND

ND = none detected; + = detectable but not quantified.

hampered studies of their growth and differentiation. Cultures of bone marrow and cord blood cells in the presence of T-lymphocyte factors, such as IL-3, have produced metachromatic cells with the characteristics of basophil leukocytes (Ishizaka et al., 1985). Human mast cells dispersed from various tissues lack IL-3-binding sites (Valent et al., 1990a). The demonstration that mast cells share certain surface membrane antigens with mononuclear phagocytic cells (gp65) that are absent on basophils and are not stained by certain myelocytic (CD11) and lymphocytic (CD25) markers expressed on basophils suggests that mast cells and basophilic leukocytes diverge early in development (Valent et al., 1989, 1990b). Recently, cocultures of cord blood mononuclear cells with mouse 3T3 fibroblasts have been found to result in the growth of mast cells, 80–90% of which are of the MC_{TC} phenotype (Furitsu et al., 1989); these findings suggest the presence in the cord blood mononuclear cell preparation of mast cell precursors that develop into the MC_{TC} type under the influence of factors derived from the mouse 3T3 fibroblasts, analogous to the development of the CTMC in the rodent system. Interestingly, addition of T-lymphocyte factors to the coculture did not alter the results such that MC_{TC} cells remained the predominant type of mast cell seen. Furthermore, these developing MC_{TC} cells did not appear to pass through an MC_T stage.

In another study, mast cells at immature stages of development were identified in newborn and adult human tissues by ultrastructure. Morphological criteria such as high nuclear/cytoplasmic ratio, small cell size, fewer and smaller granules, and lack of features of mast cell activation or regranulation indicate immaturity (Craig et al., 1989). Essentially all mast cells in foreskins of newborn infants appear immature, whereas 5–15% of the mast cells in adult lung, foreskin, bowel mucosa, and bowel submucosa appear immature. Immunogold staining with antitryptase and antichymase antibodies identifies immature mast cells as belonging to the MC_T and MC_{TC} type; their tissue distributions seem to parallel those of the mature mast cell types. Immature MC_T cells contain the same characteristic discrete scrolls found in their mature counterparts. The majority of granules in immature MC_{TC} cells have one or more amorphous electron-dense cores rather than the grating and lattice substructures characteristic of granules of mature MC_{TC} cells. However, cells of slightly higher maturity contain transitional granules with dense cores and gratings or lattices, indicating that immature and mature forms of MC_{TC} cells are developmentally related. The finding of compositional and ultrastructural differences in immature mast cells suggest that the two types of human mast cells follow distinct developmental pathways, at least from the time granule formation begins.

Evidence for the dependence of the MC_T cell on functional T lymphocytes comes from the analysis of gastrointestinal tissue from subjects with congenital or acquired disorders affecting T-lymphocyte function (AIDS and combined immunodeficiency). A selective depletion of MC_T cells is seen, while the number of MC_{TC} cells is normal or slightly increased (Irani et al., 1987b). In synovium obtained from subjects with rheumatoid arthritis, where mast cell hyperplasia has previously been documented, a mixture of MC_T and MC_{TC} cells is seen in areas of heavy lymphocytic infiltration, while MC_{TC} cells are the exclusive type of mast cells seen in the normal synovium (Irani et al., 1987a), suggesting that the lymphocytic factors present in the inflamed tissues contribute to the appearance of the MC_T cells. Similarly, recruitment of MC_T cells has been demonstrated in the acutely inflamed skin lesions of subjects with atopic dermatitis (Irani et al., 1989b), along with lymphocytic infiltration, while MC_{TC} cells account entirely for the mast cell hyperplasia seen in cutaneous lesions of subjects with mastocytosis where substantial numbers of T lymphocytes have not been observed (Irani et al., 1990). These observations extend the analogy between the human MC_T cell and the T-lymphocyte–dependent MMC, but do not indicate the specific growth factor(s) involved.

The site(s) of T-lymphocyte influence on MC_T cell development also are unknown. Progenitors present in human fetal liver, when cocultured with 3T3 fibroblasts, develop normally as MC_T cells in the presence or absence of IL-3 or T-lymphocyte–conditioned media. However, these progenitors already may be committed to develop as one or the other mast cell type. A role for T-cell factors at an earlier stage of mast cell development therefore needs to be considered. Also, a role for T-lymphocyte factors in the recruitment of a particular mast cell type to a tissue is another consideration.

Assuming a common precursor for both MC_T and MC_{TC} cells, it is likely that divergent pathways of differentiation exist in which T-lymphocyte factors facilitate the development of MC_T but not MC_{TC} cells, while the presence of factors derived from tissue fibroblasts may facilitate the development of a committed mast cell precursor from a putative stem cell as well as provide the necessary milieu for prolonged survival of both types of mast cells (Fig. 1). Compositional and ultrastructural differences seen in immature forms of the two types of mast cell, as well as the lack of identifiable transitional forms of mast cells, argue against the possibility of a linear pathway of differentiation, whereby MC_T cells would be derived from MC_{TC} cells. On the other hand, if MC_{TC} cells were derived from MC_T cells, one would expect to see a decrease in both types of mast cells in gastrointestinal tissue of subjects with defective T-lymphocyte function. Transdifferentiation, if it occurs, would involve the dedifferentiation of either type of mature mast cell into a putative precursor form followed by redifferentiation along divergent pathways into either MC_T or MC_{TC} types of mast cells. Direct interconversion between the two types of mast cell seems unlikely in light of the close proximity of MC_T and MC_{TC} cells in many tissues. The failure to detect mast cell or mast cell precursors in the circulation indicates that granule formation occurs after a tissue site of residence has been established. However, commitment of precursor cells to a particular lineage may occur prior

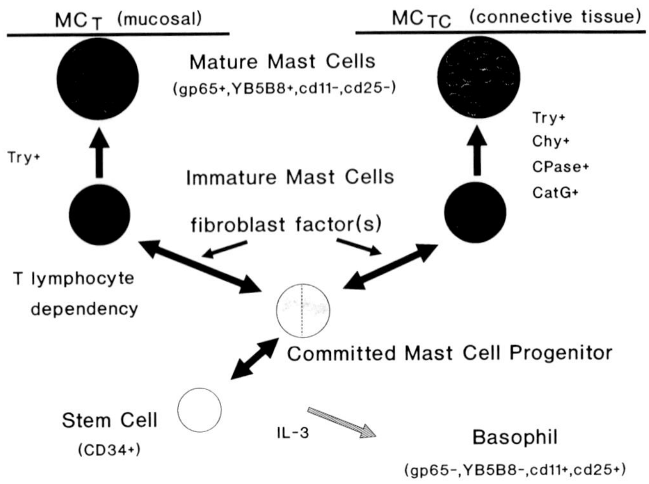

Figure 1 Development of different types of human mast cells.

to or with the onset of granule formation, as is suggested by the findings of compositional and ultrastructural differences in immature mast cells and of the predilection for mast cell progenitors in cord blood and fetal liver to develop as MC_{TC} and MC_T cells, respectively. The predominance of a particular type of mast cell in a given location may reflect selective migration of the committed precursor to that site. Alternatively, local factors may direct the maturation of precursor cells already committed to a mast cell lineage, to complete their development as either an MC_{TC} or MC_T cell type.

V. Concluding Comments

There is now strong evidence for the presence of two types of mast cell in humans. The neutral proteases of human mast cells provide a highly sensitive and selective means of identifying mast cells in human tissues and cell preparations and of recognizing the MC_{TC} and MC_T types of human mast cell. Immunohistochemical techniques provide a tool for precisely evaluating their distribution in tissues during both health and disease. Interpretation of functional and biochemical studies conducted on mast cells dispersed from various organs necessitates that the type of mast cells present be determined in each case. It is now clear that the distribution of MC_T and MC_{TC} cells can be markedly affected by pathological conditions. A factor that may affect the distribution of the two types of mast cells in dispersed cell preparations is the method of purification.

For example, dispersed human lung mast cells consist of approximately 90% MC_T cells; however, density gradient sedimentation enriches for MC_{TC} cells in the fractions of higher density (unpublished observations). The special role of each type of mast cell in biological/pathobiological events will reflect their tissue distribution and protease compositions, as well as possible differences in activation-secretion mechanisms and responses to pharmacological agents.

Discussion

Platts-Mills: Do changes in the mast cell subtypes seen in AIDs correlate with changes in eosinophils or basophils as well?
Schwartz: We have not looked.
Dvorak: What are the phenotypes in intraepithelial mast cells?
Schwartz: Intestinal and airway intraepithelial mast cells are of the MC_T type.
Hanifen: During an inflammatory response, could mast cells intraconvert?
Schwartz: It is hard to conceive of a MC_{TC} cell losing its tryptase, chymase, and cathepsin G in order to convert to a MC_T cell.
White: Is there any evidence for changes in mast cell phenotypes in relation to allergic reactions?
Schwartz: There is anecdotal information suggesting a superficial migration of MC_T during allergic nasal responses.
Lichtenstein: Do you know the mast cell phenotype of the uterus or BAL?
Schwartz: BAL cells are of MC_T type.

References

Alter, S. C., Metcalfe, D. D., Bradford, T. R., and Schwartz, L. B. (1987). Regulation of human mast cell tryptase. Effects of enzyme concentration, ionic strength and the structure and negative charge density of polysaccharides. *Biochem. J.* 248:821–827.

Alter, S. C., Kramps, J. A., Janoff, A., and Schwartz, L. B. (1990). Interactions of human mast cell tryptase with biological protease inhibitors. *Arch. Biochem. Biophys.* 276:26–31.

Befus, A. D., Dyck, N., Goodacre, R., and Bienenstock, J. (1987). Mast cells from the human intestinal lamina popria: Isolation, histochemical subtypes, and functional characterization. *Immunology* 138:2604–2610.

Benyon, R. C., Lowman, M. A., and Church, M. K. (1987). Human skin mast cells: Their dispersion, purification, and secretory characterization. *J. Immunol.* 138:861–867.

Bosso, J. V., Stevenson, D. D., and Schwartz, L. B. (1989). Tryptasemia with aspirin-induced respiratory reaction. *J. Allergy Clin. Immunol.* 83:184 (abstract).

Briggaman, R. A., Schechter, N. M., Fraki, J., and Lazarus, G. S. (1984). Degradation of the epidermal-dermal junction by a proteolytic enzyme from human skin and human polymorphonuclear leukocytes. *J. Exp. Med.* 160:1027–1042.

Broide, D. H., Eisman, S., Ramsdell, J. W., Ferguson, P., Schwartz, L. B., and Wasserman, S. I. (1990). Airway levels of mast cell-derived mediators in exercise-induced asthma. *Am. Rev. Respir. Dis.* 141:563–568.

Campbell, E. J., Silverman, E. K., and Campbell, M. A. (1989). Elastase and cathepsin G of human monocytes, quantification of cellular content, release in response to stimuli, and heterogeneity in elastase-mediated proteolytic activity. *J. Immunol.* 143:2961–2968.

Castells, M., and Schwartz, L. B. (1988). Tryptase levels in nasal-lavage fluid as an indicator of the immediate allergic response. *J. Allergy Clin. Immunol.* 82:348–355.

Castells, M. C., Irani, A. M., and Schwartz, L. B. (1987). Evaluation of human peripheral blood leukocytes for mast cell tryptase. *J. Immunol.* 138:2184–2189.

Church, M. K., and Hiroi, J. (1987). Inhibition of IgE-dependent histamine release from human dispersed lung mast cells by anti-allergic drugs and salbutamol. *Br. J. Pharmacol.* 90:421–429.

Church, M. K., Pao, G. J. K., and Holgate, S. T. (1982). Characterization of histamine secretion from mechanically dispersed human lung mast cells: Effects of anti-IgE, calcium ionophore A 23187, compound 48/80, and basic polypeptides. *J. Immunol.* 129:2116–2121.

Craig, S. S., and Schwartz, L. B. (1990). Human MC_{TC} type of mast cell granule: The uncommon occurrence of discrete scrolls associated with focal absence of chymase. *Lab. Invest.* 63:581–585.

Craig, S. S., DeBlois, G., and Schwartz, L. B. (1986). Mast cells in human keloid, small intestine, and lung by an immunoperoxidase technique using a murine monoclonal antibody against tryptase. *Am. J. Pathol.* 124:427–435.

Craig, S. S., Schechter, N. M., and Schwartz, L. B. (1988). Ultrastructural analysis of human T and TC mast cells identified by immunoelectron microscopy. *Lab. Invest.* 58:682–691.

Craig, S. S., Schechter, N. M., and Schwartz, L. B. (1989). Ultrastructural analysis of maturing human T and TC mast cells in situ. *Lab. Invest.* 60:147–157.

Enerback, L. (1966). Mast cells in rat gastrointestinal mucosa. I. Effects of fixation. *Acta Pathol. Microbiol. Scand.* 66:289–302.

Everitt, M. T., and Neurath, H. (1980). Rat peritoneal mast cell carboxypeptidase: Localization, purification and enzymatic properties. *FEBS Lett.* 110:292–296.

Flint, K. C., Leung, K. B. P., Pearce, F. L., Hudspith, B. N., Brostoff, J., and Johnson, N. M. (1985). Human mast cells recovered by bronchoalveolar lavage: Their morphology, histamine release and the effects of sodium cromoglycate. *Clin Sci.* 68:427–432.

Furitsu, T., Saito, H., Dvorak, A., Schwartz, L. B., Irani, A. A., Burdick, J. F., Ishizaka, K., and Ishizaka, T. (1989). Development of human mast cells in vitro. *Proc. Natl. Acad. Sci. USA* 86:10039–10043.

Goldstein, S. M., Kaempfer, C. E., Proud, D., Schwartz, L. B., Irani, A. M., and Wintroub, B. U. (1987). Detection and partial characterization of a human mast cell carboxypeptidase. *J. Immunol.* 139:2724–2729.

Goldstein, S. M., Kaempfer, C. E., Kealey, J. T., and Wintroub, B. U. (1989). Human mast cell carboxypeptidase: purification and characterization. *J. Clin. Invest.* 83:1630–1636.

Gruber, B. L., Marchese, M. J., Suzuki, K., Schwartz, L. B., Okada, Y., Nagase, H., and Ramamurthy, N. S. (1989). Synovial procollagenase activation by human mast cell tryptase dependence upon matrix metalloproteinase 3 activation. *J. Clin. Invest.* 84:1657–1662.

Irani, A. A., Schechter, N. M., Craig, S. S., DeBlois, G., and Schwartz, L. B. (1986). Two types of human mast cells that have distinct neutral protease compositions. *Proc. Natl. Acad. Sci. USA* 83:4464–4468.

Irani, A. A., Golzar, N., DeBlois, G., Gruber, B., and Schwartz, L. B. (1987a). Distribution of mast cell subsets in rheumatoid arthritis and osteoarthritis synovia. *Arthritis Rheum.* 30:66 (abstract).

Irani, A. M., Craig, S. S., DeBlois, G., Elson, C. O., Schechter, N. M., and Schwartz, L. B. (1987b). Deficiency of the tryptase-positive, chymase-negative mast cell type in gastrointestinal mucosa of patients with defective T lymphocyte function. *J. Immunol.* 138:4381–4386.

Irani, A. A., Bradford, T. R., Kepley, C. L., Schechter, N. M., and Schwartz, L. B. (1989a). Detection of MCT and MCTC types of human mast cells by immunohistochemistry using new monoclonal anti-tryptase and anti-chymase antibodies. *J. Histochem. Cytochem.* 37:1509–1515.

Irani, A. A., Sampson, H. A., and Schwartz, L. B. (1989b). Mast cells in atopic dermatitis. *Allergy* 44 (Suppl 9):31–34.

Irani, A. A., Garriga, M. M., Metcalfe, D. D., and Schwartz, L. B. (1990). Mast cells in cutaneous mastocytosis: Accumulation of the MCTC type. *Clin. Exp. Immunol. Clin. Exp. Allergy* 20:53–58.

Ishizaka, T., Conrad, D. H., Huff, T. F., Metcalfe, D. D., Stevens, R. L., and Lewis, R. A. (1985). Unique features of human basophilic granulocytes developed in in vitro culture. *Int. Arch. Allergy Appl. Immunol.* 77:137–143.

Jarboe, D. L., Marshall, J. S., Randolph, T. R., Kukolja, A., and Huff, T. F. (1989). The mast cell-committed progenitor. I. Description of a cell capable of IL-3 independent proliferation and differentiation without contact with fibroblasts. *J. Immunol.* 142:2405–2417.

Kanakura, Y., Thompson, H., Nakano, T., Yamamura, T., Asai, H., Kitamura, Y., Metcalfe, D. D., and Galli, S. J. (1988). Multiple bidirectional alterations of phenotype and changes in proliferative potential during the in vitro and in vivo passage of clonal mast cell populations derived from mouse peritoneal mast cells. *Blood* 72:877–885.

Kitamura, Y., Sonoda, T., Nokano, T., and Kanayama, Y. (1986). Probable dedifferentiation of mast cells in mouse connective tissues. *Current Topics Dev. Biol.* 20:325–332.

Kokkonen, J. O., and Kovanen, P. T. (1989). Proteolytic enzyme of mast cell granules degrade low density lipoproteins and promote their granule-mediated uptake by macrophages in vitro. *J. Biol. Chem.* 264:10749–10755.

Kokkonen, J. O., Vartiainen, M., and Fovanen, P. T. (1986). Low density lipoprotein degradation by secretory granules of rat mast cells: Sequential degradation of apolipoprotein B by granule chymase and carboxypeptidase A. *J. Biol. Chem.* 261:16067–16072.

Lawrence, I. D., Warner, J. A., Cohan, V. L., Hubbard, W. C., Kagey-Sobotka, A., and Lichtenstein, L. M. (1987). Purification and characterization of human skin mast cells. *J. Immunol.* 139:3062–3069.

Levi-Schaffer, F., Austen, K. F., Gravallese, P. M., and Stevens, R. L. (1986). Coculture of interleukin 3-dependent mouse mast cells with fibroblasts results in a phenotypic change of the mast cells [published erratum appears in *Proc. Natl. Acad. Sci. USA* 83(20):7805 1986]. *Proc. Natl. Acad. Sci. USA* 83:6485–6488.

Miller, J. S., Westin, E. H., and Schwartz, L. B. (1989). Cloning and characterization of complementary DNA for human tryptase. *J. Clin. Invest.* 84:1188–1195.

Miller, J. S., Moxley, G., and Schwartz, L. B. (1990). Cloning and characterization of a second complementary DNA for human tryptase. *J. Clin. Invest.* 86:864–870.

Nakano, T., Sonoda, T., Hayashi, C., Yamatodani, A., Kanayama, Y., Yamamura, T., Asai, H., Yonezawa, T., Kitamura, Y., and Galli, S. J. (1985). Fate of bone marrow-derived cultured mast cells after intracutaneous, intraperitoneal and intracenous transfer into genetically mast cell deficient W/W mice. Evidence that cultured mast cells can give rise to both connective tissue type and mucosal mast cells. *J. Exp. Med.* 162:1025–1043.

Osman, I. A. R., Garrett, J. R., and Smith, R. E. (1989). Enzyme histochemical discrimination between tryptase and chymase in mast cells of human gut. *J. Histochem. Cytochem.* 37:415–421.

Pearce, C. A., Greaves, W. M., Plummer, V. M., and Yamamoto, E. S. (1974). Effect of disodium cromoglycate on antigen-evoked histamine release from human skin. *Clin. Exp. Immunol.* 17:437–440.

Reilly, C. F., Tewksbury, D. A., Schechter, N. M., and Travis, J. (1982). Rapid conversion of angiotensin I to angiotensin II by neutrophil and mast cell proteinases. *J. Biol. Chem.* 257:8619–8622.

Reynolds, D. S., Gurley, D. S., Stevens, R. L., Sugarbaker, D. J., Austen, K. F., and Serafin, W. E. (1989). Cloning of cDNAs that encode human mast cell carboxypeptidase A, and comparison of the protein with mouse mast cell carboxypeptidase A and rat pancreatic carboxypeptidases. *Proc. Natl. Acad. Sci. USA* 86:9480–9484.

Schechter, N. M., Choi, J. K., Slavin, D. A., Deresienski, D. T., Sayama, S., Dong, G., Lavker, R. M., Proud, D., and Lazarus, G. S. (1986). Identification of a chymotrypsin-like proteinase in human mast cells. *J. Immunol.* 137:962–970.

Schechter, N. M., Sprows, J. L., Schoenberger, O. L., Lazarus, G. S., Cooperman, B. S., and Rubin, H. (1989). Reaction of human skin chymotrypsin-like proteinase chymase with plasma proteinase inhibitors. *J. Biol. Chem.* 264:21308–21315.

Schechter, N. M., Irani, A-M., A., Sprows, J. L., Abernethy, J., Wintroub, B., and Schwartz, L. B. (1990). Identification of a cathepsin G-like proteinase in the MC_{TC} type of human mast cell. *J. Immunol.* 145:2652–2661.

Schwartz, L. B. (1985). Monoclonal antibodies against human mast cell tryptase demonstrate shared antigenic sites on subunits of tryptase and selective localization of the enzyme to mast cells. *J. Immunol.* 134:526–531.

Schwartz, L. B., and Bradford, T. R. (1986). Regulation of tryptase from human lung mast cells by heparin: Stabilization of the active tetramer. *J. Biol. Chem.* 261: 7372–7379.

Schwartz, L. B., Lewis, R. A., and Austen, K. F. (1981). Tryptase from human pulmonary mast cells. Purification and characterization. *J. Biol. Chem.* 256: 11939–11943.

Schwartz, L. B., Riedel, C., Schratz, J. J., and Austen, K. F. (1982). Localization of carboxypeptidase A to the macromolecular heparin proteoglycan-protein complex in secretory granules of rat serosal mast cells. *J. Immunol.* 128:1128–1133.

Schwartz, L. B., Kawahara, M. S., Hugli, T. E., Vik, D., Fearon, D. T., and Austen, K. F. (1983). Generation of C3a anaphylatoxin from human C3 by human mast cell tryptase. *J. Immunol.* 130:1891–1895.

Schwartz, L. B., Bradford, T. R., Littman, B. H., and Wintroub, B. U. (1985). The fibrinogenolytic activity of purified tryptase from human lung mast cells. *J. Immunol.* 135:2762–2767.

Schwartz, L. B., Atkins, P. C., Bradford, T. R., Fleekop, P., Shalit, M., and Zweiman, B. (1987a). Release of tryptase together with histamine during the immediate cutaneous response to allergen. *J. Allergy Clin. Immunol.* 80:850–855.

Schwartz, L. B., Irani, A. M. A., Roller, K., Castells, C., and Schechter, N. M. (1987b). Quantitation of histamine, tryptase and chymase in dispersed human T and TC mast cells. *J. Immunol.* 138:2611–2615.

Schwartz, L. B., Metcalfe, D. D., Miller, J. S., Earl, H., and Sullivan, T. (1987c). Tryptase levels as an indicator of mast-cell activation in systemic anaphylaxis and mastocytosis. *N. Engl. J. Med.* 316:1622–1626.

Schwartz, L. B., Yunginger, J. W., Miller, J. S., Bokhari, R., and Dull, D. (1989). The time course of appearance and disappearance of human mast cell tryptase in the circulation after anaphylaxis. *J. Clin. Invest.* 83:1551–1555.

Schwartz, L. B., Bradford, T. R., Lee, D. G., and Chlebowski, J. F. (1990). Immunologic and physicochemical evidence of conformational changes occurring on conversion of human mast cell tryptase from active tetramer to inactive monomer: Production of monoclonal antibodies recognizing active tryptase. *J. Immunol.* 144:2304–2311.

Sedgwick, J. B., Calhoun, W. J., Gleich, G. J., Kita, H., Abrams, J. S., Schwartz, L. B., Volovitz, B., Ben-Jacob, M., and Busse, W. W. (1990). Localized airway eosinophil response to bronchial segmental antigen challenge. *Am. Rev. Respir. Dis.* 141:A934 (abstract).

Sekizawa, K., Caughey, G. H., Lazarus, S. C., Gold, W. M., and Nadel, J. A. (1989). Mast cell tryptase causes airway smooth muscle hyperresponsiveness in dogs. *J. Clin. Invest.* 83:175–179.

Shalit, M., Schwartz, L. B., Golzar, N., vonAllman, C., Valenzano, M., Fleekop, P., Atkins, P. C., and Zweiman, B. (1988). Release of histamine and tryptase in vivo after prolonged cutaneous challenge with allergen in humans. *J. Immunol.* 141:821–826.

Shalit, M., Schwartz, L. B., von Allmen, C., Atkins, P. C., Lavker, R. M., and Zweiman, B. (1990). Release of histamine and tryptase during continuous and interrupted cutaneous challenge with allergen in humans. *J. Allergy Clin. Immunol.* 86:117–125.

Strobel, S., Miller, H. R., and Ferguson, A. (1981). Human intestinal mucosal mast cells: Evaluation of fixation and staining techniques. *J. Clin. Pathol.* 34:851–858.

Tharp, M. D., Kagey-Sobotka, A., Fox, C. C., Marone, G., Lichtenstein, L. M., and Sullivan, T. J. (1987). Functional heterogeneity of human mast cells from different anatomic sites: In vitro responses to morphine sulfate. *J. Allergy Clin. Immunol.* 79:646–653.

Ting, S., Zweiman, B., and Lavker, R. M. (1983). Cromolyn does not modulate human allergic skin reactions in vivo. *J. Allergy Clin. Immunol.* 71:12–17.

Valent, P., Ashman, L. K., Hinterberger, W., Eckersberger, F., Majdic, O., Lechner, K., and Bettelheim, P. (1989). Mast cell typing: Demonstration of a distinct hematopoietic cell type and evidence for immunophenotypic relationship to mononuclear phagocytes. *Blood* 7:1778–1785.

Valent, P., Besemer, J., Sillaber, C. H., Butterfield, J. H., Eher, R., Majdic, O., Kishi, K., Klepetko, W., Eckersberger, F., Lechner, K., and Bettelheim, P. (1990a). Failure to detect IL-3-binding sites on human mast cells. *J. Immunol.* 145:3432–3437.

Valent, P., Majdic, O., Maurer, D., Bodger, M., Muhm, M., and Bettelheim, P. (1990b). Further characterization of surface membrane structures expressed on human basophils and mast cells. *Int. Arch. Allergy Appl. Immunol.* 91:198–203.

Vanderslice, P., Ballinger, S. M., Tam, E. K., Goldstein, S. M., Craik, C. S., and Caughey, G. H. (1990). Human mast cell tryptase: Multiple cDNAs and genes reveal a multigene serine protease family. *Proc. Natl. Acad. Sci. USA* 87:3811–3815.

Wenzel, S., Irani, A. M., Sanders, J. M., Bradford, T. R., and Schwartz, L. B. (1986). Immunoassay of tryptase from human mast cells. *J. Immunol. Methods* 86:139–142.

Wenzel, S. E., Fowler, A. A., 3d, and Schwartz, L. B. (1988). Activation of pulmonary mast cells by bronchoalveolar allergen challenge. In vivo release of histamine and tryptase in atopic subjects with and without asthma. *Am. Rev. Respir. Dis.* 137:1002–1008.

Wintroub, B. U., Schechter, N. B., Lazarus, G. S., Kaempfer, C. E., and Schwartz, L. B. (1984). Angiotensin I conversion by human and rat chymotryptic proteinases. *J. Invest. Dermatol.* 83:336–339.

Yunginger, J. W., Nelson, D. R., Squillace, D. L., Jones, R. T., Holley, K. E., Hyma, B. A., Biedrzycki, L., Sweeney, K. G., Sturner, W. Q., and Schwartz, L. B. (1991). Laboratory investigation of deaths due to anaphylaxis. *J. Forensic Sci.* 36:857–865.

7

Development of Human Mast Cells from Umbilical Cord Blood Cells by Soluble Factors from 3T3 Fibroblasts

TERUKO ISHIZAKA, TAKUMA FURITSU, NAOKI INAGAKI, and YUTAKA TAGAYA

La Jolla Institute for Allergy and Immunology
La Jolla, California

I. Introduction

A long term coculture of mononuclear cells of human umbilical cord blood with mouse skin–derived 3T3 fibroblasts resulted in the development of human mast cells. These mast cells are morphologically and functionally mature cells, containing 1.4–2.8 μg histamine per 10^6 cells and bearing approximately 10^5 $Fc_\epsilon RI$ per cell. The mast cells sensitized with human IgE released histamine and arachidonic acid upon challenge with anti-IgE. Analysis of arachidonates by radioimmunoassay and HPLC revealed that challenge with anti-IgE generated prostaglandin D_2 and leukotriene C_4. Electron microscope analysis showed that these cells were mature human mast cells and clearly different from basophilic granulocytes. Most of the cells contained some granules with regular crystalline arrays and both tryptase and chymase, resembling human skin mast cells.

When mononuclear cells of cord blood were seeded in a millicell insert that was placed on a 3T3 fibroblast monolayer, a significant number of mast cells developed in the millicells, indicating that direct contact with fibroblasts is not essential for the differentiation of human mast cell progenitors. Furthermore, development of human mast cells in the presence of concentrated culture supernatants of 3T3 fibroblasts without a fibroblast feeder layer, confirmed that soluble factors released from fibroblasts are essential and sufficient for the differentiation of human mast cell progenitors in vitro. Subsequent studies revealed that BALB/3T3 fibroblasts appeared to be the best source of the mast cell growth factors among various murine and human fibroblast cell lines. Our preliminary experiments show that mast cell growth-promoting activities in the culture supernatant of 3T3 fibroblasts were recovered in the precipitates obtained between 50 and 70% saturated ammonium sulfate. When a concentrated culture supernatant of the 3T3 fibroblasts cultured in the serum-free medium was fractionated on a Superose 12 column, the major activity was detected in the fraction of 70–100 kDa.

In the murine system, several cytokines, such as interleukin 3 (Rennick et al., 1985), 4 (Rennick et al., 1987), 9 (Renauld et al., 1990), and c-*kit* ligand (Copeland et al., 1990; Esebo et al., 1990; Anderson et al., 1990), have been shown to promote differentiation and proliferation of mast cells. In particular, suspension cultures of mouse bone marrow cells in the presence of recombinant IL-3 for 4 weeks result in the development of a pure mast cell population (Saito et al., 1987).

In the human system, recombinant human IL-3 promoted a transient increase in selective differentiation of human basophils in suspension cultures of bone marrow and cord blood cells (Saito et al., 1988; Valent et al., 1989). After 4 weeks in culture with IL-3, however, the majority of nonadherent cells in the culture became eosinophils and no mast cell was detected in the long-term culture with IL-3 (Saito et al., 1988). Contrary to the murine system, recombinant human IL-4 failed to promote differentiation of either basophils or mast cells. Our subsequent studies revealed that none of the recombinant IL-1, -2, -3, -4, -5, -6, -9, and granulocyte-macrophage colony-stimulating factors (GM-CSF), or combinations of these cytokines, facilitated differentiation of human mast cells in suspension cultures of bone marrow or cord blood cells. The results suggested that differentiation of human mast cells may require some feeder layers or some growth factors from non-T cells. To explore this possibility, we tried to develop human mast cells on both mouse and human fibroblast feeder layers.

II. Development of Human Mast Cells In Vitro and Their Morphology

We were able to develop mature human mast cells in a long-term coculture of mononuclear cells of cord blood with 3T3 fibroblasts derived from Swiss albino mouse skin (Furitsu et al., 1989). The mast cells developed in the coculture of cord blood cells with 3T3 fibroblasts are morphologically distinct from basophils developed in the culture. Electron microscopic analysis of the cultured mast cells by Dr. Ann Dvorak revealed that they have ultrastructural features characteristic for mature human mast cells. Furthermore, they contained granules of various ultrastructural patterns that had been described in human mast cells by several investigators (Dvorak, 1989). It was also found that most of the cultured mast cells contained some granules with regular crystalline arrays resembling those frequently seen in the human skin mast cells (Furitsu et al., 1989).

III. Presence of Human Mast Cell Tryptase and Chymase in Cultured Mast Cell Granules

It was found that granules in almost all mast cells obtained in the coculture were clearly stained in immunofluorescence with monoclonal antibodies specific for human mast cell tryptase (Schwartz, 1985), while granules in cultured basophils were not stained. Further examination of the cells by sequential double-staining procedures for the detection of tryptase and chymase (Castells et al., 1987) by Schwartz and Irani revealed that granules in over 85% of the mast cells contained both tryptase and chymase (Furitsu et al., 1989), suggesting that they may belong to the skin mast cell type (Irani et al., 1986).

IV. Immunological Properties of Cultured Mast Cells

Mast cells developed in the culture bear $Fc_{\epsilon}RI$, which was demonstrated by immunofluorescence and by the binding of ^{125}I-labeled human E myeloma protein. The number of $Fc_{\epsilon}RI$ was estimated to be approximately 10^5 per cell. The majority of the cells were clearly stained with monoclonal antibody YB5.B8, which recognizes surface markers on human mast cells (Mayerhofer et al., 1987), while monoclonal antibody VIM12, which recognizes a human basophil surface marker (Knapp et al., 1984), failed to stain the cultured mast cells. By contrast, mature basophils developed in the culture were stained with VIM12, but not with YB5.B8. It was also found that monoclonal antibody against $Fc_{\epsilon}RI$, H107 (Noro et al., 1986), failed to stain cultured mast cells.

Mast cells recovered after 10 weeks in culture contained 1.4–2.8 μg histamine per million cells. Furthermore, mast cells sensitized with human IgE released histamine upon challenge with anti-IgE, whereas unsensitized cells failed to do so. Challenge of the sensitized cultured mast cells with anti-IgE resulted in the release of arachidonic acid (AA) as well. Kinetics of anti-IgE-induced release of histamine and AA were similar to those of dispersed human mast cells from lung or skin tissues. Analysis of AA metabolites by radioimmunoassay and HPLC revealed that anti-IgE generated prostaglandin D_2 and leukotriene C_4 in the cultured mast cells (Table 1). The results clearly showed that mast cells developed in a long-term coculture of cord blood cells with 3T3 fibroblasts were functionally active, mature human mast cells.

Although the number of mast cells developed in the cultures greatly varied from one cord blood specimen to another, the development of mast cells is quite reproducible. When 10^6 cord blood cells were cocultured with 3T3 fibroblasts in

medium containing 5% fetal calf serum or serum-free medium, and aliquots of cord blood cells were cultured in the presence of culture supernatant of each cell line (Table 4). Culture supernatant of human fibroblasts MRC-9 promoted the development of mast cells, although a significant number of mast cells was not obtained when cord blood cells were cocultured with this cell line. Nevertheless, the results of the experiments showed that mouse BALB/3T3 cells appeared to be the best source of the mast cell growth factors.

In the preliminary experiments, a 20-fold concentrated culture supernatant of BALB/3T3 fibroblasts, containing 5% fetal calf serum, was fractionated by sequential precipitation with 50, 70, and 85% saturated ammonium sulfate at pH 7.4. Each precipitate was resuspended in and dialysed extensively against phosphate-buffered saline, followed by RPMI 1640 medium. Aliquots of a cord blood cell suspension were cultured with a ⅒th volume of each fraction for 3 weeks. As shown in Figure 1, a majority of the activity to promote differentiation of mast cells was recovered in the precipitates obtained between 50 and 70% saturated ammonium sulfate.

We were able to establish the culture of BALB/3T3 fibroblasts in serum-free culture medium. The concentrated culture supernatant of the 3T3 fibroblast cultured in the serum-free medium was fractionated on Superose 12 column (prep grade) using a Beckman HPLC system. Appropriate fractions were pooled, concentrated, and dialyzed against RPMI 1640 medium and added to cord blood cell cultures. As shown in Figure 2, major mast cell growth-promoting activity was recovered in the 100-kDa fraction. Since the activity was also detected in the

Table 4 Development of Mast Cells by Culture Supernatant of Murine and Human Fibroblasts

Concentrated[a] culture supernatant of	Mast cells developed	
	3 weeks	6 weeks
	per well	per well
BALB/3T3	7.0×10^4	9.3×10^4
ψCRE/3T3	2.6×10^4	1.4×10^4
MCR-9	2.4×10^4	1.1×10^4
MCR-9[b]	7.6×10^3	6.1×10^3
Detroit 551	1.4×10^3	1.3×10^3
Detroit 551[b]	1.0×10^3	1.2×10^3

[a]Culture supernatant of fibroblasts containing 5% fetal calf serum was concentrated to 1/20 volume and added to cord blood cells (1.5×10^6 cells/well) at the final concentration of 10%.

[b]Serum-free culture supernatant was concentrated to 1/40 volume and added to cord blood cell culture at the final concentration of 10%.

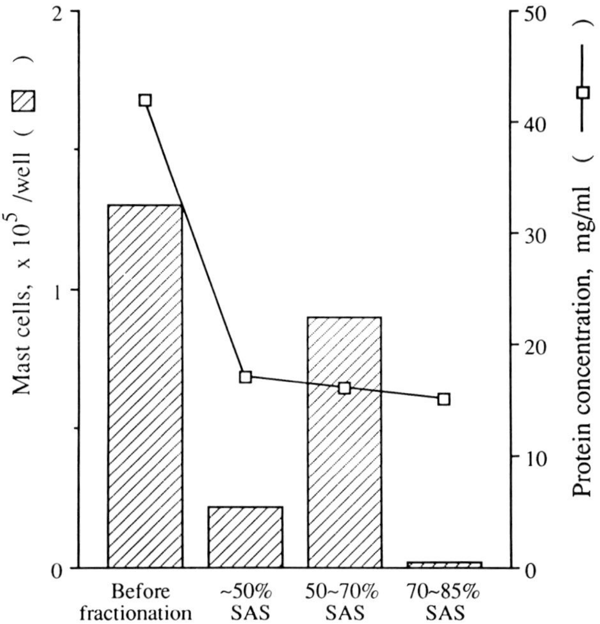

Figure 1 Fractionation of mast cell growth factor by ammonium sulfate precipitation. Culture supernatant of BALB/3T3 containing 5% FCS was fractionated by precipitation with ammonium sulfate. Each fraction was adjusted to the volume of the concentrated supernatant, and 1/10 volume of the fraction was added to cord blood cell cultures. After 3 weeks, the number of mast cells was determined by staining with May-Grumwald Giemsa and confirmed by immunofluorescence using antitryptase.

67-kDa fraction, the molecular mass of the mast cell growth factor is probably in the range of 70–100 kDa. Purification of the factor by DEAE cellulose chromatography is now underway.

Since the differentiation of precursors to human mast cells requires at least 2–3 weeks in culture, progress in purification of the growth factor(s) has been slow. However, we hope that the biochemical characteristics of human mast cell growth factors will be elucidated in the near future.

Acknowledgments

We express our sincere appreciation to Dr. J. R. Niebyl, Dr. E. Haller, Ms. O. Wilkins, and Ms. J. Garnes, of The Johns Hopkins Hospital, and Ms. V. Walborn, Scripps Memorial Hospital, for umbilical cord blood; to Dr. K. Ishizaka, La Jolla Institute for Allergy and Immunology, for his support and

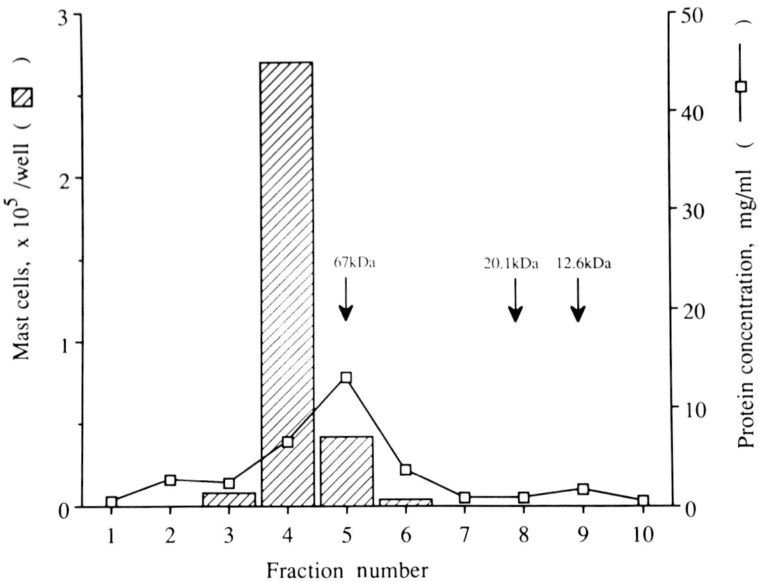

Figure 2 Gel filtration of mast cell growth factor on a Superose 12 column. Culture supernatant of BALB/3T3 in serum-free medium was concentrated 500-fold and then fractionated on a Superose 12 column (1.6 × 50 cm). Appropriate fractions were concentrated so that the final volume of each fraction was ½ the volume of the sample applied. After dialysis against RPMI 1640 medium, each fraction (5% V/U) was added to cord blood cell cultures. Mast cells were enumerated at 4 weeks.

encouragement; to Drs. L. B. Schwartz and A. M. A. Irani, Medical College of Virginia, for their collaboration on analysis of proteases; to Dr. L. Ashman, University of Adelaide; to Dr. O. Majdic, University of Vienna, and Dr. R. Andreesen, Klinikun der Albert-Ludwig-Universitat, for their generous supply of monoclonal antibodies, YB5.B8, VIM12.

Our special appreciation goes to Ms. C. G. L. Ko, The Johns Hopkins University; Ms. S. Kissell, Harvard Medical School, and Ms. M. Raygo, La Jolla Institute for Allergy and Immunology, for their outstanding technical assistance. This work was supported by Health Human Service Grants, AI 10060, AI 27517, AI 20487, and CA 28834, and research contract with DNAX Research Institute for Molecular and Cellular Biology and Gemini Science, Inc. This is Publication no. 7 from La Jolla Institute for Allergy and Immunology.

Discussion

Bienenstock: Could your 3T3-derived factor be the c-*kit* ligand (stem cell factor)?

Ishizaka: I have been helping Dr. Makio Ogawa in characterizing cells developed from cord blood cells in the presence of human c-*kit* ligand together with human IL-3. The majority of the cells are large mononuclear cells containing metachromatic granules. They bear $Fc_{\epsilon}RI$ and contain histamine. However, they are morphologically different from human mast cells developed in the coculture of cord blood cells with 3T3 fibroblasts and contain no human mast cell tryptase. Although it is too early to conclude, it seems that c-*kit* ligand may not be the major human mast cell growth factor.
Austen: Regarding the cells you begin with, have they already encountered IL-3 and are they "partially differentiated" or does IL-3 play no role?
Ishizaka: I cannot exclude the possibility that human mast cell progenitors in cord blood have already encountered IL-3. I also do not exclude the possibility that human mast cell progenitors in cord blood are in a different stage of differentiation from those in bone marrow. Our results only show that the presence or absence of IL-3 in the culture makes no difference in the development of human mast cells from their progenitors in cord blood, whereas the presence of IL-3 promotes differentiation of basophils.
Kaplan: You start with a monocyte-enriched fraction. What does the mast cell progenitor look like?
Ishizaka: At this moment, all I know is that it is a mononuclear cell.
Lichtenstein: Do your starting cells have IL-3R?
Ishizaka: We have not determined this.

References

Anderson, D. M., Lyman, S. D., Baird, A., Wignall, J. M., Eisenman, J., Rauch, C., March, C. J., Boswell, S., Gimpel, S. D., Cosman, D., and Williams, D. E. (1990). Molecular cloning of mast cell growth factors: A hematopoietin that is active in both membrane bound and soluble forms. *Cell* 63:235–243.

Castells, M. C., Irani, A. M. A., and Schwartz, L. B. (1987). Evaluation of human peripheral blood leukocytes for mast cell tryptase. *J. Immunol.* 138:2184–2189.

Copeland, N. G., Gilbert, D. J., Cho, B. C., Donovan, P. J., Jenkins, N. A., Cosman, D., Anderson, D., Lyman, S. D., and Williams, D. E. (1990). Mast cell growth factor maps near the Steel locus on mouse chromosome 10 and is deleted in a number of Steel alleles. *Cell* 63:175–183.

Danos, O., and Mulligan, R. C. (1988). Safe and efficient generation of recombinant retroviruses with amphotrophic and ecotrophic host ranges. *Proc. Natl. Acad. Sci. USA* 85:6460–6464.

Dvorak, A. M. (1989). Human mast cells. *Adv. Anat. Embryol. Cell Biol.* 114: 1–107.

Furitsu, T., Saito, H., Dvorak, A. M., Schwartz, L. B., Irani, A. M. A., Burdick, J. F., Ishizaka, K., and Ishizaka, T. (1989). Development of human mast cells in vitro. *Proc. Natl. Acad. Sci. USA* 86:10039–10043.

Irani, A. M. A., Schecter, N. M., Craig, S. S., DeBlois, G., and Schwartz, L. B. (1986). Two types of human mast cells that have distinct neutral protease compositions. *Proc. Natl. Acad. Sci. USA* 83:4464–4468.

Knapp, W., Majdic, O., Stockinger, H., Bettelheim, P., Liszka, K., Koller, U., and Peschel, C. (1984). Monoclonal antibodies to human myelomonocyte differentiation antigens in the diagnosis of acute myeloid leukemia. *Med. Oncol. Tumor Pharmacother.* 1:257–262.

Mayerhofer, G., Godd, S. J., Spargo, L. D. J., and Ashman, L. K. (1987). Specificity of a mouse monoclonal antibody raised against acute myeloid leukemia cells for mast cells in human mucosal and connective tissues. *Immunol. Cell Biol.* 65: 241–250.

Noro, N., Yoshioka, A., Adachi, M., Yasuda, K., Masuda, T., and Yodoi, J. (1986). Monoclonal antibody (H107) inhibiting IgE binding to $Fc_{\epsilon}RI(+)$ human lymphocytes. *J. Immunol.* 137:1258–1263.

Renauld, J.-C., Goethals, A., Houssiau, F., Roost, E. V., and Van Snick, J. (1990). Cloning and expression of a cDNA for the human homology of mouse T cell and mast cell growth factor P40. *Cytokine* 2:9–12.

Rennick, D. M., Lee, F. D., Yokota, T., Arai, K., Cantor, H., and Nabel, G. J. (1985). A cloned MCGF cDNA encodes a multilineage hematopoietic growth factor: Multiple activities of interleukin 3. *J. Immunol.* 134:910–914.

Rennick, D. M., Young, G., Muller-Sieburg, C., Smith, C., Arai, N., Tanabe, Y., and Gemmell, L. (1987). Interleukin 4 (B-cell stimulatory factor 1) can enhance or antagonize the factor-dependent growth of hemopoietic progenitor cells. *Proc. Natl. Acad. Sci. USA* 84:6889–6893.

Saito, H., Okajima, F., Molski, T. F. P., Sha'afi, R. I., Ui, M., and Ishizaka, T. (1987). Effects of ADP-ribosylation of GTP-binding protein by pertussis toxin on immunoglobulin E-dependent and -independent histamine release from mast cells and basophils. *J. Immunol.* 138:3927–3934.

Saito, H., Hatake, K., Dvorak, A. M., Leiferman, K. M., Donnenberg, A. D., Arai, N., Ishizaka, K., and Ishizaka, T. (1988). Selective differentiation and proliferation of hematopoietic cells induced by recombinant human interleukins. *Proc. Natl. Acad. Sci. USA* 85:2288–2292.

Schwartz, L. B. (1985). Monoclonal antibodies against human mast cell tryptase demonstrate shared antigenic sites on subunits of tryptase and selective localization of the enzyme to mast cells. *J. Immunol.* 134:526–531.

Valent, P., Ashman, L. K., Hintenberger, W., Eckersberger, F., Majdic, O., Lechner, K., and Bettelheim, P. (1989). Mast cell typing: Demonstration of a distinct hematopoietic cell type and evidence for immunophenotypic relationship to mononuclear phagocytes. *Blood* 73:1778–1785.

Zsebo, K. M., Wypych, J., McNiece, I. K., Lu, H. S., Smith, K. A., Karkare, S. B., Sachdev, R. K., Yuschenkoff, V. N., Birkett, N. C., Williams, L. R., Satyagal, V. N., Tung, W., Bosselman, R. A., Mendiaz, E. A., and Langley, K. E. (1990). Identification, purification, and biological characterization of hematopoietic stem cell factor from buffalo rat liver condition medium. *Cell* 63:195–201.

8

Molecular Characterization of Mouse Mast Cell Secretory Granule Proteases

DALE S. REYNOLDS and K. FRANK AUSTEN

Harvard Medical School
and Brigham and Women's Hospital
Boston, Massachusetts

WILLIAM E. SERAFIN

Vanderbilt University School of Medicine
Nashville, Tennessee

I. Introduction

The mature enzymes for mouse mast cell carboxypeptidase A (MC-CPA) and for six mouse mast cell proteases (MMCP) of the serine protease class, designated MMCP-1 to -6, have been resolved, and partial or full-length amino acid sequences have been determined directly from the mature enzymes or have been deduced from their cDNAs. These studies have shown that different mouse mast cell populations can express different combinations of these proteases in their secretory granules. cDNAs for MMCP-2, MMCP-4, MMCP-6, and MC-CPA were isolated from cDNA libraries prepared from Kirsten sarcoma virus-immortalized mouse mast cell lines (KiSV-MC), thereby making the mouse the first species for which mast cell proteases of each recognized category, namely, chymase (MMCP-2 and MMCP-4), tryptase (MMCP-6), and carboxypeptidase, have been molecularly characterized. Mouse MC-CPA cDNA probes were also used to isolate human MC-CPA cDNAs from two human lung cDNA libraries. The primary structures deduced from the cDNA sequences indicate that each of these proteases is synthesized as a preproenzyme, although it is the mature enzymes that are stored in the mast cell secretory granule. Mast cell chymases and carboxypeptidases may share a common mechanism for cleavage of activation peptides ending in acidic amino acid residues, whereas mast cell tryptases apparently have a separate activation mechanism. RNA blot analyses of various mouse mast cell populations using the available gene-specific cDNA probes have shown that bone marrow–derived mast cells (BMMC) cultured in WEHI-3-conditioned medium have the protease transcription phenotype MMCP-$2^-4^-6^+$, MC-CPA^+, whereas the phenotypes of the mouse tissue–derived mast cell subclasses are: MMCP-$2^-4^+6^+$, MC-CPA^+ for serosal cavity mast cells (SMC), considered to be the connective tissue mast cell (CTMC) prototype, and MMCP-$2^+4^-6^-$, MC-CPA^- for intestinal mast cells of *Nippostrongylus brasiliensis*–infected mice, designated mucosal mast cells (MMC). Well-differentiated immortalized KiSV-MC lines have a different phenotype, MMCP-2^+4^+-6^+, MC-CPA^+. Thus, BMMC are an immature mast cell population, and protease genes are attenuated or more highly expressed upon differentiation of mast cells in vivo to CTMC or MMC. The genes for proteases of each category, namely, MMCP-4 (chymase), MMCP-6 (tryptase), and human MC-CPA, have also been cloned and structurally characterized. A 44-bp apparent tryptase-specific upstream element that is highly conserved across species from mouse to human is present in the proximal 5' flanking region of the MMCP-6 gene. A distinct apparent MC-CPA-specific conserved region has also been identified through comparison of the promotor regions of the mouse and human MC-CPA genes. Such studies should lead to the identification of mechanisms that determine mast cell–specific gene expression and the differential expression of mast cell protease genes in different mast cell populations. The long-term objective of understanding the regulation of mast cell genes may have clinical applications.

The first mouse mast cell protease (MMCP) to be purified to homogeneity, termed MMCP-1 (Newlands et al., 1987), is a chymotryptic enzyme that was purified from *Trichinella spiralis*–infected mouse intestines. MMCP-1 was shown by immunohistochemistry to be expressed specifically in intestinal mucosal mast cells (MMC) (Newlands et al., 1987), and the complete amino acid sequence of the mature enzyme was determined (Le Trong et al., 1989). Diisopropylfluorophosphate (DFP)-binding proteins with proteolytic activity were described in mouse BMMC cultured in concanavalin A–stimulated splenocyte-conditioned medium (DuBuske et al., 1984). However, secretory granules in BMMC are poor in electron-dense protein cores and contain little material for molecular characterization. Small numbers of mouse connective tissue mast cells (CTMC) can be isolated by peritoneal lavage of adult animals ($\sim 2 \times 10^4$ cells/mouse), and whole cell lysates of purified peritoneal CTMC were found by Miller and colleagues (1988) to contain several highly expressed ~25–35-kDa proteins visible on a silver-stained polyacrylamide gel.

The serendipitous events that led to the identification of Kirsten sarcoma virus-immortalized mouse mast cell lines (KiSV-MC) are outlined below; these cell lines have provided the first pure source of large numbers of highly differentiated mast cells in any species. Their derivation has permitted the molecular characterization of mast cell carboxypeptidase A (MC-CPA) and of several mouse mast cell serine proteases. The identification, partial amino acid sequencing, and molecular cloning of some of these enzymes have shown that different populations of mouse mast cells express various combinations of MC-CPA and at least six distinct serine proteases in their secretory granules, and that different mouse mast cell phenotypes can be defined based on the differential transcription of protease genes.

II. Derivation and Identification of KiSV-MC Lines

Adult mouse splenocytes cultured on a monolayer of mouse 3T3 fibroblasts in standard microtiter wells were used as progenitors in initial efforts to obtain retrovirus-immortalized lymphocytic mouse cell lines (Lichtman et al., 1986). The fibroblasts were lethally irradiated to prevent proliferation and were actively producing the Kirsten sarcoma virus (KiSV), which contains the Ki-*ras* viral oncogene. Owing to incorporation of the Ki-*ras* oncogene into the retroviral genome, KiSV is replication-defective and requires packaging with a viral envelope glycoprotein provided by coinfection of the host cell with a "helper" murine leukemia virus. The envelope glycoprotein provided by the helper virus determines the host range of the viral particle, and the amphotropic helper virus that was used provided a KiSV "pseudotype" capable of infecting cells of several lineages (Lichtman et al., 1987b; Faller et al., 1988). Other than heat-inactivated fetal bovine serum and factors produced by the irradiated fibroblasts, no exogenous growth factors were provided during infection of the target splenocytes. In three independent experiments in which target splenocytes were cocultured with the retrovirus-producing fibroblasts, slowly dividing colonies of round cells appeared within 2–4 weeks in several wells. These colonies had doubling times of 1–2 weeks, and they were expanded in microwells for periods ranging from several weeks to months. Only a small fraction of the initial colonies continued to proliferate, and they eventually became established cell lines (Reynolds et al., 1988).

All 15 established cell lines grew as semiadherent cells expressing large amounts of Ki-*ras* mRNA. Phenotype analysis by immunocytochemistry and fluorescence-activated cell sorting showed that these cell lines failed to express surface-membrane markers of lymphocytes (Reynolds et al., 1988). However, they demonstrated enhanced proliferation in response to lectin-activated helper T lymphocyte type 2 (Th2) supernatants (Fig. 1). Proliferation was measured by microwell assays for [^{3}H]thymidine incorporation during a 6-hr pulse, after 72 hr of exposure to a cytokine source. Positive proliferative effects were confirmed by

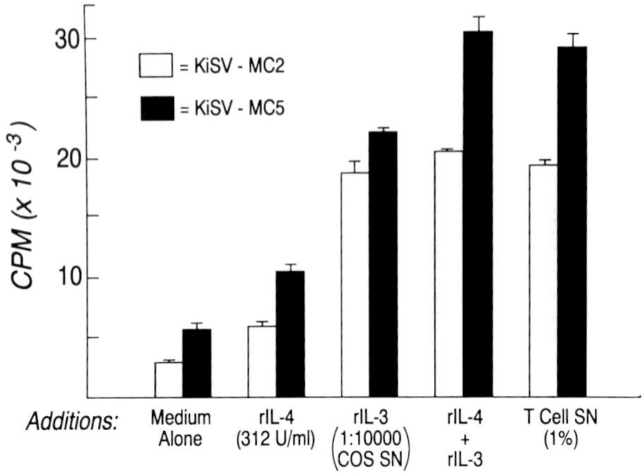

Figure 1 Enhanced [^{3}H]thymidine incorporation by KiSV-MC lines in response to recombinant (r) IL-3, rIL-4, and supernatants from concanavalin A–stimulated Th2 helper T-lymphocyte line D10.G4.1. Cells (2×10^4) from two representative KiSV-MC lines were cultured in 0.2 ml microtiter wells in enriched medium for 72 hr. Cultures were pulsed for 6 hr with 1 μCi [^{3}H]thymidine per well and then were harvested onto glass fiber filters for scintillation counting to quantitate radioactivity incorporated into DNA. rIL-4 was provided by Dr. L. Glimcher, Harvard Medical School. rIl-3 was from a transfected COS cell supernatant (SN) provided by Dr. P. Billings, Dana-Farber Cancer Institute. The T-cell supernatant was from the Th2 (Lichtman et al., 1987a) helper clone D10.G4.1 stimulated for 18 hr with 2 μg/ml concanavalin A. Responses to maximally stimulatory doses of each cytokine source are shown. Results are expressed as the mean ± standard error (error bars) of duplicate cultures.

monitoring cell numbers in 7–21-day cultures. Recombinant interleukin (IL)-1, IL-2, gamma interferon, and granulocyte/macrophage–colony-stimulating factor (GM-CSF) did not stimulate [^{3}H]thymidine incorporation at full standard-dose titrations (data not shown), whereas recombinant IL-3 and IL-4, at optimally stimulatory concentrations of each, had distinct and partial additive effects on proliferation (Fig. 1). In addition, these KiSV-immortalized cell lines exhibited a biphasic dose response to recombinant IL-3, with higher doses resulting in less than optimal proliferation, similar to the biphasic dose response exhibited to T-cell supernatants (data not shown).

Since IL-3 and IL-4 were known to have distinct and additive proliferative effects on IL-3-dependent transformed mouse mast cell lines (Smith and Rennick, 1986; Lee et al., 1986) such as the IL-3 indicator line MC/9 (Nabel et al., 1981), the KiSV-MC lines were subjected to electron microscopy and histochemical staining to identify morphological features of the mast cell lineage. Each of the KiSV-MC lines had ultrastructural features of well-differentiated mast cells and contained electron-dense secretory granules that stained metachromatic with toluidine blue (Reynolds et al., 1988). Alcian blue/safranin staining showed that the different KiSV-MC lines, taken together, represented a broad range of phenotypes, from completely safranin$^+$ to predominantly safranin$^-$ staining cell lines (Fig. 2; see colorplate). The cellular contents of histamine and MC-CPAenzymatic activity, and the level of heparin proteoglycan biosynthesis in individual cell lines correlated with the degree of safranin staining, and the most highly differentiated KiSV-MC lines contained levels of histamine and MC-CPA similar to those of peritoneal CTMC (Reynolds et al., 1988).

Rein et al. (1985) had shown that a retrovirus similar to KiSV, namely the Harvey murine sarcoma virus, which contains the Ha-*ras* viral oncogene, could immortalize mouse mast cells from adult mouse splenocyte progenitors in the presence of IL-3, resulting in the expansion of IL-3-dependent Ha-*ras*–expressing lines similar to BMMC. The experiments of Rein et al. differed from those performed with KiSV in their use of IL-3 and in their use of retrovirus-containing supernatants rather than irradiated retrovirus-producing fibroblasts. It had been shown previously that fibroblast monolayers sustain rat CTMC viability ex vivo without the requirement for exogenous cytokines (Levi-Schaffer et al., 1985). Furthermore, fibroblasts induce CTMC-like differentiation of immature mouse BMMC in vitro (Levi-Schaffer et al., 1986). Thus, the fortuitous combination in vitro of splenocyte target populations with an irradiated fibroblast monolayer producing a Ki-*ras*–containing retrovirus permitted the outgrowth of immortalized KiSV-MC lines that did not depend on IL-3 for growth and viability, and that had a well-differentiated secretory granule phenotype. Several of these cell lines have now been maintained in continuous culture for up to 4 ½ years.

Experiments in which T-cell supernatants containing IL-3 were added at the beginning of fibroblast/splenocyte immortalization cocultures later showed that the omission of a source of IL-3 during the prolonged initial expansion of the KiSV-MC colonies had been important because it avoided outgrowth (in nearly 100% of T-cell supernatant-treated wells) of rapidly dividing, IL-3-dependent KiSV-MC lines. These IL-3-dependent KiSV-MC lines stained entirely safranin$^-$ and had low levels of histamine and MC-CPA, similar to BMMC (Reynolds, 1989). Because the growth factor–independent KiSV-MC lines could be grown free of the irradiated fibroblast monolayer, they provided a unique, pure biochemical source for the isolation of sufficient mRNA to construct mast cell cDNA libraries and for the identification and molecular characterization of mouse mast cell secretory granule proteases (see below).

III. N-Terminal Amino Acid Sequencing of Mouse Mast Cell Proteases

A whole-cell lysate from a well-differentiated KiSV-MC line that contained entirely safranin$^+$-staining granules (KiSV-MC5) was subjected to sodium dodecyl sulfate–polyacrylamide gel electrophoresis (SDS-PAGE) with standard Laemmli gel electrophoresis buffers (Laemmli, 1970). Major protein species with sizes from ~28 to 36 kDa were seen in the cell lysate, and together they represented nearly 50% of total cell protein (Fig. 3). These proteins copurified with the secretory granules. In subsequent analyses of partially purified KiSV-MC5 secretory granules, a tricine-based electrophoresis buffer system (Schägger and von Jagow, 1987) was adopted, since it resolved these major KiSV-MC granule species into five discrete bands of 28, 29, 31, 32, and 36 kDa (Reynolds et al., 1990). Each of the four 28–32-kDa proteins in KiSV-MC5 bound the serine protease inhibitor [^{3}H]DFP. The 36-kDa protein, which did not bind [^{3}H]DFP, was shown to be the metalloexopeptidase MC-CPA by its selective retention on a carboxypeptidase-inhibitor affinity column (Reynolds et al., 1989a). A total of 2.6×10^6 CTMC of >95% purity were also obtained from peritoneal washes of 100 adult BALB/c mice. As in the analysis of KiSV-MC5 granules, the partly purified CTMC secretory granules were electrophoresed under reducing conditions on a 13% acrylamide tricine gel and electroblotted to Immobilon. The resolved CTMC granules on the Coomassie blue–stained membrane contained five protein species of similar size to those in KiSV-MC5 granules, plus an additional 30-kDa protein species. Each of the prominent 28–36-kDa proteins of KiSV-MC5 and CTMC was submitted for N-terminal amino acid sequence analysis, in the form of slices of the Immobilon transblots of the resolved proteins (Reynolds et al., 1989b, 1990; Serafin et al., 1990).

The sequences obtained for the KiSV-MC5 and peritoneal CTMC proteins were then compared, and the nomenclature, distribution, and partial amino acid sequences of these enzymes (Reynolds et al., 1989a, 1990) are reproduced in Table 1. MMCP-1, identified in the intestinal MMC of *T. spiralis*–infected mice (Newlands et al., 1987; Le Trong et al., 1989), was not one of the major protein species in either KiSV-MC or CTMC granules. MMCP-2 is a 28-kDa protease in KiSV-MC5 and is distinct from the similar-sized 28-kDa serine protease, designated MMCP-3, present in CTMC granules (Reynolds et al., 1990). Three distinct N-terminal amino acid sequences were obtained for the 29-, 31-, and 32-kDa KiSV-MC5 serine proteases, designated MMCP-4, MMCP-5, and MMCP-6, respectively. Identical N-terminal sequences were obtained for the similar-sized protein species in CTMC. The 30-kDa serine protease seen only in CTMC was designated MMCP-5' inasmuch as it had an N-terminal sequence

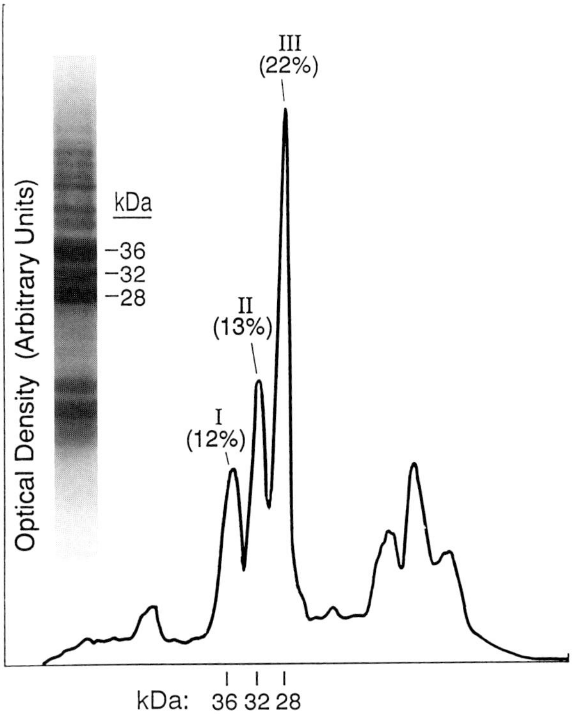

Figure 3 SDS-PAGE analysis of a whole-cell lysate of 2.5 × 10^6 KiSV-MC5 on a 7.5–15% acrylamide gradient gel under reducing conditions (inset) and optical densitometric analysis of the lane. The 36-kDa protein species in the Coomassie blue–stained gel lane is mouse MC-CPA. The broad ~32 kDa and ~28 kDa protein bands were each later resolved into two closely migrating protein species, identified as MMCP-6 and MMCP-5 for the ~32-kDa band and MMCP-4 and MMCP-2 for the ~28-kDa band. By optical densitometric analysis of the lane, peaks I, II, and III, corresponding to the ~36-, ~32-, and ~28-kDa bands, were found to represent ~12, ~13, and ~22% of total cell protein, respectively. The secretory granule proteases therefore represented ~47% of total cell protein in the safranin$^+$-staining line KiSV-MC5.

Table 1 N-Terminal Amino Acid Sequences of Mouse Mast Cell Secretory Granule Proteases

Protease	kDa	Mast cell type	Amino acid residue (1 5 10 15 20 25 30)
MMCP-1	26	MMC	I I G G V E A R P H S R P Y M A H L K I I T D R G S E D R C
MMCP-2	28	KiSV-MC5	I I G G V E A K P H S R P Y M A Y L K F T T
MMCP-3	28	CTMC	I I G G V E S R P H S R P Y M A T L E I T
MMCP-4	29	KiSV-MC5	I I G G V E S R P H S R P Y M A H L E I T[T E]
	29	CTMC	I I G G V E S R P H S R P Y M A H L E I T T E
MMCP-5'	30	CTMC	I I G G T E X I P H S R P Y M A Y L E I
MMCP-5	31	KiSV-MC5	I I G G T E X I P H S R P Y M A Y L E I V T S E
	31	CTMC	I I G G T E X I P H S R P Y M A Y L E I V T S E N Y[S]A[R]
MMCP-6	32	KiSV-MC5	I V G G H E A S E S K W P W Q V S L R F K L N
	32	CTMC	I V G G H E A S E[S]K X P X Q V
MC-CPA	36	KiSV-MC5	I A G R H S Y A K Y N D[W D]K I V – – T E K M [K/L]
		CTMC	I A G R H S Y A K Y N D W D K I

Mast cell type refers to the cellular source of the protein that was partially amino acid sequenced. Brackets indicate probable amino acid residues. An X indicates that no residue could be determined. Data for MMCP-1 are from Le Trong et al. (1989), for MMCP-2 from Serafin et al. (1990), for MMCP-3 to -6 from Reynolds et al. (1990), and for MC-CPA from Reynolds et al. (1989a).

Source: Modified from Table 1, Reynolds et al., 1990.

identical to that of the 31-kDa protein, MMCP-5, found in both cell types. MMCP-5 and MMCP-5' may represent highly similar, but distinct, gene products or they may represent the same protein with different degrees of posttranslational processing. The single amino acid difference between the N-terminal amino acid sequences of MMCP-3 and MMCP-4 was determined again when the analysis was repeated on a second series of samples. This single amino acid difference between MMCP-3 and MMCP-4 could not be attributed to allelic variation because both MMCP-3 and MMCP-4 are present in peritoneal CTMC obtained from inbred BALB/c mice. The 36-kDa protein, shown by affinity chromatography to be mouse MC-CPA, had an identical amino terminus in KiSV-MC5 and peritoneal CTMC (Reynolds et al., 1989a).

The N-terminal amino acid sequences of the mouse mast cell serine proteases were compared with those of the rat chymases, rat mast cell protease (RMCP)-I (Le Trong et al., 1987) and RMCP-II (Woodbury et al., 1978), and the human (Miller et al., 1989; Vanderslice et al., 1990) and dog (Vanderslice et al., 1989) tryptases. Based on this comparison, MMCP-1 through -5 were broadly classified as probable chymases, having N-terminal amino acid sequences with ≥65% identity with RMCP-I and RMCP-II. In contrast, the N-terminal amino acid sequence of MMCP-6 had no more than 33% identity with MMCP-1 to -5, but had 70% identity with human tryptase. Thus, the serine proteases identified in murine mast cells include five apparent chymases (MMCP-1 to -5) and one apparent tryptase (MMCP-6), and these enzymes can be expressed in different combinations in different mast cell populations (Reynolds et al., 1990).

IV. Cloning of cDNAs for MMCP-2, MMCP-4, MMCP-6, Mouse MC-CPA, and Human MC-CPA

Two mouse mast cell cDNA libraries were prepared in the vectors λ-gtll (Serafin et al., 1990) and lambda-ZAP-II (Reynolds et al., 1991) from safranin$^+$-staining KiSV-MC lines. The λ-gtll library was initially screened with an RMCP-II cDNA probe under wash conditions of low stringency (0.15 *M* NaCl, 15 m*M* Na citrate; 37°C) to isolate two recombinants containing cDNA inserts with identical restriction enzyme digestion patterns. These cDNAs were found to encode MMCP-2, based on its known N-terminal amino acid sequence (Serafin et al., 1990). The KiSV-MC cDNA libraries were also screened with synthesized oligonucleotides, based on the partial N-terminal amino acid sequences of mouse MC-CPA (Reynolds et al., 1989a), MMCP-4 (Reynolds et al., 1990), and MMCP-6 (Reynolds et al., 1990), to obtain the respective cDNAs (Reynolds et al., 1989a, 1991; Serafin et al., 1991). For mouse MC-CPA,

MMCP-4, and MMCP-6, the 5' ends of the respective transcripts were defined by primer-extension RNA sequencing. Mouse MC-CPA cDNAs were also used as probes under low-stringency conditions to obtain near full-length human MC-CPA cDNAs from two human lung cDNA libraries (Reynolds et al., 1989b).

Primer-extension RNA sequencing was again used to define the sequence on the 5' end of the human MC-CPA transcript in human lung poly(A)$^+$ RNA. This last experiment, shown in Figure 4, demonstrates the usefulness of primer-extension RNA sequencing for defining the 5' ends of rare transcripts when large quantities of poly(A)$^+$ RNA can be obtained. In screening two high-quality human lung cDNA libraries with complexities of 8.2×10^5 and 1.4×10^6 recombinants, the MC-CPA mRNA had been represented in only ~1/80,000 to ~1/100,000 of the cDNA inserts (Reynolds et al., 1989b).

The deduced amino acid sequences of the cDNAs have revealed a number of important features of the mast cell proteases. As expected, all three of the cloned mouse mast cell proteases that bound [^{3}H]DFP contained the "charge relay" His/Asp/Glu triad characteristic of serine proteases. As was suggested by their partial N-terminal amino acid sequences, MMCP-2 and MMCP-4 are chymases based on their high degree of amino acid sequence identity with RMCP-I and RMCP-II, their predicted substrate-binding regions with a serine at position 176, and their low amino acid sequence identity with mast cell tryptases. In contrast, the deduced amino acid sequence of the mature MMCP-6 has 73% identity with both the human and dog mast cell tryptases and includes the critical tryptic specificity-determining residue Asp 188.

V. Mechanisms of Activation of Mast Cell Proteases from Their Zymogen Forms

All five of the cloned mouse and human mast cell enzymes described here are predicted to be translated as preproenzymes, based on the rules of von Heijne (1984) and their known mature enzyme N-terminal amino acid sequences. The chymases MMCP-2 and MMCP-4 both have a predicted 20-amino-acid prepropeptide identical to that of the rat chymase RMCP-II (Benfey et al., 1987). This conserved 20-amino-acid prepropeptide consists of a typical 18-amino-acid hydrophobic leader sequence followed by a di-Glu activation peptide. Human and mouse MC-CPA are both predicted to have similar 15-amino-acid hydrophobic leader sequences followed by activation peptides of 94 amino acids. Although the mouse and human MC-CPA activation peptides are substantially longer than the di-Glu activation peptides of the mast cell chymases, they also end in acidic amino acid dimers (Asp-Glu for mouse MC-CPA and Glu-Asp

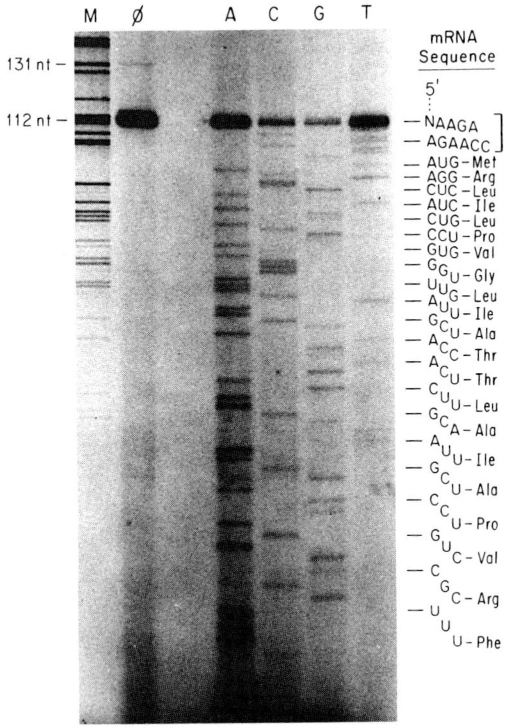

Figure 4 Primer-extension RNA sequencing of the 5' end of the human MC-CPA transcript in human lung poly(A)$^+$ RNA. Either no dideoxynucleotide (ddNTP) (lane ϕ) or ddATP (lane A), ddCTP (lane C), ddGTP (lane G), or ddTTP (lane T) was included in identical primer-extension reactions. The lengths in nucleotides (nt) of the primer-extension products (left) were determined by comparison to a standard DNA sequencing ladder (lane M). Approximately 50 μg of human lung poly(A)$^+$ RNA, selected twice by oligo-dT cellulose chromatography, was used for this experiment. The deduced mRNA sequence and translated amino acid sequences are shown on the right. The 5' untranslated region is indicated (bracket). Film was exposed to the plastic-wrapped gel at –70°C for 10 days with one enhancing screen. Although faint, the sequence was unambiguous to within one nucleotide of the major transcription initiation site. The minor population of transcripts initiating 17 nucleotides further 5' was detected in two separate experiments. The human lung RNA was obtained from a fresh surgical pathology specimen kindly provided by Dr. D. Sugarbaker, Brigham and Women's Hospital, Boston MA. (Adapted from Fig. 3, Reynolds et al., 1989b.)

for human MC-CPA). Therefore, mast cell chymases and carboxypeptidases may share a common mechanism for endopeptidase cleavage of activation peptides ending in acidic amino acid dimers. Such an endopeptidase activity has not been described previously.

As first noted for the dog tryptases (Vanderslice et al., 1989), mast cell tryptases appear to have a distinct processing mechanism. The dog, human (Miller et al., 1989, 1990; Vanderslice et al., 1990), and mouse (MMCP-6; Reynolds et al., 1991) tryptases have activation peptides ending in Gly. While each of the identified mast cell tryptases has a series of hydrophobic amino acids following the translation-initiation Met, only MMCP-6 has a readily identifiable cleavage site for a signal peptide based on the von Heijne rules (von Heijne, 1984). The dog and human tryptases may have unusual signal peptide cleavage sites, or they may be directly processed from the primary translation products to the mature enzymes without intermediate proenzyme forms (Vanderslice et al., 1989). The activation peptides of pancreatic proteases end in basic amino acids, and these enzymes are activated through cleavage of their zymogens by pancreatic trypsin. In contrast, none of the mast cell protease activities identified can account for the activities that appear to be required for processing mast cell protease zymogens. Also in contrast to the pancreatic proteases, all the mast cell proteases identified to date are stored and released as fully active mature enzymes.

VI. Charge Characteristics of Mast Cell Secretory Granule Proteases

The availability of deduced or actual amino acid sequences for a variety of mouse, rat, dog, and human mast cell proteases allows inter- and intraspecies comparisons of their charge characteristics. The estimated isoelectric points of all the described mast cell proteases are ~6.5 or above. Thus, within the secretory granules where the estimated pH is 5.5, all the proteases would be expected to be positively charged and to be ionically bound to the secretory granule proteoglycans.

However, at the extracellular pH of 7.4, the various mast cell proteases can be categorized into three charge classes. Strongly basic proteases include two of the chymases, MMCP-4 and RMCP-I, as well as mouse and human MC-CPA. These proteases have estimated charges of +15 or greater at pH 7.4 and would be expected to remain tightly bound to mast cell proteoglycans even after exocytosis into the extracellular environment. In purifying rat MC-CPA for amino acid sequencing, Cole and colleagues (1991) have shown that rat MC-CPA is fully active while remaining tightly bound in the protease/proteoglycan macromolecular complex (Everitt and Neurath, 1980; Schwartz et al., 1982). In contrast, the chymases MMCP-1, MMCP-2, and RMCP-II are weakly basic and may not remain bound to proteoglycans after secretory granule exocytosis. MMCP-1 (Newlands et al., 1987) and RMCP-II (Woodbury et al., 1978) are, in fact, readily extractable from tissues at physiological pH and ionic strength, unbound to proteoglycans. The tryptases from the three species represent a third group in that they are weakly acidic at neutral pH. The binding of human mast cell tryptase to heparin-agarose columns in vitro has been attributed to localized regions of positive charge in the protein (Vanderslice et al., 1990; Miller et al., 1990). However, based on their net negative charges at extracellular pH, tryptases may not remain bound to proteoglycans after exocytosis from the acidic granule compartment into the neutral extracellular milieu.

Following anaphylactic reactions human tryptase diffuses into the systemic circulation and can be quantitated by serum immunoassay (Schwartz et al., 1987). Tryptase, in the absence of heparin, has a very short half-life of activity (Schwartz and Bradford, 1986). This may provide a localizing regulatory mechanism. Since large heparin and chondroitin sulfate E proteoglycans released from mast cell granules would be predicted to diffuse poorly, substantial tryptase activity may be limited to the local area of mast cell activation.

VII. Development of Gene-Specific cDNA Probes for RNA Blot Analyses and Phenotyping of Mouse Mast Cell Populations Based on Their Transcription of Protease Genes

The development of antibodies specific for RMCP-I and RMCP-II allowed immunohistochemical classification of rat mast cells based on their protease contents (Gibson and Miller, 1986). Rat CTMC appear to contain RMCP-I but not RMCP-II, whereas rat MMC contain RMCP-II but not RMCP-I. Two human mast cell subclasses (Irani et al., 1986) have been described based on immunohistochemical differences in their contents of the serine proteases tryptase (Schwartz et al., 1981) and chymase (Schechter et al., 1986). One subclass, MT_{TC}, contains both tryptase and chymase in the secretory granules, and the other, MC_T, contains only tryptase. Inasmuch as mouse mast cells produce at least six distinct serine proteases, probes for more than two proteases probably will be necessary for the full classification of rat and human mast cells.

To examine the expression of proteases in different mouse mast cell populations, gene-specific cDNA probes for MMCP-2, MMCP-4, and MMCP-6 (Serafin et al., 1990, 1991; Reynolds et al., 1991) and for mouse MC-CPA (Reynolds et al., 1989a) were prepared. Specificity was confirmed by genomic

DNA blot analyses showing that each probe bound to only a single locus in restriction-digested genomic DNA. For MMCP-2 and MMCP-6, gene-specific probes were obtained by utilizing portions of the 3' untranslated regions of the respective cDNAs, where nucleotide sequences are typically poorly conserved among related members of a gene family (Tantravahi et al., 1986). However, when the 3' untranslated region of the MMCP-4 cDNA was examined for use as a gene-specific probe, two loci in genomic DNA still hybridized under conditions of high stringency (Serafin et al., 1991). A putative gene-specific probe was prepared for MMCP-4 by use of the polymerase chain reaction to amplify a short region of the translated cDNA sequence that encoded a poorly conserved region of protein sequence relative to other chymases.

RNA samples were obtained from four mouse mast cell populations for RNA blot analyses. These different mouse mast cell populations included BMMC cultured for 3–6 weeks in WEHI-3-conditioned medium, KiSV-MC cultured in the absence of growth factors other than fetal bovine serum, CTMC purified from peritoneal washes of large adult mice (retired breeders), and unpurified MMC present in the intestines of *N. brasiliensis*–infected mice. In analyzing MMC-rich intestinal tissues for apparent MMC-expressed mast cell protease transcripts, an equal amount of poly(A)$^+$ RNA from uninfected mouse intestines was examined in each case as a negative control. Each of the four mast cell populations examined expressed a distinct protease transcription phenotype, summarized in Table 2.

Conclusions can be drawn concerning mouse mast cell development based on these results. BMMC cultured in WEHI-3-conditioned medium express no MMCP-2 mRNA (Serafin et al., 1990, 1991) and no detectable MMCP-4 mRNA, whereas in vivo–derived MMC appear to contain large amounts of MMCP-2 mRNA (Table 2). Furthermore, MC-CPA mRNA is highly expressed in BMMC (Reynolds et al., 1989a) but is absent in MMC (Serafin et al., 1991), whereas MMCP-6 mRNA is present in BMMC but absent in MMC (Reynolds et al., 1991). Clearly, IL-3-containing WEHI-3-conditioned medium is not a sufficient source of differentiation factors for the development of mature MMC from mouse bone marrow progenitors. Well-differentiated KiSV-MC were initially thought to represent the CTMC subclass based on their safranin$^+$ staining, their content of histamine and MC-CPA, and their biosynthesis of heparin proteoglycans. It was found that KiSV-MC contain mRNA for MMCP-4, MMCP-6, and MC-CPA similar to CTMC, but they additionally express mRNA for MMCP-2, which was found only in MMC in vivo. Therefore, both KiSV-MC and BMMC have protease transcription phenotypes different from the in vivo–derived intestinal MMC and peritoneal CTMC populations. It is likely that progenitor mast cells exist in vivo, and it is possible that additional "mature" subclasses are also present.

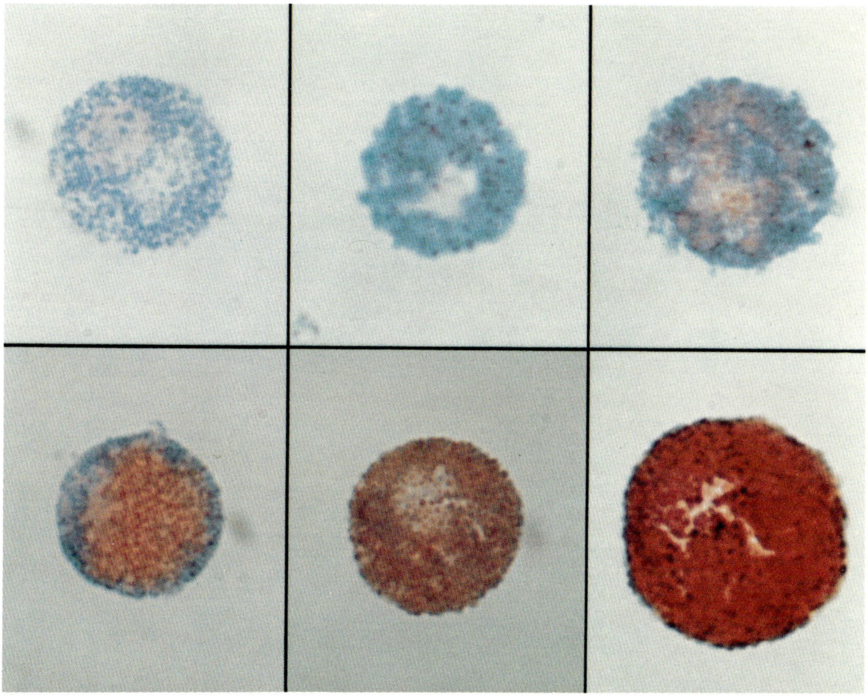

Figure 2 Alcian blue/safranin staining of KiSV-MC lines showing the full spectrum of mouse mast cell histochemical diversity. An IL-3-dependent KiSV-MC line stained completely safranin$^-$ (upper left panel), similar to mouse BBMC. Five other (IL-3-independent) KiSV-MC lines, which stained safranin$^+$ to various degrees, are also depicted. The KiSV-MC line MC5 in the lower right panel was completely safranin$^+$, similar to mouse peritoneal CTMC. (Cell lines KiSV-MC7, MC8, MC1, and MC5, in the top-middle, top-right, bottom-middle, and bottom-right panels, respectively, are those reported and illustrated in part in Fig. 2, Reynolds et al., 1988.)

Table 2 Protease Transcription in Different Mouse Mast Cell Populations

	Cell type			
Protease	BMMC	MMC	CTMC	KiSV-MC
MMCP-2	–	+++	–	+++
MMCP-4	–	–	+++	+++
MMCP-6	++	–	+++	+++
MMCP-L	–	±	–	–
MC-CPA	+++	±	+++	+++

These data were obtained using the same RNA blot that was sequentially analyzed with gene-specific cDNA probes for each protease (Serafin et al., 1991; Reynolds et al., 1991). Designations of + to +++ denote subjective scoring of the prevalence of transcripts detectable after a 16-hr autoradiographic exposure; – denotes no detectable hybridization of the probe after a 72-hr autoradiographic exposure. Barely detectable hybridization of the probe found after a 16-hr autoradiographic exposure is denoted by ±. For scoring MMC, poly(A)$^+$ RNA was extracted from the proximal small intestine of a mouse infected with *N. brasiliensis* to expand markedly the numbers of MMC; an equal amount of poly(A)$^+$ RNA from uninfected mouse intestines was used as a negative control.
Source: Modified from Table 1, Reynolds et al., 1991.

VIII. Distinct Organizations of Genes for Mast Cell Chymases and Tryptases

When mouse genomic DNA blots were analyzed with a probe derived from the 3' untranslated region of the MMCP-4 cDNA, hybridization to at least two distinct loci was found (Serafin et al., 1991). This cDNA probe was used to screen a BALB/c mouse genomic DNA library to isolate two hybridizing genomic DNA clones whose inserts had different restriction enzyme digestion patterns. Complete nucleotide sequences were obtained for the serine protease genes found within these two clones. One clone contained the gene for MMCP-4, and the second contained a highly related gene encoding an enzyme whose deduced amino acid sequence was different from all previously identified serine proteases. This gene was designated mouse mast cell protease-like (MMCP-L). The MMCP-4 and MMCP-L genes have five exons each and share identical genomic organizations with other immune/inflammatory serine proteases, including RMCP-II (Benfey et al., 1987), adipsin (a mouse adipocyte serine protease highly similar and probably identical to complement factor D) (Phillips et al., 1986; Rosen et al., 1989), and cytotoxic cell protease-I from mouse cytolytic T lymphocytes (Lobe et al., 1988). Dot matrix analyses showed that the proximal ~900 bp of the 5' flanking regions of the MMCP-4, MMCP-L, and RMCP-II genes are highly similar (Serafin et al., 1991). The corresponding introns for these three chymase genes are also similar in nucleotide sequence and have nearly identical lengths.

The genes for a human skin tryptase (Vanderslice et al., 1990) and for MMCP-6 (Reynolds et al., 1991) have also been isolated, sequenced, and found to have identical organizations. Each tryptase gene consists of six exons, with the first intron precisely separating the 5' untranslated region from the translation-initiation ATG codon. The distinct gene structure of a mouse tryptase (MMCP-6) compared to that for a mouse chymase (MMCP-4) found in the same mast cells has shown that at the gene organizational level, tryptases and chymases are distinct categories of mast cell serine proteases.

IX. Future Considerations

The availability of cDNAs and gene-specific probes for the mast cell proteases has allowed the cloning and sequencing of some of the corresponding genes, and it should now be possible to begin the delineation of promoter, suppressor, and enhancer elements that regulate these highly expressed mast cell genes. Sarid et al. (1989) have defined a *cis*-acting element within the 5' flanking region of the RMCP-II gene that interacts with a mast cell-specific *trans*-acting factor to control RMCP-II expression. By comparison with the 5' flanking region of the RMCP-II gene, a sequence with similarity to the RMCP-II enhancer has been identified in the 5' flanking region of the MMCP-4 gene (Serafin et al., 1991). Comparison of the human and mouse tryptase genes (Reynolds et al., 1991) has also identified a highly conserved sequence, consisting of 44 base pairs found in the proximal 5' flanking regions. This region is distinct from the enhancing element identified in the RMCP-II gene (Sarid et al., 1989) and may represent a tryptase-specific regulatory sequence. Likewise, when the human MC-CPA gene 5' flanking region (Reynolds et al., 1989b) was compared to a short region of the mouse MC-CPA gene 5' flank (Reynolds, 1989), the 55 nucleotides upstream of the TATA-box motifs for each gene were highly conserved across species from mouse to human (44 out of 55 matches), indicating the probable presence of MC-CPA-specific gene regulatory elements in this region.

Several mouse cytokines and presumed cytokines have been described as having mast cell growth and differentiation effects, e.g., IL-3 (Razin et al., 1984), IL-4 (Lee et al., 1986), mast cell–enhancing activity (IL-9) (Moeller et al., 1990), cytokine synthesis inhibitory factor (IL-10) (Thompson-Snipes et al., 1991), and the c-*kit* ligand (Huang et al., 1990). There have been no studies of the effects of these agents on the expression of mast cell protease genes. These studies are now possible with the available gene-specific probes and may lead to a better understanding of the mechanisms by which mast cell tropic factors, through transmembrane signals, control mast cell gene expression and phenotype.

The initial identification of MMCP-L from its gene rather than from cDNA or protein sequences leaves open the question of its expression in vivo. MMCP-L does not appear to be expressed in CTMC and is at best only minimally expressed in MMC relative to other mast cell proteases (Table 2). If MMCP-L is expressed as a major mast cell constituent in vivo, it may distinguish a subclass of mast cells that is distinct from intestinal MMC and peritoneal CTMC.

The proteases in the secretory granules of well-differentiated mast cells represent a large portion of total cell protein, yet the primary physiological substrates of these enzymes have not been definitively assigned. The substantial family of mouse chymotryptic mast cell proteases (Reynolds et al., 1990) is homologous to the substantial family of human and mouse cytolytic T lymphocyte (CTL) secretory granule serine proteases termed "granzymes" (Pasternak and Eisen, 1985; Lobe et al., 1986; Gershenfeld and Weissman, 1986; Masson and Tschopp, 1987; Jenne et al., 1988). The mast cell secretory granule serine proteases and CTL granzymes may serve related functions, although the physiological substrates of the CTL granzymes also remain unidentified. It remains to be determined whether each of the mast cell proteases has a limited number of specific protein substrates in vivo, or whether they serve collectively to degrade sequentially a wide range of protein substrates, as is the case for pancreatic trypsin, chymotrypsin, and carboxypeptidases.

The complexity of expression of mast cell protease genes in different mast cell populations should make possible investigations aimed at defining the molecular mechanisms of mast cell–specific and mast cell subset–specific gene expression. Defining the differential expression of mast cell protease genes in different phenotypic mast cell subsets in vivo by in situ hybridization and immunohistochemistry should also provide insight as to the likely different phenotype-related functions of mast cell subsets.

Acknowledgments

This work was supported by Grants HL-36110, AR-35907, and AI-22531 from the National Institutes of Health; a starter grant from the Burroughs Wellcome Fund; and the Immunology Development Fund of the Department of Medicine, Vanderbilt University.

Discussion

Bienenstock: What is the effect of activation on these cells?
Austen: Although activation results in substantial transcription as well as translation of a range of cytokines, there is no measurable increase in transcription of

secretory granule constituents during the same interval. This suggests that regranulation would have a substantial latency, and that generation of new cells from tissue precursors is certainly an alternative possibility for mast cell reconstitution.
Bienenstock: What is the significance of the Fc-gamma receptor on these cells?
Austen: Mouse bone marrow–derived mast cells have Fc-gamma receptors of class II, types 1 and 2, and of class III. These receptors were previously designated as beta-1, beta-2, and alpha. They bind immune complexes composed of mouse IgG_a, mouse IgG_b, and mouse IgG_1. They increase in number with coculture on fibroblasts.
Lichtenstein: Can TC and T mast cells of the human mature in the same microenvironment?
Austen: Although there is evidence of compartmentalization in certain settings, such as pulmonary parenchyma and intestinal mucosa, relative to skin, most other tissues do show evidence of both subclasses.
Schwartz: Does the conversion of bone marrow–derived mouse mast cells to tissue-related subclasses involve the selection and proliferation of a particular population of progenitor mast cells, or are genes turned off and turned on by the microenvironment acting on a common progenitor population?
Austen: With the availability of probes that can now be used for transcription phenotyping of various mouse mast cell populations, we have begun to address that question. We do not know whether tissue subclass specificity is defined entirely in the end tissue or also involves the selection of different intermediate mast cell populations.
Kaplan: Does the existence of five or more chymotryptic serine proteases reflect a family of isoenzymes, or is each enzyme truly different in substrate specificity and thus in function?
Austen: At present, we believe there will be different functions, because there are substantial amino acid differences for each of the consensus amino acid sequences derived from knowledge of the cDNA clones.
Kennerly: What is the role of translational events in determining differences among mast cell populations?
Austen: We have already observed that there can be substantial transcription in the IL-3-dependent bone marrow–derived mast cells, without appreciable translation, until those cells are placed in coculture with 3T3 fibroblasts. These data, for example, are quite striking with regard to carboxypeptidase A. Thus we do believe that there will be regulation by the microenvironment, in terms of both transcription and translation.

References

Benfey, P. N., Yin, F. H., and Leder, P. (1987). Cloning of the mast cell protease, RMCP II. *J. Biol. Chem.* 262:5377–5384.

Cole, K. R., Kumar, S., Le Trong, H., Woodbury, R. G., Walsh, K. A., and Neurath, H. (1991). Rat mast cell carboxypeptidase: Amino acid sequence and evidence of enzyme activity within mast cell granules. *Biochemistry* 30:648–655.

DuBuske, L., Austen, K. F., Czop, J., and Stevens, R. L. (1984). Granule-associated serine neutral proteases of the mouse bone marrow-derived mast cell that degrade fibronectin: Their increase after sodium butyrate treatment of the cells. *J. Immunol.* 133:1535–1541.

Everitt, M. T., and Neurath, H. (1980). Rat peritoneal mast cell carboxypeptidase: Localization, purification, and enzymatic properties. *FEBS Lett.* 110:292–296.

Faller, D. V., Kouvembanas, S., Ginsberg, D., Hannan, R., Collins, T., Ewenstein, B. M., Pober, J. S., and Tantravahi, R. (1988). Immortalization of human endothelial cells by murine sarcoma viruses, without morphologic transformation. *J. Cell. Physiol.* 134:47–56.

Gershenfeld, H. K., and Weissman, I. L. (1986). Cloning of a cDNA for a T cell–specific serine protease from a cytotoxic T lymphocyte. *Science* 232:854–858.

Gibson, S., and Miller, H. R. P. (1986). Mast cell subsets in the rat distinguished immunohistochemically by their content of serine proteinases. *Immunology* 58:101–104.

Huang, E., Nocka, K., Beier, D. R., Chu, T. Y., Buck, J., Lahm, H. W., Wellner, D., Leder, P., and Besmer, P. (1990). The hematopoietic growth factor KL is encoded by the Sl locus and is the ligand of the c-*kit* receptor, the gene product of the *W* locus. *Cell* 63:225–233.

Irani, A. A., Schechter, N. M., Craig, S. S., DeBlois, G., and Schwartz, L. B. (1986). Two human mast cell subsets with distinct neutral protease compositions. *Proc. Natl. Acad. Sci. USA* 83:4464–4468.

Jenne, D., Rey, C., Masson, D., Stanley, K. K., Herz, J., Plaetinck, G., and Tchopp, J. (1988). cDNA cloning of granzyme C, a granule-associated serine protease of cytolytic T lymphocytes. *J. Immunol.* 140:318–323.

Laemmli, U. K. (1970). Cleavage of structural proteins during the assembly of the head of bacteriophage T4. *Nature* 227:680–685.

Lee, F., Yokota, T., Otsuka, T., Meyerson, P., Villaret, D., Coffman, R., Mosmann, T., Rennick, D., Roehm, N., Smith, C., Zlotnick, A., and Arai, K-I. (1986). Isolation and characterization of a mouse interleukin cDNA clone that expresses B-cell stimulatory factor 1 activities and T-cell- and mast-cell–stimulating activities. *Proc. Natl. Acad. Sci. USA* 83:2061–2065.

Le Trong, H., Parmelee, D. C., Walsh, K. A., Neurath, H., and Woodbury, R. G. (1987). Amino acid sequence of rat mast cell protease I (chymase). *Biochemistry* 26:6988–6994.

Le Trong, H., Newlands, G. F. J., Miller, H. R. P., Charbonneau, H., Neurath, H., and Woodbury, R. G. (1989). Amino acid sequence of a mouse mucosal mast cell protease. *Biochemistry* 28:391–395.

Levi-Schaffer, F., Austen, K. F., Caulfield, J. P., Hein, A., Bloes, W. F., and Stevens, R. L. (1985). Fibroblasts maintain the phenotype and viability of the rat heparin-containing mast cell in vitro. *J. Immunol.* 135:3454–3462.

Levi-Schaffer, F., Austen, K. F., Gravallese, P. M., and Stevens, R. L. (1986). Coculture of interleukin 3-dependent mouse mast cells with fibroblasts results in a phenotypic change of the mast cells. *Proc. Natl. Acad. Sci. USA* 83:6485–6488.

Lichtman, A. H., Reynolds, D. S., Faller, D. V., and Abbas, A. K. (1986). Mature murine B lymphocytes immortalized by Kirsten sarcoma virus. *Nature* 324:489–491.

Lichtman, A. H., Kurt-Jones, E. A., and Abbas, A. K. (1987a). B-cell stimulatory factor 1 and not interleukin 2 is the autocrine growth factor for some helper T lymphocytes. *Proc. Natl. Acad. Sci. USA* 84:824–827.

Lichtman, A. H., Williams, M. E., Ohara, J., Paul, W. E., Faller, D. V., and Abbas, A. K. (1987b). Retrovirus infection alters growth factor responses of T lymphocytes. *J. Immunol.* 138:3276–3283.

Lobe, C. G., Finlay, B. B., Paranchych, W., Paetkau, V. H., and Bleakley, R. C. (1986). Novel serine proteases encoded by two cytotoxic T-lymphocyte–specific genes. *Science* 232:858–861.

Lobe, C. G., Upton, C., Duggan, B., Ehrman, N., Letellier, M., Bell, J., McFadden, G., and Bleackley, R. L. (1988). Organization of two genes encoding cytotoxic T lymphocyte–specific serine proteases CCPI and CCPII. *Biochemistry* 27:6941–6946.

Masson, D., and Tschopp, J. (1987). A family of serine esterases in lytic granules of cytolytic T lymphocytes. *Cell* 49:679–685.

Miller, H. R. P., Huntley, J. F., Newlands, G. F. J., Mackellar, A., Lamma, D. A., and Wakelin, D. (1988). Granule proteinases define mast cell heterogeneity in the serosa and the gastrointestinal mucosa of the mouse. *Immunology* 65:559–566.

Miller, J. S., Westin, E. H., and Schwartz, L. B. (1989). Cloning and characterization of complementary DNA for human tryptase. *J. Clin. Invest.* 84:1188–1195.

Miller, J. S., Moxley, G., and Schwartz, L. B. (1990). Cloning and characterization of a second complementary DNA for human tryptase. *J. Clin. Invest.* 86: 864–870.

Moeller, J., Hültner, L., Schmitt, E., Breuer, M., and Dörmer, P. (1990). Purification of MEA, a mast cell growth-enhancing activity, to apparent homogeneity and its partial amino acid sequencing. *J. Immunol.* 144:4231–4234.

Nabel, G., Galli, S. J., Dvorak, A. M., Dvorak, H. F., and Cantor, H. (1981). Inducer T lymphocytes synthesize a factor that stimulates proliferation of cloned mast cells. *Nature* 291:332–334.

Newlands, G. F. J., Gibson, S., Knox, D. P., Grencis, R., Wakelin, D., and Miller, H. R. P. (1987). Characterization and mast cell origin of a chymotrypsin-like proteinase isolated from intestines of mice infected with *Trichinella spiralis*. *Immunology* 62:629–634.

Pasternak, M. S., and Eisen, H. N. (1985). A novel serine esterase expressed by cytotoxic T lymphocytes. *Nature* 314:743–745.

Phillips, M., Djian, P., and Green, H. (1986). The nucleotide sequence of three genes participating in the adipose differentiation of 3T3 cells. *J. Biol. Chem.* 261:10821–10827.

Razin, E., Ihle, J. N., Seldin, D., Mencia-Huerta, J-M., Katz, H. R., LeBlanc, P. A., Hein, A., Caulfield, J. P., Austen, K. F., and Stevens, R. L. (1984). Interleukin 3: A differentiation and growth factor for the mouse mast cell that contains chondroitin sulfate E proteoglycan. *J. Immunol.* 132:1479–1486.

Rein, A., Keller, J., Schultz, A. M., Holmes, K. L., Medicus, R., and Ihle, J. N. (1985).

Infection of immune mast cells by Harvey sarcoma virus: Immortalization without loss of requirement for interleukin-3. *Mol. Cell. Biol.* 5:2257–2264.

Reynolds, D. S. (1989). Development of immortalized mouse mast cell lines and molecular characterization of mast cell secretory granule proteases. Ph.D. thesis, Harvard University.

Reynolds, D. S., Serafin, W. E., Faller, D. V., Wall, D. A., Abbas, A. K., Dvorak, A. M., Austen, K. F., and Stevens, R. L. (1988). Immortalization of murine connective tissue-type mast cells at multiple stages of their differentiation by coculture of splenocytes with fibroblasts that produce Kirsten sarcoma virus. *J. Biol. Chem.* 263:12783–12791.

Reynolds, D. S., Stevens, R. L., Gurley, D. S., Lane, W. S., Austen, K. F., and Serafin, W. E. (1989a). Isolation and molecular cloning of mast cell carboxypeptidase A: A novel member of the carboxypeptidase gene family. *J. Biol. Chem.* 264:20094–20099.

Reynolds, D. S., Gurley, D. S., Stevens, R. L., Sugarbaker, D. J., Austen, K. F., and Serafin, W. E. (1989b). Cloning of human mast cell carboxypeptidase A, and comparison of the protein with mouse mast cell carboxypeptidase A and rat pancreatic carboxypeptidase. *Proc. Natl. Acad. Sci. USA* 86:9480–9484.

Reynolds, D. S., Stevens, R. L., Lane, W. S., Carr, M. H., Austen, K. F., and Serafin, W. E. (1990). Different mouse mast cell populations express various combinations of at least six distinct mast cell serine proteases. *Proc. Natl. Acad. Sci. USA* 87:3230–3234.

Reynolds, D. S., Gurley, D. S., Austen, K. F., and Serafin, W. E. (1991). Cloning of the cDNA and gene of mouse mast cell protease-6: Transcription by progenitor mast cells and mast cells of the connective tissue subclass. *J. Biol. Chem.* 266:3847–3853.

Rosen, B. S., Cook, K. S., Yaglom, J., Groves, D. L., Volanakis, J. E., Damm, D., White, T., and Spiegelman, B. M. (1989). Adipsin and complement factor D activity: An immune-related defect in obesity. *Science* 244:1483–1487.

Sarid, J., Benfey, P. N., and Leder, P. (1989). The mast cell-specific expression of a protease gene, RMCP II, is regulated by an enhancer element that binds specifically to mast cell trans-acting factors. *J. Biol. Chem.* 264:1022–1026.

Schägger, H., and von Jagow, G. (1987). Tricine-sodium dodecyl sulfate–polyacrylamide gel electrophoresis for the separation of proteins in the range from 1 to 100 kDa. *Anal. Biochem.* 166:368–379.

Schechter, N. M., Choi, J. K., Slavin, D. A., Deresienski, D. T., Sayama, S., Doug, G., Lavker, R. M., Proud, D., and Lazarus, G. S. (1986). Identification of a chymotrypsin-like proteinase in human mast cells. *J. Immunol.* 137:962–970.

Schwartz, L. B., and Bradford, T. M. (1986). Regulation of tryptase from human lung mast cells by heparin: Stabilization of the active tetramer. *J. Biol. Chem.* 261:7372–7379.

Schwartz, L. B., Lewis, R. A., Seldin, D., and Austen, K. F. (1981). Acid hydrolases and tryptase from secretory granules of dispersed lung mast cells. *J. Immunol.* 126:1290–1294.

Schwartz, L. B., Riedel, C., Schratz, J. J., and Austen, K. F. (1982). Localization of carboxypeptidase A to the macromolecular heparin proteoglycan-protein complex in secretory granules of rat serosal mast cells. *J. Immunol.* 128:1128–1133.

Schwartz, L. B., Metcalfe, D. D., Miller, J. S., Earl, H., and Sullivan, T. (1987). Tryptase levels as an indicator of mast cell activation in systemic anaphylaxis and mastocytosis. *N. Engl. J. Med.* 316:1622–1626

Serafin, W. E., Reynolds, D. S., Rogelj, S., Lane, W. S., Conder, G., Johnson, S. S., Austen, K. F., and Stevens, R. L. (1990). Identification and molecular cloning of a novel mouse mucosal mast cell serine protease. *J. Biol. Chem.* 265:423–429.

Serafin, W. E., Sullivan, T. P., Conder, G. A., Ebrahimi, A., Marcham, P., Johnson, S. S., Austen, K. F., and Reynolds, D. S. (1991). Cloning of the cDNA and gene for mouse mast cell protease-4: Demonstration of its late transcription in mast cell subclasses and analysis of its homology to subclass-specific neutral proteases of the mouse and rat. *J. Biol. Chem.* 266:1934–1941.

Smith, C. A., and Rennick, D. M. (1986). Characterization of a murine lymphokine distinct from interleukin 2 and interleukin 3 (IL-3) possessing a T-cell growth factor activity and a mast-cell growth factor activity that synergizes with IL-3. *Proc. Natl. Acad. Sci. USA* 83:1857–1861.

Tantravahi, R. V., Stevens, R. L., Austen, K. F., and Weis, J. H. (1986). A single gene in mast cells encodes the core peptides of heparin and chondroitin sulfate proteoglycans. *Proc. Natl. Acad. Sci. USA* 83:9207–9210.

Thompson-Snipes, L., Dhar, V., Bond, M. W., Mosmann, T. R., Moore, K. W., and Rennick, D. M. (1991). Interleukin 10: A novel stimulatory factor for mast cells and their progenitors. *J. Exp. Med.* 173:507–510.

Vanderslice, P., Craik, C. S., Nadel, J. A., and Caughy, G. H. (1989). Molecular cloning of dog mast cell tryptase and a related protease: Structural evidence of a unique mode of serine protease activation. *Biochemistry* 28:4148–4155.

Vanderslice, P., Ballinger, S. M., Tam, E. K., Goldstein, S. M., Craik, C. S., and Caughey, G. H. (1990). Human mast cell tryptase: Multiple cDNAs and genes reveal a multigene serine protease family. *Proc. Natl. Acad. Sci. USA* 87:3811–3815.

von Heijne, G. (1984). How signal sequences maintain cleavage specificity. *J. Mol. Biol.* 173:243–251.

Woodbury, R. G., Katunuma, N., Kobayashi, K., Titani, K., and Neurath, H. (1978). Covalent structure of a group-specific protease from rat small intestine. *Biochemistry* 17:811–819.

9

Modulation of Mediator Release from Mast Cells

ROBERT J. HOHMAN and THOMAS HULTSCH

National Institute of Allergy and Infectious Diseases
National Institute of Health
Bethesda, Maryland

I. Introduction

A. Activation of Mast Cells

Mast cells can be stimulated to secrete by a wide variety of stimuli (Table 1). The classic allergic reactions occurs when antigen-specific IgE bound to the high-affinity IgE receptor ($Fc_\epsilon RI$) on the surface of mast cells is aggregated by binding to a multivalent antigen (Fig. 1). The crosslinking of cell-bound IgE, in turn, aggregates the $Fc_\epsilon RI$ that activates the mast cell. Activation of mast cells leads to three different responses: (1) exocytosis of secretory granules containing histamine and other preformed mediators of immediate hypersensitivity; (2) synthesis and secretion of newly formed eicosanoid mediators (such as prostaglandins and leukotrienes); and (3) synthesis and secretion of cytokines. The first two events occur within minutes of stimulation. The majority of cytokines secreted by mast cells represent newly synthesized protein and, therefore, appear several hours after stimulation. However, it has recently been reported that tumor necrosis factor α is preformed and stored in secretory granules; thus, this cytokine appears within minutes.

The generation of eicosanoids and production of cytokines in response to aggregation of IgE receptors are covered in another chapter of this book. This

Table 1 Stimuli that Can Activate Mast Cells

Complement
Major basic protein
Opioids
Cytokines
Chymotrypsin
Polysaccharides
Neuropeptides
Polyamines (compound 48/80)
Ca^{2+}-ionophores (A23187)
Histamine-releasing factors (HRF's)
Aggregation of IgE receptors

chapter will focus on the control of the release of preformed mediators from mast cells.

B. Role of the IgE Receptor in Activation of Mast Cells

Activation of mast cells via $Fc_\epsilon RI$, like activation of T and B lymphocytes by antigen-specific receptors, requires *aggregation* of cell surface receptors; the binding of monomeric IgE to its receptor does not result in activation (Fewtrell and Metzger, 1980; Ishizaka, 1982; Ishizaka et al., 1979; Ishizaka and Ishizaka, 1984). The mast cell does, however, have a system for distinguishing occupied from unoccupied receptors. The half-life of the IgE receptor bound to monomeric IgE is longer than that for empty receptors (Furuichi et al., 1985, 1986; Rivera et al., 1986; Isersky et al., 1983). Studies by a number of workers have demonstrated that a dimer of IgE receptors is the minimum signaling unit for activation, and that the rate of activation is proportional to both the size and number of IgE receptor aggregates (Kagey-Sobotka et al., 1981; Fewtrell and Metzger, 1980; Maeyama et al., 1986; Segal et al., 1977). Any mechanism that results in aggregation of IgE receptors activates mast cells. This includes (1) addition of antigen to cells sensitized with specific IgE; (2) addition of anti-IgE to cells sensitized with any IgE; (3) direct aggregation of $Fc_\epsilon RI$ with antireceptor antibody; (4) addition of preformed oligomers of IgE to cells containing vacant receptors; and (5) addition of lectins (such as concanavalin A) that aggregate cell surface glycoproteins (including the IgE receptor). Not only is receptor aggregation necessary for activation, but continued activation requires persistent aggregation. If receptors are disaggregated at any time during secretion, exocytosis and all other IgE receptor-mediated events (see below) are immediately halted or reversed.

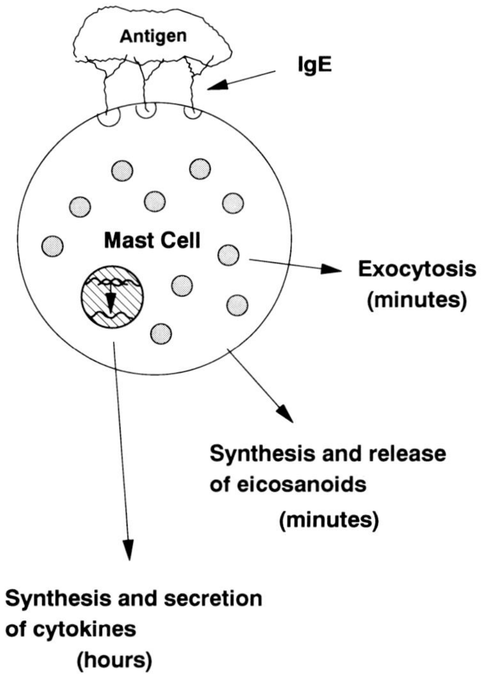

Figure 1 IgE receptor-mediated activation of mast cells results in three different responses.

The affinity of the IgE receptor for IgE is 10^{-10} *M*. This high affinity is primarily due to a very slow rate of dissociation (Metzger et al., 1986; Kulczycki and Metzger, 1974). In other words, the binding of IgE to its receptor is, for all practical purposes, irreversible. There are 10^5 to 10^6 IgE receptors per cell, and a detectable response is observed when as few as 100 receptors are aggregated. Moreover, maximum secretion occurs when only 10% of the receptors are aggregated. Therefore, the mast cell is an extremely efficient system for binding IgE, being activated by antigen, and releasing mediators of immediate hypersensitivity.

Although the structure of $Fc_{\epsilon}RI$ is now known in detail (Kinet et al., 1989; Blank et al., 1989), the mechanism by which aggregation of this receptor triggers a cellular response remains unknown. The major question is, "What activity do aggregated receptors exhibit that unaggregated receptors do not?" Aggregated receptors may possess two "types" of activity: intrinsic (the receptors themselves express an activity) or extrinsic (the aggregated receptors interact with distal components in a signal transduction cascade) (Metzger et al., 1986). Examples of receptors possessing an intrinsic activity are the insulin and epidermal growth factor receptors, which are tyrosine kinases, and the nicotinic cholinergic receptor, which is an ion channel. Other receptors possess no intrinsic activity themselves, but interact with separate components. For example, when the β-adrenergic receptor binds its ligand, the hormone-receptor complex then interacts with a GTP-binding protein (G protein) that, in turn, activates adenylate cyclase. Despite an extensive search, no intrinsic activities have yet been ascribed to the IgE receptor. Efforts are now being directed at identifying an extrinsic activity such as interaction with a G protein or with a tyrosine kinase.

C. Biochemical Events that Occur When IgE Receptors Are Aggregated

A number of IgE receptor-mediated events have been identified (reviewed in Metzger et al., 1986; Ishizaka and Ishizaka, 1984; Oliver et al., 1988; Beaven and Cunha-Melo, 1988), some of which are listed in Table 2. Although there is reasonable evidence that these events occur when mast cells are activated, the precise role of these events in exocytosis is, for the most part, poorly understood. In addition, virtually nothing is known about the interaction of these events with each other. This field is complicated by the fact that it is likely that aggregation of $Fc_{\epsilon}RI$ initiates several different (and perhaps unrelated) parallel sequences of events, all of which are necessary for secretion.

It is noteworthy that most of the IgE receptor-mediated biochemical events identified to date that have been proposed to be involved in activation of the mast cell have also been proposed to mediate signal transduction in T cells, B cells, neutrophils, and other cell types. This observation has several implications. First, new information gained in the study of mast cell activation can likely be

Table 2 Biochemical Events that Occur When IgE Receptors Are Aggregated

1. Ruffling of the plasma membrane
2. Immobilization of the aggregated IgE receptors
3. Association of the IgE receptor with the membrane cytoskeleton
4. Activation of a serine esterase-like enzyme
5. Activation of protein tyrosine kinases
6. Phosphorylation of myosin by protein kinase C (PKC)
7. Activation of adenylate cyclase (rise in cAMP)
8. Activation of phospholipase C (PLC) and phospholipase D (PLD)
9. Influx of Ca^{2+} into the cell
10. Rise in the concentration of Ca^{2+} in the cytosol

applied to other cells in the immune system, and vice versa. Unfortunately, this also means that it will be difficult to produce drugs to inhibit mast cell functions without affecting other cell types.

II. Modulation of Mediator Release

Therapies designed to control allergic diseases attempt to prevent either the degranulation of mast cells or the biological effects of the released mediators. For example, immunotherapy is useful in allergic rhinitis in part by suppressing the biosynthesis of specific IgE and/or by producing IgG-blocking antibodies. In addition, a limited number of pharmacological agents, such as cromolyn, are currently being used to modulate secretion, but their mechanism of action is only poorly understood.

As our knowledge of mast cell activation and the structure of $Fc_{\epsilon}RI$ grows, the prospects of designing agents to specifically prevent IgE receptor-mediated activation of mast cells are improving. The rest of this chapter will deal with the most promising new areas of research with respect to developing clinically important agents that might act by preventing activation of mast cells.

A. Prevention of the Binding of IgE to Its Receptor

The genes coding for the high-affinity receptor for IgE in both the rat and human have recently been cloned, sequenced, and expressed in non-$Fc_{\epsilon}RI$-bearing cells (Miller et al., 1989; Blank et al., 1989). These advances make it now possible to study, at the molecular level, the protein-protein interactions between IgE and its receptor (Kinet, 1989; Varin-Blank and Metzger, 1990; Metzger and Kinet, 1988; Metzger, 1988). The goal of these studies is to develop a peptide or some other appropriate reagent that can block the binding of IgE to its receptor on mast cells (Dreskin and Metzger, 1988). If mast cells are not sensitized, they cannot be activated by allergen. Considerable progress is being made toward characterizing the interaction between IgE and its receptor; however, in addition to the cost and logistic problems with the use of peptides as drugs, there are considerable obstacles (discussed below) that must be overcome before "blocking peptides" will be clinically useful.

IgE binds to its receptor with a very high affinity ($K_d = 10^{-10}$ M). Although there is nothing remarkable about the association constant, IgE dissociates very slowly from the receptor. The half-life of skin-sensitizing activity of IgE is 8–14 days (Dreskin and Metzger, 1988). Therefore, blocking peptides must be used prophylactically. Moreover, the blocking agent must be continuously present since, once sensitized with IgE, the mast cell is not easily desensitized. In addition to the high affinity of the IgE receptor for its ligand, the mast cell requires aggregation of very few receptors to activate the cell. In fact, maximum degranulation occurs when only 10% of the receptors are aggregated. Thus, although these studies are providing valuable information on receptor-ligand interactions, the development of a clinically useful drug may be problematic.

Given the inherent problems with preventing activation of mast cells by blocking the binding of IgE to its receptors, strategies are being developed to pharmacologically prevent mast cells from degranulating. In addition to potential therapeutic benefits, these studies are slowly unraveling the complicated series of events leading from aggregation of the IgE receptor to exocytosis.

B. Pharmacological Modulation of Secretion

Diisopropylfluorophosphate

In 1960, Austen and Brocklehurst reported that if mast cells were activated in the presence of diisopropylfluorophosphate (DFP), an irreversible inhibitor of serine esterases, secretion was inhibited (Austen and Brocklehurst, 1960). In fact, all IgE receptor-mediated events are inhibited by DFP; however, if mast cells are incubated with DFP and then washed, resuspended in DFP-free buffer, and then activated, degranulation proceeds normally. These results have led to the following model (Ishizaka and Ishizaka, 1984). A very early step in the activation of mast cells involves a DFP-sensitive enzyme that exists in an inactive, DFP-resistant form in resting cells. When IgE receptors are aggregated, the DFP-sensitive enzyme is activated, binds DFP, and is irreversibly inhibited. Despite an intensive search, the DFP-sensitive enzyme has never been identified. DFP itself could never be used clinically since it is a potent neurotoxin. However, by defining the intracellular target for this inhibitor, more specific (and less toxic) drugs can possibly be developed.

Sodium Cromoglycate

Topical applications (to upper airways, eye) of sodium cromoglycate are currently being used extensively to treat symptoms of immediate hypersensitivity. In vitro, this drug has been shown to prevent degranulation of mast cells and, therefore, is commonly referred to as a "mast cell stabilizer." Despite its importance clinically, very little is known about its mechanism of action.

In the early 1980s, an exciting series of papers published by Pecht and co-workers claimed to have purified a cromolyn-binding protein from the plasma membrane of mast cells (Mazurek et al., 1980, 1984). They proposed that this binding protein was the Ca^{2+} channel-forming protein whose activity is coupled to the IgE receptor. Unfortunately, there were several shortcomings to this work (reviewed in Metzger et al., 1986), and the identity of the cromolyn-binding protein as well as the mechanism of action of this drug remains to be established.

Other Modulators

Other pharmacological modulators of mast cell secretion are either reviewed in other chapters of this book or have recently been reviewed in detail (cAMP modulators; see Winslow and Austen, 1984).

III. Immunosuppressive Compounds

A. Immunosuppressive Compounds and Their Intracellular Binding Proteins

The remainder of this chapter will deal with modulation of mast cell activation by a series of immunosuppressive drugs called immunophilin ligands. Until recently, these drugs were thought to specifically inhibit T-cell-receptor–mediated activation of T lymphocytes; however, it is now obvious that these compounds are potent inhibitors of receptor-mediated functions in other cells. The first report of an effect of immunsuppressive drugs on secretion of mast cells was by Pedersen et al. (1985).

The structures of the four known immunophilin ligands are shown in Figure 2.

Cyclosporin A

Cyclosporin A (CsA) is a neutral, lipophilic, cyclic, endecapeptide (MW = 1203) isolated from the fungus *Tolypocladium inflatum*. In 1976, Borel reported that CsA was a potent immunosuppressive drug when tested in a murine model of graft rejection (Borel, 1976; Borel et al., 1976). Because of this immunosuppressive property, CsA has revolutionized the field of organ transplantation. Therapeutic concentrations of CsA dramatically reduce both the rate and severity of episodes of rejection for renal, cardiac, hepatic, heart-lung, and lung transplantation (Cohen et al., 1984; Shevach, 1985; Lorber, 1988; Kahan, 1989).

In addition to its use in organ transplantation, CsA is being tested for efficacy in a variety of diseases with an immunological component, including psoriasis (Biren and Barr, 1986; Ellis et al., 1986, 1991; Ho et al., 1990; Borel, 1990), diabetes (Stiller et al., 1984; Bougneres et al., 1988), rheumatoid arthritis (Weinblatt et al., 1987), severe atopic dermatitis (Biren and Barr, 1986; Nakagawa et al., 1988; De Prost et al., 1989a), and autoimmune uveitis (Nussenblatt et al., 1983a,b). Unfortunately, CsA has significant side effects that limits its systemic application to severe disease; the most prominent side effect is nephrotoxicity (Kahan, 1989; Schmitz-Schumann, 1986).

FK506

A new immunosuppressive compound, called FK506, has recently been described (Thomson, 1989). FK506 (MW = 822) is a lipophilic macrolide and,

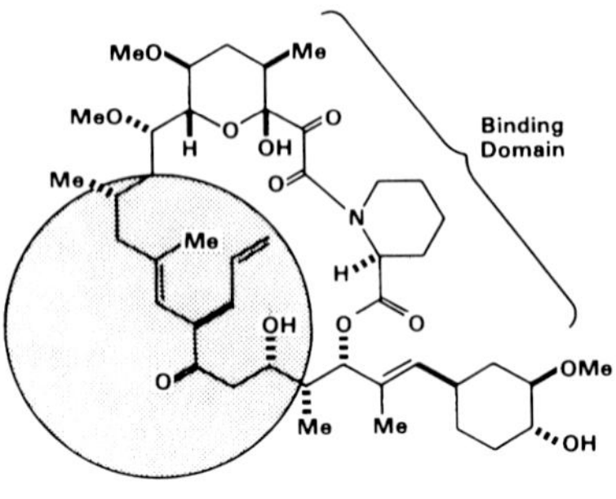

FK506

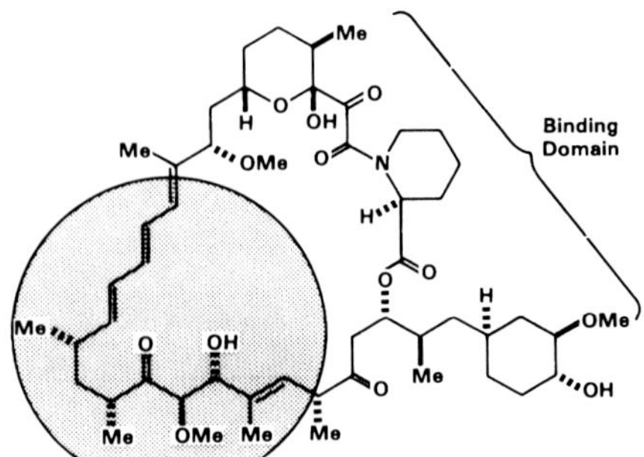

Rapamycin

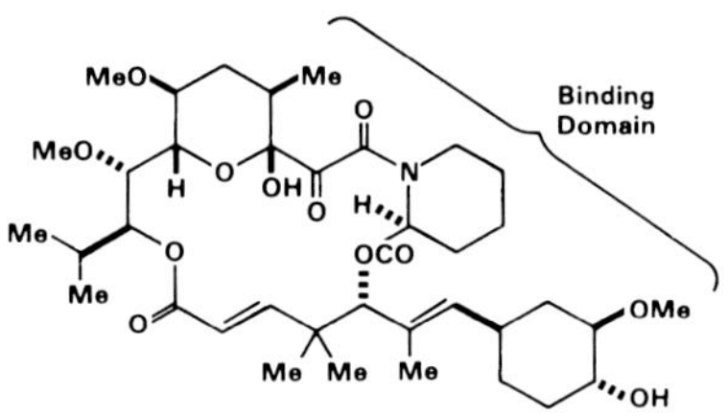

506BD

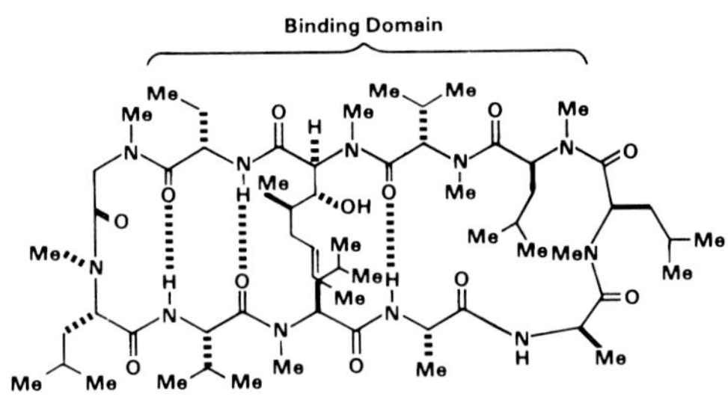

Cyclosporin A (CsA)

Figure 2 Structure of immunophilin ligands (Schreiber, 1991). The structures of CsA, FK506, rapamycin, and 506BD are shown with their "binding domains" (the part of the molecule that interacts with the respective binding protein) labeled. Note that the binding domains of FK506 and rapamycin (the two natural ligands for FKBP) and the binding domain for 506BD (the synthetic ligand) are nearly identical. The shaded areas of FK506 and rapamycin represent the proposed "effector domains" of these two molecules (see text). 506BD has no effector domain.

thus, shares no structural homology to CsA. Nevertheless, FK506 (which is produced by *Streptomyces tsukubaenis*) shares interesting functional similarities to CsA. In both in vivo models of graft rejection and in vitro models of receptor-mediated signal transduction, the effects of FK506 are indistinguishable from those of CsA, with the exception that FK506 is 10–100 times more potent than CsA.

Rapamycin

Rapamycin (MW = 914) is another new immunosuppressive drug that is structurally very similar to FK506 (Martel et al., 1977). Like FK506, rapamycin is produced by a species of *Streptomyces (S. hygroscopicus)* (Sehgal et al., 1975; Vezina et al., 1975). In vivo, rapamycin has identical immunosuppressive properties to those of CsA and FK506, with a potency close to that of FK506. Interestingly, despite this similarity in vivo, rapamycin targets different receptor-signaling pathways in vitro (see below).

506BD

Schreiber and colleagues (Bierer et al., 1990a; Schreiber, 1991) compared the x-ray structure of FK506 and rapamycin and observed that parts of the molecules were structurally nearly identical whereas other parts were different (see legend to Fig. 2). They reasoned that the homologous regions were the domains by which these two compounds bind to a common binding protein, and that the domains that were different represented different effector functions. Schreiber then synthesized a compound, called 506BD, that preserved the binding domain but lacked the effector domain. 506BD binds tightly to the FK506 and rapamycin binding protein (FKBP; K_d=20 nM), although with a lower affinity than that of FK506 (K_d = 0.4 nM) and rapamycin (K_d=0.2 nM). FK506, rapamycin, and 506BD compete with one another for the binding to FKBP, presumably by sharing a common binding site on the protein.

B. Immunophilins Are the Intracellular Targets for Immunosuppressive Compounds

In the mid-1980s, radiolabeled CsA was used to identify (Handschumacher et al., 1984) and purify (Harding et al., 1986) a 17-kDa, cytoplasmic, CsA-binding protein from human spleen and bovine thymus. This protein, called cyclophilin, had a high affinity for CsA (K_d = 30 nM) and was present in large amounts (0.1–0.4% to total soluble protein) (Harding and Handschumacher, 1988). Since CsA was thought to be specific for T lymphocytes, the initial isolation of cyclophilin was from lymphoid tissue; however, cyclophilin is very ubiquitous. In fact, cyclophilin has been found in all mammalian tissue and cell lines that have been tested, as well as in other eukaryotic cells (Merker, 1984; Koletsky et al., 1986). Moreover, CsA-binding proteins of comparable size (17–18 kDa) have been found in mollusks, arthropods, trematodes, fungi, yeasts, plants, and marine sponges. The structure of cyclophilin is highly conserved between species. There is >98% identity between the amino acid sequences of cyclophilin from bovine and human tissues. Moreover, an antiserum raised against bovine cyclophilin cross-reacts with cyclophilin from human and murine tissue as well as marine sponges (Harding and Handschumacher, 1988).

Not only is cyclophilin found in all mammalian cells, but most cells contain multiple isoforms of the protein. For example, extracts from T cells were subjected to affinity chromatography using a matrix with covalently attached

CsA. Cyclophilins of 18, 19, 20, 31, 42, and 80 kDa were specifically eluted with CsA (Fretz et al., 1991). Similar results have been obtained using extracts from mast cells (see below). Therefore, cyclophilin apparently is involved in the control of very basic cellular functions, and different isoforms of cyclophilin may control different functions.

In analogy with the CsA-cyclophilin complex, FK506 (as well as rapamycin and 506BD) binds to an intracellular binding protein called FKBP (Harding et al., 1989; Rosen et al., 1990; Standaert et al., 1990; Fretz et al., 1991; Siekierka et al., 1989; Dumont et al., 1990a; Tropschug et al., 1990; Hohman and Hultsch, 1990). Although cyclophilin and FKBP share no sequence homology at either the DNA or protein level, they share several interesting properties. Like cyclophilin, FKBP is ubiquitous and abundant. FKBP is found in all mammalian cells, and it accounts for up to 0.4% of total cellular protein. The concentration of FKBP in Jurkat cells is 5 nM. The major isoforms of both cyclophilin and FKBP are small (<20 kDa), have basic isoelectric points, and exhibit an intrinsic rotamase activity (see below).

FKBP binds FK506, rapamycin, and 506BD with similar affinities: 0.4 nM, 0.2 nM, and 20 nM, respectively (Bierer et al., 1990a,b). Each ligand competitively inhibits the binding of the other, presumably because they share a common binding site. The relative affinity of FKBP for FK506 (K_d = 0.4 nM) is much higher than the affinity of cyclophilin for CsA (K_d = 30 nM). This probably accounts for the fact that FK506 is 10–100 times more potent than CsA both in vitro and in vivo.

C. All Immunophilins Have Peptidyl-Prolyl *cis-trans* Isomerase Activity

During studies on protein folding, an enzyme that catalyzes the *cis-trans* isomerization of proline-containing peptide bonds was identified and named peptidyl-prolyl *cis-trans* isomerase (PPlase) (Fischer and Bang, 1985; Fischer et al., 1984; Lang et al., 1987). The presence of a proline residue in a polypeptide has two important implications for its tertiary structure. Unlike all the other amino acids found in proteins that have a primary amino group attached to the α carbon, the side group in proline is bound to both the α carbon and the nitrogen attached to the α carbon. Therefore, the amino group in proline is secondary, whereas all the other amino acids have a primary amino group.

As shown in Figure 3, the presence of proline in a polypeptide chain produces a marked "kink" in its secondary structure. Moreover, the configuration of the proline-containing peptide bonds *(cis* versus *trans)* dramatically changes the structure of the peptide backbone. When this bond is in the *cis* configuration, the protein doubles back on itself, whereas in the *trans* configuration, there is a much gentler kink (see Fig. 3). In addition to distorting the

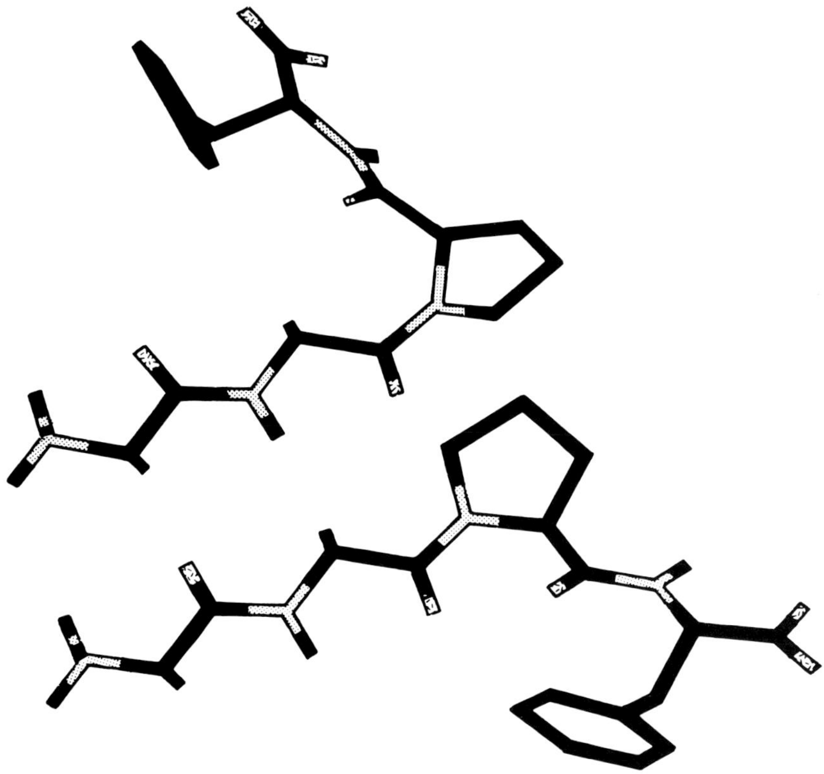

Figure 3 The configuration *(cis* versus *trans)* of a proline-containing peptide bond dramatically affects the structure of the peptide backbone. The peptide Ala-Ala-Pro-Phe is shown with the Ala-Pro bond in the *cis* configuration (upper structure) and *trans* configuration (lower configuration). Notice the sharp kink in the upper structure versus the gentler bend in the lower. (From Hohman and Hultsch, 1990.)

peptide chain, the proline-containing peptide bond is more rigid than other peptide bonds. Since the configuration *(cis* versus *trans)* of this bond has a dramatic effect on the structure of the protein, an enzyme that catalyzes this isomerization may have an important role in protein folding (Baechinger, 1987; Fischer and Bang, 1985; Lang et al., 1987; Lung-Nan et al., 1988).

In a search for enzymes that might be important for protein folding, PPIase (which is also referred to as rotamase) was purified and characterized. In vitro, this enzyme catalyzes both the *cis-trans* isomerization of proline-containing peptide bonds and the refolding of several proteins, such as RNase λ1, after denaturation in urea; however, a role for this enzyme in protein folding in vivo has yet to be demonstrated.

Table 3 Inhibition of Receptor-Mediated Signaling in T Cells and Mast Cells by Immunophilin Ligands

	T cell		Mast cell	
Ligand	TCR	IL-2 R	IgE R	IL-3 R
CSA	+		+	
FK506	+	−	+	−
Rapamycin	−	+	−	+
506BD	−	−	−	

506BD, which comprises only the binding domain common to FK506 and rapamycin and lacks the effector domain (see above), binds to FKBP and inhibits its PPlase activity. As for the functional assay, 506BD has no effect on receptor signaling by either the TCR or IL-2 receptor and, in fact, prevents inhibition by either FK506 or rapamycin (see Table 3).

A model for the mechanism of action of CsA, FK506, rapamycin, and 506BD on receptor-mediated signaling that accounts for all these results is presented below.

CsA Inhibits Degranulation of Cytotoxic T Cells

Until recently, immunosuppressive drugs were thought to specifically inhibit TCR-mediated production of IL-2; however, Trenn et al. (1989) demonstrated that both TCR-mediated degranulation and lysis of antigen-bearing target cells are inhibited by 0.2 μg/ml CsA, the same concentration that inhibits production of IL-2. TCR-mediated hydrolysis of phosphatidylinositol was not affected by the drug. This was the first demonstration that a T-cell function other than cytokine production was inhibited by CsA.

E. CsA and FK506 Inhibit IgE Receptor-Mediated Exocytosis from Mast Cells

In addition to inhibition of TCR-mediated degranulation of cytotoxic T cells, IgE receptor-mediated degranulation of mast cells is also inhibited by CsA. The first report of an effect of CsA on activation of mast cells was by Pedersen et al. (1985).

As shown in Figure 4, IgE receptor-mediated degranulation of RBL cells, a tumor analog of rat mucosal mast cells, is inhibited in a dose-dependent manner by CsA and FK506, with an IC_{50} of 200 nM and 2 nM, respectively. Inhibition occurs over the same range of concentrations of CsA and FK506 that inhibits TCR-mediated production of IL-2, and the same concentrations are found in the

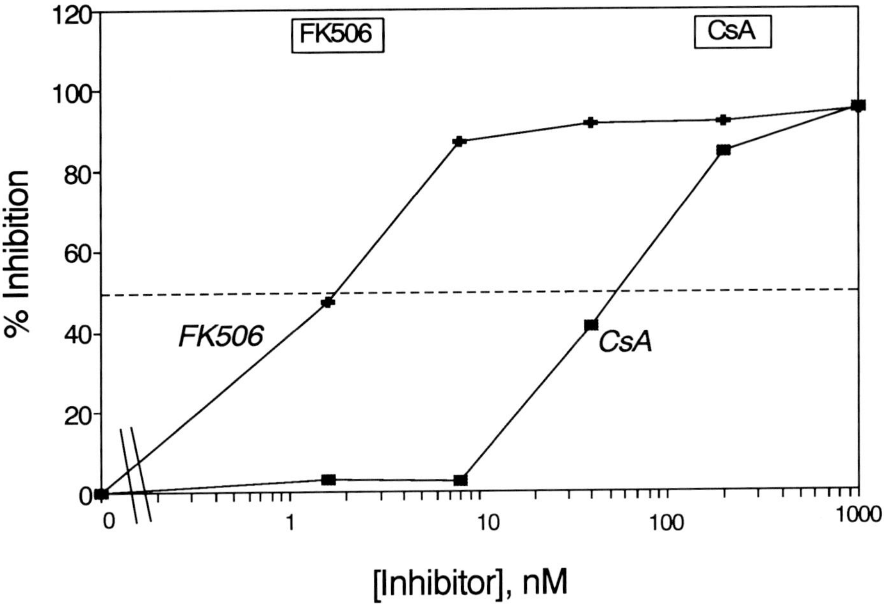

Figure 4 CsA and FK506 inhibit IgE receptor-mediated exocytosis from mast cells. RBL-2H3 cells were preincubated for 5 min with the indicated concentrations of CsA or FK506, stimulated by the addition of oligomeric IgE, incubated for an additional 10 min, and the percent exocytosis determined. The bars at the top of the graph represent the concentrations of CsA and FK506 found in the sera of patients undergoing immunosuppressive therapy with these drugs. (From Hultsch et al., 1990, 1991.)

serum of patients undergoing immunosuppressive therapy with these drugs. The kinetics of inhibition are very rapid. In a 10-min assay, a 5-min preincubation with CsA results in maximum inhibition, and a 2-min preincubation is nearly maximum (Fig. 5). Moreover, if CsA and FK506 are added after the IgE receptors are aggregated, subsequent release is inhibited (De Paulis et al., 1991; Triggiani et al., 1989). Taken together, these results demonstrate that inhibition of exocytosis is not a secondary effect due to inhibition of cytokine production (or some other macromolecule) and indicate that these drugs have a direct effect on some step in exocytosis.

In addition to inhibiting IgE receptor-mediated exocytosis, degranulation in response to the Ca^{2+}-ionophore A23187 is inhibited by the same concentration of CsA that inhibits receptor-mediated release. This suggests that inhibition occurs at a later step in exocytosis, rather than an early step in signal transduction. This hypothesis is supported by studies that directly examined the effect of CsA and FK506 on a variety of IgE receptor-mediated events. At suboptimal

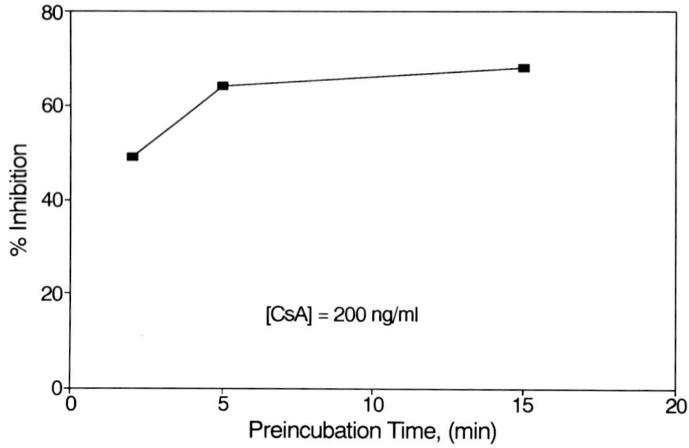

Figure 5 Inhibition by CsA requires only a short preincubation. RBL-2H3 cells were preincubated for the indicated times with 0.2 μg/ml CsA (approximately the IC_{50} for this drug), triggered with oligomeric IgE, incubated an additional 10 min, and the percent exocytosis measured. (Graph constructed from data in Hultsch et al., 1990.)

concentrations of receptor aggregation, the rate of Pl hydrolysis is proportional to both the number and size of IgE receptor aggregates. Hultsch et al. (1990) demonstrated that CsA has no effect on receptor-mediated Pl hydrolysis in RBL cells, even at suboptimal concentrations of oligomeric IgE. Therefore, this drug has no effect on either the binding of IgE to the receptor or aggregation of IgE receptors. In addition, experiments performed with $^{45}Ca^{2+}$ (to measure receptor-mediated influx of Ca^{2+} into the cell) and with quin 2 (to measure the rise in the $[Ca^{2+}]_i$) revealed that CsA does not inhibit these Ca^{2+} fluxes. In fact, CsA causes a small potentiation of both these responses (Hultsch et al., 1990). Besides receptor-mediated Pl hydrolysis and Ca^{2+} fluxes, concentrations of CsA that result in total inhibition of degranulation have no effect on the polymerization of actin or the phosphorylation of myosin by protein kinase C. Moreover, in RBL cells, CsA and FK506 have no effect on the release of arachidonic acid and metabolites from [^{14}C]-arachidonic acid–labeled cells or the release of LTC_4. The lack of an effect of CsA and FK506 on arachidonic acid metabolism is somewhat different than those reported by Marone and colleagues (Triggiani et al., 1989; De Paulis et al., 1991). These authors found that both CsA and FK506 inhibit the generation of LTC_4 from human basophils in response to anti-IgE. This is the only significant difference between the responses of human basophils and RBL cells to CsA and FK506. This difference may be explained by the purity of the cell populations used for the experiments. RBL cells are a cloned cell line, whereas the experiments of Marone and colleagues were performed on a mixture of leukocytes containing 0.5% basophils. Whether the differences between the response to RBL and human basophils are due to the cells themselves or interaction of the drugs with other cells in the suspension of basophils awaits experiments with a more purified population of human basophils.

F. CsA Inhibits Cytokine Production in Mast Cells

As summarized in another chapter in this book, activated mast cells produce a variety of cytokines. Similar to what has been reported in the T cell, transcription of some, but not all, cytokines is blocked by CsA.

G. Inhibition of Degranulation by FK506, but Not Inhibition by CsA, is Prevented by Rapamycin and 506BD

The effects of the FKBP ligands FK506, rapamycin, and 506BD on IgE receptor-mediated exocytosis were studied, and the results revealed striking similarities between TCR- and IgE receptor-mediated signaling pathways (Hultsch et al., 1991). As discussed above, all three drugs bind to FKBP and inhibit the isomerase activity of this enzyme. Yet, FK506, rapamycin, and 506BD have antagonistic effects on receptor-mediated signaling in the T cell. As summarized in Table 3, FK506 inhibits TCR-mediated transcription of IL-2, and this inhibition is prevented by rapamycin. Rapamycin inhibits IL-2 receptor-mediated proliferation, and this inhibition is prevented by FK506. 506BD by itself has no effect of either signaling pathway and, in addition, prevents inhibitory effect of either FK506 or rapamycin.

The inhibition of $Fc_\epsilon RI$-mediated exocytosis by FK506 is prevented in a dose-dependent manner by rapamycin (Fig. 6A). The concentration of rapamycin required to prevent inhibition reflects the relative affinity of these two drugs for FKBP. Equimolar concentrations of rapamycin and FK506 reverse approximately two-thirds of the inhibition by FK506. This 2:1 ratio is equivalent to the ratio of affinities for FK506 and rapamycin for FKBP (0.4 nM and 0.2 nM, respectively). Rapamycin alone has no effect on secretion; moreover, consistent with the specificity of rapamycin for FKBP and CsA for cyclophilin, rapamycin has no effect on inhibition of secretion due to CsA.

As shown in Figure 6B, 506BD alone has no effect on $Fc_\epsilon RI$-mediated secretion, but prevents the inhibition by FK506. As was observed with rapamycin, the concentration of 506BD required to reverse inhibition reflects the relative affinity of these drugs for FKBP (K_d for 506BD = 20 nM). As is shown in Figure 6B, 506BD has no effector inhibition of secretion by CsA.

Rapamycin inhibits IL-3 receptor-mediated proliferation of mast cells (T.H. and R.J.H., unpublished observation). Certain mast cell lines, such as PT18, require the presence of exogenous IL-3 for growth and proliferation.

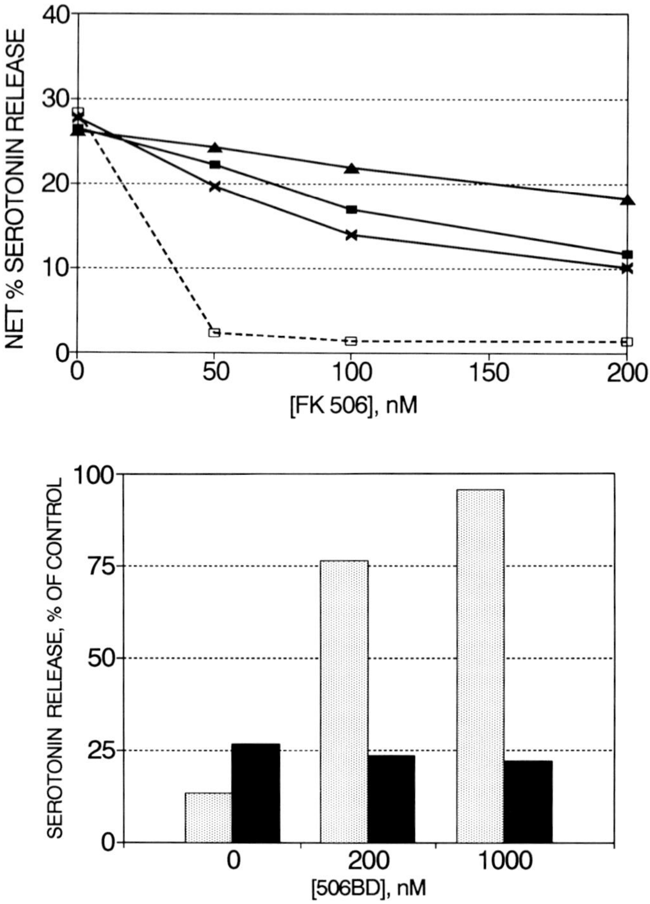

Figure 6 Inhibition of exocytosis by FK506 is prevented by either rapamycin or 506BD. (A) RBL-2H3 cells were preincubated for 10 min with 0 nM (open squares), 50 nM (X), 100 nM (filled squares), or 200 nM (triangles) rapamycin before addition of the indicated concentrations of FK506. The cells were incubated for an additional 5 min before addition of oligomeric IgE. The release of serotonin was measured after an additional 10 min of incubation. Note that rapamycin by itself (the data points where FK506 = 0 nM) has no effect on IgE receptor-mediated exocytosis. (B) 506BD prevents inhibition of IgE receptor-mediated mast cell activation by FK506 (gray bars) but not by CsA (black bars). RBL cells were preincubated for 10 min with the indicated concentration of 506BD before FK506 (3.2 nM) or CsA (330 nM) was added. After an additional 5 min of incubation, the cells were triggered with oligomeric IgE, and serotonin release was measured as described. (Data taken from Hultsch et al., 1991.)

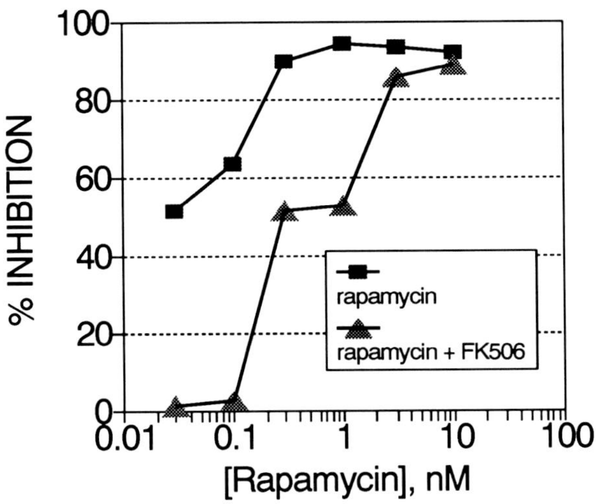

Figure 7 FK506 prevents the inhibition of proliferation of mast cells by rapamycin. Rapamycin or rapamycin plus 10 nM FK506 was added at $t = 0$ to PT 18 cells (2×10^5 cells/ml) in RPMI supplemented with 2 ng/ml recombinant IL-3. The cells were then seeded in a 96-well cluster place (200 μl/well). After 6 hr ($t = 6$ hr), a second addition of rapamycin and FK506 (same concentration as the first dose) was added along with 25 nCi/well of [^{3}H]-thymidine. After an additional 24 hr of incubation, the cellular DNA was harvested, and the [^{3}H]-thymidine incorporation was measured.

Proliferation is generally measured either by counting cell numbers or by following the incorporation of [^{3}H] thymidine into DNA. IL-3-driven proliferation of PT-18 cells is inhibited by rapamycin (Fig. 7). FK506, which by itself has no effect on proliferation, prevents the inhibition by rapamycin. It is interesting to note that these two drugs have an opposite effect on $Fc_\epsilon RI$-mediated secretion from mast cells (see Table 3).

H. Similarities Between $Fc_\epsilon RI$- and TCR-Mediated Signaling

Until recently, it appeared that TCR- and $Fc_\epsilon RI$-mediated signaling appear to have little in common. However, the results of experiments examining the effects of CsA, FK506, rapamycin, and 506BD on TCR- and IL-2 receptor-mediated activation of T cells and $Fc_\epsilon RI$ and IL-3 receptor-mediated signaling in mast cells (summarized in Table 3) reveal striking similarities. These drugs have identical effects on antigen receptor-mediated (TCR and $Fc_\epsilon RI$) signaling pathways, and these effects are very different from those of the drugs on lymphokine-receptor mediated pathways (IL-2 in T cells and IL-3 in mast cells). Therefore, these immunosuppressive drugs are not specific for certain cell types, but rather specifically inhibit certain receptor-signaling pathways and provide a basis for categorizing signal transduction from various receptors based on their sensitivity to CsA/FK506 or rapamycin. In addition, these results suggest there may be a step common to TCR-mediated transcription of IL-2- and $Fc_{\epsilon}RI$-mediated secretion.

In addition to their identical susceptibilities to immunosuppressive drugs, there are a number of other interesting similarities between TCR- and IgE receptor-mediated signaling:

1. Activation in both signaling pathways requires aggregation of receptors; monovalent interactions are not sufficient.
2. Aggregation of both receptors results in the same spectrum of activities. Although the usual readout for TCR activation is cytokine production, activation of cytotoxic T cells results in degranulation that is inhibited by CsA. Aggregation of IgE receptors results not only in exocytosis but also in production of cytokines that is inhibited by CsA.
3. Aggregation of either receptor induces the phosphorylation of phospholipase $C_{\gamma}1$. This may be the mechanism that couples receptor aggregation to Pl hydrolysis.
4. Both TCR and IgE receptors are coupled to similar sequences of events, including Pl hydrolysis, influx of Ca^{2+} into the cell, and a rise in the intracellular Ca^{2+}.
5. Upon aggregation, both receptors become associated with the membrane cytoskeleton.
6. Consistent with these functional similarities, there is a 60% homology between the γ chain of the IgE receptor and the ζ chain of the TCR. Both these subunits have been proposed to be important for signal transduction for these two receptors, suggesting that the TCR and $Fc_{\epsilon}RI$ may be coupled to common signal transduction machinery.

Additional similarities between T cells and mast cells were revealed upon an examination of the pattern of immunophilins found in these two cell types. Extracts from RBL cells were passed over affinity columns of either FK506 or CsA, washed, and proteins were eluted by adding FK506 or CsA, respectively, to the buffer. The proteins were eluted and analyzed by SDS-PAGE. As shown in Figure 8, FKBP of MW 12, 13, 14, and 60 kDa were eluted from the FK506 affinity matrix, and proteins of 17, 18, 19, 20, 21, and 60kDa were eluted from the CsA matrix. This pattern of immunophilins is very similar to that found in the T-cell line Jurkat (Fretz et al., 1991). The function of these multiple isoforms of cyclophilin and FKBP remains to be established.

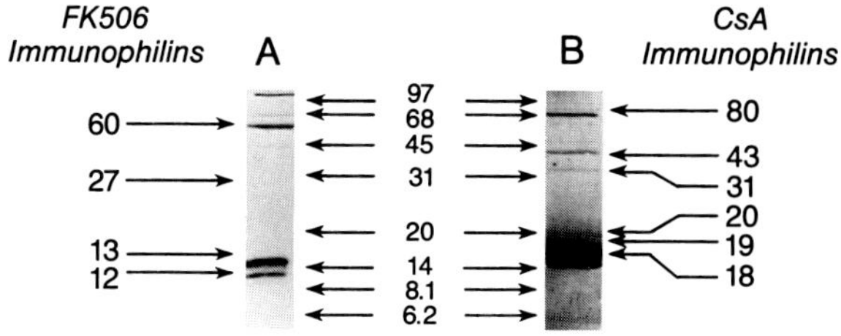

Figure 8 A similar pattern of immunophilins is present in mast cells and T cells. Extracts of RBL-2H3 cells were passed over affinity matrices of covalently-bound FK506 (A) or CsA (B). The matrices were washed and proteins were eluted with either FK506 (A) or CsA (B). The eluted proteins were separated by SDS-PAGE and detected by silver stain. The apparent molecular masses (kDa) of the retained proteins from the FK506 matrix are indicated at left and those from the CsA matrix at right. Positions of molecular mass markers are indicated in the center. The band of 58 kDa is BSA, a component of the lysis buffer. (From Hultsch et al., 1991.)

I. Model to Explain the Inhibition of Receptor-Mediated Signaling by Immunosuppressive Drugs

An early model to explain the inhibition of receptor-mediated signaling by CsA focused on the PPlase activity of this protein. According to this model, some step in signal transduction requires the folding (or refolding) of a protein to its proper tertiary structure. When cyclophilin binds CsA, PPlase activity is inhibited and, therefore this critical protein folding event cannot occur; hence, receptor-mediated activation is blocked. This model was strengthened when it was discovered that FKBP is also a PPlase, and this enzymatic activity is blocked by FK506. In fact, all cyclophilins and FKBPs isolated possess a PPlase activity that is blocked when the protein binds its respective ligand.

Although this was an attractive model, more recent data have demonstrated that it cannot be correct. Both FK506 and rapamycin bind FKBP and inhibit its PPlase activity; however, these two drugs have antagonistic effects on signaling pathways in both the mast cell and T cell (see Table 3). Therefore, the mere inhibition of isomerase activity, by itself, is not sufficient to explain the effects of these drugs on receptor-mediated signaling.

A new model was proposed that called for the formation of an "active inhibitor" rather than the inhibition of an activator (Fig. 9). In other words, a complex is formed between cyclophilin and CsA, or between FKBP and either FK506 or rapamycin, which "poisons" some step in receptor-mediated signaling. In the case of complexes involving FKBP, the specificity (antigen receptor versus lymphokine receptor) comes from the effector domain (see Fig. 2) of FK506 or rapamycin. While this model accounts for most of the data generated

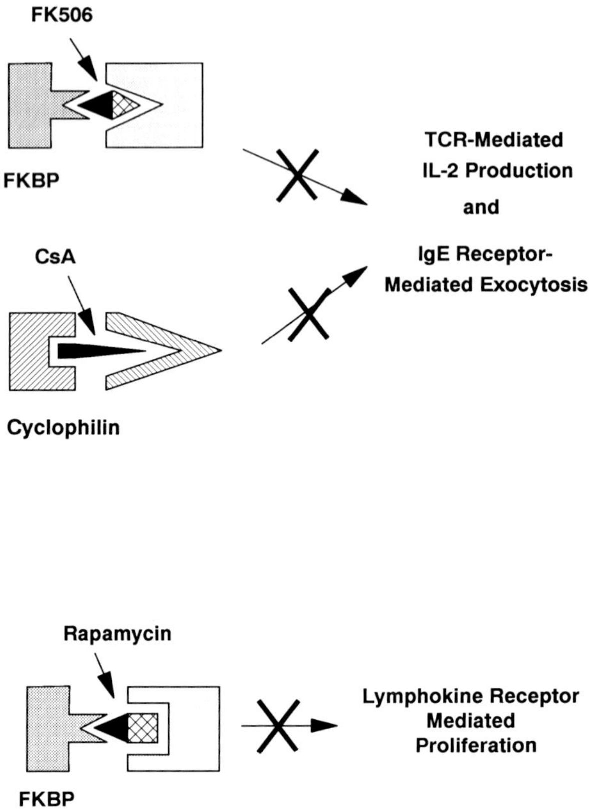

Figure 9 The "inhibitory complex" model proposed to explain the inhibition by CsA, FK506, and rapamycin on receptor-mediated signaling. According to this model, a complex is formed between the inhibitor and its respective binding protein that interacts with some as yet unidentified cellular component that blocks a critical step in signal transduction. See text for details.

in both the T-cell and mast cell system, it does not account for the fact that all cyclophilins and all FKBPs possess PPlase activity. Although inhibition of the PPlase activity, by itself, is not sufficient for these drugs to inhibit receptor-mediated cellular functions, this enzymatic activity might still be an important part of the physiological function of cyclophilin and FKBP. In light of those considerations, we present a modification of the "active inhibitor" model that incorporates the PPlase activity.

The precedent for this modification is the GTPase activity of the γ subunit of G proteins (Casey and Gilman, 1988; Gilman, 1989). In this system, a tertiary "active complex" is formed between the γ subunit, GTP, and adenylate cyclase. In this complex, adenylate cyclase (an enzyme that converts ATP to cAMP) is active. The γ subunit possesses an intrinsic GTPase activity. This activity is not involved in the formation of the active complex, but instead controls the lifetime of the complex. The hydrolysis of GTP (to GDP + Pi) results in the dissociation of the tertiary complex, and the adenylate cyclase is no longer active (adenylate cyclase activity is expressed only when it is part of the complex).

As mentioned above, this GTPase activity associated with the γ subunit is not necessary for the formation of the complex. If GTP is replaced by GTP-γ-s (a nonhydrolyzable analog of GTP), GTPase activity is blocked. Under such conditions, not only does the complex still form, but it cannot dissociate; hence, the adenylate cyclase in the complex becomes locked in the "on" position.

Using the γ subunit as a precedent, consider the following modification (see Fig. 10) of the "active complex" model proposed to explain the action of immunophilin ligands. This modifications makes two assumptions: (1) CsA and FK506 mimic endogenously produced ligands that temporarily shut down receptor-signaling pathways. For example, there may be times when it is disadvantageous for a cell to respond to external stimuli. At these times, the cell

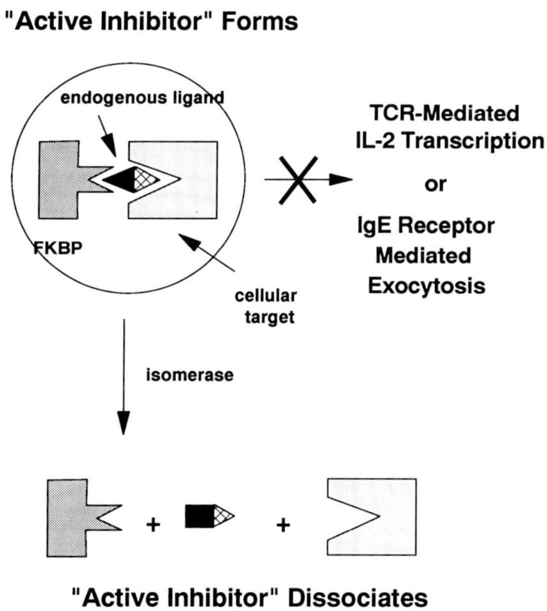

Figure 10 Modification of the model shown in Figure 9 that takes into account the fact that all immunophilins exhibit an intrinsic PPlase activity. See text for details.

would produce an endogenous immunophilin ligand to prevent activation. (2) The rotamase activity of the immunophilins would isomerize the ligand, which in turn would cause dissociation of the complex; hence, receptor-mediated signaling can continue. According to this model, in analogy to GTP-γ-s, FK506 and CsA mimic an as yet unidentified, endogenous immunophilin ligand that blocks the rotamase activity of immunophilins. This causes the immunophilin-ligand inhibitory complex to become locked in the "on" position, resulting in persistent inhibition of TCR- and $Fc_{\epsilon}RI$-mediated signaling. This model is consistent with all the results obtained in both the T cell and mast cell, as well as recently published structural data suggesting that FK506 is a transition-state analog for the *cis-trans* isomerization of a proline-containing peptide bond.

IV. Clinical Aspects

The main clinical application for CsA and FK506 is in the field of organ transplantation, but there are also a variety of immunological diseases that are driven by an overreactive (or inadequately reactive) immune system. Examples are diabetes (type I) (Stiller et al., 1984; Bougneres et al., 1988), autoimmune uveoretinitis (Nussenblatt et al., 1983a), psoriasis (Ellis et al., 1986; Ho et al., 1990), and pyoderma gangrenosum (as reported at the 1st International Congress on FK506, Pittsburgh, PA, 1991), all of which could potentially be treated with CsA or FK506 in humans.

In addition, in light of the dramatic effects of FK506 and CsA on $Fc_{\epsilon}RI$-mediated activation of mast cells and basophils, atopic diseases may become candidates for treatment. Systemic CsA or FK506 therapy in patients with severe asthma could provide a corticosteroid-sparing alternative, similar to methotrexate (Dyer et al., 1991; Shiner et al., 1990; Mullarkey et al., 1990). In fact, in vitro data have shown inhibition of $Fc_{\epsilon}RI$-mediated activation of human lung mast cells by CsA (Triggiani et al., 1989). Moreover, a pilot study in patients with severe, corticosteroid-dependent asthma revealed a corticosteroid-sparing effect of CsA, preferentially in patients with an atopic background (Szczeklik et al., 1991).

Topical application of CsA and more so FK506, which is 100 times more potent than CsA on a molar basis, could provide an important alternative in the clinical management of allergic rhinitis and bronchitis. In the eye, topical CsA has already been shown to be useful for allergic conjunctivitis (vernal) (Secchi et al., 1990) and ligneous conjunctivitis (Rubin et al., 1991). The use of FK506 instead of CsA may even improve the clinical results.

As to topical dermatitis, a number of clinical trials with topical application of CsA have shown positive results (Nakagawa et al., 1988; De Prost et al., 1989a,b; Biren and Barr, 1986; Van Joost et al., 1987; Sowden et al., 1991; Ross and Camp, 1990). A major limiting factor has been that CsA did not penetrate in sufficient amounts to the basal layers of the epidermis and the dermis. The fact that FK506 is 100 times more potent than CsA gives rise to the hope that the absorption problems of CsA can be overcome with FK506.

Discussion

Sullivan: In contrast to other observers, we see no effect of cyclosporin on wheal-and-flare reactions in the skin, but do see a decrease in late-phase reactions. Galli has report that CSA can inhibit antigen-activated mast cell gene expression. CSA did have a beneficial effect on asthma in one open trial of which I am aware. Can you comment on this apparent discrepancy between in vivo effects of CSA on late reactions and your in vitro effects on immediate reactions?
Hohman: Several groups, including ours, have failed to demonstrate an effect in vivo of CSA and related drugs on immediate hypersensitivity. It may be that while histamine release is inhibited, other mediators such as eicosanoids are still produced by activated mast cells.
Galli: Have you looked to see what effects CSA has on the secretion of mast cell enzymes?
Hohman: Yes. IgE-mediated secretion of B-glucuronidase is also inhibited by CSA.
Kaplan: Can you achieve a sufficient concentration of CSA in vivo to affect mast cells?
Hohman: Yes. These agents work on mast cells at their average peak plasma concentration.
Schwartz: Are CSA and FK-506 binding proteins found in plasma?
Hohman: No, but both CSA and FK-506 are hydrophobic and readily enter cells where the binding proteins are ubiquitous.

References

Austen, K. F., and Brocklehurst, W. E. (1960). Anaphylaxis in chopped guinea pig lung. Effect of peptidase substrates and inhibitors. *J. Exp. Med.* 113:521–539.

Baechinger, H. P. (1987). The influence of peptidyl-prolyl cis-trans isomerase on the in vitro folding of type III collagen. *J. Biol. Chem.* 262:17144–17148.

Beaven, M. A., and Cunha-Melo, J. R. (1988). Membrane phosphoinositide-activated signals in mast cells and basophils. *Prog. Allergy* 42:1–62.

Bierer, B. E., Mattila, P. S., Standaert, R. F., Herzenberg, L. A., Burakoff, S. J., Crabtree, G. R., and Schreiber, S. L. (1990a). Two distinct signal transmission pathways in T lymphocytes are inhibited by complexes formed between an immunophilin and either FK506 or rapamycin. *Proc. Natl. Acad. Sci. USA* 87:9231–9235.

Bierer, B. E., Somers, P. K., Wandless, T. J., Burakoff, S. J., and Schreiber, S. L. (1990b). Probing immunosuppressant action with a nonnatural immunophilin ligand. *Science* 250:556–559.

Biren, C. A., and Barr, R. J. (1986). Dermatologic applications of cyclosporine. *Arch. Dermatol.* 122:1028–1032.

Blank, U., Ra, C., Miller, L., White, K., Metzger, H., and Kinet, J.-P. (1989). Complete structure and expression in transfected cells of high affinity IgE receptor. *Nature* 337:187–189.

Borel, J. F. (1976). Comparative study of in vitro and in vivo drug effects on cell-mediated cytotoxicity. *Immunology* 31:631–641.

Borel, J. F. (1990). Mechanism of action rationale for cyclosporin A in psoriasis. *Br. J. Dermatol.* 36:5–12.

Borel, J. F., Feurer, C., Gubler, H. U., and Stahelin, H. (1976). Biological effects of Cyclosporin A: A new antilymphocytic agent. *Agents Actions* 6:468–475.

Bougneres, P. F., Carel, J. C., Castano, L., Boitard, C., Gardin, J. P., Landais, P., Hors, J., Mihatsch, M. J., Paillard, M., Chaussain, J. L., and Bach, J. F. (1988). Factors associated with early remission of type I diabetes in children treated with cyclosporine. *N. Engl. J. Med.* 318:663–670.

Casey, P. J., and Gilman, A. G. (1988). G protein involvement in receptor-effector coupling. *J. Biol. Chem.* 263:2577–2580.

Cohen, D. J., Loertscher, R., Rubin, M. F., Tilney, N. L., Carpenter, C. B., and Strom, T. B. (1984). Cyclosporine: A new immunosuppressive agent for organ transplantation. *Ann. Intern. Med.* 101:667–682.

De Paulis, A., Cirillo, R., Ciccarelli, A., Condorelli, M., and Marone, G. (1991). FK-506, a potent novel inhibitor of the release of proinflammatory mediators from human FcERI+ cells. *J. Immunol.* 146:2374–2381.

De Prost, Y., Bodemer, C., and Teillac, D. (1989a). Randomised double-blind placebo-controlled trial of local cyclosporin in atopic dermatitis. *Acta Dermatol. Venerol. (Stockh.)* 144(Suppl.):136–138.

De Prost, Y., Bodemer, C., and Teillac, D. (1989b). Randomised double-blind placebo-controlled trial of local cyclosporin in atopic dermatitis. *Acta Dermatol. Venereol. (Stockh.)* 144(Suppl.):136–138.

Dreskin, S. C., and Metzger, H. (1988). The high-affinity receptor for immunoglobulin E. Prospects for the therapy of immediate hypersensitivity reactions. *JAMA* 260:1265–1268.

Dumont, F. J., Melino, M. R., Staruch, M., Koprak, S. L., Fischer, P. A., and Sigal, N. H. (1990a). The immunosuppressive macrolides FK-506 and rapamycin act as reciprocal antagonists in murine T cells. *J. Immunol.* 144:1418–1424.

Dumont, F. J., Staruch, M. J., Koprak, S. L., Melino, M. R., and Sigal, N. H. (1990b). Distinct mechanisms of suppression of murine T cell activation by the related macrolides FK-506 and rapamycin. *J. Immunol.* 144:251–258.

Dyer, P. D., Vaughan, T. R., and Weber, R. W. (1991). Methotrexate in the treatment of steroid-dependent asthma. *J. Allergy Clin. Immunol.* 88:208–212.

Elliott, J. F., Lin, Y., Mizel, S. B., Bleackley, R. C., Harnish, D. G., and Paetkau, V. (1984). Induction of interleukin 2 messenger RNA inhibited by cyclosporin A. *Science* 226:1439–1441.

Ellis, C. N., Gorsulowsky, D. C., Hamilton, T. A., Billings, J. K., Brown, M. D., Headington, J. T., Cooper, K. D., Baadsgaard, O., Duell, E. A., Annesley, T. M., Turcotte, J. G., and Voorgees, J. J. (1986). Cyclosporine improves psoriasis in a double-blind study. *JAMA* 256:3110–3116.

Ellis, C. N., Fradin, M. S., and Messana, J. M. (1991). Cyclosporine for plaque-type psoriasis. *N. Engl. J. Med.* 324:277–284.

Emmel, E. A., Verweij, C. L., Durand, D. B., Higgins, K. M., Lacy, E., and Crabtree, G. R. (1989). Cyclosporin A specifically inhibits function of nuclear proteins involved in T cells activation. *Science* 246:1617–1620.

Fewtrell, C., and Metzger, H. (1980). Larger oligomers of IgE are more effective than dimers in stimulating rat basophilic leukemia cells. *J. Immunol.* 125:701–710.

Fischer, G., and Bang, H. (1985). The refolding of urea-denatured ribonuclease A is catalyzed by peptidyl-prolyl *cis-trans* isomerase. *Biochim. Biophys. Acta* 828:39–42.

Fischer, G., Bang, H., and Mech, C. (1984). Nachweis einer Enzymkatalyse für die *cis-trans*-Isomerisierung der Peptidbindung in prolinhaltigen Peptiden. *Biomed. Biochim. Acta* 43:1101–1111.

Fischer, G., Wittmann-Liebold, B., Kiefhaber, T., Schmid, F. X., and Lang, K. (1989). Cyclophilin and peptidyl-prolyl cis-trans isomerase are probably identical proteins. *Nature* 337:476–478.

Flanagan, W. M., Corthesy, B., Bram, R. J., and Crabtree, G. R. (1991). Nuclear association of a T-cell transcription factor blocked by FK506 and cyclosporin A. *Nature* 352:803–807.

Fretz, H., Albers, M. W., Galat, A., Standaert, R. F., Lane, W. S., Burakoff, S. J., Bierer, B. E., and Schreiber, S. L. (1991). Rapamycin and FK506 binding proteins (immunophilins). *J. Am. Chem. Soc.* 113:1409–1411.

Furuichi, K., Rivera, J., Triche, T., and Isersky, C. (1985). The fate of IgE bound to rat basophilic leukemia cells. IV. Functional association between the receptors for IgE. *J. Immunol.* 134:1766–73.

Furuichi, K., Rivera, J., Buonocore, L. M., and Isersky, C. (1986). Recycling of receptor-bound IgE by rat basophilic leukemia cells. *J. Immunol.* 136:1015–1021.

Gilman, A. G. (1989). G proteins and regulation of adenylyl cyclase. *JAMA* 262:1819–1825.

Handschumacher, R. E., Harding, M. W., Rice, J., and Drugge, R. J. (1984). Cyclophilin: A specific cytosolic binding protein for cyclosporin A. *Science* 226:544–547.

Harding, M. W., and Handschumacher, R. E. (1988). Cyclophilin, a primary molecular target for cyclosporin. *Transplantation* 46:29S–35S.

Harding, M. W., Handschumacher, R. E., and Speicher, D. W. (1986). Isolation and amino acid sequence of cyclophilin. *J. Biol. Chem.* 261:8547–8555.

Harding, M. W., Galat, A., Uehling, D. E., and Schreiber, S. L. (1989). A receptor for the immunosuppressant FK506 is a *cis-trans* peptidyl-prolyl isomerase. *Nature* 341:758–760.

Harrison, R. K., and Stein, R. L. (1990). Mechanistic studies of peptidyl prolyl *cis-trans* isomerase: Evidence for catalysis by distortion. *Biochemistry* 29:1684–1689.

Hess, A. D., Tutschka, P. J., and Santos, G. W. (1982). Effect of cyclosporin A on human lymphocyte responses in vitro. *J. Immunol.* 128:355–359.

Ho, V. C., Griffiths, C. E. M., Ellis, C. N., Gupta, A. K., McCuaig, C. C., Nickoloff, B. J., Cooper, K. D., Hamilton, T. A., and Voorhees, J. J. (1990). Intralesional cyclosporine in the treatment of psoriasis. *J. Am. Acad. Dermatol.* 22:94–100.

Hohman, R. J., and Hultsch, T. (1990). Cyclosporin A: New insights for cell biologists and biochemists. *New Biologist* 2:663–672.

Hultsch, T., Rodriguez, J. L., Kaliner, M. A., and Hohman, R. J. (1990). Cyclosporin A inhibits degranulation of rat basophilic leukemia cells and human basophils. Inhibition of mediator release without affecting Pl hydrolysis or CA^{++} fluxes. *J. Immunol.* 144:1000–1001.

Hultsch, T., Albers, M. W., Schreiber, S. L., and Hohman, R. J. (1991). Immunophilin ligands demonstrate common features of signal transduction leading to exocytosis or transcription. *Proc. Natl. Acad. Sci. USA* 88:6229–6233.

Isersky, C., Rivera, J., Segal, D. M., and Triche, T. (1983). The fate of IgE bound to rat basophilic leukemia cells II. Endocytosis of IgE oligomers and effect on receptor turnover. *J. Immunol.* 131:388–396.

Ishizaka, T. (1982). Biochemical analysis of triggering signals induced by bridging of IgE receptors. *Fed. Proc.* 14:17–21.

Ishizaka, T., and Ishizaka, K. (1984). Activation of mast cells for mediator release through IgE receptors. *Prog. Allergy* 34:188–235.

Ishizaka, T., Foreman, J. C., Sterk, A. R., and Ishizaka, K. (1979). Induction of calcium flux across the rat mast cell membrane by bridging IgE receptors. *Proc. Natl. Acad. Sci. USA* 76:5858–5862.

Kagey-Sobotka, A., Dembo, M., Goldstein, B., Metzger, H., and Lichtenstein, L. M. (1981). Qualitative characteristics of histamine release from human basophils by covalently cross-linked IgE. *J. Immunol.* 127:2285–91.

Kahan, B. D. (1989). Cyclosporine. *N. Engl. J. Med.* 321:1725–1738.

Kinet, J-P. (1989). Antibody-cell interactions: Fc receptors. *Cell* 57:351–354.

Kinet, J-P., Metzger, H., Alber, G., Blank, U., Huppi, K., Jouvin, M-H., Kuster, H., Miller, L., Ra, C., Rivera, J., and Varin-Blank, N. (1989). The high affinity receptor for immunoglobulin E: New developments. *Prog. Immunol.* 7:716–723.

Kofron, J. L., Kuzmic, P., Kishore, V., Colon-Bonilla, E., and Rich, D. H. (1991). Determination of kinetic constants for peptidyl prolyl *cis-trans* isomerases by an improved spectrophotometric assay. *Biochemistry* 30:6127–6134.

Koletsky, A. J., Harding, M. W., and Handschumacher, R. E. (1986). Cyclophilin: Distribution and variant properties in normal and neoplastic tissues. *J. Immunol.* 137:1054–1059.

Kronke, M., Leonard, W. J., Depper, J. M., Arya, S. K., Wong-Stall, F., Gallo, R. C., Waldmann, T. A., and Greene, W. C. (1984). Cyclosporin A inhibits T-cell growth factor gene expression at the level of mRNA transcription. *Proc. Natl. Acad. Sci. USA* 81:5214–5218.

Kulczycki, A., Jr., and Metzger, H. (1974). The interaction of IgE with rat basophilic leukemia cells. II. Quantitative aspects of the binding reaction. *J. Exp. Med.* 140:1676–1695.

Lang, K., Schmid, F. X., and Fischer, G. (1987). Catalysis of protein folding by prolyl isomerase. *Nature* 329:268–270.

Lorber, M. I. (1988). The mechanism of ciclosporin immunosuppression. *Year in Immunol.* 4:253–263.

Lung-Nan, L., Hasumi, H., and Brandts, J. F. (1988). Catalysis of proline isomerization during protein-folding reactions. *Biochim. Biophys. Acta* 956:256–266.

Maeyama, K., Hohman, R. J., Metzger, H., and Beaven, M. A. (1986). Quantitative relationships between aggregation of IgE receptors, generation of intracellular signals, and histamine secretion in rat basophilic leukemia (2H3) cells. *J. Biol. Chem.* 261:2583–92.

Martel, R. R., Klicius, J., and Galet, S. (1977). Inhibition of the immune response by rapamycin, a new antifungal antibiotic. *Can. J. Physiol. Pharmacol.* 55:48–51.

Mazurek, N., Berger, G., and Pecht, I. (1980). A binding site on mast cells and basophils for the anti-allergic drug cromolyn. *Nature* 286:722–723.

Mazurek, N., Schindler, H., Schurholz, T. L., and Pecht, I. (1984). The cromolyn binding protein constitutes the Ca^{++} channel of basophils opening upon immunological stimulus. *Proc. Natl. Acad. Sci. USA* 81:6841–6845.

Merker, M. M. (1984). Uptake and nature of the intracellular binding of cyclosporin A in a murine thymoma cell line BW5147. *J. Immunol.* 132:3064–3070.

Metzger, H. (1988). Molecular aspects of receptors and binding factors for IgE. *Adv. Immunol.* 43:277–312.

Metzger, H., and Kinet, J-P. (1988). How antibodies work: focus on Fc receptors. *FASEB J.* 2:3–11.

Metzger, H., Alcaraz, G., Hohman, R. J., Kinet, J. P., Pribluda, V., and Quarto, R. (1986). The receptor with high affinity for immunoglobulin E. *Annu. Rev. Immunol.* 4:419–70.

Miller, L., Blank, U., Metzger, H., and Kinet, J-P. (1989). Expression of high affinity binding of human immunoglobulin E by transfected cells. *Science* 244:334–337.

Mullarkey, M. F., Lammert, J. K., and Blumenstein, B. A. (1990). Long-term methotrexate treatment in corticosteroid-dependent asthma. *Ann. Intern. Med.* 112:577–581.

Nakagawa, S., Oka, D., Jinno, Y., Takei, Y., Bang, D., and Ueki, H. (1988). Topical application of cyclosporine on guinea pig allergic contact dermatitis. *Arch. Dermatol.* 124:907–910.

Nussenblatt, R. B., Palestine, A. G., and Chan, C-C. (1983a). Cyclosporine A therapy in the treatment of intraoccular inflammatory disease resistant to systemic corticosteroids and cytotoxic agents. *Am. J. Ophthalmol.* 96:275–282.

Nussenblatt, R. B., Rook, A. H., Wacker, W. B., Palestine, A. G., Scher, I., and Gery, I. (1983b). Treatment of intraocular inflammatory disease with cyclosporin A. *Lancet* 2:235–238.

Oliver, J. M., Seagrave, J., Stump, R. F., Pfeiffer, J. R., and Deanin, G. G. (1988). Signal transduction and cellular response in RBL-2H3 mast cells. *Prog. Allergy* 42:185–245.

Pedersen, C., Permin, H., Stahl Skov, P., Norn, S., Svenson, M., Mosbech, H., and Bendtzen, K. (1985). Inhibitory effect of cyclosporin A on histamine release from human leukocytes and rat mast cells. *Allergy* 409:103–107.

Rivera, J., Mullins, J. M., Furuichi, K., and Isersky, C. (1986). Endocytosis of aggregated immunoglobulin G by rat basophilic leukemia cells; rate, extent, and effects on the endocytosis of immunoglobulin E. *J. Immunol.* 136:623–627.

Rosen, M. K., Standaert, R. F., Galat, A., Nakatsuka, M., and Schreiber, S. L. (1990). Inhibition of FKBP rotamase activity by immunosuppressant FK506: Twisted amide surrogate. *Science* 248:863–866.

Ross, J. S., and Camp, R. D. (1990). Cyclosporin A in atopic dermatitis. *Br. J. Dermatol.* 122(Suppl. 36):41–45.

Rubin, B. I., Holland, E. J., DeSmet, M. D., Belfort, R., and Nussenblatt, R. B. (1991). Response of reactivated ligneous conjunctivitis to topical cyclosporin. *Am. J. Ophthalmol.* 112:95–96.

Schmitz-Schumann, M. (1986). Interim report of clinical studies presented at the International Symposium on Ciclosporin in Auto-Immune Diseases, Basel, March 18–20, 1985. *Prog. Allergy* 38:436–446.

Schreiber, S. L. (1991). Chemistry and biology of the immunophilins and their immunosuppressive ligands. *Science* 251:283–287.

Secchi, A. G., Tognon, M. S., and Leonardi, A. (1990). Topical use of cyclosporin in the treatment of vernal keratoconjunctivitis. *Am. J. Ophthalmol.* 110:641–645.

Segal, D. M., Taurog, J. D., and Metzger, H. (1977). Dimeric immunoglobulin E serves as a unit signal for mast cell degranulation. *Proc. Natl. Acad. Sci. USA* 74:2993–2997.

Sehgal, S. N., Baker, H., and Vezina, C. (1975). Rapamycin(AY-22,989), a new antifungal antibiotic. II. Fermentation, isolation and characterization. *J. Antibiotics* 28:727–731.

Shevach, E. M. (1985). The effects of cyclosporin A on the immune system. *Annu. Rev. Immunol.* 3:397–423.

Shiner, R. J., Nunn, A. J., Chung, K. F., and Geddes, D. M. (1990). Randomised, double-blind, placebo-controlled trial of methotrexate in steroid-dependent asthma. *Lancet* 336:137–140.

Siekierka, J. J., Hung, S. H. Y., Poe, M., Lin, C. S., and Sigal, N. H. (1989). A cytosolic binding protein for the immunosuppressant FK506 has peptidyl-prolyl isomerase activity but is distinct from cyclophilin. *Nature* 341:755–757.

Sowden, J. M., Berth-Jones, J., Ross, J. S., Motley, R. J., Marks, R., Finlay, A. Y., Salek, M. S., Graham-Brown, R. A., Allen, B. R., and Camp, R. D. (1991). Double-blind, controlled, crossover study of cyclosporin in adults with severe refractory atopic dermatitis. *Lancet* 338:137–140.

Standaert, R. F., Galat, A., Verdine, G. L., and Schreiber, S. L. (1990). Molecular cloning and overexpression of the human FK506-binding protein FKBP. *Nature* 346:671–674.

Stiller, C. R., Dupre, J., Gent, M., Jenner, M. R., Keown, P. A., Laupacis, A., Martell, R., Rodger, M. W., Graffenried, B. V., and Wolfe, B. M. J. (1984). Effects of Cyclosporine immunosuppression in insulin-dependent diabetes mellitus of recent onset. *Science* 223:1362–1367.

Szczeklik, A., Nizankowska, E., Dworski, R., Domagala, B., and Pinis, G. (1991). Cyclosporin for steroid-dependent asthma. *Allergy* 46:312–315.

Takahashi, N., Hayano, T., and Suzuki, M. (1989). Peptidyl-prolyl *cis-trans* isomerase is the cyclosporin A-binding protein cyclophilin. *Nature* 337:473–475.

Thomson, A. W. (1989). FK-506—How much potential? *Immunol. Today* 10:6–9.

Trenn, G., Taffs, R., Hohman, R. J., Kincaid, R., Shevach, E. M., and Sitkovsky, M. (1989). Biochemical characterization of the inhibitory effect of CsA on cytolytic T lymphocyte effector functions. *J. Immunol.* 142:3796–3802.

Triggiani, M., Cirillo, R., Lichtenstein, L. M., and Marone, G. (1989). Inhibition of histamine and prostaglandin D2 release from human lung mast cells by cyclosporin A. *Int. Arch. Allergy Appl. Immunol.* 88:253–255.

Tropschug, M., Wachter, E., Mayer, S., Schonbrunner, E. R., and Schmid, F. X. (1990). Isolation and sequence of an FK506-binding protein from *N. crassa* which catalyses protein folding. *Nature* 346:674–676.

Van Joost, T., Stolz, E., and Heule, F. (1987). Efficacy of low-dose cyclosporine in severe atopic skin disease. *Arch. Dermatol.* 123:166–167.

Varin-Blank, N., and Metzger, H. (1990). Surface expression of mutated subunits of the high affinity mast cell receptor for IgE. *J. Biol. Chem.* 265:15685–15694.

Vezina, C., Kudelski, A., and Sehgal, S. N. (1975). Rapamycin (AY-22,989), a new antifungal antibiotic. I. Taxonomy of the producing streptomycete and isolation of the active principle. *J. Antibiotics* 28:725–726.

Weinblatt, M. E., Coblyn, J. S., Fraser, P. A., Anderson, R. J., Spragg, J., Trentham, D. E., and Austen, K. F. (1987). Cyclosporin a treatment of refractory rheumatoid arthritis. *Arthritis Rheum.* 30:11–17.

Wicker, L. S., Boltz, R. C., Matt, V., Nichols, E. A., Peterson, L. B., and Sigal, N. H. (1990). Suppression of B cell activation by cyclosporin A, FK506 and rapamycin. *Eur. J. Immunol.* 20:2277–2283.

Winslow, C. M., and Austen, K. F. (1984). Role of cyclic nucleotides in the activation-secretion response. *Prog. Allergy* 34:236–270.

10

Lipid Metabolism and Mast Cell Activation

DONALD KENNERLY

University of Texas Southwestern Medical Center at Dallas
Dallas, Texas

I. Introduction

A. Scope

In addition to its importance in the pathogenesis of both IgE-dependent and IgE-independent hypersensitivity disorders, the mast cell serves as an excellent model for studying receptor-initiated cell activation. Dramatic and rapid exocytosis is initiated by physical approximation of the high-affinity IgE receptor ($Fc_\epsilon RI$), as the result of multivalent antigens recognized by receptor-associated IgE. A number of other physiologically relevant or irrelevant secretagogues can cause exocytosis in some, but not all, mast cell phenotypes and permanent cell lines, but the discussion that follows will deal principally with stimulation occurring in response to crosslinking $Fc_\epsilon RI$.

In addition to exocytosis, $Fc_\epsilon RI$ stimulation is associated with the genesis of a heterogeneous group of newly synthesized inflammatory mediators. First, receptor-dependent release of arachidonic acid from cellular lipid stores, coupled with its subsequent conversion to a variety of important eicosanoids (prostaglandins, leukotrienes, thromboxanes, and HETEs), has been the focus of a number of investigations. Second, the synthesis of platelet-activating factor

(PAF) in stimulated mast cells is also likely to be of significant importance in a number of immunopathological reactions involving mast cells. Third, an increasing number of groups have shown that $Fc_{\epsilon}RI$ stimulation of mast cells also results in the robust formation of extremely potent protein cytokines typically associated with T_{H2} "phenotype" (reviewed by Gordon et al., 1990). The role of these agents may be critical in perpetuating chronic inflammation involving mast cells.

Most investigators examining the intracellular regulatory pathways contributing to mast cell activation have thus far employed exocytosis as a functional end-point, and the focus of material presented subsequently will similarly relate to the biochemical processes associated with secretion of preformed mast cell granules. Although the mechanisms involved in regulating new mediator synthesis (eicosanoids, PAF, and cytokines) likely have much in common with the regulation of exocytosis, they almost certainly have certain unique features that are beyond the scope of the current discussion.

Much information has evolved as the result of both the ability to purify rat serosal mast cells and the development of the immortal RBL cell lines and IL-3-dependent, bone marrow–derived mast cell lines. These models have permitted careful examination of highly purified populations of $Fc_{\epsilon}RI$-bearing cells, all of which can be triggered to undergo exocytosis. The current review seeks to stress important common findings and will endeavor to explore in more depth the evolution during the last few years of information related to a single class of second messengers, effectors, and mediators—those that are themselves lipids or derived from membrane lipids.

B. Structural and Effector Functions of Membrane Lipids: Membrane Fusion During Exocytosis

Biologically relevant membranes are formed from phospholipids and cholesterol and have a characteristic bilayer structure as a consequence of their amphipathic nature (the result of the energy favoring the interaction of hydrophobic fatty acid side chains with each other and avoid contact with an aqueous environment). Hydrophilic phospholipid head groups face and are readily solubilized by the aqueous milieu on either side of the bilamellar membrane. Although rotational and lateral movement of phospholipids in a membrane is rapid, "flipflop" of a phospholipid from one leaflet to the other is energetically unfavorable and occurs only very slowly. Membranes are important biochemical barriers in the cell—allowing functional compartmentalization within and between cells—but also obstruct the flow of information from the extracellular environment to the interior of the cell. The evolution of transmembrane receptor proteins and/or transmembrane signal transducing proteins likely occurred in response to the need of cells to recognize and respond to changes in the extracellular milieu.

Mast cells and basophils share with all secretory cells the regulated ability to release preformed secretory granule constituents to the extracellular environment as the result of fusion of the perigranule membranes with the plasma membrane. Because this process is energetically highly unfavorable, it takes place only at a very slow rate in unstimulated cells. During exocytosis, granules not only must come into close proximity to the plasma membrane (perhaps facilitated by cytoskeletal elements), but also must overcome the thermodynamic barrier to membrane fusion. To overcome this energy hurdle, cells must synthesize locally either specialized proteins or lipids that can form nonbilayer membrane structures capable of facilitating membrane fusion, but which do not result in loss of integrity of either the plasma membrane or granule membrane, a feat of some consequence. As illustrated in Figure 1, the fusion of adjacent membranes can be promoted by endogenous lipids termed "fusogens" that facilitate the formation of transition structures necessary for exocytosis (Ellens et al., 1989).

C. Brief Relevant Historical Perspective

Although the concept of second messengers began with the description of the role of cAMP in the regulation hepatic glycogenolysis many years ago, the existence and relevance of *lipid* or *lipid-derived* second messengers has only been known for just over a decade. The ubiquity of receptor-dependent phosphoinositide metabolism has been extensively developed after its initial description in pancreas (Hokin and Hokin, 1953). The relevance of this pathway (Fig. 2) was not appreciated until the description by Nishizuka of the existence of protein kinase K (PKC), a family of homologous protein kinases that are activated by the presence in membranes of 1,2-diacylglycerol (DAG) and Ca^{2+} (reviewed by Bell and Burns, 1991). The subsequent description of the ability of phosphoinositide derived IP_3 to participate importantly in cytosolic Ca^{2+} homeostasis (Fein et al., 1984) propelled a large number of studies examining the role of phospho-

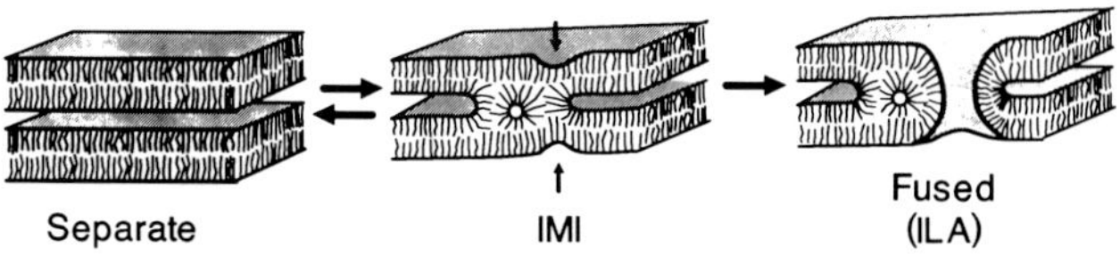

Figure 1 Mechanism of membrane fusion. Accumulation of fusion-promoting lipids (fusogens) having small hydrophilic head groups results in the reversible formation of inverted micellar intermediates (IMIs) that facilitate the formation of fusion pores termed interlaminar attachments (ILAs) (1).

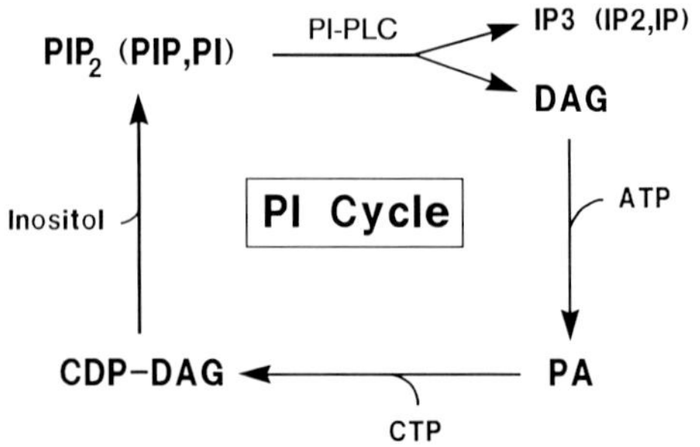

Figure 2 Phosphoinositide metabolism and the PI cycle. PIP_2, phosphatidylinositol 4,5-bisphosphate; PIP, phosphatidylinositol 4-phosphate; PI, phosphatidylinositol; DAG, 1,2-diacylglycerol; PA, phosphatidic acid; CDP-DAG, cytidyl-DAG.

inositide-specific phospholipase C (PI-PLC) in regulating cellular activation in a number of model systems.

D. Overview of Components of Intracellular Signaling

A critical feature of multicellular organisms is the exquisite coordination achieved between different cells and tissues. The need for well-regulated communication between and within cells is obvious and is largely achieved by bioinformational small molecules synthesized by one cell and subsequently recognized by itself or by other cells. Structural and functional diversity demands that each cell have the ability to recognize a large subset of these molecules in the extracellular milieu and translate an extracellular binding event into an amplified intracellular biochemical signal causing an appropriate cellular response.

Responsiveness to such communication requires a variety of structures and/or mechanisms. First, recognition by the target cells requires an appropriate cell surface or intracellular receptor. For the most part, cells must distinguish between receptors that are occupied by the ligand or agonist and those that are not, presumably the result of conformational changes in an intracellular signal-transducing domain of the receptor—a process termed signal transduction. In contradistinction to this mechanism, the capacity of each mast cell to respond vigorously to a variety of different antigens requires the existence of $Fc_{\epsilon}RI$, which both allows antigen specificity to be conferred by tightly associated IgE and initiates exocytotic signals in response to the physical approximation (often referred to as "crosslinking") of IgE-bearing $Fc_{\epsilon}RI$ by multivalent antigen (Ishizaka and Ishizaka, 1978). Thus, the degree of receptor-receptor interaction rather than the frequency of ligand binding to receptors is the physiologically relevant parameter causing antigen-specific mast cell activation.

The translation of receptor occupancy or receptor-receptor association into a meaningful response involves three broad categories of mechanisms that involve: (1) direct translation of signals because the receptors either have endogenous protein kinase activity that phosphorylate target proteins or are intracellular receptors that alter transcription of one or more genes; (2) changing the activity of ion channels or pumps that contribute to changes in membrane potential and/or the concentration of intracellular ions with second-messenger activity; and (3) interaction of receptors with an intermediate transducer such as GTP-binding proteins (G proteins; vide infra).

Many receptors translate information regarding ligand occupancy by utilizing a translation mechanism employing G proteins that possess intrinsic GTPase activity (reviewed by Reed, 1990). Classical G proteins involved in receptor signaling represent a family of similar oligomeric heterotrimers each consisting of one alpha, beta, and gamma subunit that interact with the intracellular signal-transducing domain of plasma membrane–associated receptors. The beta and gamma subunits are structurally very similar and functionally interchangeable among members of the G-protein family. The alpha subunit not only contains the guanine nucleotide binding region and GTPase activities, but provides specificity with regard to the ability of a given G protein to interact with both specific receptors and specific second-messenger-generating proteins (vide infra). As a result, classification of G proteins is based on the identity of the distinct alpha subunits (G_α). The mechanism by which various G_α subunits are freed from the beta-gamma complex and convey signals from receptors to second-messenger-regulating proteins and potential pharmacological alteration of this process is complex and outside the scope of the current discussion.

By one or more of the mechanism described above, plasma membrane receptor activation causes rapid changes in the intracellular levels of regulatory molecules termed second messengers. Second messengers function both to amplify receptor-mediated signals and to exert their influence by rapidly altering the activity of one or more enzymes or nonenzymatic proteins critical to the appropriate targeted function of the cell. Intracellular concentrations of second messengers are tightly regulated by the balance of rates of second-messenger formation and destruction. In contrast to the wide variety of extracellular bioinformation molecules and their respective receptors, the repertoire of second-messenger molecules is somewhat restricted, although new second messengers will undoubtedly be described in the future. The most extensively studied second messengers include: cyclic-AMP (cAMP), cyclic-GMP (cGMP), inositol 1,4,5-trisphosphate (IP_3), diacylglycerol (DAG), Ca^{2+}, arachidonic acid (AA), and phosphatidic acid (PA). Most commonly, second messengers function by changing the activity of one or more members of an increasingly large family of second-messenger-specific protein kinases, enzymes that alter the activity of a subset of target proteins as the result of phosphorylating them. Changes in a discreet subset of target proteins together effect a specific cellular response (examples include exocytosis, cytokine synthesis, differentiation, and proliferation).

Although a variety of protein kinases exist and have been characterized in significant detail, the needs of the current discussion require a brief description of protein kinase C (PKC). PKC was found to be responsive to two different second messengers: 1,2-diacylglycerol (DAG) and Ca^{2+} (reviewed by Bell and Burns, 1991). Given an appropriate membrane surface containing phosphatidylserine (PS), membrane-associated DAG causes PKC to translocate from the cytosol to the membrane and increase its affinity for Ca^{2+} (for most PKC isoforms), so that physiologically relevant $[Ca^{2+}]_{cytosol}$ are permissive and PKC becomes active. That DAG is an intermediate in the PI cycle (Fig. 2) led to the attractive hypothesis during the early 1980s that the importance of the PI cycle was to generate DAG in order to regulate PKC. In addition to PI, the family of phosphoinositides was known for some time to also include phosphorylated isomers of PI, such as PI 4-phosphate (PIP) and PI 4,5-bisphosphate (PIP_2). The potential importance of the minor phosphoinositide PIP_2 was brought to the fore by the description in 1984 (Fein et al., 1984) of the ability of PI-PLC hydrolysis of PIP_2 not only to form DAG, but also to form the water-soluble product, inositol 1,4,5-trisphosphate (IP_3)—a compound able to act as a second messenger as the result of its capacity to control $[Ca^{2+}]_{cytosol}$ by the IP_3 receptor-dependent liberation of calcium sequestered in specific intracellular sites.

In a specific cell type, activation of a single receptor causes the genesis of a "signal" that is defined by a specific pattern of changes in the levels of a subset of the available second messengers and effectors. Because different patterns of changes of second messenger levels likely result in different cellular responses, knowledge regarding the mechanisms of signal transduction is important to an adequate understanding of the regulation of the mast cell and provides an important framework for developing strategies of pharmacological modulation of excessive mast cell activity in hypersensitivity states.

II. Phosphoinositides and the "PI Cycle"

Since the initial description of receptor-enhanced labeling of phosphoinositides and phosphatidic acid (PA) by $^{32}P_i$ in pancreas, virtually all cells have been shown to have this capacity in response to stimulation by one or more appropriate receptors (reviewed by Rana and Hokin, 1991). Although the mechanism by which enhanced activity of this cyclic pathway (PI $\rightarrow$ DAG $\rightarrow$ PA $\rightarrow\rightarrow$ PI; Fig. 2) might contribute to cell activation was uncertain, our work and that of others demonstrated enhanced activity in mast cells (Kennerly et al., 1979b; Cockcroft and Gomperts, 1979; Ishizuka et al., 1984; Beaven and Cunha-Melo, 1988).

Because PIP_2 hydrolysis resulted in the formation of two second messengers that synergistically activated PKC [DAG, and Ca^{2+} (via IP_3)], receptor-dependent PI-PLC activity was felt by many to be both necessary and sufficient for activating mast cells.

As described in detail subsequently, recent studies have forced reevaluation of certain aspects of this hypothesis. First, the quantitative presence of PIP_2 and PIP in many tissues was not sufficient to explain the increases in DAG that were observed as the result of receptor stimulation. Second, the recent description of a variety of isoenzymes of PKC having the ability to respond to arachidonic acid and others to be Ca^{2+} independent suggested that PKC activation was not necessarily completely dependent on products exclusively derived directly or indirectly from PI-PLC. Finally, analysis of DAG in several model systems demonstrated that it was likely to be derived in large part from phosphatidylcholine (PC) and, to a lesser extent, from phosphoinositides (vide infra).

III. Role of Phosphatidylcholine Metabolism in Mast Cells

Recently, increasing attention has focused on metabolism of PC because it can potentially generate several second messengers (DAG and PA) and/or requisite substrates for the synthesis of newly formed lipid mediators (lyso-PAF and arachidonic acid).

A. Phospholipase D (PLD) Mediates Phosphatidylcholine Hydrolysis: An Emerging Pathway of Regulatory Importance

The Role of PC in DAG Accumulation

Although the PI cycle had been assumed to be responsible for receptor-dependent changes in DAG content, several lines of evidence in the mast cell suggest that hydrolysis of PC was likely of greater quantitative importance during $Fc_{\epsilon}RI$ activation. Molecular species analysis, a method used to evaluate the precursor-product relationship of glycerol-based lipids, showed that most of the DAG accumulating after $Fc_{\epsilon}RI$ stimulation could not be derived principally from PI (Kennerly, 1987). Figure 3 demonstrates that DAG accumulating as the result of $Fc_{\epsilon}RI$ stimulation bears striking resemblance to PC, an observation suggesting that $Fc_{\epsilon}RI$-dependent PC hydrolysis is more important than PI hydrolysis in $Fc_{\epsilon}RI$-dependent DAG accumulation. These findings have been extended to other cells (Pessin and Raben, 1989), and it is now evident that many of the hormones that induce PI turnover also cause PC hydrolysis (reviewed by Exton, 1990). The mechanisms by which different phospholipases act on PC are illustrated in Figure 4.

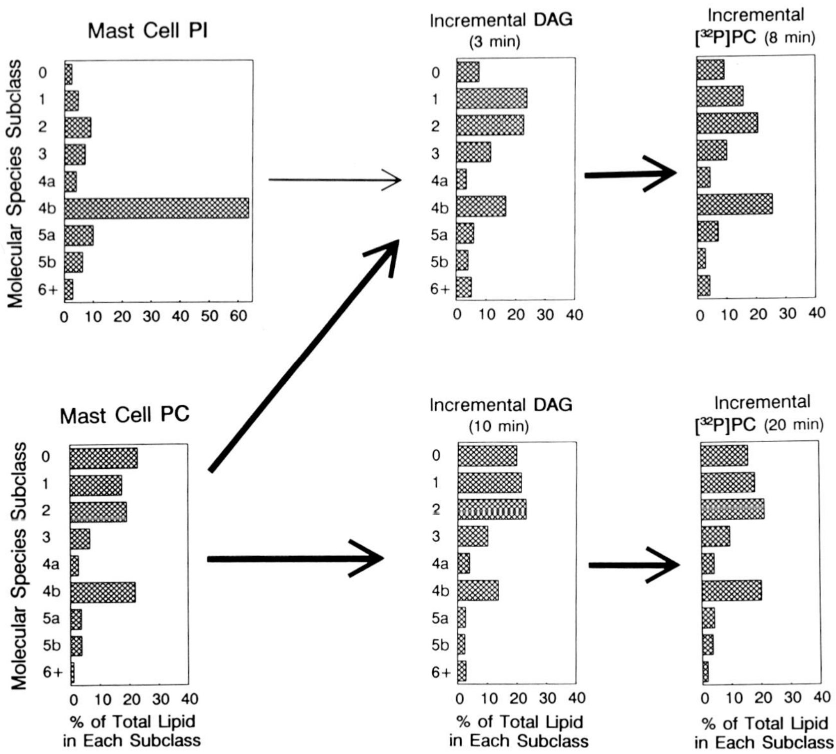

Figure 3 Molecular species analysis of the metabolic origin of DAG in $Fc_{\epsilon}RI$-stimulated mast cells. Cellular phospholipids and DAG were isolated and separated into different molecular species subclasses based on degree of unsaturation of fatty acids. DAG mass in $Fc_{\epsilon}RI$-stimulated cells doubled at 3 min and was increased threefold at 10 min. The similar patterns of DAG and PC (versus PI compared to DAG) indicate that DAG accumulating in $Fc_{\epsilon}RI$-stimulated mast cells is primarily derived from PC. The similarity of patterns of [^{32}P]PC and DAG (in $^{32}P_i$-prelabeled mast cells) indicates the existence of $Fc_{\epsilon}RI$-dependent PC resynthesis.

Potential Mechanisms of PC Conversion to DAG: PC-PLD Versus PC-PLD

Figure 5 illustrates that two mechanisms might be involved in the formation of DAG from PC—a *direct pathway* involving PC-PLC and/or an *indirect pathway* initiated by PC-PLD. Several lines of evidence support the primary importance of PC-PLD and the indirect pathway in mast cells. First, kinetic analysis demonstrated, in fatty acid prelabeled mast cells, that accumulation of labeled PA preceded slightly that of DAG, an observation most consistent with the PA acting as a substrate for DAG formation (by PA-PHase) rather than a product of

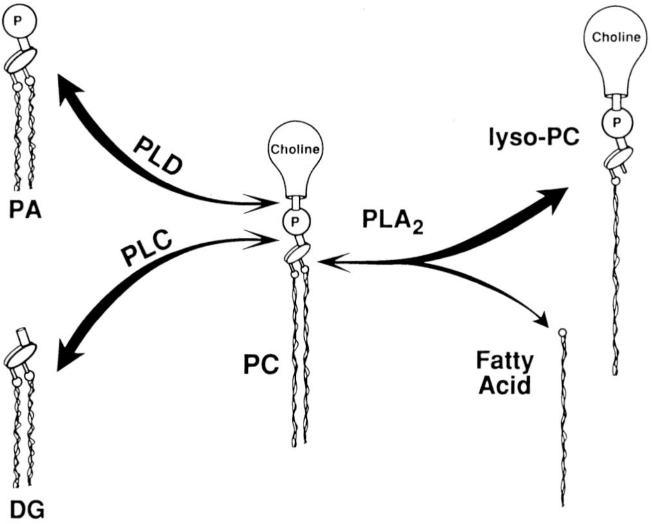

Figure 4 Mechanisms of PC hydrolysis by phospholipases. PLD, phospholipase D; PLC, phospholipase C.

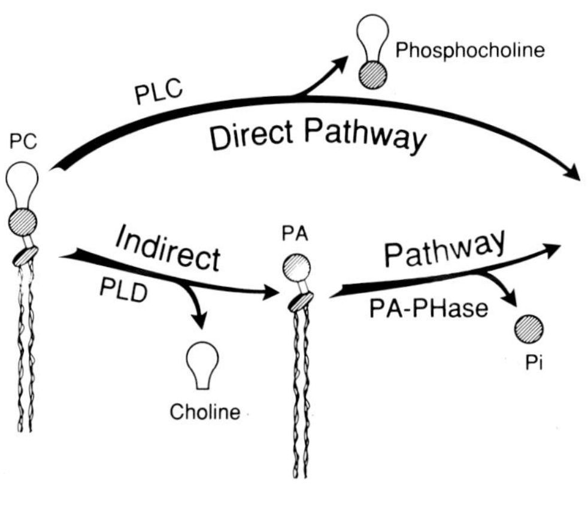

Figure 5 Potential pathways of DAG formation from PC. The "direct pathway" generates DAG in a single step by the action of PLC. The "indirect pathway" of DAG formation involves two steps: (1) PLD-mediated formation of choline and PA and (2) subsequent conversion of PA to DAG by phosphatidic acid phosphohydrolase (PA-PHase).

the phosphorylation of DAG (Dinh and Kennerly, 1991). Second, $Fc_{\epsilon}RI$ stimulation of fatty acid prelabeled mast cells in the presence of low concentrations of ethanol was accompanied by receptor-dependent formation of the phosphatidylethanol (PEt)—the transphosphatidylation product catalyzed solely by activation of a cellular PLD (Gruchalla et al., 1990).

Most recently, methods were developed to assess the relative importance of PC-PLD versus PC-PLC during mast cell activation by examining the water-soluble products of these reactions (Murray et al, 1990). Specifically, sensitive methods were developed to assess the intracellular levels of the water-soluble products of PC-PLC and PC-PLD, phosphocholine and choline, respectively. Figure 6 demonstrates that $Fc_{\epsilon}RI$ stimulation was associated with a rapid and dramatic increase in the levels of intracellular choline, the product of PC-PLD activation (Dinh and Kennerly, 1991). Although the intracellular levels of choline increased in stimulated cells, phosphocholine mass (a measure of PC-PLC) declined with stimulation—an observation undermining the importance of PC-PLC in the genesis of receptor dependent DAG generation. Recent unpublished observations from our laboratory in the mast cell indicate that PC-PLD activity appears to be regulated by both Ca^{2+} and PKC.

Further encouraging the importance of PC-PLD in receptor-dependent DAG accumulation is our observation of significant phosphatidate phosphohydrolase (PA-PHase) activity, the second and necessary element in the formation of DAG from PC via the indirect pathway (Fig. 5; Duffy and Kennerly, unpublished observations).

A Potentially Independent Regulatory Role for PA Generated by PC-PLD

PC-PLD may be important not only from the perspective of generating DAG via the indirect pathway, but also as the result of the potential importance of PA as a second messenger and/or effector. In certain cell models, adding PA has been associated with cell activation, including: Ca^{2+}-dependent membrane phase changes (Boughriet et al., 1988), increased membrane permeability to Ca^{2+} in membranes containing PA (Blau and Weissmann, 1988), substitution of PA for PS for PKC binding to membranes (Oishi et al., 1988), activation of a PA-dependent protein kinase that may be distinct from PKC (Bocckino et al., 1991), and regulation of the activity of a protein that regulates the activity of cellular *ras* (Tsai et al., 1989). In recent experiments, lyso-PA, the product of PLA_2-catalyzed hydrolysis of PA (a frequent contaminant of commercial preparations of PA; unpublished observations), has been shown to act as a second messenger by liberating Ca^{2+} from intracellular sites and to be mitogenic (Jalionk et al., 1990) at concentrations well below those causing cytotoxicity. In the mast cell, evidence implicating lyso-PA include $Fc_{\epsilon}RI$-dependent increases in the

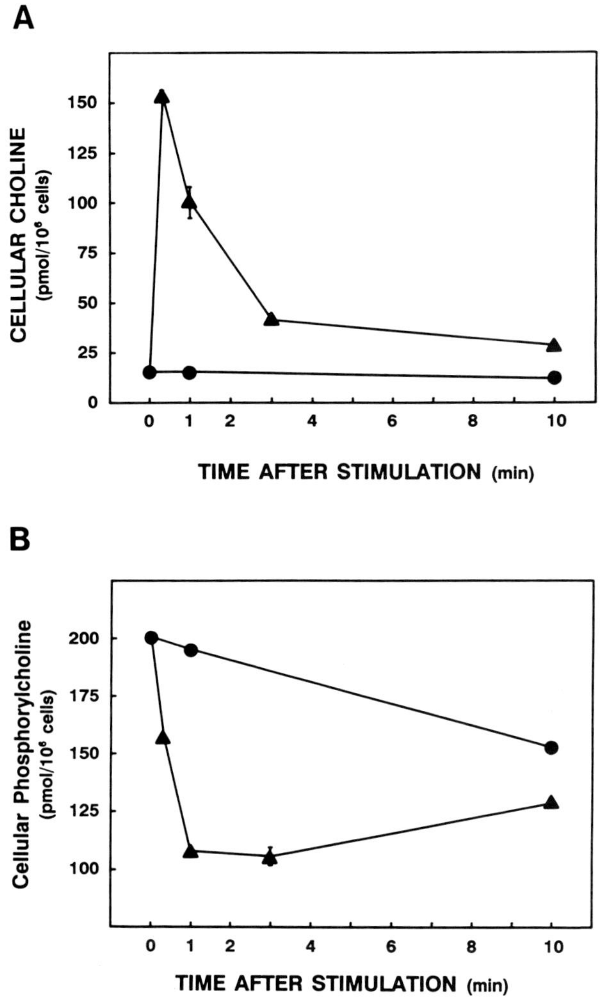

Figure 6 Assessment of the relative activities of PC-PLD and PC-PLC by evaluating the water-soluble products of these reactions. Unstimulated mast cells are indicated by the circles; $Fc_{\epsilon}RI$-stimulated cells are indicated by triangles. (A) The receptor-dependent increase in the mass of intracellular choline is consistent with increased activity of PC-PLD. (B) The failure to see a $Fc_{\epsilon}RI$ increase in cell-associated phosphocholine is likely due to the absence of receptor-dependent PC-PLC activity. The transience of the increase in choline and the decrease in phosphocholine mass in stimulated cells is likely the result of consumption of these compounds during $Fc_{\epsilon}RI$-dependent PC resynthesis (data not shown).

accumulation of labeled lyso-PA in $^{32}P_i$ prelabeled cells (Fagan, Kennerly, and Sullivan, unpublished observations) and the ability of lyso-PA to cause mast cell exocytosis (Fagan and Sullivan, personal communication).

Phosphatidylcholine Resynthesis: A Potential Mechanism of DAG Removal

Although the principal focus of investigators has been on the mechanisms responsible for the formation of second-messenger molecules, the level of a given regulatory molecule is dependent on the balance of pathways of formation and removal. Figure 2 illustrates the mechanism by which DAG formed from phosphoinositides can be reutilized in the resynthesis of these phospholipids. PC resynthesis from DAG is more direct, as illustrated in Figure 7. A major biochemical difference of the PC cycle is that the CDP-linked, high-energy intermediate is of the water-soluble group destined for the phospholipid head group (CDP-choline) rather than of the lipid portion of the molecule (CDP-DAG for the PI cycle). $Fc_\epsilon RI$ stimulation in $^{32}P_i$-prelabeled mast cells results in a dramatic increase in the rate of PA and PI synthesis (via the PI cycle), but also a 5–10-fold increase in the PC synthesis as well (Kennerly et al., 1979b). As a result of specific activity arguments beyond the scope of this review, it is likely that PC resynthesis is quantitatively the most vigorous pathway of DAG removal in mast cells. Figure 3 demonstrates that PC resynthesized after $Fc_\epsilon RI$ stimulation bears a molecular species "fingerprint" very similar to that of the DAG derived from unlabeled PC as the result of the PLD-initiated indirect pathway.

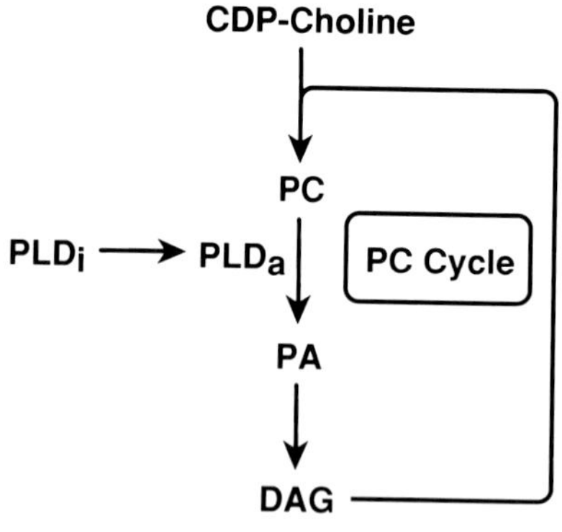

Figure 7 The PC cycle. In contrast to the PI cycle, which utilizes PI-PLC, the PC cycle is initiated by activation of PLD (PLD_i-inactive PLD, PLD_a = active PLD) and activates the water-soluble component in the resynthesis reaction (CDP-choline). Additionally, DAG formation requires the activity of phosphatidic acid phosphohydrolase (PA-PHase).

Interestingly, molecular species analysis of the [^{32}P]PA and [^{32}P]PI formed as the result of $Fc_{\epsilon}RI$ stimulation of mast cells indicates that these lipids are formed from DAG derived from phosphoinositides (Kennerly, 1987; Kennerly, unpublished observations). Taken together, these observations indicate that while these two pathways (the PI and PC cycles) are capable of both producing and removing DAG in the mast cell, they appear to generate/utilize DAG having distinct molecular species fingerprints, an observation that strongly suggests that they are active in spatially distinct sites.

B. Phospholipase A_2 (PLA_2) Activation: A Role in Lipid Mediator Biosynthesis and Signal Transduction

Although PLA_2 was initially principally associated with a role in eicosanoid biosynthesis, it may play a variety of roles during mast cell activation: (1) genesis of the platelet-activating factor substrate (1,alkyl-2,lyso-PC), (2) formation of fusogenic lysophospholipids that may contribute to exocytosis, (3) formation of products that have regulatory significance, and (4) release of arachidonate for the biosynthesis of inflammatory and/or regulatory eicosanoids.

PLA_2 and New Mediator Biosynthesis

Although mast cells have the capacity to liberate AA from DAG (via a two-step reaction involving DAG lipase and monoglyceride lipase; Kennerly et al., 1979a), the bulk of arachidonate is likely released as the result of activation of PLA_2. Recent labeling studies in mast cells (Nakamura et al., 1991) and mass spectroscopic studies in neutrophils (Chilton, 1989) suggest that 1,ether-2,arachidonoyl forms of PE may be a more important substrates for PLA_2 than are diacyl forms of PC and PE. The hydrolysis of 1,alkyl-2,arachidonoyl-PC by PLA_2 is also of considerable importance inasmuch as this reaction generates the potential PAF precursor (1,alkyl-2,lyso-PC or lyso-PAF).

PLA_2 and Regulation of Exocytosis

In addition to a role for PLA_2 hydrolysis of PC in the genesis of AA and lyso-PAF for receptor-dependent biosynthesis of lipid mediators, recent evidence from Ishizaka's group (personal communication) suggests that PLA_2 may mediate hydrolysis of lipids in addition to PC and may play a potentially important role in exocytosis. Baird's group has shown in disrupted cells a Ca^{2+}- and GTP[S]-augmented PLA_2 activity that increases as the result of $Fc_{\epsilon}RI$ stimulation (Narasimhan et al., 1990). Additionally, Marquardt has shown that noncytotoxic concentrations of lyso-PC, a potential product of PLA_2 activation, augments $Fc_{\epsilon}RI$-induced exocytosis and PKC activation (Marquardt and Walker, 1991).

Several mechanisms may contribute to the importance of PLA_2 activation

mediated increase in the PLD-initiated indirect pathway will trigger an accelerative cycle (DAG → ↑ PKC → ↑ PLD → ↑ PA → ↑ DAG, etc.). We suggest that perhaps this explosive *local* production of DAG may represent the "biochemical commitment" of any given granule to undergo fusion/exocytosis as the result of rapid accumulation of fusogenic lipids such as DAG (Siegel et al., 1989). This hypothesis could explain the morphological observation that granules display an "all or none" swelling response in $Fc_{\epsilon}RI$-stimulated mast cells (Schmauder-Chock and Chock, 1990). This concept is consistent with Chock's data and proposals relating to the assembly of lipids stored in the granule matrix into membrane that is integrated into the perigranule membrane during mast cell activation (Chock and Schmauder-Chock, 1990).

Two attractive corollaries of this model emerge. First, exocytosis of secretory granules might usefully be viewed in probabilistic terms. In an unstimulated cell, the frequency of granules exceeding the concentration of DAG required for self-sustaining DAG formation (by the PKC-augmented, PLD-initiated indirect pathway) is low, though not zero—consistent with the observed existence of a low rate of spontaneous exocytosis. Receptor-dependent enhancement of *granule-associated* DAG formation by the PLD-initiated indirect pathway could increase the probability that any given granule will exceed its threshold for irreversible "commitment" and thus drives secretion. Second, delivery of DAG to the plasma membrane by exocytosis of DAG-rich secretory granules might provide appropriate negative feedback by reducing proexocytotic signals generated in the plasma membrane, perhaps as the result of direct or indirect PKC-mediated down-regulation of $Fc_{\epsilon}RI$ responsiveness or the responsiveness of signal transduction elements linking activation of $Fc_{\epsilon}RI$ with that of PLD.

Discussion

Hohman: Mast cells have multiple G proteins. Is it safe to interpret your experiments to indicate that PLC is not involved in exocytosis from mast cells?
Kennerly: Although PI hydrolysis by PLC may have some role in regulating some functions within mast cells, the capacity of IgE-mediated exocytosis to proceed normally in the absence of detectable PI hydrolysis strongly suggests that PI is not essential for exocytosis.
Austen: Many people have shown that activation of mast cells with peptide ligands proceeds without the production of PGD_2. Thus, the role of PLA_2 in phospholipase D activation may be minimal.
Kennerly: Your point is valid. The absence of eicosanoid products implies that activation occurs without involvement of PLA_2.
Platts-Mills: Formation of reverse micelles with diacylglycerol would equally

favor fusion between individual granules or between granules and the membrane. However, have you considered whether diacylglycerol might favor bleb formation and piecemeal degranulation?

Kennerly: No good model for piecemeal degranulation exists in which to test this hypothesis. However, I think it possible that diacylglycerol could participate in this process. Perhaps phosphatidic acid, which can be distributed unequally in the leaflets of membranes, can participate in bled formation.

Ishizaka: Could you comment on how your findings relate to Chock's ultrastructural observations in mast cell granules?

Kennerly: Chock's high-resolution EM demonstration of membrane vesicles emerging from the dense granule matrix is in keeping with our observations. The ability to acutely increase the surface area of the granule membrane by such a process suggests that fusogenic lipids might be involved.

Kaplan: Do you know whether PLD exists in the various types of mast cells?

Kennerly: PLD has not been studied in human mast cells or basophil, to my knowledge. Receptor-dependent PLD activity has, however, been seen in other human tissues, and I am confident that PLD will be shown in human mast cells as well.

References

Beaven, M. A., and Cunha-Melo, J. R. (1988). Membrane phosphoinositide-activated signals in mast cells and basophils. *Prog. Allergy* 42:123.

Bell, R. M., and Burns, D. J. (1991). Lipid activation of protein kinase C. *J. Biol. Chem.* 266:4661.

Blau, L., and Weissmann, G. (1988). Transmembrane calcium movements mediated by ionomycin and phosphatidic acid in liposomes with Fura-2 entrapped. *Biochemistry* 27:5661.

Bocckino, S. B., Wilson, P. B., and Exton, J. H. (1991). Phosphatidate-dependent protein phosphorylation. *Proc. Natl. Acad. Sci. USA* 88:6210.

Boughriet, A., Ladjadj, M., and Bicknell-Brown, E. (1988). Calcium-induced condensation-reorganization phenomena in multilamellar vesicles of phosphatidic acid. *Biochem. Biophys. Acta* 939:523.

Chalifour, R., and Kanfer, J. N. (1982). Fatty acid activation and temperature perturbation of rat brain microsomal phospholipase D. *J. Neurochem.* 39:299.

Chilton, F. H. (1989). Potential phospholipid sources of arachidonate used for the synthesis of leukotrienes by the human neutrophil. *Biochem. J.* 258:327.

Chock, S. P., and Schmauder-Chock, E. A. (1990). A new model for the mechanism of stimulus-secretion coupling. *BioFactors* 2:133.

Cockcroft, S., and Gomperts, B. D. (1979). Evidence for a role of phosphatidylinositol turnover in stimulus-secretion coupling: studies with rat peritoneal mast cells. *Biochem. J.* 178:681.

Dennis, E. A., and Davidson, F. F. (1990). Phospholipase A_2 and lipocortin effects. *Prog. Clin. Biol. Res.* 349:47.

Dinh, T. T., and Kennerly, D. A. (1991). Assessment of receptor dependent activation of phosphatidylcholine hydrolysis by both phospholipase D and C. *Cell Regulation* 2:229.

Ellens, H., Siegel, D. P., Alford, D., Yeagle, P. L., Boni, L., Lis, L. J., Quinn, P. J., and Bentz, J. (1989). Membrane fusion and inverted phases. *Biochemistry* 28:3692.

Exton, J. H. (1990). Signaling through phosphatidylcholine breakdown. *J. Biol. Chem.* 265:1.

Fein, A., Payne, R., Corson, D. W., Berridge, M. J., and Irvine, R. F. (1984). Photoreceptor excitation and adaptation by inositol 1,4,5-trisphosphate. *Nature* 311:157.

Flower, R. J. (1990). Lipocortin. *Prog. Clin. Biol. Res.* 349:11.

Gilfillan, A. M., Wiggan, G. A., and Welton, A. F. (1990). The effects of protein kinase C inhibitors staurosporine and H7 on the IgE dependent mediator release from RBL-2H3 cells. *Agents Actions* 30:418.

Gordon, J. R., Burd, P. R., and Galli, S. J. (1990). Mast cells as a source of multifunctional cytokines. *Immunol. Today* 11:458.

Gruchalla, R. S., Dinh, T. T., and Kennerly, D. A. (1990). An indirect pathway of receptor-mediated 1,2-diacylglycerol formation in mast cells I: IgE receptor-mediated activation of phospholipase D. *J. Immunol.* 144:2336.

Heiman, A. S., and Crews, F. T. (1985). Characterization of the effects of phorbol esters on rat mast cell secretion. *J. Immunol.* 134:548.

Hokin, R. R., and Hokin, L. E. (1953). Enzyme secretion and the incorporation of ^{32}P into the phospholipids of pancreas slices. *J. Biol. Chem.* 203:967.

Ishizaka, T., and Ishizaka, K. (1978). Triggering of histamine release from rat mast cells by divalent antibodies against IgE receptors. *J. Immunol.* 120:800.

Ishizuka, Y., Imai, A., and Nozawa, Y. (1984). Polyphosphoinositide turnover in rat mast cells stimulated by antigen. *Biochem. Biophys. Res. Commun.* 123:875.

Jalionk, K., van Corven, E. J., and Moolenaar, W. H. (1990). Lysophosphatidic acid, but not phosphatidic acid, is a potent Ca^{2+}-mobilizing stimulus for fibroblasts. *J. Biol. Chem.* 265:12232.

Kennerly, D. A. (1987). Diacylglycerol metabolism in mast cells—Analysis of lipid metabolic pathways using molecular species analysis of intermediates. *J. Biol. Chem.* 262:16305.

Kennerly, D. A., Parker, C. W., and Sullivan, T. S. (1979a). Diacylglycerol metabolism in mast cells: a potential role in membrane fusion and arachidonic acid release. *J. Exp. Med.* 150:1039.

Kennerly, D. A., Sullivan, T. J., and Parker, C. W. (1979b). Activation of phospholipid metabolism during mediator release from stimulated rat mast cells. *J. Immunol.* 122:152.

Marquardt, D. L., and Walker, L. L. (1989). Pretreatment with phorbol esters abrogates adenosine responsiveness. *J. Immunol.* 142:1268.

Marquardt, D. L., and Walker, L. L. (1991). Lysophosphatidylcholine induces mast cell secretion and protein kinase C activation. *J. Allergy Clin. Immunol.* 88:721.

Murray, J., Dinh, T. T., Truett, A. P., and Kennerly, D. A. (1990). Isolation and enzymic assay of choline and phosphocholine present in cellular extracts with picomole sensitivity. *Biochem. J.* 270:63.

Nakamura, T., Fonteh, A. N., Hubbard, W. C., Trigianni, M., Inagaki, N., Ishizaka, T., and Chilton, F. H. (1991). Arachidonic acid metabolism during antigen and ionophore activation of the mouse bone marrow derived mast cell. *Biochim. Biophys. Acta* 1085:191.

Narasimhan, V., Holowka, D., and Baird, B. (1990). A guanine nucleotide-binding protein participates in IgE receptor-mediated activation of endogenous and reconstituted phospholipase A2 in a permeabilized cell system. *J. Biol. Chem.* 265:1459.

Oishi, K., Raynor, R. L., Charp, P. A., and Kuo, J. F. (1988). Regulation of protein kinase C by lysophospholipids, potential role in signal transduction. *J. Biol. Chem.* 263:6865.

Pessin, M. S., and Raben, D. M. (1989). Molecular species analysis of 1,2-diglycerides stimulated by alpha thrombin in cultured fibroblasts. *J. Biol. Chem.* 264:8729.

Rana, R. S., and Hokin, L. E. (1991). Role of phosphoinositides in transmembrane signaling. *Physiol. Rev.* 70:115.

Reed, R. R. (1990). G protein diversity and the regulation of signaling pathways. *New Biologist* 2:957.

Saito, H., Ishizaka, K., and Ishizaka, T. (1989). Effects of nonhydrolyzable guanosine phosphate on IgE-mediated activation of phospholipase C and histamine release from rodent mast cells. *J. Immunol.* 143:250.

Schmauder-Chock, E. A., and Chock, S. P. (1990). Mechanism of secretory granule exocytosis: Can granule enlargement precede pore formation? *Histochem. J.* 19:413.

Siegel, D. P., Banschbach, J., Alford, D., Ellens, H., Lis, L. J., Quinn, P. J., Yeagle, P. L., and Bentz, J. (1989). Physiological levels of diacylglycerols in phospholipid membranes induce membrane fusion and stabilize inverted phases. *Biochemistry* 28:3703.

Tsai, M. H., Yu, C. L., Wei, F. S., and Stacey, D. W. (1989). The effect of GTPase activating protein upon ras is initiated by mitogenically responsive lipids. *Science* 243:522.

11

Histamine

DIANA K. CAVANAH AND THOMAS B. CASALE

University of Iowa College of Medicine
Iowa City, Iowa

I. Introduction

Histamine (β-imidazolyl-ethylamine) was first synthesized by Windaus and Vogt (1907). It was Dale and Laidlaw (1910, 1919), however, who initially demonstrated the potential importance of histamine as a mediator when they observed anaphylaxis and respiratory distress in laboratory animals after histamine infusion. A subsequent landmark in the understanding of the role of histamine in human disease occurred in 1927 when Best and colleagues (1927) demonstrated a high concentration of histamine in lung tissues. In 1937 Bovet and Staub (1937) synthesized the first effective antagonist of histamine, facilitating research efforts to better understand the complex pathophysiological actions of histamine.

Histamine is of universal biological occurrence. In humans, histamine is produced and stored predominantly in tissue mast cells, with concentrations of 4–10 pg/cell and in circulating basophils, in a concentration of about 1 pg/cell (Casale, 1988). It is found in varying concentrations in different organs of the human body, including brain, lung, stomach, small and large intestine, uterus, and ureters. Under physiological conditions, the tissue content of histamine corresponds closely to the number of mast cells (Metcalfe et al., 1981). Histamine release from mast cells and basophils may be triggered by a variety of stimuli, including specific IgE and antigen as well as nonspecific degranulating factors. Nonspecific degranulating factors include calcium ionophore, complement fragments C3a, C4a, and C5a, cytokines, histamine-releasing factors, neuropeptides, opiates, and other drugs. In addition, physical factors such as cold, pressure, or vibration may trigger histamine release in certain individuals (Joad and Casale, 1988). The release of histamine occurs within 30–45 sec after an inciting stimulus, with the onset of action on local vasculature occurring within 1–5 min (Theoharides, 1989). Once released from mast cells or basophils, histamine is metabolized via two major pathways (Ring et al., 1986; Joad and Casale, 1987). Metabolism by diamine oxidase (histaminase) leads to imidazole acetic acid, and metabolism via *N*-methyltransferase leads to *N*-methylhistamine and *N*-methylimidazole acetic acid. High concentrations of histamine ($>10\ \mu M$) have been reported to inhibit these major metabolizing enzymes; however, this inhibition can be reversed by antihistamines (Joad and Casale, 1987, 1988). Thus, antihistamines may function both to block the histamine receptor and to reduce the concentration of extracellular histamine available to bind to receptors.

II. Histamine Receptors

There currently are known to be at least three specific histamine receptor types. The existence of more than one specific type of histamine receptor was initially proposed by Ash and Schild (1966) after the observation that some of the known effects of histamine, such as gastric acid secretion and rat uterus relaxation, could not be blocked by the conventional (H_1) antihistamines. In 1972, Black and colleagues synthesized a compound, burimamide, that competitively and selectively blocked gastric acid secretion and rat uterus relaxation. The receptors antagonized by burimamide were designated H_2 receptors. A third specific histamine receptor type was discovered by Arrang et al. (1983) and has subsequently been confirmed by studies involving the use of selective agonists and antagonists (Arrang et al., 1987; Schwartz, 1990).

Histamine receptors, like all hormone receptors, perform two vital functions. First, they recognize specific molecular structures by a process of high-affinity binding. Second, when bound by an agonist they initiate a cascade of biological reactions that culminate in biochemical and physiological responses. Better characterization of the biological and physiological activities mediated by the three specific histamine receptors has resulted from the development of receptor-specific agonists and antagonists. In addition, radioligand binding assays have allowed localization and quantification of H_1, H_2, and H_3 receptors.

A. H_1 Receptors

Although numerous highly potent and specific antagonists for the H_1 receptor have been successfully developed, histamine remains the most potent agonist known for this receptor type. Small variations in the histamine molecule have resulted in agonists with greater specificity for the H_1 receptor type, but not enhanced potency. *N*-methyl histamine, 2-(2-thiazolyl)ethylamine, and 2-methyl histamine are analogs of histamine and are highly specific H_1 receptor agonists (Casale, 1988; Haaksma et al., 1990). In contrast, numerous highly potent H_1 antagonists that are structurally different from histamine have been formulated and used with good clinical success. Broad categories of H_1 antagonists include the ethanolamines, alkylamines, ethylenediamines, and piperazines (Table 1). Problems with these agents have included antimuscarinic activity when used in high doses and sedation due to central nervous system H_1-receptor blockade. Because of these clinically limiting factors, new structurally dissimilar H_1 antagonists without sedating side effects and with mast cell–stabilizing properties have been formulated. A review of H_1 antagonists is contained in Section IV.

Table 1 Histamine Receptors

	H_1	H_2	H_3
Agonists	*N*-methylhistamine 2-(2-thiazolyl)-ethylamine 2-methylhistamine	4-methylhistamine Dimaprit Impromidine	α-methylhistamine
Antagonists	Ethanolamines Alkylamines Ethylenediamines Piperazines Phenothiazines Piperidines Tricyclic Anti-depressants Second-generation drugs	Burimamide Cimetidine Ranitidine Famotidine Nizatidine Tiotidine Metiamide	Thioperamide Impromidine *N*-α(4-phenyl-butanoyl) histamine
2nd messenger(s)	Inositol triphosphate Diacylglycerol Cyclic GMP	Cyclic AMP	?
Radioligand	[^{3}H]-mepyramine	[^{3}H]-cimetidine [^{3}H]-tiotidine	[^{3}H]α-methylhistamine

As previously mentioned, the second function of histamine receptors is to initiate a cascade of biochemical reactions that result in a physiological or biological response. The primary action of H_1 agonists on all cell types is to increase the intracellular concentration of free calcium ions, probably through inositol triphosphate and diacyclglycerol-mediated effects (Carswell et al., 1985; Joad and Casale, 1987; Haaksma et al., 1990). The peak rise in cytosolic calcium concentration occurs 15–30 sec after histamine stimulation and represents mobilization from intracellular stores. Sustained calcium elevation, however, is dependent on an influx of extracellular calcium, which may be regulated via protein kinase C (Chakravarty, 1990; Haaksma et al., 1990). In the lung, histamine receptor stimulation also results in changes in cyclic nucleotide concentrations, with H_1 receptor stimulation resulting in a rise in cyclic guanosine monophosphate (cGMP) (Platshon and Kaliner, 1978; Casale et al., 1985; Joad and Casale, 1987; Sertl et al., 1987; Casale, 1988).

Methods useful in localizing and quantifying H_1 receptors include radioligand binding and immunohistochemical techniques. Radioligand binding assays with $[^3H]$-mepyramine have shown that H_1 receptors may exhibit multiple binding states (Casale et al., 1985). Employing monoclonal antibodies directed at cGMP, immunohistochemical techniques have been used to identify specific cells responding to histamine H_1 receptor stimulation with increases in cGMP (Sertl et al., 1987). Both techniques have been used to better characterize the role of H_1 receptors in histamine-mediated lung responses (Casale et al., 1985; Sertl et al., 1987).

B. H_2 Receptors

Formulation of specific agonists has been much more successful for H_2 receptors than for H_1 receptors (Table 1). The first relatively selective agent was 4-methylhistamine, a histamine derivative that possessed 70% of the activity of histamine and was 40 times more active for H_2 receptors than for H_1 receptors (Haaksma et al., 1990). Further formulation has led to improved agonists, including dimaprit, which exhibits 70% of the activity of histamine and is almost 100% H_2 receptor selective, and impromidine, which is 4810 times more active than histamine and is a weak antagonist for H_1 and H_3 receptors (Haaksma et al., 1990).

Since the introduction of burimamide by Black et al. (1972), a large number of selective H_2 antagonists have been described. Although cimetidine and ranitidine have gained the most use clinically, other H_2 receptor antagonists include tiotidine and metiamide, as well as the recently introduced famotidine and nizatidine.

An important intracellular second messenger for H_2 receptors is cyclic adenosine monophosphate (cAMP). In fact, levels of cAMP are of sufficient sensitivity to be used as a biological marker for histamine H_2 receptor activity (Platshon and Kaliner, 1978). The characteristics of the histamine H_2 receptor have been further defined by use of radioligand binding assays. These assays initially used [^{3}H]-cimetidine as a probe. However, there has been some controversy over the reliability of [^{3}H]-cimetidine as a radioligand for H_2 receptors. [^{3}H]-tiotidine has been more recently used, but it too may not meet all the requirements for a desirable radioligand (Haaksma et al., 1990). Due to discrepant data on the affinities of various ligands for H_2 receptors, the possibility of the existence of H_2-receptor subtypes has been raised. Careful review of the data controlling for differing experimental conditions, however, does not support evidence for H_2 receptor subtypes (Haaksma et al., 1990). With the development of new highly specific H_2 radioligands, better characterization of this receptor can be expected.

C. H_3 Receptors

Within the past few years, immunocytochemical and biochemical studies have shown that histamine is a neurotransmitter that is present in nerve endings and synthesized from l-histidine (Steinbusch and Mulder, 1985; Watanabe et al., 1985; Haaksma et al., 1990). The postsynaptic receptors for this system are either H_1 or H_2 subtypes. Further investigation of this system revealed a class of presynaptic receptors that respond to histamine stimulation by inhibiting both the synthesis of histamine from histidine and its release. These presynaptic inhibitory autoreceptors have been designated H_3 receptors (Table 1) (Arrang et al., 1983; Haaksma et al., 1990). The H_3 receptor has subsequently been found to be more multifunctional and widespread than initially believed (van der Werf and Timmerman, 1989; Haaksma et al., 1990; Schwartz et al., 1990).

Alpha-methylhistamine is currently the best H_3 receptor agonist, with 15 times greater potency for the H_3 receptor than histamine itself. It also is very selective, with only weak activity at H_1 and H_2 receptor sites (van der Werf and Timmerman, 1989; Haaksma et al., 1990; Schwartz et al., 1990). The most potent and selective H_3 antagonist is thioperamide, though impromidine and N_α-(4 phenylbutanoyl) histamine function as less potent and less selective antagonists (van der Werf and Timmerman, 1989; Haaksma et al., 1990; Schwartz et al., 1990). Radioligand binding assays for evaluation of the H_3 receptor have been successfully performed using [^{3}H]-α-methylhistamine as the radioligand. These and other ligand specific studies have shown the presence of H_3 receptors in the human brain as well as in peripheral tissues, including guinea pig ileum and enteric ganglia, lung, and vascular smooth muscle (van der Werf and Timmerman, 1989; Schwartz et al., 1990).

III. Histamine Receptor-Mediated Effects

The physiological consequences of stimulating histamine receptors are numerous and are widespread through many organ systems. These histamine-mediated responses will be further discussed by organ system.

A. Respiratory System

One of the most striking effects initially observed with infusion of histamine was respiratory distress, and the possible role of histamine in asthma has subsequently been extensively evaluated (Fig. 1). Stimulation of H_1 receptors has been shown to produce bronchial smooth muscle contraction, both via direct effects on smooth muscle and through stimulation of vagal afferent nerve fibers (Dunlop et al., 1977; Eiser et al., 1981; Casale, 1988; Rafferty and Holgate, 1989). The effects of H_2 receptor stimulation on bronchial smooth muscle tone

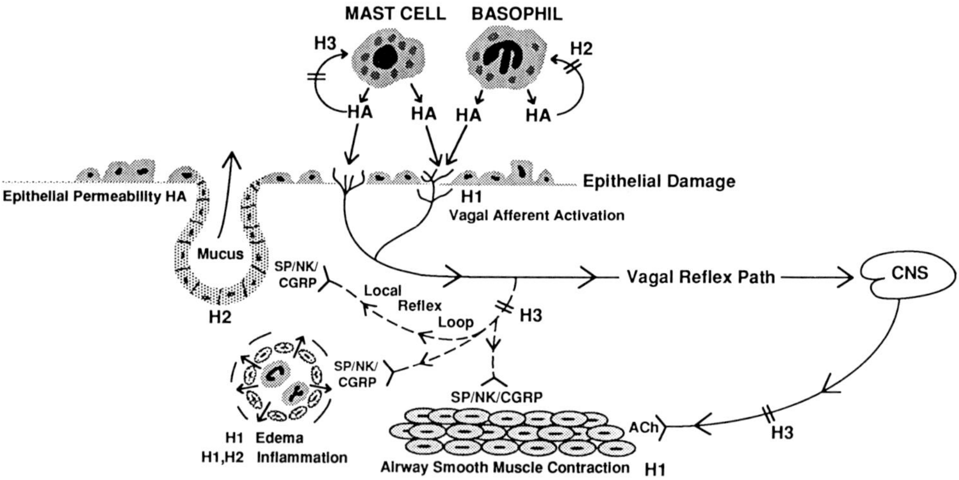

Figure 1 Histamine's effects in asthma. Mast cell and basophil degranulation results in histamine (HA) release. Histamine through the indicated receptors can cause epithelial permeability, vagal afferent nerve activation, airway smooth muscle contraction, edema and mucus release, and modulate inflammatory responses. Stimulation of vagal afferents results in activation of the vagal reflex path and the antidromic release (dashed lines) of substance P (SP), neurokinin A (NK), and calcitonin gene-related peptide (CGRP). These neuropeptides can then also lead to the above effects. Stimulation of H_2 receptors on basophils and H_3 receptors on mast cells may inhibit further histamine release. H_3 receptor activation can also inhibit both vagal reflex and local reflex loop-mediated release of acetylcholine (ACh) and neuropeptides, respectively.

are unclear. Some reports show H_2 receptor-mediated bronchodilation (Dunlop et al., 1977), whereas others show bronchoconstriction (Eiser et al., 1981). The predominant effect of histamine, however, appears to be H_1 receptor-mediated bronchoconstriction. Histamine also appears to have a dual action on the pulmonary vasculature bed, mediating pulmonary vasoconstriction via H_1 receptors and pulmonary vasodilation via H_2 receptors (Casale, 1988; Rafferty and Holgate, 1989). Other histamine-mediated effects that may be important in asthma include increased capillary permeability and serous fluid secretion mediated via H_1 receptors, as well as increased mucus secretion mediated by H_2 receptors (Shelhamer et al., 1980; Casale, 1988; Rafferty and Holgate, 1989). Histamine has also been shown to increase airway epithelial permeability. In addition, histamine has been shown via H_1 receptors to induce prostaglandin and thromboxane production and release, which could lead to multiple airway effects (Platshon and Kaliner, 1978; Steel et al., 1979; Casale, 1988; Rafferty and Holgate, 1989). H_2 receptors have been shown to modulate the function of T lymphocytes, neutrophils, and basophils, thereby influencing the inflammatory response. Finally, the H_3 receptor has recently been shown to mediate airway effects in a manner that may prove clinically useful in the management of asthma. Ichinose and colleagues (1989) have shown that H_3 receptors inhibit cholinergic neurotransmission both in isolated guinea pig and in human airways. Moreover, H_3 receptor agonists strongly inhibit the nonadrenergic, noncholinergic bronchoconstriction caused by neurokinin A and other neuropeptides (Barnes and Ichinose, 1989; Rafferty and Holgate, 1989). In preliminary unpublished studies, Barnes and colleagues have also provided evidence for H_3 receptor-mediated inhibition of lung mast cell degranulation.

The importance of histamine in mediating upper airway diseases such as allergic rhinitis has long been appreciated. Most of the symptoms of rhinitis appear to be mediated via H_1 receptors. The nasal pruritus and sneezing associated with rhinitis are due to stimulation of H_1 receptors on sensory nerves. Mucosal edema secondary to H_1 receptor stimulation is clinically manifest as nasal congestion. Rhinorrhea due to increased mucus secretion results largely from H_1-mediated stimulation of vagal reflex pathways causing muscarinic-induced mucus gland discharge. Thus, it is not surprising that H_1 antagonists have been used so successfully for the management of rhinitis.

B. Cardiovascular System

The cardiovascular effects of histamine include both peripheral vascular responses and direct cardiac responses (Table 2). As initially noted by Dale and Laidlaw (1910, 1919), histamine infusion causes shock with flushing and hypotension. This occurs primarily via vasodilation of the smaller peripheral vessels. A study by Kaliner and colleagues (1981) has shown this vasodilatory

Table 2 Histamine Receptor-Mediated Effects on the Cardiovascular System

1. H_1 receptor
   A. Peripheral vasodilation
   B. Increased vasopermeability
   C. Positive chronotropy
   D. Coronary artery vasoconstriction
2. H_2 receptor
   A. Peripheral vasodilation
   B. Positive chronotropy
   C. Positive ionotropy
   D. Arrhythmias

effect to be predominantly mediated via H_1 receptors; however, H_2 receptors also play a minor role. Histamine also acts by the H_1 receptor to cause increased vasopermeability leading to peripheral edema formation (Casale, 1988).

Determination of the in vivo effects of histamine on the heart has been difficult owing to the problem of distinguishing between direct cardiac effects of histamine and indirect cardiac effects of histamine such as catecholamine release and reflex responses to hypotension. Both positive chronotropy and ionotropy have been consistently observed with excessive histamine (Casale, 1988). Coronary artery vasoconstriction has also been a consistent effect of histamine, mediated by the H_1 receptor. Various arrhythmias occur during histaminemia and appear to be largely H_2 receptor mediated, though the H_1 receptor may also play a role.

C. Gastrointestinal System

The effects of histamine in stimulating gastric acid secretion via the H_2 receptor have resulted in the widespread clinical use of H_2 antagonists for the treatment of peptic ulcer disease and Zollinger-Ellison syndrome. H_2 receptor stimulation may also result in very weak, and probably not physiologically important, contraction of the lower esophageal sphincter (Casale, 1988). Gastrointestinal effects of histamine that are mediated via the H_1 receptor include spasmodic contractions of the stomach, intestine, and gallbladder. These H_1-mediated responses may be responsible for the abdominal cramping, pain, and diarrhea that are clinically observed during allergic or anaphylactic reactions to food (Table 3). Finally, there is evidence that H_3 receptors presynaptically inhibit acetylcholine release at nicotinic synapses at the level of enteric ganglia in guinea pigs. This effect may be responsible for the inhibition of guinea pig ileum

Table 3 Histamine Receptor-Mediated Effects on the Gastrointestinal System

1. H_1 receptor
   A. Spasmodic contraction of the stomach
   B. Spasmodic intestinal contraction
   C. Spasmodic contraction of the gallbladder
2. H_2 receptor
   A. Gastric acid secretion
   B. Lower esophageal sphincter contraction
3. H_3 receptor
   A. Inhibition of guinea pig ileum contraction
   B. Inhibition of pentagastrin-stimulated gastric acid secretion

contraction and pentagastrin-stimulated gastric acid secretion in cats that is observed with use of H_3 agonists (Schwartz et al., 1990).

D. Cutaneous Responses

The exact role of histamine and H_1, H_2, and H_3 receptors in urticaria and atopic dermatitis remains somewhat unclear. Intradermal injection of histamine results in the "triple response of Lewis," which includes: (1) the formation of a small localized area of erythema caused by vasodilation; (2) a flare response caused by an axonal reflex leading to vasodilation and extension of the flare beyond the original area of erythema; and (3) an area of edema due to increased vasopermeability (Lewis, 1927). Both H_1 and H_2 agonists have been reported to induce these cutaneous responses, which are reminiscent of urticarial lesions (Summers et al., 1981). In addition, H_1 receptor stimulation can cause sensory nerve–induced pruritus and flare responses through the release of neuropeptides. The released neuropeptides, especially substance P, can enhance these responses by directly causing vasodilation and edema and by degranulating cutaneous mast cells (Fig. 2). H_1 antagonists alone or in combination with H_2 antagonists are able to suppress histamine-induced skin responses. H_2 antagonists alone have not been effective in inhibiting histamine-induced cutaneous responses and appear to add little to the therapeutic efficacy of H_1 antagonists for urticaria (Theoharides, 1989). Thus, stimulation of H_1 receptors is likely an important factor in the pathogenesis of urticaria.

E. Hematological/Immunological System

Histamine has also been shown in multiple studies to have significant effects on immune responses and the hematological system in general, largely via H_2 receptors (Table 4). Both H_1 and H_2 receptors have been identified on a number

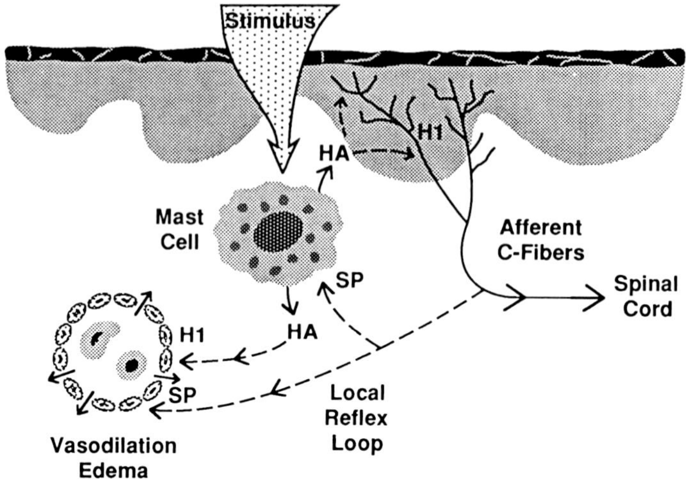

Figure 2 Histamine's effects in the skin. A stimulus causes mast cell degranulation with the release of histamine (HA) from mast cells. Histamine then causes vadodilation and edema through direct H_1 receptor-mediated effects on cutaneous blood vessels and through H_1 receptor-mediated stimulation of afferent C-fibers. Stimulation of C-fibers results in the release of neuropeptides, including substance P (SP) via a local reflex loop. The released neuropeptides such as SP can directly cause vasodilation and edema and can degranulate cutaneous mast cells, causing additional histamine release.

Table 4 Histamine Receptor-Mediated Effects on the Hematological and Immunological Systems

Effect	Receptor
1. Inhibition of basophil and cutaneous mast cell release	H_2
2. Inhibition of delayed hypersensitivity responses	H_2
3. Inhibition of in vitro generation of cytotoxic T lymphocytes	H_2
4. Inhibition of neutrophil lysosomal enzyme release	H_2
5. Modulation of neutrophil and eosinophil chemotaxis	H_1, H_2
6. Effects mediated by H2 receptor-bearing lymphocytes	
A. Inhibition of antigen-stimulated B-cell maturation	H_2
B. Inhibition of antibody secretion by mature plasma cells	H_2
C. Inhibition of immunoglobulin production by mononuclear cells	H_2
D. Lymphokine production including histamine suppressive factor	H_2

of inflammatory cells. H_2 receptors mediate inhibition of basophil release (Tung et al., 1982), delayed hypersensitivity skin test responses (Rocklin, 1976), and in vitro generation of cytotoxic T lymphocytes (Schwartz et al., 1980). In addition, stimulation of H_2 receptors on neutrophils and eosinophils results in inhibition of neutrophil lysosomal enzyme release and modulation of eosinophil and neutrophil migration, respectively (Casale, 1988). Histamine stimulation of H_2 receptor-bearing lymphocytes has also been shown to cause inhibition of antigen-stimulated B-cell maturation (Fallah et al., 1975), antibody secretion by mature plasma cells (Casale, 1988), and immunoglobulin production by human mononuclear cells (Lima and Rocklin, 1981). H_2 receptor stimulation of T lymphocytes can also lead to the production of cytokines, including histamine suppressive factor, which has numerous activities, as reviewed by White and Kaliner (1988).

IV. Antihistamines

After review of the numerous and varied effects of histamine, it becomes evident why antihistamines can be used clinically with such effectiveness for allergic diseases. As mentioned, the first antihistamine was developed in 1937 by Bovet and Staub (1937), and currently a number of H_1 and H_2 antagonists are available. These drugs all act as competitive antagonists for the H_1 or H_2 receptor site; however, unlike the agonists, they do not elicit a physiological response. Most antihistamines have a higher affinity for the H_1 and H_2 receptor than histamine or receptor-specific agonists. Binding of the antihistamines to the receptor site is generally reversible.

A. H_1 Antihistamines

The general formula for classic H_1 antihistamine drugs is shown in Figure 3. Based on the atom (X) connecting the aromatic rings to the ethylamine group, the classic H_1 antihistamines can be divided into six major subclasses (Ennis and Lorenz, 1984; Flowers et al., 1986; Popa, 1986; Simons, 1989) (see Table 5).

The first major subclass of H_1 antihistamines are the ethylenediamine derivatives, which contain a nitrogen atom in the X position. Members of this group include tripelennamine (Pyribenzamine), pyrilamine, methapyrilene, and antazoline (in Vasocon-A). As a whole, this group has relatively weak central nervous system (CNS) effects; however, adverse gastrointestinal effects are commonly seen with the ethylenediamine derivatives (Ennis and Lorenz, 1984; Flowers et al., 1986; Popa, 1986; Simons, 1989).

The second major subclass of H_1 antihistamines are the ethanolamine derivatives or aminoalkyl ethers. This group of antihistamines has an oxygen molecule in the X position and contains commonly used antihistamines such as

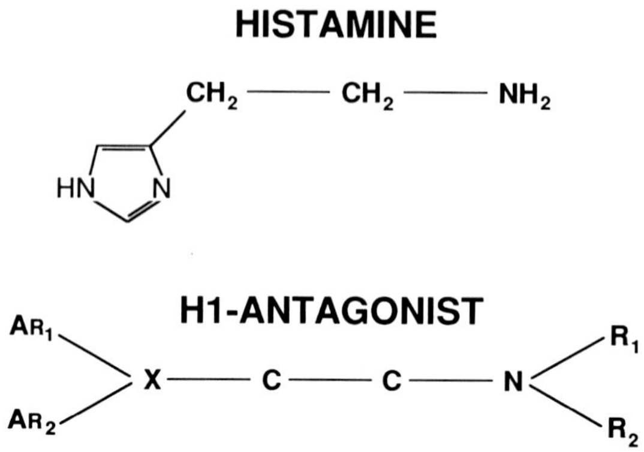

Figure 3 The structure of histamine and the classic H_1 antagonists. The aromatic rings (AR) are responsible for the hydrophilic nature of H_1 antagonists. The position (X) contains a nitrogen, carbon, or oxygen molecule and divides the classic H_1 antihistamines into six major subclasses. The R groups are variable, but antihistamines containing methyl or cyclic moieties at these positions are more active.

clemastine (Tavist), diphenhydramine (Benadryl), phenytoloxamine (in Sinutab), and carbinoxamine (in Rondec). This group of drugs frequently causes CNS depression and sedation, with greater than 50% of patients experiencing some drowsiness. The incidence of adverse gastrointestinal effects is low, but anticholinergic side effects occur with moderate frequency (Ennis and Lorenz, 1984; Flowers et al., 1986; Popa, 1986, Simons, 1989).

The third subclass of H_1 antihistamines are the alkylamines or the propylamine derivatives. This class of drugs has a carbon atom in the X position. They include such commonly used antihistamines as chlorpheniramine (Chlor-Trimeton, Teldrin), brompheniramine (Dimetane, Bromfed), triprolidine (Actidil and Triafed), and dexchlorpheniramine (Dexchlor, Polaramine). These antihistamines have only very weak CNS effects and thereby cause less drowsiness, making them a more suitable choice for daytime use. In addition, they have weak anticholinergic side effects and only rare gastrointestinal side effects (Ennis and Lorenz, 1984; Flowers et al., 1986; Popa, 1986; Simons, 1989).

The phenothiazine derivatives are a class of H_1 antihistamines containing nitrogen in the X position. They include promethazine (Phenergan), trimeprazine (Temaril), and methdilazine (Tacaryl). The most common uses for this class of drugs are as antiemetics or sedatives. They have very strong CNS effects and are thus very sedating and also have strong anticholinergic effects (Ennis and Lorenz, 1984; Flowers et al., 1986; Popa, 1986; Simons, 1989).

The piperazines also contain nitrogen as part of a piperazine nucleus in the X position of the classic antihistamine structure. This group of drugs includes

Table 5 The Classic H_1 Antihistamines

Group	Members	CNS effects	Comments
Ethylenediamine derivatives	Tripelennamine Pyrilamine Methapyrilene Antazoline	Weak	Adverse gastrointestinal effects common
Ethanolamine derivatives (aminoalkyl ethers)	Clemastine Diphenhydramine Phenytoloxamine Carbinoxamine	Common	Moderate anticholinergic effects
Alkylamines (propylamine derivatives)	Chlorpheniramine Brompheniramine Triprolidine Dexchlorpheniramine	Weak	Weak anticholinergic effects
Phenothiazine derivatives	Promethazine Trimeprazine Methdilazine	Strong	Antiemetic and sedative effects Strong anticholinergic effects
Piperazines	Hydroxyzine Meclizine Cyclizine Buclizine	Moderate	Antiemetic and antimotion sickness effects Moderate anticholinergic effects
Piperidines	Phenindamine Cyproheptadine	Mild Strong	Strong anticholinergic and antiserotoninergic effects

hydroxyzine (Atarax, Vistaril), as well as meclizine (Antivert), cyclizine (Marezine), and buclizine (Bucladin). Hydroxyzine is commonly used as an antipruritic, antiemetic, or sedative. The other drugs in this class are used most frequently for their antiemetic effects for motion sickness. This class of drugs has moderate CNS effects and moderate anticholinergic side effects, but a low incidence of gastrointestinal side effects (Ennis and Lorenz, 1984; Flowers et al., 1986; Popa, 1986; Simons, 1989).

The final subclass of classic H_1 antihistamines are the piperidines, which also contain a nitrogen atom in the X position. This group includes phenindamine (in Nolamine), which has only mild CNS side effects but may cause excitability in children. Cyproheptadine (Periactin), also a piperidine derivative, has strong CNS, anticholinergic, and antiserotoninergic properties. Cyproheptadine is often used as an antipruritic agent (Ennis and Lorenz, 1984; Flowers et al., 1986; Popa, 1986; Simons, 1989).

Other drugs that exhibit high affinity for the H_1 receptor and have strong H_1 antihistamine properties are the tricyclic antidepressants. Doxepin (Sinequan) and amitriptyline (Elavil) exhibit particularly strong antihistamine effects. They also, however, have strong anticholinergic and CNS side effects with sedation.

The major adverse effects noted with the use of H_1 antihistamines include CNS depression and sedation, occasionally CNS stimulation, gastrointestinal disturbances, and anticholinergic effects. The anticholinergic effects include suppression of salivary and lacrimal secretions, urinary retention or dysuria, impotence, vertigo, visual disturbances, and tachycardia. It is because of these adverse effects, primarily sedation and anticholinergic effects, that the newer, "nonsedating" antihistamines were formulated. The "second generation" H_1 antihistamines include terfenadine, astemizole, cetirizine, loratadine, levocabastine, acrivastine, ketotifen, and azelastine. The lower incidence of side effects attributed to these drugs relates to their poor penetration into the CNS due to their lipophobic nature and their preferential affinity for peripheral H_1 receptors (Kaliner and Check, 1988; Simons and Simons, 1988; de Vos, 1989; Mann et al., 1989; Rohr, 1989; Simons, 1989) (see Table 6).

Terfenadine (Seldane) was introduced in the United States in 1985 and was the first nonsedating antihistamine marketed in this country. It is a butyrophenone derivative and is structurally unrelated to other currently available antihistamines. It has essentially no CNS side effects and no appreciable anticholinergic or antiserotoninergic effects (Mann et al., 1989; McTavish et al., 1990).

Astemizole (Hismanal) is a piperidine derivative that is a long-acting, selective H_1 antagonist with antiserotoninergic properties. It has very poor CNS penetration and thus produces no substantial sedation. Astemizole is very long-acting, with a half-life of 20–60 hr, and is able to suppress cutaneous responses to histamine for 6–12 weeks (Mann et al., 1989).

Cetirizine (Reactine) is a carboxylic acid metabolite of the classical piperazine antihistamine, hydroxyzine. It is unique among the antihistamines because it does not undergo hepatic metabolism and is excreted primarily unchanged in the urine. Because of this, dosage adjustments may need to be made for patients with renal impairment. Cetirizine, like the other nonsedating second generation antihistamines, has poor penetration into the CNS but does have mild CNS effects at high doses (Rohr, 1989; Meltzer, 1990).

Loratidine (Claritin), a piperidine derivative, is structurally related to azatidine and cyproheptadine. It also is chemically similar to the tri-

Table 6 The Second-Generation H_1 Antihistamines

Drug	Structure	CNS effect	Comments
Terfenadine	Butyrophenone derivative	None	First nonsedating antihistamine marketed in U.S.
Astemizole	Piperidine derivative	None	Long-acting Antiserotoninergic properties
Cetirizine	Piperazine derivative	Mild	Metabolite of hydroxyzine Renal excretion
Loratidine	Piperidine derivative	None	Antiserotoninergic activity
Levocabastine	Piperidine derivative	None	Topical antihistamine Long-acting
Acrivastine	Alkylamine derivative	Mild	Metabolite of triprolidine
Ketotifen	Piperidine derivative	Mild	Multiple antiallergic effects
Azelastine	Phthalazinone	Mild	Multiple antiallergic effects

cyclic antidepressants imipramine, nortriptyline, and doxepin. Loratidine has no substantial central or autonomic nervous system effects but does have antiserotoninergic activity in high doses (Mann et al., 1989; Rohr, 1989; Meltzer, 1990).

Levocabastine is a topical piperidine derivative. In animal studies it is 15,000 times more potent than chlorpheniramine, 1500 times more potent than terfenadine, and 65 times more potent than astemizole in inhibiting histamine-induced responses. It is effective when applied topically to the nasal mucosa or conjunctiva, and some systemic absorption is observed after topical mucosal application. Levocabastine also is very long-acting, with a serum elimination half-life of 35 hr (Simons and Simons, 1988).

Acrivastine (Prolert and in DuAct) is a side-chain-reduced metabolite of triprolidine, one of the classic alkylamine antihistamines. It penetrates the CNS poorly and lacks anticholinergic effects even at high doses (Mann et al., 1989; Meltzer, 1990).

There are also several H_1 receptor antagonists that have additional antiallergic effects. These antihistamines include ketotifen (Zaditen), which is a

role of histamine in human diseases. Three specific histamine receptor types have been identified, and the role of these receptors in mediating effects on various organ systems is becoming increasingly understood. In addition, the armamentarium of H_1 and H_2 receptor antagonists continues to broaden with increasing improvement in clinical efficacy and side effect profiles. With further evaluation and understanding of the autoinhibitory role of the H_3 receptor, therapeutic manipulation of histamine-mediated effects through specific H_3 agonists may prove to be of clinical utility as well.

Acknowledgment

This work was supported in part by a Veterans Administration Merit Review Award and an Asthma and Allergic Diseases Center Award (AI 19093) from the National Institutes of Health. The authors thank Gary Beck for help in preparing this manuscript.

Discussion

Hanafin: Has histamine been found in endothelial cells?
Casale: No.
Platts-Mills: Is it important which antihistamine you use to treat asthmatics, taking into account the anticholinergic properties of some?
Casale: The classic, but not the newer, nonsedating, antihistamines have anticholinergic effects that might be useful in asthma. The nonsedating antihistamines can be given in higher doses because of the lack of sedation and are somewhat beneficial in asthma.
Kaliner: At least the nonsedating antihistamines are certainly not contraindicated in asthma, as some old (and probably inaccurate) studies suggested.
Lee: We have recently examined the duration of skin reactions to intradermal histamine in patients with chronic urticaria. The lesions were greatly prolonged in the urticaria patients, suggesting that histamine clearance or metabolism might be abnormal.
Casale: Histamine-induced wheals that are prolonged might be attributed to several factors: (1) decreased catabolism of histamine or (2) activation of sensory nerves by histamine with the recruitment of neuropeptide release into the skin. Certain neuropeptides, such as substance P and CGRP, can have effects on blood vessels and even reactivate mast cells.
Claman: How is histamine bound to the secretory granule and how is it released?
Casale: Histamine is bound to the granule by ionic charges and is eluted from these charges by exchange with interstitial fluid ions.

Kennerly: Can you comment on histidine decarboxylase activation in the synthesis of histamine during the regranulation of previously stimulated mast cells?
Casale: Recent work has suggested that histamine acting through an H_3 receptor might reduce histamine resynthesis, perhaps by affecting histidine decarboxylase. No other work on regulation of this enzyme has been reported.
Metcalfe: Have any histamine receptors been cloned?
Casale: I know of work in progress but not published reports on histamine receptor cloning.

References

Abramowicz, M., ed (1987). Famotidine (Pepcid). *Med. Lett. Drugs Ther.* 29:17–18.

Arrang, J. M., Garbarg, M., and Schwartz, J. C. (1983). Autoinhibition of brain histamine release mediated by a novel class (H_3) of histamine receptor. *Nature* 302:832–837.

Arrang, J. M., Garbarg, M., Lancelot, J. C., LeComte, J. M., Pollard, H., Robba, M., Schunack, W., and Schwartz, J. C. (1987). Highly potent and selective ligands for histamine H_3-receptors. *Nature* 327:117–123.

Ash, A. S., and Schild, H. O. (1966). Receptors mediating some actions of histamine. *Br. J. Pharmacol.* 27:427–439.

Barnes, P. J., and Ichinose, M. (1989). H_3 receptors in airways. *Trends Pharmacol. Sci.* 10:264.

Best, C. H., Dale, H. H., Dudley, H. W., and Thorpe, W. V. (1927). The nature of the vasodilator constituents of certain tissue extracts. *J. Physiol.* 62:397–417.

Black, J. W., Duncan, W. A., Durant, C. J., Ganellin, C. R., and Parsons, E. M. (1972). Definition and antagonism of histamine H_2 receptors. *Nature* 236:385–390.

Bovet, D., and Staub, A. (1937). Action protectrice des ethers phenoliques au cours de l'intoxication histaminique. *Comp. Rend. Soc. Biol.* 124:547–549.

Carswell, H., Daum, P. R., and Young, J. M. (1985). Histamine H_1-agonist stimulated breakdown of inositol phospholipids. In *Frontiers in Histamine Research.* Edited by C. R. Ganellin and J. C. Schwartz. New York, Pergamon Press, pp. 27–38.

Casale, T. B. (1988). Histamine H_1 and H_2 receptors. In *H_1 and H_2 Histamine Receptors.* Edited by G. Settipane. Providence, RI, Ocean Side Publications, pp. 14–20.

Casale, T. B., Rodbard, D., and Kaliner, M. (1985). Characterization of histamine H-1 receptors on human peripheral lung. *Biochem. Pharmacol.* 34:3285–3292.

Chakravarty, N. (1990). Mechanism of histamine secretion. *Agents Actions* 30:5–12.

Craps, L. P. (1985). Immunologic and therapeutic aspects of ketotifen. *J. Allergy Clin. Immunol.* 76:389–393.

Dale, H. H., and Laidlaw, P. P. (1910). The physiological action of beta-imidazolylethylamine. *J. Physiol.* 41:318–344.

Dale, H. H., and Laidlaw, P. P. (1919). Histamine shock. *J. Physiol.* 52:355–390.

de Vos, C. (1989). New antihistamines. *Clin. Exp. Allergy* 19:503–507.

Dunlop, L. S., Smith, A. P., and Piper, P. J. (1977). The effect of histamine antagonists on antigen-induced contractions of sensitized human bronchus in vitro. *Br. J. Pharmacol.* 59:475P (proceedings).

Eiser, N. M., Mills, J., Snashall, P. D., and Guz, A. (1981). The role of histamine receptors in asthma. *Clin. Sci.* 60:363–370.

Ennis, M., and Lorenz, W. (1984). Histamine receptor antagonists in discoveries. In *Discoveries in Pharmacology*. Vol. 2: *Hemodynamics, Hormones and Inflammation*. Edited by M. J. Parnham and J. Bruinvels. New York, Elsevier.

Fallah, H. A., Maillard, J. L., and Voison, G. A. (1975). Regulatory mast cells. I. Suppressive action of their products on an in vitro primary immune reaction. *Ann. Immunol. (Paris)* 126:669–682.

Flowers, F. P., Araujo, O. E., and Nieves, C. H. (1986). Antihistamines. *Int. J. Dermatol.* 25:224–231.

Haaksma, E. E. J., Leurs, R., and Timmerman, H. (1990). Histamine receptors: Subclasses and specific ligands. *Pharmacol. Ther.* 47:73–104.

Ichinose, M., and Barnes, P. J. (1989). Inhibitory histamine H_3-receptors on cholinergic nerves in human airways. *Eur. J. Pharmacol.* 163:383–386.

Ichinose, M., Stretton, C. D., Schwartz, J. C., and Barnes, P. J. (1989). Histamine H_3-receptors inhibit cholinergic bronchoconstriction in guinea pig airways. *Br. J. Pharmacol.* 97:13–15.

Joad, J. P., and Casale, T. B. (1987). Airway histamine H_1 receptors. In *Current Topics in Pulmonary Pharmacology and Toxicology*. Vol. 3. Edited by M. A. Hollinger. New York, Elsevier, pp. 95–121.

Joad, J., and Casale, T. B. (1988). Histamine and airway caliber. *Ann. Allergy* 61:1–7.

Kaliner, M. A., and Check, W. A. (1988). Non-sedating antihistamines. *Allergy Proc.* 9:649–663.

Kaliner, M., Sigler, R., Summers, R., and Shelhamer, J. H. (1981). Effects of infused histamine: Analysis of H_1 and H_2 histamine receptor antagonists on cardiovascular and pulmonary responses. *J. Allergy Clin. Immunol.* 68:365–371.

Lewis, T. (1927). *The Blood Vessels of the Human Skin and Their Responses*. London, Shaw.

Lima, M., and Rocklin, R. E. (1981). Histamine modulates in vitro IgG production by pokeweed mitogen-stimulated human mononuclear cells. *Cell. Immunol.* 64:324–336.

Lipsy, R. J., Fennerty, B., and Fagan, T. C. (1990). Clinical review of histamine$_2$ receptor antagonists. *Arch. Intern. Med.* 150:745–751.

Little, M. M., and Casale, T. B. (1989). Azelastine inhibits IgE-mediated human basophil histamine release. *J. Allergy Clin. Immunol.* 83:862–865.

Little, M. M., Wood, D. R., and Casale, T. B. (1989). Azelastine inhibits stimulated histamine release from human lung tissue in vitro but does not alter cyclic nucleotide content. *Agents Actions* 28:16–21.

Mann, K. V., Crowe, J. P., and Tietze, K. J. (1989). Nonsedating histamine H_1-receptor antagonists. *Clin. Pharm.* 8:331–344.

McTavish, D., and Sorkin, E. M. (1989). Azelastine: A review of its pharmacodynamic and pharmacokinetic properties, and therapeutic potential. *Drugs* 38:778–800.

McTavish, D., Goa, K. L., and Ferrill, M. (1990). Terfenadine: An updated review of its pharmacological properties and therapeutic efficacy. *Drugs* 39:552–574.

Meltzer, E. O. (1990). Performance effects of antihistamines. *J. Allergy Clin. Immunol.* 86(4 Part 2):613–619.

Metcalfe, D. D., Kaliner, M., and Donlon, M. A. (1981). The mast cell. *CRC Crit. Rev. Immunol.* 3:23–74.

Platshon, L. F., and Kaliner, M. (1978). The effects of the immunologic release of histamine upon human lung cyclic nucleotide levels and prostaglandin generation. *J. Clin. Invest.* 62:1113–1121.

Popa, V. (1986). The classic antihistamines (H_1 blockers) in respiratory medicine. *Clin. Chest Med.* 7:367–382.

Rafferty, P., and Holgate, S. T. (1989). Histamine and its antagonists in asthma. *J. Allergy Clin. Immunol.* 84:144–151.

Ring, J., Sedlmeier, F., von der Helm, D., Mayr, T., Walz, U., Ibel, H., Riepel, H., Przybilla, B., Reimann, H. J., and Dorsch, W. (1986). Histamine and allergic dieases. In *New Trends in Allergy II*. Edited by J. Ring and G. Burg. Berlin, Springer-Verlag, pp. 44–77.

Rocklin, R. E. (1976). Modulation of cellular-immune responses in vivo and in vitro by histamine receptor-bearing lymphocytes. *J. Clin. Invest.* 57:1051–1058.

Rohr, A. S. (1989). Non-sedating antihistamines: A selective review of terfenadine, astemizole, cetirizine and loratidine. *Immunol. Allergy Pract.* 11:17–20.

Schwartz, A., Askenase, P. W., and Gershon, R. K. (1980). Histamine inhibition of the in vitro induction of cytotoxic T-cell responses. *Immunopharmacology* 2: 179–190.

Schwartz, J. C., Arrang, J. M., Garbarg, M., and Pollard, H. (1990). A third histamine receptor subtype: Characterization, localization and functions of the H_3 receptor. *Agents Actions* 30:13–23.

Sertl, K., Casale, T. B., Wescott, S. L., and Kaliner, M. A. (1987). Immunohistochemical localization of histamine-stimulated increases in cyclic GMP in guinea pig lung. *Am. Rev. Respir. Dis.* 135:456–462.

Shelhamer, J. H., Marom, Z., and Kaliner, M. (1980). Immunologic and pharmacologic stimulation of mucous glycoprotein release from human airways in vitro. *J. Clin. Invest.* 66:1400–1408.

Simons, F. E. R. (1989). H_1 receptor antagonists: Clinical pharmacology and therapeutics. *J. Allergy Clin. Immunol.* 84:845–862.

Simons, F. E. R., and Simons, K. J. (1988). New H_1-receptor antagonists: A review. *Am. J. Rhinol.* 2:21–25.

Simons, F. E. R., Leciuk, G. H., Becker, A. B., and Gillespie, C. A. (1982). Ketotifen: A new drug for prophylaxis of asthma in children. *Ann. Allergy* 48:145–150.

Steel, L., Platshon, L., and Kaliner, M. (1979). Prostaglandin generation by human and guinea pig lung tissue: Comparison of parenchymal and airway responses. *J. Allergy Clin. Immunol.* 64:287–293.

Steinbusch, H. W. M., and Mulder, A. H. (1985). Localization and projections of histamine immunoreactive neurons in the central nervous system of the rat. In *Frontiers in Histamine Research*. Edited by C. R. Ganellin and J. C. Schwartz. Oxford, Pergamon Press, pp. 119–130.

Summers, R., Sigler, R., Shelhamer, J. H., and Kaliner, M. (1981). Effects of infused histamine on asthmatic and normal subjects: Comparison of skin test responses. *J. Allergy Clin. Immunol.* 67:456–464.

Theoharides, T. C. (1989). Histamine$_2$-receptor antagonists in the treatment of urticaria. *Drugs* 37:345–355.

Tung, R., Kagey-Sobotka, A., Plaut, M., and Lichtenstein, L. M. (1982). H_2 antihistamines augment antigen-induced histamine release from human basophils in vitro. *J. Immunol.* 129:2113–2115.

van der Werf, J. F., and Timmerman, H. (1989). The histamine H_3 receptor: A general presynaptic histaminergic regulatory system? *Trends Pharmacol. Sci.* 10:159–162.

Watanabe, T., Taguchi, Y., Takeda, N., Shiosaka, S., Tokyama, M., and Wada, H. (1985). Purification of and antibodies against 1-histidine decarboxylase. In *Frontiers in Histamine Research*. Edited by C. R. Ganellin and J. C. Schwartz. Oxford, Pergamon Press, pp. 91–102.

White, M. V., and Kaliner, M. A. (1988). Histamine. In *Inflammation: Basic Principles and Clinical Correlates*. Edited by J. I. Gallin, I. M. Goldstein, and R. Snyderman. New York, Raven Press, pp. 169–193.

Windaus, A., and Vogt, W. (1907). Synthese des Imidazolyläthylamins. *Berl. Dtsch. Chem. Ges.* 40:3691–3695.

12

Mast Cell Proteases

SANFORD M. GOLDSTEIN and BRUCE U. WINTROUB

University of California, San Francisco
San Francisco, California

I. Introduction

Mast cell neutral proteases are preformed enzymes, stored and released from mast cell secretory granules in fully active form and not as zymogens. In the last 10 years our knowledge of human mast cell proteases has grown tremendously, and it is not surprising that current concepts of their potential biological role have also greatly expanded. Although at least seven proteases have been described in mast cells from various species, most reports have concentrated on tryptase, chymase, and carboxypeptidase, and we have indisputable evidence that these enzymes are contained in and released from mast cell secretory granules. Because this book centers on the mast cell in health and disease, and because one must extrapolate from data using nonhuman species with caution, we will concentrate on the enzymes from humans, unless animal studies illustrate a point or mechanism not yet investigated in humans.

II. Tryptase

A. Introduction

Tryptase has been the subject of recent reviews (Schwartz 1987, 1990; Schwartz and Austen, 1984; Caughey, 1989, 1990). First detected in human cutaneous and gingival mast cells (Chiu and Langunoff, 1972; Glenner and Cohen, 1960; Hopsu and Glenner, 1963; Lagunoff and Benditt, 1963), tryptase was identified and purified from human skin (Fraki, 1977) and pulmonary mast cells over a decade ago (Schwartz et al., 1981a,b) and subsequently from human lung (Smith et al., 1984), skin (Harvima et al., 1988a), and a human mast cell line (Butterfield et al., 1990). A protease that is probably tryptase was also identified in the human uterine cervix (Ito et al., 1980). There is evidence for both functional (Tanaka et al., 1983) and structural (Cromlish et al., 1987) heterogeneity among tryptases extracted from different human tissues. It has since been purified from dog mastocytoma cells (Caughey et al., 1987) and rat mast cells (Kido et al., 1985) and is homologous with these enzymes. Tryptase is the most abundant mast cell neutral protease, present at up to 35 pg/mast cell in foreskin mast cells (Schwartz et al., 1987a). At 12 pg/lung mast cell, it accounts for 23% or more of total pulmonary mast cell protein. It is a unique serine endopeptidase of tetrameric structure with four active sites (Schwartz et al., 1981a). Although tryptase has been cloned (Miller et al., 1989b; Vanderslice et al., 1990a; Miller et al., 1990), it is still unknown how it is assembled as an active enzyme. It binds in vitro and presumably in vivo to anionic sulfated mast cell proteoglycans by ionic interactions.

B. Tryptase Measurement and Control of Activity

Tryptase may be measured or detected by spectrophotometric assay (Schwartz and Bradford, 1986), commercially available radioimmunoassay, ELISA (Wenzel et al., 1986), immunohistochemistry (Smith et al., 1984; Craig et al., 1986), or histochemistry (Caughey et al., 1988d; Osman et al., 1989; Harvima et al., 1989a). Its pH optimum is ~8.0 for TAME esterase activity and ~7.4 for peptidase activity, and it is inhibited by DFP, PMSF, leupeptin, and TLCK, but not by TPCK (Schwartz et al., 1981b). Salt concentrations, specifically NaCl (Alter et al., 1987a), KCl, and ammonium sulfate, affect the kinetics of tryptase activity in vitro (Harvima et al., 1988b; Cromlish et al., 1987). The peptidase activity of tryptase exhibits much more substrate selectivity than trypsin. This is largely due to subsite interactions with the extended binding site of tryptase, which favors substrates with two adjacent basic amino acids (Cromlish et al., 1987) and is especially inhibited by a proline in the P_3 position (Tanaka et al., 1983). On the other hand, tryptase tends to cleave after arginines or lysines that follow proline by four to six residues (Cromlish et al., 1987).

Tryptase has no known endogenous inhibitor (Schwartz et al., 1981a; Caughey et al., 1987). Unlike bovine trypsin, human tryptase is not inhibited by aprotinin, LBTI, SBTI, C1 esterase inhibitor, ovomucoid trypsin inhibitors, α_2 macroglobulin or α_1 trypsin inhibitor (Smith et al., 1984; Schwartz and Bradford, 1986; Caughey et al., 1987; Cromlish et al., 1987; Schwartz et al., 1981b).

Tryptase is inhibited by ovoinhibitor and Ca^{2+} (Smith et al., 1984). Although unpublished data noted inhibition with mucous proteinase inhibitor (antileukoprotease) (Fritz, 1988), recent studies demonstrate a lack of inhibition of tryptase by antileukoprotease and human lung low-molecular-weight elastase inhibitor, hiruden, and antithrombin III (Alter et al., 1990). However, purified tryptase dissociates in vitro at physiological ionic strength into inactive monomers (Schwartz and Bradford, 1986; Alter et al., 1987a) that cannot be reassembled into active enzyme. This process is associated with changes in secondary and tertiary structures (Schwartz et al., 1990) and is inhibited by binding of tryptase to glycosaminoglycans and proteoglycans, correlating with their charge density and not their carbohydrate composition. Since heparin bound tryptase appears to be stable and does not dissociate below 0.75 *M* NaCl, it is not clear when and where this occurs in vivo. Monoclonal antibodies have been made that distinguish between inactive and active enzyme (Schwartz et al., 1990), and it is possible that they may be used in vivo in the future to investigate this question. It has been proposed, however, that tryptase dissociates in vivo from mast cell proteoglycans after exocytosis and becomes inactivated by dissociation of its quaternary structure. It was suggested, using antithrombin III as an in vitro model, that proteins that compete with tryptase for heparin binding might displace tryptase from heparin and thereby promote its destabilization (Alter et al., 1990).

In the rat, tryptase may be regulated by association with the low-molecular-weight endogenous mast cell inhibitor trypstatin and is not bound to heparin (Kido et al., 1985). In humans, trypstatin has not been identified.

Recently, histamine, 1-methyl histamine, and histadine, as well as divalent cation (especially Zn^{2+}), have been shown to inhibit tryptase cleavage of Tosyl-Gly-Pro-Lys-*p*-nitroanalide (Alter and Schwartz, 1989). Competitive inhibition of tryptase by calcium was seen with possibly a K_i of 30 mM. At 5 mM, Ca^{2+} caused a 50% loss of activity with time, presumably by destabilizing tryptase, but not by displacing it from heparin. Histamine inhibition of tryptase in vitro exhibited different kinetics from calcium ion and had no effect on destabilization of tryptase. It is not clear how these results are reflected in vivo, but histamine might function in vivo in controlling tryptase activity in the secretory granule (Alter and Schwartz, 1989).

C. Protein Structure and Molecular Biology

SDS-PAGE of purified tryptase indicated that the active tetramer was comprised of two different monomer subunits, of M_r from ~31 to 36 kDa that varies from tissue to tissue (Schwartz and Bradford, 1986; Schwartz et al., 1981a; Cromlish et al., 1987). It was not known whether these differences were due to glycosylation or other posttranslational processing or to amino acid structural differences.

However, some of the heterogeneity appeared due to N-linked glycosylation when human pituitary was digested with *N*-glycosidase F. Such heterogeneity was not found when lung tryptase was so treated (Cromlish et al., 1987).

The Number of Tryptase Genes

Tryptase from dog mastocytoma cells has been cloned (Vanderslice et al., 1989), and recent reports have described mouse (Chu et al., 1990) and human tryptase cDNAs. Several overlapping partial cDNAs have been isolated from a human lung mast cell cDNA library and yielded a deduced sequence of 244 amino acids for the coding region of a monomer called α tryptase with a molecular weight of 27,423 (Miller et al., 1989b). Two putative N-linked glycosylation sites were identified. Recently three different cDNAs, predicting a 245-residue catalytic region and M_r of 27,449, have been reported from a human skin cDNA library (Vanderslice et al., 1990b). They are 98% identical. The differences among them in sequence outside the 3' untranslated regions are limited to a single redundant base substitution at bp 6, and single substitutions at nucleotides 152, 155, 158, and 396, resulting in aa changes at residues 21, 22, 23, and at 102, eliminating one of two consensus N-linked glycosylation sites. A second lung cDNA was reported and called beta tryptase (Miller et al., 1990). β tryptase and clone II from skin seem to be identical to each other (except several nucleotides in the 3' untranslated region) and contain only one glycosylation site. cDNA cloning has therefore apparently explained differences in M_r of tryptase protein subunits that are due to glycosylation. Clone III from skin and α tryptase from lung share several distinct amino acid substitutions at positions 21, 22, 23 but are not identical (Miller et al., 1989b; Vanderslice et al., 1990b).

The presence of several tryptase genes was suggested by Southern blotting (Vanderslice et al., 1990b) along with the identification of α and β clone specific genomic PCR fragments in 10 unrelated individuals (Miller et al., 1990). However, the PCR fragments reported cannot distinguish between α and III cDNAs or among β, I, and II cDNAs, which share the same sequences in the amplified segments. Therefore, while the PCR fragments document at least two gene products, they do not exclude more than two tryptase genes. Tryptase genes have been assigned to chromosome 16 (Miller et al., 1990). One tryptase gene that was cloned and sequenced is comprised of six introns and five small introns (Vanderslice et al., 1990b) and is identical to cDNA clone I. A second genomic clone is 98% identical to cDNA I, but its exons have some sequence differences from clone I. Therefore, it appears that α tryptase represents one gene product; β tryptase and skin II tryptase represent a second gene; and skin I tryptase and the genomic clone are a probable third gene. Skin III tryptase cDNA represents a possible fourth gene product. It has not yet been elucidated how these different genes are expressed, and these findings do not yet shed light on the exact composition of the active tetrameric protein or how subunits in different tissues correspond to cDNAs. Interestingly, a preliminary report noted that one of the cDNAs from skin mast cells has been expressed in *Escherichia coli* as an active ~28,000-dalton protein monomer that bound antihuman lung tryptase antibodies (Vanderslice et al., 1990b) and was inhibited with DFP and TLCK. These findings raise questions about what in vivo posttranslational modifications are required for tetramer assembly in humans and suggest that these modifications might be responsible for the loss of activity of monomers upon dissociation from the native human enzyme (Vanderslice et al., 1990b).

Structure of Human Tryptase

The cloning of human tryptase has demonstrated several other features that may have physiological implications (Miller et al., 1989b, 1990; Vanderslice et al., 1990b). First, the activation peptide of tryptase ends in glycine, unlike the serine pancreatic proteases, which end in a basic residue such as arginine, or the dog and rodent mast cell chymases (reviewed and references in Caughey et al., 1990) and human mast cell carboxypeptidase (Reynolds et al., 1989), which end in acidic residues such as glutamic acid or aspartic acid. These findings suggest that the enzymatic activation of tryptase in the mast cell is likely to be different from that of chymase and carboxypeptidase. However, the site and mechanism by which tryptase and the other neutral proteases are activated are not known. Second, the different clones encode subunits with slight variations in substrate binding sites and net charge, perhaps accounting for some of the functional differences in tryptases extracted from different tissues (Schwartz, 1990). Finally, the cloning and sequencing of the human tryptase gene has revealed a region homologous to the enhancer of pancreatic serine proteases that might be involved in regulating the levels of gene expression in mast cells (references in Vanderslice et al., 1990b). It was also noted that the intron-exon structure of human tryptase is closer to that of trypsin and kallikrein than to rodent chymase, leukocyte proteases, or coagulation proteins (Vanderslice et al., 1990b).

D. The Role of Tryptase in Health and Disease

Investigations that attempt to delineate the role of tryptase and the other mast cell proteases in human physiology and pathophysiology have progressed along three paths. The first is to identify protein and peptide substrates in vitro that are hydrolyzed by the proteases. The second is to study the effects of these enzymes on animal or tissue models to identify novel physiological phenomena. Finally, studies in humans have attempted to document protease release in situ and to correlate the presence or activity of proteases with disease states. While multiple studies have identified many intriguing potential roles for mast cell proteases,

matrix, and this was partially inhibited by TLCK (Gruber and Schwartz, 1990). Preliminary evidence suggests that fibronectin is released from human fibroblast-generated matrix proteins and is subsequently degraded by human lung tryptase. A gelatinase/type IV procollagenase-like enzyme was also digested by tryptase (Lohi et al., 1990).

G. Involvement of Tryptase in In Vitro Pathophysiological Responses

Airway Contractility

Released dog mastocytoma supernatants and purified tryptase increased the contractile response of dog airway smooth muscle to histamine, KCl, and serotonin, but not acetylcholine (Sekizawa et al., 1989). This effect was prevented by tryptase inhibition, nifedipine, and verapamil, suggesting that tryptase amplifies airway contractility that is directly or indirectly mediated via calcium channels. Tryptase may also promote bronchoconstriction via a second pathway (Franconi et al., 1989). Ferret trachial rings were precontracted with serotonin and then relaxed with vasoactive intestinal peptide (VIP). Tryptase, and to a lesser extent chymase, paralleling their in vitro relative rates of hydrolysis of VIP, reversed this relaxation. Neither enzyme affected relaxation caused by isoproterenol. Interestingly, rat serosal mast cells appear to make VIP and VIP peptide fragments (Goetzl et al., 1989). However, these peptide fragments are different from those generated by human tryptase (Caughey et al., 1988b; Tam and Caughey, 1990). Human mast cell production of VIP has not been reported. The overall effect of tryptase in situ, therefore, may be to possibly promote airway constriction by these mechanisms.

In Vitro Mast Cell Activation and Mediator Release

A number of studies using protease inhibitors have attempted to dissect out the contribution of proteases to mast cell granule release. Results using inhibitors have suggested several protease-mediated steps in mast cell activation. While the effects of these inhibitors may be related to inhibition of phospholipid methylation (Ishizaka, 1981), the concentrations required for inhibition of histamine release are 1000-fold lower. Tryptase, unlike chymase, has not been shown to directly activate mast cells. In human pulmonary mast cells, but not rat peritoneal mast cells, DFP and TPCK, but not TLCK, caused a dose-dependent inhibition of histamine release by A23187 (Hultsch et al., 1988), implicating the involvement of chymase- and not tryptase-like activity. However, in rat mast cells, 48/80 release of histamine was inhibited by PMSF and TLCK and not inhibited by antichymase F(ab')2 or chymostatin (Vassimon and Rothschild, 1990), suggesting tryptase involvement. Tryptase inhibitors had no effect on anti-IgE or A23187-induced release in rat mast cells (Katunuma et al., 1986).

Because these studies are based solely on inhibitors, the exact proteases that are involved and their location have not been further definitively characterized.

As a Mitogen for Fibroblasts

A recent study demonstrated that human lung mast cell and dog mastocytoma tryptase stimulates DNA synthesis in cultured Chinese hamster lung (CCL39 line) fibroblasts and rat-1 fibroblasts up to 29-fold (Ruoss et al., 1991). This response is equivalent to that seen with 10 nM thrombin or 15% fetal calf serum and was synergistic with EGF, basic FGH, and insulin and additive with thrombin. The response was half-maximal at 15 nM. Tryptase stimulated the amiloride-sensitive Na/H-antiporter, but not production of inositol phosphates or a transient increase in cytoplasmic Ca^{2+} or cAMP. It was not inhibited by pertussis toxin and appears not to use a G-protein-coupled mechanism, unlike thrombin. CCL39 cells demonstrated a sevenfold increase in cell number 5 days after treatment with 7.5 nM tryptase. These data are consistent with a preliminary report suggesting that unidentified factors, in addition to histamine in released supernatants of human lung mast cells, stimulated human fibroblast proliferation (Dahodawala et al., 1990).

H. Involvement of Tryptase In Vivo

Experimental Release of Tryptase by Antigen Challenge

The following release studies are important in several respects. First, they document mast cell activation in vivo by detection of tryptase in biological fluids. Second, they document that the time course of tryptase secretion and clearance cannot be predicted solely by the stimulus or challenge. Finally, they suggest that not all "allergic" phenomena necessarily involve mast cell activation.

Skin

Skin chamber assays have demonstrated maximal release of histamine at 0–30 min and then tryptase at 30–60 min at levels of 25 ng and 95 ng, respectively, after antigen challenge of sensitized individuals (Schwartz et al., 1987b). Tryptase, but not histamine, declined to baseline 4 hr after a 1-hr challenge. Longer-term release studies were performed with continuous challenge, and mediators were assayed at hourly intervals. Tryptase protein identified by Elisa had tryptase activity using tosyl-glycyl-L-prolyl-lysine *p*-nitroanilide at a specific activity close to that of purified tryptase, suggesting that it was not being rapidly inactivated. This finding is the strongest suggestive evidence to date that active tryptase, perhaps bound to proteoglycans, can diffuse through tissue. Tryptase release peaked at 60 min and decreased to baseline at 5–9 hr postchallenge

(Shalit et al., 1988). Histamine peaked at 1 hr but then persisted at a low constant concentration from 2 through 9 hr. This pattern was constant and showed no peak in tryptase with late repeat challenge except when very low doses of antigen were used initially or when one antigen was followed by an unrelated antigen at 4 hr. This system was altered to compare continuous 6-hr challenge with two 1-hr challenges separated by 4 hr (Shalit et al., 1990). Continuous antigen challenge resulted in the patterns of histamine and tryptase release described above. An additional release was seen after subsequent codeine challenge.

With interrupted antigen challenge, a peak in release of mediators was followed by a sharp decrease of histamine and a slower decline of tryptase activity between challenges. On antigen rechallenge after 4 hr, histamine but not tryptase was detected, but both peaked on rechallenge with codeine. Rechallenge with codeine after initial codeine challenge caused no additional histamine or tryptase release, and constant codeine challenge did not cause the plateau histamine release seen with antigen. Mast cells were degranulated in the upper dermis but appeared not to be degranulated in the lower dermis. Basophils were not increased over blood levels in chamber fluids and in touch preparations from the dermis and were not found in tissue. However, it is felt that the plateau levels of histamine and late release of histamine or antigen rechallenge may be related to basophils, and not to mast cells that become desensitized to the initial challenge. Initial codeine or antigen challenge differs in the ability to elicit this plateau level of histamine or late response to antigen rechallenge. The data in these studies are also likely to reflect the various mechanisms of diffusion, binding, and metabolism of mediators in tissue, in addition to mast cell activation or desensitization in situ (Schwartz et al., 1987b).

I. Pulmonary Challenge

Bronchoalveolar lavage fluids (BALF) from atopic asthmatics before antigen challenge contained increased tryptase, but not histamine, compared to normals, suggesting ongoing mast cell activation (Wenzel et al., 1988). Atopic nonasthmatics and atopic asthmatics had 6–12-fold increases in lavage fluid histamine, and atopic asthmatics had fivefold increased tryptase levels after challenge, but nonatopic asthmatic controls did not. There were no differences in mast cells in BALF among the groups. The presence of tryptase in nonatopic asthmatics during an acute episode is not known. When lavage fluids from cigarette smokers in their late 20s were examined, 4/12 contained increased levels of tryptase and 6/12 had increased histamine (Kalenderian et al., 1988). In atopics with exercise-induced asthma, no differences were found between pre- and postexercise histamine, tryptase, LTC_4, and PGD_2 levels (Broide et al., 1990). Thus, these data demonstrate the release of mast cell tryptase in the airways of sensitized individuals and some smokers. However, it is not known whether the enzyme is active in the airways. Tryptase may not be released in all cases of bronchoconstriction.

Allergic Rhinitis

TAME esterase activity was noted in nasal secretions after allergen challenge (Baumgarten et al., 1986). Gel filtration of these secretions suggested that 25% of this activity is due to tryptase, and the rest to activated plasma kallikrein. After atopics were challenged (Castells and Schwartz, 1988), tryptase protein levels increased 7.5–60-fold. Antigen doses that caused maximum tryptase release caused maximal clinical responses. In contrast, histamine increases were lower (three- to sixfold); in one subject histamine levels actually decreased and in one subject increased by only 50%. Maximal histamine levels did not correlate with maximal clinical symptoms in three of seven subjects. However, histamine and clinical symptoms rose at low challenge doses in two subjects, whereas tryptase increased only at the highest doses. In another study immunoreactive tryptase was detected at twofold elevated levels in nasal lavage in subjects immediately after exposure to ozone (Koren et al., 1990). In nasal and bronchoalveolar lavage studies, it is not known how tryptase is transported or secreted, or whether it is present as an inactive monomer, as a tetramer bound to heparin, or in its unbound active form, as the ELISA assay measures tryptase monomer immunoreactive protein (Castells and Schwartz, 1988).

J. Release into the Circulation in Anaphylaxis and Mastocytosis

Tryptase is released into the circulation during mast cell activation. Plasma tryptase protein levels were elevated in 11/17 patients with mastocytosis (4–88 ng/ml) or with anaphylaxis from different causes (9–75 ng/ml range). Levels were normal (<5 ng/ml) in patients with myocardial disease, sepsis, and controls (Schwartz et al., 1987c). In three patients with experimentally induced anaphylaxis due to bee stings, tryptase levels peaked at 1–2 hr, whereas histamine peaked at 5–10 min (Schwartz et al., 1989). The levels of tryptase protein in subjects and patients with hypersensitivity reactions declined with a half-life of 1.5–2.3 hr and histamine declined by 15–60 min. However, endogenous tryptase present in serum removed from the subjects had a longer half-life in vitro of ~4 days. Purified exogenous tryptase protein added to serum had a half-life of ~2 days with or without heparin. In plasma at 37°C, added purified tryptase without heparin had a half-life of ~5–6 hr, which was slowed by heparin. This is contrasted with an activity half-life of 6–8 min under physiological conditions (Schwartz and Bradford, 1986). Therefore, tryptase may be a useful marker in cases of mast cell release and may suggest a mast cell–associated disease if not suspected already (Schwartz et al., 1989).

K. Involvement of Tryptase in Clinical Diseases

Aside from the assessment of tryptase release, the study of tryptase in vivo has been limited to detecting increased numbers of tryptase-containing mast cells or altered levels of tryptase activity or immunologically detected tryptase protein. Its definitive pathophysiological role in disease, although likely, remains to be demonstrated.

Psoriasis

The presence of tryptase-positive mast cells was examined in lesions of psoriasis (Harvima et al., 1989a). Involved skin demonstrated increased numbers of cells in the superficial dermis. In 4/12 subjects some granular epidermal staining for tryptase was noted in lesional skin. The significance of these findings is not known.

Rheumatoid Arthritis

Tryptase was immunohistochemically localized to mast cells in the synovium of patients with rheumatoid arthritis (Gruber et al., 1988). Purified tryptase or mast cell lysates were added to latent collagenase from synovial fluid or from cultured synoviocytes. Activation of collagenase by tryptase was demonstrated by SDS-PAGE and autoradiography of ^{3}H-labeled collagen. It was later shown that tryptase activates procollagenase indirectly through the activation of matrix metalloproteinase 3 (stromolysin) (Gruber et al., 1989).

Gingivitis and Periodontis

Tryptase-like, as well as cathepsins B- and L-, elastase-, trypsin- and dipeptidyl peptidase IV-like, activities are measurable from gingiva using fluorescent substrates (Cox and Eley, 1989a,b). Enzyme activities show wide variations in patients with periodontal disease. Activities were also measured in tissue samples from such patients. While chymotrypsin-like activity correlated with increasing pocket depth and other clinical parameters, tryptase activity did not correlate with disease state (Eley and Cox, 1990). Both activities were higher in gingival tissue compared to granulomata.

Scleroderma

Multiple studies have implicated mast cells in the skin lesions of scleroderma (Claman, 1989), as discussed in another chapter. The finding that tryptase is a fibroblast mitogen in vitro suggests a potential role for this protease in the sclerotic lesions of skin and other organ systems.

III. Chymase

A. Introduction

Chymase has been recently reviewed (Miller et al., 1989a; Caughey, 1989, 1990; Woodbury et al., 1989; Schechter, 1990). Mast cell chymases were first identified and were localized to mast cell granules (Benditt and Arase, 1959; Lagunoff and Pritzl, 1976; Chiu and Lagunoff, 1972) and purified in the rat (Yurt and Austen, 1977; Woodbury et al., 1981). Two different chymotryptic proteases, rat mast cell proteinase (RMCP) I, or chymase I, from connective tissue mast cells, and RMCP II, from mucosal mast cells, have been purified and extensively characterized (Woodbury and Neurath, 1980; Yoshida et al., 1980; Powers et al., 1985; LeTrong et al., 1987a). RMCP II has been cloned (Benfey et al., 1987). Dog chymase has also been identified and purified (Powers et al., 1985; Caughey et al., 1988c; Schechter et al., 1988) and cloned (Caughey et al., 1990). Human mast cells, like dog mast cells, appear to express only one chymase, and only a subset of mast cells contain this enzyme (Irani et al., 1986). In humans, chymase was first described as an extractable chymotrypic proteinase from human skin (Jansen and Hopsu-Havu, 1969; Fraki and Hopsu-Havu, 1975). Chymase was purified from human skin and did not immunologically cross-react with an anti-RMCP-1 antibody (Schechter et al., 1983; Johnson et al., 1986). This enzyme was found at 15-fold higher levels in extracts of skin from patients with mastocytosis, and it was suspected that this was of mast cell origin (Schechter et al., 1983). Several years ago chymase was identified biochemically as a secretory granule mediator of human lung mast cells (Wintroub et al., 1986). It was shown, by immunohistochemical studies, to be localized to mast cells in skin and lung (Schechter et al., 1986; Irani et al., 1986, 1989; Login et al., 1987; Osman et al., 1989) and, by immunological methods, to be distinct from cathepsin G, elastase, and tryptase (Schechter et al., 1983, 1986, 1990).

Chymase is positively charged and tends to remain tightly bound to mast cell proteoglycans (Sayama et al., 1987) and the mast cell after release, requiring treatment in higher than physiological NaCl concentrations to dissociate it from plasma membrane of the mast cell (Hammel et al., 1988; Schwartz et al., 1981c). Chymase incubated in vitro with skin appears to bind to skin and possibly to heparan sulfate by electrostatic interaction at the dermoepidermal junction (Sayama et al., 1987). This has not yet been demonstrated in situ in skin from disease states. Compared to other proteases, human chymase is present at low levels (~4 pg/mast cell in adult foreskins). It migrates as a single broad band on SDS PAGE of M_r ~30,000 Da. Cleavage with *N*-glycosidase F resolves the microheterogeneity in size on SDS-PAGE and identifies dog (Raymond and Caughey, 1989), human (Schechter, 1990), but not rat chymase as a glycopro-

Factor IX Nagoya

Rat mast cell chymase activated factor IX Nagoya in vitro (Suchiro et al., 1989), but the physiological relevance of this finding is likely to be limited.

Neuropeptides

Like tryptase, dog mastocytoma chymase digests VIP but, unlike tryptase, also hydrolyzes substance P. Thus, unlike tryptase, which promotes bronchoconstriction, chymase inactivates a potential bronchoconstrictor (SP) and a bronchodilator (VIP) (Caughey et al., 1988b). Human skin chymase also digests substance P (Wintroub and Kaempfer, unpublished observations, 1987).

Gelatinase

A protease from rat peritoneal mast cells similar to rat mast cell chymase activated human granulocyte gelatinase (Sopata et al., 1986).

Matrix Proteins

Rat chymase was shown to hydrolyze purified human type IV collagen in vitro (Sage et al., 1979) and fibronectin (Vartio et al., 1981), but not types I, II, and III collagen. The intercellular matrix proteoglycans (Seppa et al., 1979) also demonstrated changes after incubation with rat chymase. Several other studies have reported matrix degradation associated with rat mast cell degranulation, but have not employed specific inhibitors (Dabbous et al., 1986; Patrick et al., 1988). These findings should be extrapolated with caution, as human skin strips incubated with human chymase demonstrated no immunohistochemical or morphological changes in type IV collagen, laminin, bullous pemphigoid antigen, or type VII collagen (Briggaman et al., 1984), as discussed below.

Myelin Proteins

Released supernatants from rat serosal mast cells degraded bovine myelin protein P_0 and myelin basic protein, releasing fragments that were secretagogues for rat mast cells. However, no inhibitors were used to identify the protease(s) involved (Johnson et al., 1988).

F. Chymase as Secretagogue

Whereas tryptase has anticoagulant properties and may be important as a mitogen and potentiator of bronchoconstriction, chymase has unique properties in inducing secretion from several cell types, a potentially important role in vivo.

Activation of Mast Cells

Rat chymase binds to rat mast cells at 1°C without inducing release. However, it induces activation of rat mast cells with 50% net percent dose-dependent release of β-hexosaminidase and generation of PGD_2 when chymase in solution is removed and the temperature is raised to 25°C (Schick et al., 1984; Schick and Austen, 1986). Heparin blocked this release. The release was Ca^{2+} but not Mg^{2+} dependent, although chymase binding at 1°C was cation independent. DFP and LBTI block this reaction if added within the first 10 min of interaction of mast cells and chymase at 1°C (Schick and Austen, 1986, 1989). Evidence suggests that chymase activation might be mediated by the chymase-specific cleavage of a trypsin-sensitive 90-kDa membrane protein on rat serosal mast cells (Schick, 1990). This system has allowed the separation of stimulation and exocytosis stages of rat mast cell activation by rat chymase. It has not been investigated using human materials. It may be relevant clinically, but must be studied in a species-specific manner. Injection of rat chymase into human, rabbit, or rat skin induced wheals and pruritus (Hagermark et al., 1972; Fraki, 1977; Seppa, 1980; Hatcher et al., 1977). However, injection of dog chymase into dog skin does not result in wheals (Rubenstein et al., 1990), and injection of human chymase into human skin caused erythema after 10–20 min and slight induration at several hours (Fraki, 1977).

Aside from its role as secretagogue, chymase or a chymase-like enzyme may be involved in exocytosis caused by other mast cell activators, as discussed earlier. Chymase inhibitors or antichymase F(ab)2 inhibited histamine release induced by antigen, but chymostatin alone inhibited calcium ionophore-induced histamine release from dispersed rat mast cells (Katunuma et al., 1986). The inhibition correlated with the amounts of inhibitors of chymase that accumulated in rat mast cell secretory granules (Katunuma and Kido, 1988; Kido et al., 1988). This inhibitory effect was also demonstrated for human lung mast cells after ionophore-induced release (but not for rat peritoneal mast cells) using DFP and TPCK, but not TLCK (Hultsch et al., 1988). However, the presence of chymase in only a small percentage of human pulmonary mast cells suggests that another protease, and not chymase, may be involved.

Secretion of Airway Gland Serous Cells

Dog chymase, but not tryptase, induces secretion of ^{35}S-labeled mucopolysaccharides, mainly chondroitin sulfate proteoglycans, from cultured bovine tracheal gland serous cells (Sommerhoff et al., 1989). Chymase is a more potent secretagogue for cultured bovine tracheal gland serous cells than histamine or bradykinin, but is not mediated through the second messengers cAMP, inositol phosphates, protein kinase C, or cytoplasmic Ca^{2+} (Sommerhoff et al., 1990).

Chymase-Induced Release of Tracheal Epithelial Cell Sulfated Macromolecular Glycoconjugates

Dog mast cell chymase and several other mammalian and bacterial proteases increase the release of sulfated macromolecular glycoconjugates from dog tracheal epithelial cells in culture. The conjugates are synthesized by the cells and are then transported to apical cell surfaces and are released when these surfaces are exposed to extracellular proteases (Varsano et al., 1987). The contribution of protease-mediated release of glycoconjugates to airway inflammation remains to be studied in vivo in humans.

LDL and Cholesterol Uptake into Macrophages

The uptake of cholesterol into mouse macrophages in culture is facilitated by binding of LDL to proteoglycans from rat mast cells (Kokkonen and Kovanen, 1987a,b, 1989). Apolipoprotein B is digested in LDL by chymase. Carboxypeptidase further digests chymase-generated peptides, but inhibition of chymase and not carboxypeptidase prevents the hydrolysis of LDL (Kokkonen et al., 1986). Mast cell granules inhibited by SBTI increase macrophage LDL accumulation 10-fold, but enzymatically active granules increase the uptake 50-fold. This uptake correlates with apolipoprotein degradation and LDL fusion into larger particles by fusion of lipid cores. These results were replicated in vivo in the peritoneal cavity of rats stimulated by 48/80 and coinjected with ^{14}C-labeled LDL (Kokkonen, 1989). Preliminary data suggested that released human mast cell supernatants also degrade Apo B-100 (Gonen et al., 1987). This hydrolysis was only partly inhibited by SBTI and was augmented by heparin, suggesting a possible role for mast cell tryptase as well.

It is not known whether this phenomenon occurs in humans, but receptor-mediated pathways for oxidized LDL and acetylated cholesterol uptake into macrophages have been identified (Parthasarthy et al., 1989). These are much more active systems than the LDL receptor-mediated uptake of cholesterol, as they are not down-regulated by uptake of LDL. Although mast cell protease-mediated uptake of cholesterol has not been demonstrated in human macrophages, one might speculate that protease digestion of apolipoprotein could be a mechanism for altering LDL for alternative pathways of uptake. Alternatively, the increased uptake of macrophages may be due to the aggregation of proteolytically altered LDL (Kokkonen and Kovanen, 1989) and has also been documented after experimental aggregation induced by vortexing (Khoo et al., 1988).

Effect of Chymase on Fibroblasts

Murine mast cell chymase has been implicated in the effects of released mouse mast cells cocultured with fibroblasts on subsequent fibroblast morphology (Ginsburg et al., 1989). However, the effect of activated mast cells was inhibited by SBTI but not PMSF, both of which inhibit chymase. Purified human chymase from skin (0.2 μg/ml) inhibited protein synthesis in cultured human fibroblasts and was cytotoxic (Hatcher et al., 1977).

G. Effects on Model Systems

Blistering in the Skin

Human skin strips were incubated with purified human skin chymase (Briggaman et al., 1984). After 4–6 hr in 70–100 nM or 6–8 hr with 10–25 nM enzyme, loss of anchoring filaments and widening of the lamina lucida of the dermo-epidermal junction was seen, followed by separation of the epidermis and dermis at the lamina lucida. The epidermis showed few changes and the dermis was not affected. It is interesting that no changes in type IV collagen were seen, as would be predicted by the in vitro studies using rat chymase and purified human type IV collagen discussed above, emphasizing again the need for caution in extrapolating from studies using nonhuman materials and purified preparations. It has been thought that mast cell chymase may contribute to blistering in diseases such as bullous pemphigoid, but thus far proteases isolated from blister fluid do not fit the inhibitor profile of chymase (Naito et al., 1982). Chymase has been proposed, but not yet demonstrated, to possibly cause the blistering seen occasionally in children with cutaneous mastocytosis (Schwartz, 1989).

Airway Responsiveness

Efferent peptidergic neurons release VIP in the airways, mediating nonadrenergic airway smooth muscle relaxation. Chymase was able to reverse the effect of VIP relaxation of ferret trachial rings precontracted by serotonin. Tryptase was more potent in reversing the effect of VIP (Franconi et al., 1989). Chymase also cleaves substance P, a potential bronchoconstrictor (Caughey et al., 1988b). However, the importance of chymase in modulating pulmonary neuropeptide effects remains to be determined because of the scarcity of MC_{TC}-type mast cells in lung and the unresponsiveness of lung mast cells to substance P (Caughey, 1989).

Neutrophil Chemotaxis

Neither chymase nor heparin isolated from rat mast cell granules appears to cause chemoattraction of rat neutrophils in vitro using a microchemotaxis chamber assay (LeManske et al., 1987). However, purified human chymase caused infiltration of polymorphonuclear cells after injection into rabbit skin (Hatcher et al., 1977; Fraki, 1977), and injection of chymase is followed by infiltration of neutrophils in rat skin (Katunuma et al., 1986). In addition, proteolytic chymase-induced fragments of rat IgG were chemotactic to human neutrophils in a chamber assay, but chymase alone was not.

Muscle Cell Regulation

In fasting diabetic rats, mast cell granules were seen by immunofluorescence in the extracellular space and inside some myofibers and their cytoplasm, suggesting that muscle cells may take up mast cell granules (Stauber et al., 1986). Chymase activity increased by 150% in rat skeletal muscle after rats fasted for 3 days (Kuehn et al., 1988). This was due to a lowering of a chymase inhibitor, chymostatin. The significance of mast cell chymase activity in muscle wasting in rats or in human muscle tissue is speculative.

H. In Vivo Reactions

Regulation of Neuropeptides Released Locally

In vivo evidence has been presented that demonstrates the ability of mast cell proteases to regulate neuropeptide activity in skin (Brain and Williams, 1988). The long-lasting erythema caused by calcitonin gene related peptide (CGRP) injected into human skin in vivo was decreased six-fold by coinjection of SP, but not by neurokinins A or B (which cannot activate mast cells) or histamine, implicating mast cell release caused by SP. Coinjection of 48/80 with CGRP to locally activate mast cells also inhibited the erythema, but 48/80 and SBTI (which inhibits mast cell chymase) has no effect on CGRP-induced erythema. These experiments postulated that the release of SP, colocalized with CGRP, from sensory nerves would be capable of activating immediately adjacent mast cells, which in turn would release neutral proteases (tryptase and chymase) capable of hydrolyzing, and thereby down-regulating, the released neuropeptides. This study was a key observation of the potential homeostatic regulation of cutaneous nerve function by mast cell proteases in situ.

Wheal Formation and Vasopermeability

Chymase from dog skin mastocytomas augments the size of histamine-, antigen-, and 48/80-induced wheals in dog skin, although chymase alone does not cause wheals. Chymase caused wheal formation with subthreshold histamine doses. This effect is inhibited by prior incubation of chymase with SBTI or preinjection with SBTI and/or an H1 antihistamine (Rubenstein et al., 1990). Thus chymase, like tryptase, may act as a modulator of the effects of histamine. While rat chymase induces vasopermeability after injection into rat skin (Seppa, 1980), as did human enzyme injected into rabbit skin (Fraki, 1977), the mechanism for these effects is not clear.

I. Diseases

Cystic Fibrosis

A preliminary study reported an increase in MC_{TC} in bronchial epithelium from patients with cystic fibrosis (Schwartz et al., 1987d). Since chymase can promote in vitro hypersecretion of serous gland cells and epithelial cells in this location in vivo, it was speculated that mast cell proteases might contribute to the pathophysiology of this disease and to hypersecretion in vivo (Nadel, 1989).

Asthma

Since (1) tryptase potentiates the smooth muscle contractility of histamine (Sekizawa et al., 1989) and (2) tryptase and chymase reverse the contractility of VIP (Franconi et al., 1989), it has been speculated that these proteases may play a role in controlling bronchial airway tone and contribute to bronchospasm in disease (Nadel, 1989). As discussed above, tryptase protein has been identified in bronchoalveolar lavage fluids in atopic asthmatics but not nonatopic asthmatics reacting to antigen challenge. Studies are still required to determine the release, fate, and effect of mast cell proteases on tissue in nonatopic asthmatics, with bronchospasm.

Endotoxic Shock

Inhibition of chymase, cathepsin G, and leukocyte elastase by Eglin C reduced the extravasation of protein after endotoxin shock in pigs (Siebeck, et al., 1989). However, it is not clear whether mast cells are released in endotoxin shock in humans, as tryptase was not detected in serum in septic shock in humans (Schwartz et al, 1987c). Which of these enzymes, if any, plays a predominant role in this condition is not known.

Pruritus

Injection of various non–mast cell proteases induced itch without other cutaneous sign (Arthur and Shelley, 1955). Rat mast cell chymase caused pruritus, wheal, and flare in human skin (Hagermark et al., 1972).

IV. Mast Cell Carboxypeptidase

A. Introduction

Carboxypeptidase (CP) activities were first detected in rat liver (Haas et al., 1979), rat peritoneal mast cells (Everitt and Neurath, 1980), and rat skeletal muscle (Bodwell and Meyer, 1981). Mast cell CP was also detected in mouse bone marrow mast cells (BMMC) and in BALB/c serosal mast cells (Serafin et al., 1987). Because spectrophotometric assays using synthetic dipeptide substrates are too insensitive to detect CP activity in crude extracts or released supernatants of mast cells, human mast cell CP was first detected in preparations of dispersed lung mast cells using a sensitive HPLC assay of the cleavage of the carboxyterminal His^9–Leu^{10} bond of angiotensin I (AI), yielding des-Leu^{10} AI (Goldstein et al., 1987). Mast cell CP activity was demonstrated in >99% pure dispersed mast cells from lung. Its net percent release after immunological stimulation correlated with the net percent release of histamine, localizing CP to lung mast cell secretory granules. CP activity was also detected in whole skin extracts and preparations of dispersed skin cells that contained fibroblasts,

F. Release of Mast Cell Proteases and Relation to the Macromolecular Heparin Proteoglycan-Protein Complex in Mast Cell Secretory Granules

Although the various proteases from mast cells have been studied in their purified form, several investigators have demonstrated that they are released from mast cells of all studied species in the form of a high-molecular-weight complex of protein and proteoglycans (Serafin et al., 1987; Schwartz et al., 1981c, 1982). The CP from rat serosal mast cells is released as part of a macromolecular complex that contains chymase, β-hexosaminidase, and presumably other unidentified constituents ionically linked to heparin proteoglycan (Schwartz et al., 1982). This complex remains bound to the extracellular surface of mast cells after release from secretory granules, while histamine readily diffuses away (Schwartz et al., 1981c, 1982). Conditions using high salt concentrations are required to dissociate this complex from mast cells and to extract its individual constituents. Using sucrose density gradient sedimentation and Dowex chromatography as assays of complex dissociation, β-hexosaminidase, chymase, CP, and heparin progressively dissociated after treatment of the complex with 0.15 *M* NaCl up to 3 *M* NaCl (Schwartz et al., 1982).

^{35}S-labeled mouse bone marrow mast cells activated by calcium ionophore release a macromolecular complex of $>10^7$ MW, which eluted in the void volume of Sepharose CL-2B gel filtration (Serafin et al., 1987). The complex comprised 65% of the released CP from these cells, with the remainder of CP eluting in a broad peak of somewhat $>$200,000 MW, probably bound to chondroitin sulfate E proteoglycans.

In human mast cells as well, it appears that CP and chymase are the most tightly bound of the neutral proteases (Goldstein et al., 1992). The large number of basic residues in human and rat mast cell CP and its basic isoelectric point contribute to the high affinity of CP for heparin proteoglycans in the complex (Everitt and Neurath, 1980; Goldstein et al., 1989a,b; Serafin et al., 1987; Reynolds et al., 1989). Sonication of human mast cells from lung or skin in the presence of physiological salt concentrations results in the release of a high-MW complex consisting of tryptase, chymase, and CP, which elutes just after the void volume using Sephacryl S-200 gel filtration (Goldstein et al., 1989b). CP progressively dissociates from this complex after treatment with 1–4 *M* NaCl, appearing at a MW between 30,000 and 35,000 Da. The CP from skin mast cells appears to require higher salt concentrations than the CP from lung mast cells for full dissociation. Recent studies using human skin mast cells demonstrate that mast cell carboxypeptidase and chymase are exocytoses in complexes that are distinct from and of higher molecular weight than complexes containing tryptase (Goldstein et al. 1992).

G. Carboxypeptidase as a Marker of Mast Cell Heterogeneity

When cocultured with 3T3 fibroblasts (Serafin et al., 1987), mouse bone marrow mast cells (BMMC), which are mucosal-like mast cells, assume a morphology and chemical profile that is similar to serosal mast cells with respect to safranin staining and histamine and proteoglycan content. In this system $\approx$50% of the BMMC are serosal-like after 28 days in culture. At the same time, CP levels increase from $\approx$0.004 U to 0.36 U/10^6 mast cells, compared to 1.4 U for pure BALB/c serosal mast cells. Thus, CP in mouse mast cells may be a marker for the differentiated serosal-like mast cell phenotype. The study of carboxypeptidase gene expression in mouse mast cells is reviewed in another chapter.

The levels of CP in human mast cells vary with respect to age and donor site (Goldstein et al., 1989a). Activity levels of CP have been measured in mast cells from adult lung, neonatal and adult foreskin, and adult facial skin. These are 15, 17, 564, and 173 U/10^6 mast cells, respectively, where 1 U = 1 nmol des-Leu 10 AI generated per minute. CP activity was measured as 406 U/10^6 mast cells from the foreskin of an 11-month old child, suggesting that CP activity in skin mast cells increases from a low level to that approaching the adult within the first year of life (Goldstein et al., unpublished observations, 1988). Using a specific activity of 36 U/μg of protein for purified skin mast cell CP, the amount of CP in human mast cells was estimated to be 0.4, 0.5, 5, and 16 μg/10^6 for adult lung, neonatal foreskin, adult facial skin, and foreskin mast cells, respectively. The levels in adult foreskin fall between that of chymase (4.5 μg) and tryptase (35 μg) per 10^6 adult foreskin mast cells (Schwartz et al., 1987a). The distribution of human mast cell CP with age and donor site correlates closely with that reported for mast cell chymase and has recently been established by in situ localization by immunohistochemistry (Irani et al., 1991), as described in another chapter.

V. Concluding Comments

The fact that mast cells, like pancreatic acinar cells, contain enzymes with tryptic and chymotryptic activities, as well as a carboxypeptidase, suggests analogous roles for mast cells and the pancreas as physiological effectors of protein and peptide digestion, although the storage of enzymes (active versus zymogen), route of delivery, and site of action are certainly different (Austen, 1989). This analogy is further highlighted by the homology of consensus regulatory sequences in RMCP II (Sarid et al., 1989) and human tryptase (Vanderslice et al., 1990a) to pancreatic CPs, and by the homology of human mast cell carboxypeptidase with pancreatic CPA and CPB (Reynolds et al., 1989; Natsuaki et al., 1992). Research over the last decade has revealed that these proteases also have the potential for modulating humoral and cellular events in tissue, including regulation of vascular and airway tone, vasopermeability, inflammatory cell response, secretion, growth regulation, neuropeptide modulation, coagulation, lipoprotein metabolism, tissue destruction, intercellular protein and peptide processing, and hydrolysis of inflammatory mediators. Understanding the role of these proteases in vivo will require elucidating the multiple biochemical, cellular, and tissue events that converge to cause the clinical spectrum of complex diseases affecting tissues such as the airways, gut, and skin. For example, understanding what mediators actually cause baseline vascular airway tone in health and disease will help determine how mast cells modify that state. Conversely, determining the release, activity, fate, and time course of release of mast cells proteases in each tissue in different disease states is also an essential goal of future studies. Models will also have to be developed to study specific microenvironments where subsets of mast cells may function. The current development and future use in vivo of specific inhibitors of these proteases will play a significant role in facilitating our understanding of their function.

Discussion

Austen: Have you identified a human mast cell aminopeptidase?
Goldstein: We are looking for it and have identified such an activity in unpurified dispersed mast cells but do not know whether its release correlates with histamine release.
Hanifin: Trypsin injected into skin causes itch. What is the relationship of tryptase to trypsin and does tryptase cause itch or mast cell degranulation?
Goldstein: No study has been performed to study the pruritogenic potential of tryptase. Rat chymase does cause itch when injected into human skin.
Schwartz: Is there sequential activity between chymase and carboxypeptidases on protease substrates?
Goldstein: Yes. The best evidence comes from the study of Kokkonen et al. (1986) where rat chymase hydrolyzes the lipoprotein B of LDL and carboxypeptidase releases free amino acids from chymase-induced fragments.
Casale: Do mast cells have any peptidases that break down the tachykinins?
Goldstein: Caughey could not demonstrate cleavage of neurokinin A or B by tryptase. Chymase, but not tryptase, hydrolyzes substance P.
Austen: Please review the evidence for four human tryptase genes.
Goldstein: All the skin cDNA clones came from a library made from the skin from a single individual. cDNA I and a genomic clone are identical and represent one gene. β and II are identical with one N-glycosylation site and represent a second gene product. A third gene product, α, has 244 amino acids and amino acid substitutions at positions 21–23. cDNA III is similar to α in these sub-

stitutions, but has 245 amino acids and two N-linked glycosylation sites like I, and represents a fourth possible gene product. III and α have 32 nucleotide differences between them in the catalytic portion alone.

References

Alter, S. C., and Schwartz, L. B. (1989). Effect of histamine and divalent cations on the activity and stability of tryptase from human mast cells. *Biochim. Biophys. Acta.* 991:426–430.

Alter, S. C., Metcalfe, D. D., Bradford, T. R., and Schwartz, L. B. (1987a). Regulation of human mast cell tryptase. Effects of enzyme concentration, ionic strength and the structure and negative charge density of polysaccharides. *Biochem. J.* 248:821–827.

Alter, S. C., Yates, P., Margolius, H. S., and Schwartz, L. B. (1987b). Tryptase and kinin generation: tryptase from human mast cells does not activate human urinary prokallikrein. *Int. Arch. Allergy Appl. Immunol.* 83:321–324.

Alter, S. C., Lammle, B., Griffin, J. H., and Schwartz, L. B. (1988). Tryptase from human mast cells does not activate purified human Hageman factor. *Clin. Allergy* 18:151–155.

Alter, S. C., Kramps, J. A., Janoff, A., and Schwartz, L. B. (1990). Interactions of human mast cell tryptase with biological protease inhibitors. *Arch. Biochem. Biophys.* 276:26–31.

Arthur, R. P., and Shelley, W. B. (1955). Experimental evidence for an enzymatic basis for itching in man. *Nature* 175:901–902.

Austen, K. F. (1989). In *IgE, Mast Cells and the Allergic Response*. New York, Wiley, p. 46.

Baumgarten, C. R., Nichols, R. C., Naclerio, R. M., Lichtenstein, L. M., Norman, P. S., and Proud, D. (1986). Plasma kallikrein during experimentally induced allergic rhinitis: role in kinin formation and contribution to TAME-esterase activity in nasal secretions. *J. Immunol.* 137:977–982.

Benditt, E. P., and Arase M. (1959). An enzyme in mast cells with properties like chymotrypsin. *J. Exp. Med.* 110:451–460.

Benfey, P. N., Yin, F. H., and Leder, P. (1987). RMCP II. Evidence for cell-specific expression and a multigene family. *J. Biol. Chem.* 262:5377–5384.

Bodwell, J. E., and Meyer, W. L. (1981). Purification and characterization of carboxypeptidase A from rat skeletal muscle. *Biochemistry* 20:2767–2777.

Brain, S. D., and Williams, T. J. (1988). Substance P regulates the vasodilator activity of calcitonin gene-related peptide. *Nature* 135:73–75.

Briggaman, R. A., Schechter, N. M., Fraki, J., and Lazarus, G. S. (1984). Degranulation of the epidermal dermal junction by proteolytic enzymes from human skin and human polymorphonuclear leukocytes. *J. Exp. Med.* 160:1027–1042.

Broide, D. H., Eisman, S., Ramsdell, J. W., Ferguson, P., Schwartz, L. B., and Wasserman, S. I. (1990). Airway levels of mast cell-derived mediators in exercise-induced asthma. *Am. Rev. Respir. Dis.* 141:563–568.

Bunnett, N. W., Goldstein, S. M., and Nakazato, P. (1992). Neuropeptide-degrading enzymes in human gastric tissue. Isolation of a carboxypeptidase-24.11 and aminopeptidase activity *Gastroenterology*. 102:76–87.

Butterfield, J. H., Weiler, D. A., Hunt, L. W., and Roche, P. C. (1990). Purification of tryptase from a human mast cell line. *J. Leuk. Biol.* 47:409–419.

Castells, M., and Schwartz, L. B. (1988). Tryptase levels in nasal-lavage fluid as an indicator of the immediate allergic response. *J. Allergy Clin. Immunol.* 82(3 pt 1):348–355.

Caughey, G. H. (1989). Roles of mast cell tryptase and chymase in airway function. *Am. J. Physiol.* 257:L39–L46.

Caughey, G. H. (1990). Tryptase and chymase in dog mast cells. *Monogr. Allergy* 27:67–89.

Caughey, G. H., Viro, N. F., Ramachandran, J., Lazarus, S. C., Borson, D. B., and Nadel, J. A. (1987). Dog mastocytoma tryptase: affinity purification, characterization, and amino-terminal sequence. *Arch. Biochem. Biophys.* 258:555–563.

Caughey, G. H., Viro, F., Calonico, D., McDonald, D. M., Lazarus, S. C., and Gold, W. M. (1988a). Chymase and tryptase in dog mastocytoma cells: asynchronous expression as revealed by enzyme cytochemical staining. *J. Histochem. Cytochem.* 36:1053–1060.

Caughey, G. H., Leidig, F., Viro, F., and Nadel, J. A. (1988b). Substance P and vasoactive intestinal peptide degradation by mast cell tryptase and chymase. *J. Pharmacol. Exp. Ther.* 244:133–137.

Caughey, G. H., Viro, N. F., Lazarus, S. C., and Nadel, J. A. (1988c). Purification and characterization of dog mastocytoma chymase: Identification of an octapeptide conserved in chymotryptic leukocyte proteinases. *Biochim. Biophys Acta* 952:142–149.

Caughey, G. H., Lazarus, S. C., Viro, N. F., Gold, W. M., and Nadel, J. A. (1988d). Tryptase and chymase: Comparison of extraction and release in two dog mastocytoma lines. *Immunology* 63:339–344.

Caughey, G. H., Raymond, W. W., and Vanderslice, P. (1990). Dog mast cell chymase: molecular cloning and characterization. *Biochemistry* 29:5166–5171.

Caughey G. H., Zerweck E. H., and Vanderslice P. (1991). Structure, chromosomal assignment, and deduced amino acid sequence of a human gene for mast cell chymase. *J. Biol. Chem.* 266:12956–12963.

Chiu, H., and Lagunoff, D. (1972). Histochemical comparison of vertebrate mast cells. *Histochem. J.* 4:135–144.

Chu, W., Johnson, D. A., and Musich, P. R. (1990). Identification and molecular cloning of a mouse mast cell tryptase. *FASEB J.* 4:A2159.

Claman, H. N. (1989). On scleroderma, mast cells, endothelial cells, and fibroblasts. *JAMA* 262:1206–1209.

Cochrane, D. E., Carraway, R. E., and Boucher. (1990). Degradation of neurotensin (NT) by mast cells. *J. Cell Biol.* 3:309a.

Cox, S. W., and Eley, B. M. (1989a). Identification of a tryptase-like enzyme in extracts of inflamed human gingiva by affector and gel-filtration studies. *Arch. Oral Biol.* 34:219–221.

Cox, S. W., and Eley, B. M. (1989b) Detection of cathepsin B- and L-, elastase-, tryptase-, trypsin-, and dipeptidyl peptidase IV-like activities in crevicular fluid from gingivitis and periodontitis patients with peptidyl derivatives of 7-amino-4-trifluoromethyl coumarin. *J. Peridont. Res.* 24:353–361.

Craig, S. S., DeBlois, G., and Schwartz, L. B. (1986). Mast cells in human keloid, small intestine, and lung by an immunoperoxidase technique using a murine monoclonal antibody against tryptase. *Am. J. Pathol.* 124:427–435.

Cromlish, J. A., Seidah, N. G., Marcinkiewicz, M., Hamelin, J., Johnson, D. A., and Chretien, M. (1987). Human pituitary tryptase: molecular forms, NH2-terminal sequence, immunocytochemical localization, and specificity with prohormone and fluorogenic substrates. *J. Biol. Chem.* 262:1363–1373.

Dabbous, M. K. L., Walker, R., Haney, L., Carter, L. M., Nicolson, G. L., and Woolley, D. E. (1986). Mast cells and matrix degradation at sites of tumour invasion in rat mammary adenocarcinoma. *Br. J. Cancer* 54:459–465.

Dahodawala, I., Schulman, E. S., Raible, D. G., Post, T. J., and Scavicchio, K. (1990). Histamine and human lung mast cell supernatants stimulate human fibroblast proliferation. *FASEB J.* 4:A1941.

Eley, B. M., and Cox, S. W. (1990). A biochemical study of serine proteinase activities at local gingival tissue sites in human chronic periodontitis. *Arch. Oral. Biol.* 35:23–27.

Everitt, M. T., and Neurath, H. (1980). Rat peritoneal mast cell carboxypeptidase: Localization, purification and enzymatic properties. *FEBS Lett.* 110:292.

Fraki, J. E. (1977). Human skin proteases: Effect of separated proteases on vascular permeability and leukocyte emigration in skin. *Acta Dermatovenereol.* 57:393–398.

Fraki, J. E., and Hopsu-Havu, V. (1975). Human skin proteases. Separation and characterization of two alkaline proteases, one splitting trypsin nd other chymotrypsin substrates. *Arch. Dermatol. Res.* 253:261.

Franconi, G. M., Graf, P. D., Lazarus, S. G., Nadel, J. A., and Caughey, G. H. (1989). Mast cell tryptase and chymase reverse airway smooth muscle relaxation induced by vasoactive intestinal peptide in the ferret. *J. Pharmacol. Exp. Ther.* 248:947–951.

Fritz, H. (1988) Human mucus proteinase inhibitor (human MPI). Human seminal inhibitor I (HUSI-I), antileukoprotease (ALP), secretory leukocyte protease inhibitor (SLPI). *Biol. Chem. Hoppe-Seyler* 369(Suppl):79–82.

Gervasoni, J. E., Jr., Conrad, D. H., Hugli, T. E., Schwartz, L. B., and Ruddy, S. (1986). Degradation of human anaphylatoxin C3a by rat peritoneal mast cells: A role for the secretory granule enzyme chymase and heparin proteoglycan. *J. Immunol.* 136:285–292.

Ginsburg, H., Amiro, M., Padawar, J., and Davidson, S. (1989). Structural alterations in fibroblast monolayers caused by mast cell degranulation. *J. Leukocyt. Biol.* 45:491–497.

Glenner, C. G., and Cohen, L. A. (1960). Histochemical demonstration of a species-specific trypsin like enzyme in mast cells. *Nature* 185:846–847.

Glenner, G. G., Hopsu, V. K., and Cohen, L. A. (1982). Histochemical demonstration of a trypsin-like esterase activity in mast cells. *J. Histochem. Cytochem.* 10:109–110.

Goetzl, E. J., Finch, R. J., Peterson, K. E., Turck, C. W., and Sreedharan, S. P. (1989).

Mast cell and basophil mediation of lymphocyte functions. In *Mast Cell and Basophil Differentiation and Function in Health and Disease*. Edited by S. J. Galli and K. F. Austen. New York, Raven Press, pp. 247–254.

Goldstein, S. M., Kaempfer, C. E., Proud, D., Schwartz, L. B., Irani, A. M., and Wintroub, B. U. (1987). Identification and partial characterization of human mast cell carboxypeptidase. *J. Immunol.* 139:2724–2729.

Goldstein, S. M., Kaempfer, C. E., Kealy, J. P., and Wintroub, B. U. (1989a). Human mast cell carboxypeptidase. Purification and characterization. *J. Clin. Invest.* 83:1630–1636.

Goldstein, S. M., Kaempfer, C. E., and Wintroub, B. U. (1989b). Proteoglycan binding of human skin mast cell carboxypeptidase and other secretory granule proteases. *J. Invest. Dermatol.* 92:435.

Goldstein, S. M., Leong, J., and Bunnett, N. (1991). Human mast cell proteases hydrolyze neurotensin, kinetensin and [Leu^5] enkephalin. *Peptides* 12:995–1000.

Goldstein, S. M. Leong, J., Schwartz, L. B., and Cooke D. (1992). The protease composition of exocytosed human skin mast cell protease—proteoglycan complexes: tryptase resides in a complex distinct from chymase and carboxypeptidase. *J. Immunol.* (in press).

Gonen, B., Post, T. J., Quinn, T. J., and Schulman, E. J. (1987). Enzymes released by human mast cells can digest apoprotein B of low density lipoprotein. *Artherosclerosis* 7:499a.

Gruber, B. L., and Schwartz, L. B. (1990). The mast cell as an effector of connective tissue degradation: A study of matrix susceptibility to human mast cells. *Biochem. Biophys. Res. Commun.* 171:1272–1278.

Gruber, B. L., Schwartz, L. B., Ramamurthy, N. S., Irani, A. M., and Marchese, M. J. (1988). Activation of latent rheumatoid synovial collagenase by human mast cells tryptase. *J. Immunol.* 140:3936–3942.

Gruber, B. L., Marchese, M. J., Suzuki, K., Schwartz, L. B., Okada, Y., Nagase, H., and Ramamurthy, N. S. (1989). Synovial procollagenase activation by human mast cell tryptase dependence upon matrix metalloproteinase 3 activation. *J. Clin. Invest.* 84:1657–1662.

Haas, R., Heinrich, P. C., and Sasse, D. (1979). Proteolytic enzymes of rat liver mitochondria. Evidence for a mast cell origin. *FEBS Lett.* 103:168.

Hagermark, O., Rajka, G., and Bergvist, V. (1972). Experimental itch in human skin by rat mast cell chymase. *Acta Dermatovenereol.* 52:125–128.

Hammel, I., Shiloh-Rabinovich, H., and Nir, I. (1988). Two populations of mast cells on fibroblast monolayers: Correlation of quantitative microscopy and functional activity. *J. Cell Sci.* 91:13–19.

Harvima, I. T., Schechter, N. M., Harvima, R. J., and Fraki, J. E. (1988a). Human skin tryptase: Purification, partial characterization and comparison with human lung tryptase. *Biochim. Biophys. Acta.* 957:71–80.

Harvima, I. T., Harvima, R. J., Eloranta, T. O., and Fraki, J. E. (1988b). The allosteric effect of salt on human mast cell tryptase. *Biochim. Biophys. Acta.* 956: 133–139.

Harvima, I. T., Naukkarinen, A., Harvima, R. J., and Horsmanheimo, M. (1989a). Enzyme-and immunohistochemical localization of mast cell tryptase in psoriatic skin. *Arch. Dermatol. Res.* 281(6):387–391.

Harvima, I. T., Harvima, R. J., Penttila, I. M., Eloranta, T. O., Horsmanheimo, M., and Fraki, J. E. (1989b). Effect of human mast cell tryptase on human plasma proenzymes. *Int. Arch. Allergy Appl. Immunol.* 90:104–108.

Hatcher, V. B., Lazarus, G. S., Levine, N., Burk, P. G., and Yost, F. J., Jr. (1977). Characterization of a chemotactic and cytotoxic proteinase from human skin. *Biochim. Biophys. Acta.* 483:160–171.

Hopsu, V. K., and Glenner, G. G. (1963). A histochemical enzyme kinetic system applied to the trypsin-like amidase and esterase activity in human mast cells. *J. Cell Biol.* 17:503–520.

Hultsch, T., Ennis, M., and Heidtmann, H. H. (1988). The effect of serine esterase inhibitors on ionophore-induced histamine release from human pulmonary mast cells. *Agents Actions* 23:198–200.

Irani, A. M., Schechter, N. M., Craig, S. S., DeBlois, G., and Schwartz, L. B. (1986). Two types of human mast cells that have distinct neutral protease compositions. *Proc. Natl. Acad. Sci. USA* 83:4464–4468.

Irani, A. M., Bradford, T. R., Kepley, C. L., Schechter, N. M., and Schwartz, L. B. (1989). Detection of MCT and MCTC types of human mast cells by immunohistochemistry using new monoclonal anti-tryptase and anti-chymase antibodies. *J. Histochem. Cytochem.* 37:1509–1515.

Irani, A. A., Goldstein, S. M., Wintroub, B. U., Bradford, T., and Schwartz, L. B. (1991). Human mast cell carboxypeptidase: selective localization to MC_{TC} cells. *J. Immunol.* 147:247–253.

Ishizaka, T. (1981). Analysis of triggering events in mast cells for immunoglobin E–mediated histamine release. *J. Allergy Clin. Immunol.* 67:90–96.

Ito, A., Ihara, H., and Mori, Y. (1980). Partial purification and characterization of a novel neutral proteinase from human uterine cervix. *Biochem. J.* 185:443–450.

Jansen, C. T., and Hopsu-Havu V. (1969). Proteolytic enzymes in the skin. II. A comparative study of homogenates of five mammalian species. *Acta Dermatovenerol.* 49:468–475.

Johnson, D., Seeldrayers, P. A., and Weiner, H. L. (1988). The role of mast cells in demyelination. 1. Myelin proteins are degraded by mast cell proteases and myelin basic protein and P2 can stimulate mast cell degranulation. *Brain Res.* 444:195–198.

Johnson, D. A., and Cawston, T. E. (1985). Human lung mast cell tryptase fails to activate procollagenase or degrade connective proteoglycan. *Biochem. Biophys. Res. Commun.* 132:453–459.

Johnson, L. A., Moon, K. E., and Eisenberg, M. (1986). Purification to homogeneity of the human skin chymotryptic proteinase "chymase." *Anal. Biochem.* 155:358–364.

Kalenderian, R., Raju, L., Roth, W., Schwartz, L. B., Gruber, B., and Janoff, A. (1988). Elevated histamine and tryptase levels in smokers' bronchoalveolar lavage fluid. Do lung mast cells contribute to smokers' emphysema? *Chest* 94:119–123.

Katunuma, N., and Kido, H. (1988). Biological functions of serine proteases in mast cells in allergic inflammation. *J. Cell. Biochem.* 38:291–301.

Katunuma, N., Fukusen, N., and Kido, H. (1986). Biological functions of serine proteases in the granules of rat mast cells. *Adv. Enzyme Reg.* 25:241–255.

Kerouac, R., St.-Pierre, S., and Rioux, F. (1984). Histamine release by neurotensin in the rat hindquarter: Structure-activity studies. *Peptides* 5:695–699.

Khoo, J. C., Miller, E., McLoghlin, P., and Steinberg, D. (1988). Enhanced macrophage uptake of low-density lipoprotein after self-aggregation. *Artherosclerosis* 8:348–358.

Kido, H., Fukusen, N., and Katunuma, N. (1985). Chymotrypsin- and trypsin-type serine proteases in rat mast cells: properties and functions. *Arch. Biochem. Biophys.* 239:436–443.

Kido, H., Fukusen, N., and Katunuma, N. (1988). Antibodies and inhibitor of chymase are incorporated into mast cell granules and inhibit histamine release. *Biol. Chem. Hoppe-Seyler* 369 (Suppl):95–100.

Kokkonen, J. O. (1989). Stimulation of rat peritoneal mast cells enhances uptake of low density lipoproteins by rat peritoneal macrophages in vivo. *Arteriosclerosis* 79:213–223.

Kokkonen, J. O., and Kovanen, P. T. (1987a). Low-density-lipoprotein binding by mast-cell granules. Demonstration of binding of apolipoprotein B to heparin proteoglycan of exocytosed granules. *Biochem. J.* 241:583–589.

Kokkonen, J. O., and Kovanen, P. T. (1987b). Stimulation of mast cells leads to cholesterol accumulation in macrophages in vitro by a mast cell granule-mediated uptake of low density lipoprotein. *Proc. Natl. Acad. Sci. USA* 84:2287–2291.

Kokkonen, J. O., and Kovanen, P. T. (1989). Proteolytic enzymes of mast cell granules degrade low density lipoproteins and promote their granule-mediated uptake by macrophages in vitro. *J. Biol. Chem.* 264:10749–10755.

Kokkonen, J. O., Vartiainen, M., and Kovanen, P. T. (1986). Low density lipoprotein degradation by secretory granules of rat mast cells. Sequential degradation of apolipoprotein B by granule chymase and carboxypeptidase. *J. Biol. Chem.* 261:16067–16072.

Koren, H. S., Hatch, G. E., and Graham, D. E. (1990). Nasal lavage as a tool in assessing acute inflammation in response to inhaled pollutant. *Toxicology* 60:15–25.

Kuehn, L., Dahlmann, B., Heath, R., and Kay, J. (1988). Changes in proteinase/proteinase inhibitor levels in rat skeletal muscle tissue during diabetes and fasting. *Biol. Chem. Hoppe-Seyler* 369 (Suppl):299–305.

Lagunoff, D., and Benditt, E. P. (1963). Proteolytic enzymes of mast cells. *Ann. NY Acad. Sci.* 103:185–198.

Lagunoff, D., and Pritzl, P. (1976). Characterization of rat mast cell granule proteins. *Arch. Biochem. Biophys.* 173:554–563.

LeManske, R. F., Jr., Esser, B., Kopp, D., Asperheim, M., Junk, P., and Tashoff, T. (1987). The biologic activity of mast cell granules. VIII. In in vivo and in vitro characterization of mast cell granule-derived inflammatory factors involved in rat late phase reactions. *J. Allergy Clin. Immunol.* 79:32–39.

LeTrong, H., Neurath, H., and Woodbury, R. G. (1987a) Substrate specificity of the chymotrypsin-like protease in secretory granules isolated from rat mast cells. *Proc. Natl. Acad. Sci. USA* 84:364–367.

LeTrong, H., Parmelee, D. C., Walsh, K. A., Neurath, H., and Woodbury, R. G. (1987b). Aminoacid sequence of rat protease I (chymase). *Biochemistry* 26:6988–6994.

Login, G. R., Galli, S. J., Morgan, E., Arizono, N., Schwartz, L. B., and Dvorak,

A. M. (1987). Rapid microwave fixation of rat mast cells. I. Localization of granule chymase with an ultrastructural postembedding immunogold technique. *Lab. Invest.* 57:592–599.

Lohi, J., Harvima, I., and Keski-Oja, J. (1990). Pericellular substrates of human mast cell tryptase: 66 kDa gelatinase and fibronectin. *J. Cell Biol.* 111:16a.

Meier, H. L., Heck, L. W., Schulman, E. S., and MacGlashan, D. W., Jr. (1985). Purified human mast cells and basophils release human elastase and cathepsin G by an IgE-mediated mechanism. *Int. Arch. Allergy Appl. Immunol.* 77:179–183.

Meier, M., Spragg, J., and Schwartz, L. B. (1983). Inactivation of human high molecular weight kininogen by human mast cell tryptase. *J. Immunol.* 130:2352–2356.

Miller, H. R. P., Huntley, J. F., and Newlands, G. F. J., Mackellar, A., Irvine, J., Haig, D. M., MacDonald, A., Lammas, A. D., Wakelin, D., and Woodbury, R. G. (1989a). Mast cell granule proteases in mouse and rat: a guide to mast cell heterogeneity and activation in the gastrointestinal tract. In *Mast Cell and Basophil Differentiation and Function in Health and Disease*. Edited by S. J. Galli and K. F. Austen. New York, Raven Press, pp. 81–91.

Miller, J. S., Westin, E. H., and Schwartz, L. B. (1989b). Cloning and characterization of complementary DNA for human tryptase. *J. Clin. Invest.* 84:1188–1195.

Miller, J. S., Moxley, G., and Schwartz, L. B. (1990). Cloning and characterization of a second complementary DNA for human tryptase. *J. Clin. Invest.* 86:864–870.

Moreau, I., Gutman, N., Faucher, D., and Gauthier, F. (1989). Limited proteolysis of I-kininogen (thiostatin). Release of comparable fragments by different endopeptidases. *J. Biol. Chem.* 284:4299–4303.

Nadel, J. A. (1989). Roles of mast cell proteases in airways. *Drugs* 37:51–55.

Naito, K., Morioka, S., and Ogawa, H. (1982). The pathogenic mechanisms of blister formation in bullous pemphigoid. *J. Invest. Dermatol.* 79:303–306.

Natsuaki, M., Stewart C-B., Vanderslice, P., Schwartz, L. B., Natsuaki, M., Wintroub, B. U., Rutter, W. J., and Goldstein, S. M. (1992). Human skin mast cell carboxypeptidase: functional characterization, cDNA cloning, and genealogy. *J. Invest. Dermatol.* (in press).

Osman, I. A., Garrett, J. R., and Smith, R. E. (1989). Enzyme histochemical discrimination between tryptase and chymase in mast cells of human gut. *J. Histochem. Cytochem.* 37:415–421.

Patrick, M. K., Dunn, I. J., Buret, A., Miller, H. R. P., Huntley, J. F., Gibson, S., and Gall, D. G. (1988). Mast cell protease release and mucosal ultrastructure during intestinal anaphylaxis in the rat. *Gastroenterology* 94:1–9.

Parthasarathy, S., Quinn, M. T., Schwenke, D. C., Carew, T. E., and Steinberg, D. (1989). Oxidative modification of beta-very low density lipoprotein. Potential role in monocyte recruitment and foam cell formation. *Arteriosclerosis* 9:398–404.

Powers, J. C., Tanaka, T., Harper, J. W., Minematsu, Y., Barker, L., Lincoln, D., Crumley, K. V., Fraki, J. E., Schechter, N. M., Lazarus, G. G., Nakajima, K., Nakashino, K., Neurath, H., and Woodbury, R. G. (1985). Mammalian chymotrypsin-like enzymes. Comparative reactivities of rat mast cell proteases, human and dog skin chymases, and human cathepsin G with peptide 4-nitroanilide substrates and with peptide chloromethyl ketone and sulfonyl fluoride inhibitors. *Biochemistry* 24:2048–2058.

Proud, D., Siekierski, E. S., and Bailey, G. S. (1988). Identification of human lung mast cell kininogenase as tryptase and relevance of tryptase kininogenase activity. *Biochem. Pharmacol.* 37:1473–1480.

Raymond, W. W., and Caughey, G. H. (1989). N-glycosylation of dog mast cell chymase and tryptase. *FASEB J.* 3:A1333 (abstract).

Reilly, C. F., Schechter, N. B., and Travis, J. (1985). Inactivation of bradykinin and kallidin by cathepsin G and mast cell chymase. *Biochem. Biophys. Res. Commun.* 127:443–449.

Reynolds, D. S., Gurley, D. S., Stevens, R. L., Sugarbaker, D. J., Austen, K. F., and Serafin, W. E. (1989). Cloning of cDNA encoding human mast cell carboxypeptidase A, and comparison with mouse mast cell carboxypeptidase A and rat pancreatic carboxypeptidases. *Proc. Natl. Acad. Sci. USA* 86:9480–9484.

Reynolds, D. S., Gurley, D. S., and Austen, K. S. (1992). Cloning and characterization of the novel gene for mast cell carboxypeptidase *A. J. Clin. Invest.* 89:273–282.

Rubenstein, I., Nadel, J. A., Graf, P. D., and Caughey, G. H. (1990). Mast cell chymase potentiates histamine induced wheal formation in the skin of ragweed allergic dogs. *J. Clin. Invest.* 86:555–559.

Ruoss, S. J., Hartmann, T., and Caughey, G. H. (1991). Mast cell tryptase is a mitogen for cultured fibroblasts. *J. Clin. Investig.* 88:493–499.

Sage, H., Woodbury, R. G., and Bornstein, P. (1979). Structural studies on human type IV collagen. *J. Biol. Chem.* 254:9893–9900.

Sarid, J., Benfey, P. N., and Leder, P. (1989). The mast cell-specific expression of a protease fene, RMCPII, is regulated by an enhancer element that binds specifically to mast cell transacting factors. *J. Biol. Chem.* 264:1022–1026.

Sayama, S., Iozzo, R. V., Lazarus, G. S., and Schechter, N. M. (1987). Human skin chymotrypsin-like proteinase chymase. Subcellular localization to mast cell granules and interaction with heparin and other glycosaminoglycans. *J. Biol. Chem.* 262:6808–6815.

Schechter, N. M. (1990). Human chymase. *Monogr. Allergy* 27:114–131.

Schechter, N. M., Fraki, J. E., Geesin, J. C., and Lazarus, G. S. (1983). Human skin chymotryptic proteinase. Isolation and relation to cathepsin G and rat mast cell proteinase. *J. Biol. Chem.* 258:2973–2978.

Schechter, N. M., Choi, J. K., Slavin, D. A., Deresienski, D. T., Sayama, S., Dong, G., Lavker, R. M., Proud, D., and Lazarus, G. S. (1986). Identification of a chymotrypsin-like proteinase in human mast cells. *J. Immunol.* 137:962–970.

Schechter, N. M., Slavin, D., Fetter, R. D., Lazarus, G. S., and Fraki, J. E. (1988). Purification and identification of two serine class proteinases from dog mast cells biochemically and immunologically similar to human proteinaess tryptase and chymase. *Arch. Biochem. Biophys.* 262:232–244.

Schechter, N. M., Sprows, J. L., Schoenberger, O. L., Lazarus, G. S., Cooperman, B. S., and Rubin, H. (1989). Reaction of human skin chymotrypsin-like proteinase chymase with plasma proteinase inhibitors. *J. Biol. Chem.* 264:21309–21319.

Schechter, N. M., Irani, A. A., Sprows, J. L., Abernathy, J., Wintroub, B. U., and Schwartz, L. B. (1990). Identification of a cathepsin G-like antigen in human tryptase/chymase containing mast cells.

Schick, B. (1990). Cleavage of a rat serosal mast cell membrane component during degranulation mediated by chymase, a secretory granule protease. *Immunology* 69:423–428.

Schick, B., and Austen, K. F. (1986). Rat serosal mast cell degranulation mediated by chymase, an endogenous secretory granule protease. Active site-dependent initiation at 1oC. *J. Immunol.* 136:3812–3818.

Schick, B., and Austen, K. F. (1989). Modulation of chymase-mediated serosal mast cell degranulation by trypsin or diisopropyl fluorophosphate. *Immunology* 68: 434–439.

Schick, B., Austen, K. F., and Schwartz, L. B. (1984). Activation of rat serosal mast cells by chymase; an endogenous secretory granule protease. *J. Immunol.* 132:2571–2577.

Schoenberger, O. L., Sprows, J. L., Schechter, N. M., Cooperman, B. S., and Rubin, H. (1989). Limited proteolysis of CI-inhibitor by chymotrypsin-like proteinases. *FEBS Lett.* 259:185–187.

Schwartz, L. B. (1987) Mediators of human mast cells and human mast cell subsets. *Ann. Allergy* 58:226–235.

Schwartz, L. B. (1989). Heterogeneity of mast cells in humans. In *Mast Cell and Basophil Differentiation and Function in Health and Disease*. Edited by S. J. Galli and K. F. Austen, New York, Raven Press, pp. 93–105.

Schwartz, L. B. (1990). Tryptase from human mast cells: Biochemistry, biology and clinical utility. *Monogr. Allergy* 27:70–113.

Schwartz, L. B., and Austen, K. F. (1984). Structure and function of the chemical mediators of mast cells. In *Progress in Allergy: Mast Cell Activators and Mediator Release*. Vol. 34. Edited by K. Ishizaka, P. Kallos, H. Waksman, and A. L. deWeck. Basel, Karger, pp. 271–321.

Schwartz, L. B., and Bradford, T. R. (1986). Regulation of tryptase from human lung mast cells by heparin. Stabilization of the active tetramer. *J. Biol. Chem.* 261:7372–7379.

Schwartz, L. B., Lewis, R. A., and Austen, K. F. (1981a). Tryptase from human pulmonary mast cells: purification and characterization. *J. Biol. Chem.* 256:11939–11943.

Schwartz, L. B., Lewis, R. A., Seldin, D., and Austen, K. F. (1981b). Acid hydrolases and tryptase from secretory granules of dispersed human lung mast cells. *J. Immunol.* 126:1290–1294.

Schwartz, L. B., Riedel, C., Caulfield, J. P., Wasserman, S. I., and Austen, K. F. (1981c). Cell association of complexes of chymase, heparin proteoglycan, and protein after degranulation by rat mast cells. *J. Immunol.* 126:2071–2078.

Schwartz, L. B., Riedel, C., Schratz, J. J., and Austen, K. F. (1982). Localization of carboxypeptidase A to the macromolecular heparin proteoglycan-protein complex in secretory granules of rat serosal mast cells. *J. Immunol.* 128:1128.

Schwartz, L. B., Kawahara, M. S., Hugli, T. E., Vik, D., Fearon, D. T., and Austen, K. F. (1983). Generation of C3a anaphylatoxin from human C3 by human mast cell tryptase. *J. Immunol.* 130:1891–1895.

Schwartz, L. B., Bradford, T. R., Littman, B. H., and Wintroub, B. U. (1985). the fibrinolytic activity of purified tryptase from human lung mast cells. *J. Immunol.* 135:2762–2767.

Schwartz, L. B., Maier, M., and Spragg, J. (1986). *Adv. Exp. Med. Biol.* 198(pt.A):105–111.

Schwartz, L. B., Irani, A. A., Roller, K., Castells, M. C., and Schechter, N. M. (1987a). Quantitation of histamine tryptase and chymase in dispersed human T and TC mast cells. *J. Immunol.* 138:2611–2615.

Schwartz, L. B., Atkins, P. C., Bradford, T. R., Fleekop, P., Shalit, M., and Zweiman, B. (1987b). Release of tryptase together with histamine during the immediate cutaneous response to allergen. *J. Allergy Clin. Immunol.* 80:850–855.

Schwartz, L. B., Metcalfe, D. D., Miller, J. S., Earl, H., and Sullivan, T. (1987c). Tryptase levels as an indicator of mast-cell activation in systemic anaphylaxis and mastocytosis. *N. Engl. J. Med.* 316:1622–1626.

Schwartz, L. B., Irani, A. A., Mroveh, S., and Spock, A. (1987d). Reversed ratio of T/TC types of human mast cells in cystic fibrosis. *Clin. Res.* 35:255A.

Schwartz, L. B., Yunginger, J. W., Miller, J., Bokhari, R., and Dull, D. (1989). Time course of appearance and disappearance of human mast cell tryptase in the circulation after anaphylaxis. *J. Clin. Invest.* 83:1551–1555.

Schwartz, L. B., Bradford, T. R., Lee, D. C., and Chlebowski, J. F. (1990). Immunologic and physicochemical evidence for conformational changes occurring on conversion of human mast cells tryptase from active tetramer to inactive monomer. Production of monoclonal antibodies recognizing active tryptase. *J. Immunol.* 144:2304–211.

Sekizawa, K., Caughey, G. H., Lazarus, S. C., Gold, W. M., and Nadel, J. A. (1989). Mast cell tryptase causes airway smooth muscle hyperresponsiveness in dogs. *J. Clin. Invest.* 83:175–179.

Seppa, H. E. J. (1980). The role of chymotrypsin-like protease of rat mast cell in inflammatory vasopermeability and fibrinolysis. *Inflammation* 4:1–8.

Seppa, H. E. J., Vaananen, H. K., and Korhonen, L. K. (1979). Effects of mast cells chymase of rat skin on intercellular matrix: a histochemical study. *Acta Histochem.* 64:64.

Serafin, W. E., Dayton, E. T., Gravallese, R. M., Austen, K. F., and Stevens, R. L. (1987). Carboxypeptidase A in mouse mast cells. Identification, characterization and use as a differentiation marker. *J. Immunol.* 139:3771.

Shalit, M., Schwartz, L. B., Golzar, N., von Allman, C., Valenzano, M., Fleekop, P., Atkins, P. O., and Zweiman, B. (1988). Release of histamine and tryptase in vivo after prolonged cutaneous challenge with allergen in humans. *J. Immunol.* 141:821–826.

Shalit, M., Schwartz, L. B. von Allmen, C., Atkins, P. C., Lavker, R. M., and Zweiman, B. (1990). Release of histamine and tryptase during continuous and interrupted cutaneous challenge with allergen in humans. *J. Allergy Clin. Immunol.* 86:117–125.

Siebeck, M., Hoffmann, H., Weipert, J., and Spannagl, M. (1989). Therapeutic effects of the combination of two proteinase inhibitors in endotoxin shock of the pig. *Prog. Clin. Biol. Res.* 308:937–943.

Smith, T. J., Hougland, M. W., and Johnson, D. A. (1984). Human lung tryptase. Purification and characterization. *J. Biol. Chem.* 259:11046–11051.

Sommerhoff, C. P., Caughey, G. H., Finkbeiner, W. E., Lazarus, S. C., Basbaum, C.

B., and Nadel, J. A. (1989). Mast cell chymase. A potent secretogogue for airway gland serous cells. *J. Immunol.* 142:2450–2456.

Sommerhoff, C. P., Caughey, G. H., and Nadel, J. A. (1990). Classical second messengers are not involved in the stimulation-secretion coupling of chymase-induced degranulation of airway gland serous cells. *FASEB J.* 4:A1940.

Sopata, I., Wojteka-Lukasik, E., and Maslinski, S. (1986). Activation of latent human granulocyte gelainase by rat mast cell protease. *Folia Histochem. Cytobiol.* 24:133–137.

Stauber, U. T., Fritz, U. K., Dahlman, B., and Reinaver, H. (1986). Immunofluorescent localization of an alkaline proteinase in skeletal muscles from diabetic rats. *Basic Appl. Histo.* 30:147–152.

Suchiro, K., Kawabata, S., Miyota, I., Takeya, Takamatsu, J., Ogata, K., Kamiya, I., Saito, H., Niho, Y., and Iwanaga, S. (1989). Substitution of arginine 180 by tryptophan and its activation by alpha-chymotrypsin and rat mast cell chymase. *J. Biol. Chem.* 284:21257–21289.

Tam, E. K., and Caughey, G. H. (1990). Degradation of airway neuropeptides by human lung tryptase. *Am. J. Respir. Cell. Mol. Biol.* 3:27–32.

Tanaka, T., McRae, B. J., Cho, K., Cook, R., Fraki, J. E., Johnson, D. A., and Powers, J. C. (1983). Mammalian tissue trypsin-like enzymes: Comparative reactions of human skin tryptase, human lung tryptase, and bovine tryptsin with peptide 4-nitroanilide and thioester substrates. *J. Biol. Chem.* 258:13552–13557.

Vanderslice, P., Craik, C. S., Nadel, J. A., and Caughey, G. H. (1989). Molecular cloning of dog mast cell tryptase and a related protease: Structural evidence of a unique mode of serine protease activation. *Biochemistry* 28:4148–4155.

Vanderslice, P., Ballinger, S. M., Tam, E. K., Goldstein, S. M., Craik, C. S., and Caughey, G. H. (1990a). Human mast cell tryptase: multiple cDNAs and genes reveal a multigene serine protease family. *Proc. Natl. Acad. Sci. USA* 87:3811–1815.

Vanderslice, P., Craik, C., and Caughey, G. H. (1990b). Expression of a recombinant human mast cell tryptase as an active monomer in *E. coli*. *FASEB J.* 4: 1945.

Van Nostrand, W. E., Wagner, S. L., Farrow, J. S., and Cunningham, D. D. (1990). Immunopurification and protease inhibitory properties of protease nexin-2/amyloid beta-protein precursor. *J. Biol. Chem.* 289:9591–9594.

Varsano, S., Basbaum, C. B., Forsberg, S., Borson, D. B., Caughey, G., and Nadel, J. A. (1987). Dog tracheal epithelial cells in culture synthesize sulftated macromolecular glycoconjugates and release them from the cell surface upon exposure to extracellular proteinases. *Exp. Lung Res.* 13:157–184.

Vartio, T., Seppa, H., and Vaheri, A. (1981). Susceptibility of soluble and matrix fibronectins to degradation by tissue proteinases, mast cell chymase, and cathepsin G. *J. Biol. Chem.* 256:1171–1181.

Vassimon, C. S., and Rothschild, A. M. (1990). Compound 48/80-induced secretion of histamine from rat peritoneal mast cells depends on a tryptase controlled step also leading to chymase activity. *Agents Actions* 30:150–152.

Wenzel, S. E., Irani, A. M., Sanders, J. M., Bradford, T. R., and Schwartz, L. B.

(1986). Immunoassay of tryptase from human mast cells. *J. Immunol. Methods* 86:139–142.

Wenzel. S. E., Fowler, A. A., 3d, and Schwartz, L. B. (1988). Activation of pulmonary mast cells by bronchoalveolar allergen challenge. In vivo release of histamine and tryptase in atopic subjects with and without asthma. *Am. Rev. Respir. Dis.* 137(5):1002–1008.

Wintroub, B. U., Schechter, N. M., Lazarus, G. S., Kaempfer, C. E., and Schwartz, L. B. (1984). Angiotensin I conversion by human and rat chymotryptic proteinases. *J. Invest. Dermatol.* 83:336–339.

Wintroub, B. U., Kaempfer, C. E., Schechter, N. M., and Proud, D. (1986). A human lung mast cell chymotrypsin-like enzyme. Identification and partial characterization. *J. Clin. Invest.* 77:196.

Woodbury, R. G., and Neurath, H. (1980). Structure, specificity and localization of the serine proteases of connective tissue. *FEBS Lett.* 114:189–195.

Woodbury, R. G., Everitt, M. T., and Neurath, H. (1981). Mast cell proteases. *Methods Enzymol.* 80c:588–609.

Woodbury, R. G., LeTrong, H., Cole, K., Neurath, H., and Miller, H. R. P. (1989). Rat mast cell proteases. In *Mast Cell and Basophil Differentiation and Function in Health and Disease*. Edited by S. J. Galli and K. F. Austen. New York, Raven Press, pp. 71–81.

Yoshida, N., Everitt, M. T., Neurath, H., Woodbury, R. G., and Powers, J. C. (1980). Substrate specificity of two chymotrypsin-like proteases from rat mast cells. Studies with peptide 4 nitroanilides and comparison with cathepsin G. *Biochemistry* 19:5799–5804.

Yurt, R. W., and Austen, K. F. (1977). Preparative purification of rat mast cell chymase. Characterization and interaction with granule components. *J. Exp. Med.* 146:1405–1419.

13

Mast Cell Proteoglycans

RICHARD L. STEVENS

Harvard Medical School
Boston, Massachusetts

I. Introduction

The reason why the population of mast cells that resides in the serosal cavity of rats and mice can be so easily stained with a number of cationic dyes is because these cells have abundant amounts of heparin proteoglycans stored in their cytoplasmic granules. By the late 1970s, rat serosal mast cell–derived heparin proteoglycan was clearly shown to be a unique molecule whose peptide core contained a glycosaminoglycan attachment region that consisted of alternating serines and glycines (Yurt et al., 1977; Robinson et al., 1978; Metcalfe et al., 1980). Because serosal mast cells and mucosal mast cells could be distinguished histochemically, Enerback (1966) and Tas and Berndsen (1977) speculated that non–heparin-containing proteoglycans were present in mucosal mast cells. Although the major proteoglycan in these cells was not isolated and characterized until 20 years later (Stevens et al., 1986), it is now clear that different populations of mast cells store in their secretory granules proteoglycans that possess varied types of glycosaminoglycan side chains.

were prepared from different populations of mast cells to determine which type(s) of mast cells transcribe this proteoglycan peptide core gene. Irrespective of the type of glycosaminoglycan found in the secretory granule, all populations of mast cells contain large amounts of the same proteoglycan peptide core transcript (Tantravahi et al., 1986). Because only one gene appears to encode the peptide cores of all mast cell secretory granule proteoglycans, the glycosaminoglycan heterogeneity of these proteoglycans is likely to be a consequence of differential posttranslational modification of a common peptide core.

The genes that encode the mouse (Avraham et al., 1989a) and human (Stevens et al., 1988a; Nicodemus et al., 1990) secretory granule proteoglycan peptide cores have recently been isolated and characterized. Except for the size of the second intron, the exon/intron organizations of these genes are the same in both species. The mouse gene spans ~18 kb and consists of three exons. An 8-kb intron separates exons 1 and 2, and a 4-kb intron separates exons 2 and 3. Exon 1 encodes the 26-amino-acid hydrophobic signal peptide that is predicted to be cleaved off the translated protein in the endoplasmic reticulum. Exon 2 encodes a 48-amino-acid sequence that is predicted to be the N-terminus of the peptide core before the proteoglycan interacts with its proteases in the secretory granule. Because exon 2 is the most conserved exon, the 48-amino-acid sequence that it encodes is probably important for targeting and/or subsequent posttranslational modification of the peptide core. Exon 3 is the largest exon, and it encodes the rest of the peptide core, including the glycosaminoglycan attachment, serine-glycine repeat region. Despite the fact that the overall amino acid sequence homology of the exons is only 48%, the 300-bp nucleotide sequence that is immediately upstream of the transcription-initiation site in the human and mouse genes is nearly identical. Therefore, *cis*-acting elements are probably present in this 5' flanking region that are critical for transcription of the gene.

An 18-kb genomic clone containing the mouse secretory granule proteoglycan peptide core gene was transfected into rat-1 fibroblasts to determine whether nonhematopoietic cells could transcribe the gene. Because detectable amounts of mouse proteoglycan peptide core mRNA were found in two of the transfected rat fibroblast cell lines, it was concluded that the mouse genomic clone used in the transfections contained the gene's promoter, and that fibroblasts possess at least one *trans*-acting factor that stimulates transcription of this gene.

To determine the precise nucleotide sequences that regulate transcription of the gene in different cell types, rat-1 fibroblasts, mouse 3T3 fibroblasts, mouse WEHI-3 myelomonocytic cells, and rat basophilic leukemia-1 cells were transiently transfected with chimeric constructs containing various regions of the 5' flanking region of the mouse proteoglycan gene ligated to the human growth hormone gene (Avraham et al., 1990). Based on the amount of growth hormone in the culture medium of the transfected cells, it was concluded that there are at least two *cis*-acting elements in the 200-bp sequence flanking the 5' end of this gene that enhance its transcription. A *cis*-acting element was found slightly further upstream that suppressed transcription of the gene in fibroblasts. It appears that the secretory granule proteoglycan peptide core gene is not normally transcribed in fibroblasts primarily because these mesenchymal cells have abundant amounts of a *trans*-acting factor that suppresses its transcription.

V. Transcription of the Secretory Granule Proteoglycan Gene During the Differentiation and Immunological Activation of Mast Cells

RNA blots have been prepared from starting bone marrow cells, and from 1-, 2-, and 3-week-old cultures of mouse BMMC. When these blots were probed with cDNAs that encode carboxypeptidase A, $Fc_{\epsilon}RI_{\alpha}$, mouse mast cell protease (MMCP)-2, and the peptide core of secretory granule proteoglycans, a specific order of transcript expression emerged (Thompson et al., 1990; Stevens, unpublished observation). The proteoglycan peptide core is an abundant transcript in the starting bone marrow cells and appears to be one of the earliest expressed genes. As assessed by in situ hybridization, all of the mast cells in the cultures contained large amounts of proteoglycan peptide core mRNA (Gurish et al., 1991). Small amounts of carboxypeptidase A mRNA and $Fc_{\epsilon}RI_{\alpha}$ mRNA were found in 1-week-old cultures; maximal mRNA levels were not obtained until the second and third weeks of culture. In contrast, MMCP-2 mRNA was not detected in any of the mast cells derived by this culture technique. The finding that the proteoglycan peptide core gene is expressed before the carboxypeptidase A gene was expected, based on the assumption that the function of this proteoglycan is to package basically charged proteases in the secretory granule. The lack of MMCP-2 mRNA in these cells was surprising because it was expected that mast cells would coordinately express carboxypeptidase A and this chymotryptic protease. Recently, it has been discovered that mouse mast cells can express any one of at least five chymotryptic proteases (Le Trong et al., 1989; Reynolds et al., 1990). MMCP-5 mRNA and/or protein has been detected in BMMC, in Kirsten sarcoma virus-immortalized mast cells, and in serosal mast cells (Reynolds et al., 1990, 1991). Because MMCP-5 is the only serine protease expressed in all populations of mast cells that contain heparin proteoglycans and carboxypeptidase A (McNeil, unpublished observation), transcription of the carboxypeptidase A and MMCP-5 genes may occur concomitantly when the secretory granule proteoglycan peptide core begins to be posttranslationally modified with heparin glycosaminoglycans.

Several laboratories have recently reported that BMMC and other immature mouse mast cell lines increase their levels of cytokine mRNAs when they are activated by calcium ionophore treatment or by crosslinking of their $Fc_{\epsilon}RI$ receptors (Young et al., 1987; Plaut et al., 1989; Wodnar-Filipowicz et al., 1989; Burd et al., 1989; Ohno et al., 1990; Gordon and Galli, 1990; Gurish et al., 1991). In contrast to the cytokine transcripts, there was no appreciable change in the levels of the transcripts that encode carboxypeptidase A, a generic serine protease, and the peptide core of secretory granule proteoglycans (Gurish et al., 1991). Therefore, restoration of the high levels of heparin and chondroitin sulfate proteoglycans in the secretory granules of degranulated mast cells is probably a slow process that does not occur by substantially increasing the rate of transcription of the proteoglycan peptide core gene.

VI. Future Directions of Mast Cell Proteoglycan Research

Using a site-directed mutagenesis/transfection approach, it should be possible for investigators to identify all the *cis*-acting elements in the secretory granule proteoglycan peptide core gene that regulate its transcription. Introns often contain important regulatory elements, and therefore the nucleotide sequence of the two introns within the secretory granule proteoglycan peptide core gene will have to be studied in depth before all the *trans*-acting factors in mast cells and nonhematopoietic cells that interact with the *cis*-acting elements in this gene can be identified. No doubt, the significance of the conserved amino acid sequence that precedes the glycosaminoglycan attachment region will be addressed experimentally, as well as specific interaction of different glycosaminoglycans with the diverse types of proteases that are present in various populations of mast cells.

Discussion

Kaliner: There is substantial morphological evidence that mast cell granules undergo "activation" in situ prior to release. In rats, the granules swell, while in humans, the granules change from a dense homogeneous pattern to scrolls or lattices and appear to dissolve prior to release. Thus, it appears that the granules are changed in vivo. Could it be that the enzymes are added to the granule at release and not before?

Stevens: Histochemical studies first demonstrated that proteoglycans and proteases were stored in the secretory granule. Subsequent activation/secretion studies, electron microscopic studies, and characterization studies of isolated granules confirmed that the proteoglycans and proteases were packaged together in the granule. The only evidence that I am aware of that demonstrates that the proteoglycan binds the proteases in the granule is the fact that the N-terminus and C-terminus of the proteoglycan are cleaved when it is stored in the granule. The

only way this could occur is for the bound proteases to attack the protease-susceptible region of the core.
Metcalfe: If the primary function of proteoglycans is to bind to and stabilize proteases, why do most mast cells have heparin to do this, and other cells accomplish this with chondroitin sulfate?
Stevens: The nature of the glycosaminoglycan chain bound to the proteoglycan peptide core is probably a consequence of what type of protease the proteoglycan has to interact with inside the secretory granule.
Bienenstock: Is there any evidence that any of these proteoglycans synthesized by live mast cells are incorporated into the membrane?
Stevens: No. There is no lipid-spanning domain in the peptide core. However, it is possible that the proteoglycan could have covalently linked lipid bound to it. This has not been examined.
Kennerly: Are any of the proposed regulatory elements that you have identified for the core protein also associated with the mast cell protease genes?
Stevens: I am unaware of any genomic information on the *cis*-acting regulatory elements in any of the genes that encode mast cell proteases. Thus, it is impossible to determine whether the regulatory regions I talked about for the secretory granule proteoglycan peptide core gene are also present in the mast cell–specific serine protease genes.
Schwartz: What portion of the proteoglycan core regulatory region best accounts for its tissue specificity? Does the 3' end of the gene contain a regulatory region?
Stevens: This proteoglycan peptide core gene is expressed in many hematopoietic cells. Thus there is no mast cell–specific regulatory region.
Platts-Mills: Do heparin glycosaminoglycans have to be released from the peptide core to be active?
Stevens: No.

References

Avraham, S., Stevens, R. L., Gartner, M. C., Austen, K. F., Lalley, P. A., and Weis, J. H. (1988). Isolation of a cDNA that encodes the peptide core of the secretory granule proteoglycan of rat basophilic leukemia-1 cells and assessment of its homology to the human analogue. *J. Biol. Chem.* 263:7292–7296.

Avraham, S., Austen, K. F., Nicodemus, C. F., Gartner, M. C., and Stevens, R. L. (1989a). Cloning and characterization of the mouse gene that encodes the peptide core of secretory granule proteoglycans and expression of this gene in transfected rat-1 fibroblasts. *J. Biol. Chem.* 264:16719–16726.

Avraham, S., Stevens, R. L., Nicodemus, C. F., Gartner, M. C., Austen, K. F., and Weis, J. H. (1989b). Molecular cloning of a cDNA that encodes the peptide core of a mouse mast cell secretory granule proteoglycan and comparison with the analogous rat and human cDNA. *Proc. Natl. Acad. Sci. USA* 86:3763–3767.

Avraham, S., Avraham, H., Austen, K. F., and Stevens, R. L. (1992). Negative and positive *cis*-acting regulatory elements in the 5' flanking region of the mouse gene that encodes the serine/glycine-rich peptide core of secretory granule proteoglycans. *J. Biol. Chem.* 267:610–617.

Bourdon, M. A., Oldberg, A., Pierschbacher, M., and Rouslahti, E. (1985). Molecular cloning and sequence analysis of a chondroitin sulfate proteoglycan cDNA. *Proc. Natl. Acad. Sci. USA* 82:1321–1325.

Bourdon, M. A., Shiga, M., and Ruoslahti, E. (1986). Identification from cDNA of the precursor form of a chondroitin sulfate proteoglycan core protein. *J. Biol. Chem.* 261:12534–12537.

Burd, P. R., Rogers, H. W., Gordon, J. R., Martin, C. A., Jayaraman, S., Wilson, S. D., Dvorak, A. M., Galli, S. J., and Dorf, M. E. (1989). Interleukin 3-dependent and -independent mast cells stimulated with IgE and antigen express multiple cytokines. *J. Exp. Med.* 170:245–257.

Davidson, S., Gilead, L., Amira, M., Ginsburg, H., and Razin, E. (1990). Synthesis of chondroitin sulfate D and heparin proteoglycans in murine lymph node derived mast cells. The dependency on fibroblasts. *J. Biol. Chem.* 265:12324–12330.

Dayton, E. T., Pharr, P., Ogawa, M., Serafin, W. E., Austen, K. F., Levi-Schaffer, F., and Stevens, R. L. (1988). 3T3 fibroblasts induce cloned interleukin 3-dependent mouse mast cells to resemble connective tissue mast cells in granular constituency. *Proc. Natl. Acad. Sci. USA* 85:569–572.

Eliakim, R., Gilead, L., Ligumsky, M., Okon, E., Rachmilewitz, D., and Razin, E. (1986). Possible presence of E-mast cells in the human colon. *Proc. Natl. Acad. Sci. USA* 83:461–467.

Enerbäck, L. (1966). Mast cells in rat gastrointestinal mucosa. 2. Dye-binding and metachromatic properties. *Acta. Pathol. Microbiol. Scand.* 66:303–312.

Galli, S. J., Dvorak, A. M., Marcum, J. A., Ishizaka, T., Nabel, G., Der Simonian, H., Pyne, K., Goldin, J. M., Rosenberg, R. D., Cantor, H., and Dvorak, H. F. (1982). Mast cell clones: A model for the analysis of cellular maturation. *J. Cell Biol.* 95:435–444.

Gordon, J. R., and Galli, S. J. (1990). Mast cells as a source of both preformed and immunologically inducible TNF-α/cachectin. *Nature* 346:274–276.

Gurish, M. F., Ghildyal, N., Arm, J., Austen, K. F., Avraham, S., Reynolds, D., and Stevens, R. L. (1991). Cytokine mRNAs are preferentially increased relative to secretory granule protein mRNAs in mouse bone marrow-derived mast cells that have undergone IgE-mediated activation and degranulation. *J. Immunol.* 146:1527–1533.

Katz, H. R., Austen, K. F., Caterson, B., and Stevens, R. L. (1986). Secretory granules of heparin-containing rat serosal mast cells also possess highly sulfated chondroitin sulfate proteoglycans. *J. Biol. Chem.* 261:13393–13396.

Le Trong, H., Newlands, G. F. J., Miller, H. R. P., Charbonneau, H., Neurath, H., and Woodbury, R. G. (1989). Amino acid sequence of a mouse mucosal mast cell protease. *Biochemistry* 28:391–395.

Levi-Schaffer, F., Austen, K. F., Gravallese, P. M., and Stevens, R. L. (1986). Coculture of interleukin 3–dependent mouse mast cells with fibroblasts results in a phenotypic change of the mast cells. *Proc. Natl. Acad. Sci. USA* 83:6485–6488.

Levi-Schaffer, F., Dayton, E. T., Austen, K. F., Hein, A., Caulfield, J. P., Gravallese, P. M., Liu, F-T., and Stevens, R. L. (1987). Mouse bone marrow derived-mast cells cocultured with fibroblasts: Morphology and stimulation-induced release of histamine, leukotriene B_4, leukotriene C_4, and prostaglandin D_2. *J. Immunol.* 139:3431–3441.

McNeil, H. P., Austen, K. F., Somerville, L. L., Gurish, M. F., and Stevens, R. L. (1991). Molecular cloning of the mouse mast cell protease-5 gene. A novel secretory granule protease expressed early in the differentiation of serosal mast cells. *J. Biol. Chem.* 266:20316–20322.

Metcalfe, D. D., Smith, J. A., Austen, K. F., and Silbert, J. E. (1980). Polydispersity of rat mast cell heparin. *J. Biol. Chem.* 255:11753–11758.

Nabel, G., Galli, S. J., Dvorak, A. M., Dvorak, H. F., and Cantor, H. (1981). Inducer T lymphocytes synthesize a factor that stimulates proliferation of cloned mast cells. *Nature* 291:332–334.

Nicodemus, C. F., Avraham, S., Austen, K. F., Purdy, S., Jablonski, J., and Stevens, R. L. (1990). Characterization of the human gene that encodes the peptide core of secretory granule proteoglycans in promyelocytic leukemia HL-60 cells, and analysis of the translated product. *J. Biol. Chem.* 265:5889–5896.

Ohno, I., Tanno, Y., Yamauchi, K., and Takishima, T. (1990). Production of tumour necrosis factor by mastocytoma P815 cells. *Immunology* 69:312–315.

Plaut, M., Pierce, J. H., Watson, C. J., Hanley-Hyde, J., Nordan, R. P., and Paul, W. E. (1989). Mast cell lines produce lymphokines in response to cross-linkage of $Fc_{\epsilon}RI$ or to calcium ionophores. *Nature* 339:64–67.

Razin, E., Cordon-Cardo, C., and Good, R. A. (1981). Growth of a pure population of mouse mast cells in vitro with conditioned medium derived from concanavalin A–stimulated splenocytes. *Proc. Natl. Acad. Sci. USA* 78:2559–2561.

Razin, E., Stevens, R. L., Akiyama, F., Schmid, K., and Austen, K. F. (1982). Culture from mouse bone marrow of a subclass of mast cells possessing a distinct chondroitin sulfate proteoglycan with glycosaminoglycans rich in *N*-acetylgalactosamine-4,6-disulfate. *J. Biol. Chem.* 257:7229–7236.

Razin, E., Ihle, J. N., Seldin, D., Mencia-Huerta, J-M., Katz, H. R., LeBlanc, P. A., Hein, A., Caulfield, J. P., Austen, K. F., and Stevens, R. L. (1984). Interleukin 3: A differentiation and growth factor for the mouse mast cell that contains chondroitin sulfate E proteoglycan. *J. Immunol.* 132:1479–1486.

Reynolds, D. S., Serafin, W. E., Faller, D. V., Wall, D. A., Abbas, A. K., Dvorak, A. M., Austen, K. F., and Stevens, R. L. (1988). Immortalization of murine connective tissue-type mast cells at multiple stages of their differentiation by coculture of splenocytes with fibroblasts that produce Kirsten sarcoma virus. *J. Biol. Chem.* 263:12783–12791.

Reynolds, D. S., Stevens, R. L., Lane, W. S., Carr, M. H., Austen, K. F., and Serafin, W. E. (1990). Different mouse mast cell populations express various combinations of at least six distinct mast cell serine proteases. *Proc. Natl. Acad. Sci. USA* 87:3230–3234.

Robinson, H. C., Horner, A. A., Höök, M., Ogren, S., and Lindahl, U. (1978). A proteoglycan form of heparin and its degradation to single-chain molecules. *J. Biol. Chem.* 253:6687–6693.

Schrader, J. W., Lewis, S. J., Clark-Lewis, I., and Culvenor, J. G. (1981). The persisting (P) cell: Histamine content, regulation by a T cell–derived factor, origin from a bone marrow precursor, and relationship to mast cells. *Proc. Natl. Acad. Sci. USA* 78:323–327.

Schwartz, L. B., Riedel, C., Caulfield, J. P., Wasserman, S. I., and Austen, K. F. (1981). Cell association of complexes of chymase, heparin proteoglycan, and protein after degranulation by rat mast cells. *J. Immunol.* 126:2071–2078.

Schwartz, L. B., Riedel, C., Schratz, J. J., and Austen, K. F. (1982). Localization of carboxypeptidase A to the macromolecular heparin proteoglycan-protein complex in secretory granules of rat serosal mast cells. *J. Immunol.* 128:1128–1133.

Seldin, D. C., Seno, N., Austen, K. F., and Stevens, R. L. (1984). Analysis of polysulfated chondroitin disaccharides by high performance liquid chromatography. *Anal. Biochem.* 141:291–300.

Seldin, D. C., Austen, K. F., and Stevens, R. L. (1985). Purification and characterization of protease-resistant secretory granule proteoglycans containing chondroitin sulfate di-B and heparin-like glycosaminoglycans from rat basophilic leukemia cells. *J. Biol. Chem.* 260:11131–11139.

Serafin, W. E., Katz, H. R., Austen, K. F., and Stevens, R. L. (1986). Complexes of heparin proteoglycans, chondroitin sulfate E proteoglycans, and [^{3}H]diisopropyl fluorophosphate-binding proteins are exocytosed from activated mouse bone marrow-derived mast cells. *J. Biol. Chem.* 261:15017–15021.

Serafin, W. E., Dayton, E. T., Gravallese, P. M., Austen, K. F., and Stevens, R. L. (1987). Carboxypeptidase A in mouse mast cells: Identification, characterization, and use as a differentiation marker. *J. Immunol.* 139:3771–3776.

Serafin, W. E., Reynolds, D. S., Rogelj, S., Lane, W. S., Conder, G. A., Johnson, S. S., Austen, K. F., and Stevens, R. L. (1990). Identification and molecular cloning of a novel mouse mucosal mast cell serine protease. *J. Biol. Chem.* 265:423–429.

Stevens, R. L., Razin, E., Austen, K. F., Hein, A., Caulfield, J. P., Seno, N., Schmid, K., and Akiyama, F. (1983). Synthesis of chondroitin sulfate E glycosaminoglycan onto *p*-nitrophenyl-*β*-*D*-xyloside and its localization to the secretory granules of rat serosal mast cells and mouse bone marrow-derived mast cells. *J. Biol. Chem.* 258:5977–5984.

Stevens, R. L., Otsu, K., and Austen, K. F. (1985). Purification and analysis of the core protein of the protease-resistant intracellular chondroitin sulfate E proteoglycan from the interleukin 3-dependent mouse mast cell. *J. Biol. Chem.* 260:14194–14200.

Stevens, R. L., Lee, T. D. G., Seldin, D. C., Austen, K. F., Befus, A. D., and Bienenstock, J. (1986). Intestinal mucosal mast cells from rats infected with *Nippostrongylus brasiliensis* contain protease-resistant chondroitin sulfate di-B proteoglycans. *J. Immunol.* 137:291–295.

Stevens, R. L., Avraham, S., Gartner, M. C., Bruns, G. A. P., Austen, K. F., and Weis, J. H. (1988a). Isolation and characterization of a cDNA that encodes the peptide core of the secretory granule proteoglycan of human promyelocytic leukemia HL-60 cells. *J. Biol. Chem.* 263:7287–7291.

Stevens, R. L., Fox, C. C., Lichtenstein, L. M., and Austen, K. F. (1988b). Identification of chondroitin sulfate E proteoglycans and heparin proteoglycans in the secretory granules of human lung mast cells. *Proc. Natl. Acad. Sci. USA* 85:2284–2287.

Tantravahi, R. V., Stevens, R. L., Austen, K. F., and Weis, J. H. (1986). A single gene in mast cells encodes the core peptides of heparin and chondroitin sulfate proteoglycans. *Proc. Natl. Acad. Sci. USA* 83:9207–9210.

Tas, J., and Berndsen, R. G. (1977). Does heparin occur in mucosal mast cells of the rat small intestine? *J. Histochem. Cytochem.* 25:1058–1062.

Tertian, G., Yung, Y-P., Guy-Grand, D., and Moore, M. A. S. (1981). Long-term in vitro culture of murine mast cells. I. Description of a growth factor–dependent culture technique. *J. Immunol.* 127:788–794.

Thompson, H. L., Schulman, E. S., and Metcalfe, D. D. (1988). Identification of chondroitin sulfate E in human lung mast cells. *J. Immunol.* 140:2708–2713.

Thompson, H. L., Metcalfe, D. D., and Kinet, J-P. (1990). Early expression of high-affinity receptor for immunoglobulin E ($Fc_{\epsilon}RI$) during differentiation of mouse mast cells and human basophils. *J. Clin. Invest.* 85:1227–1233.

Wodnar-Filipowicz, A., Heusser, C. H., and Moroni, C. (1989). Production of the haemopoietic growth factor GM-CSF and interleukin-3 by mast cells in response to IgE receptor-mediated activation. *Nature* 339:150–152.

Young, J.D-E., Liu, C-C., Butler, G., Cohn, Z. A., and Galli, S. J. (1987). Identification, purification, and characterization of a mast cell-associated cytolytic factor related to tumor necrosis factor. *Proc. Natl. Acad. Sci. USA* 84:9175–9179.

Yurt, R. W., Leid, R. W., Jr., Austen, K. F., and Silbert, J. E. (1977). Native heparin from rat peritoneal mast cells. *J. Biol. Chem.* 252:518–521.

14

Leukotrienes

PANDORA E. CHRISTIE, JONATHAN P. ARM, and TAK H. LEE

Guy's Hospital
London, England

It has been suggested for many years that the sulfidopeptide leukotrienes may play a role in the pathogenesis of asthma. The recent evidence that leukotriene receptor antagonists and leukotriene synthesis inhibitors attenuate asthmatic attacks provoked by antigen (Hendeles et al., 1990), exercise (Manning et al., 1990), and hyperventilation (Israel et al., 1990) supports the role for these mediators in the disease.

I. Synthesis and Metabolism

A. Biochemistry of the Leukotrienes

Arachidonic acid is a polyunsaturated, 20-carbon fatty acid (5, 8, 11, 14-*cis*-eicosatetraenoic acid) and is released from membrane phospholipids during cell activation by the action of phospholipase A_2 (Samuelsson, 1983). The arachidonic acid released may be oxidatively metabolised by the cyclooxygenase and lipoxygenase pathways (Borgeat and Samuelsson, 1979a). The cyclooxygenase pathway generates prostaglandins and thromboxane A_2. The 5-lipoxygenase pathway generates 5*S*-hydroperoxy-6-*trans*-8,11,14-*cis*-eicosatetraenoic acid (5-HPETE) (Borgeat and Samuelsson, 1979b). This is converted en-

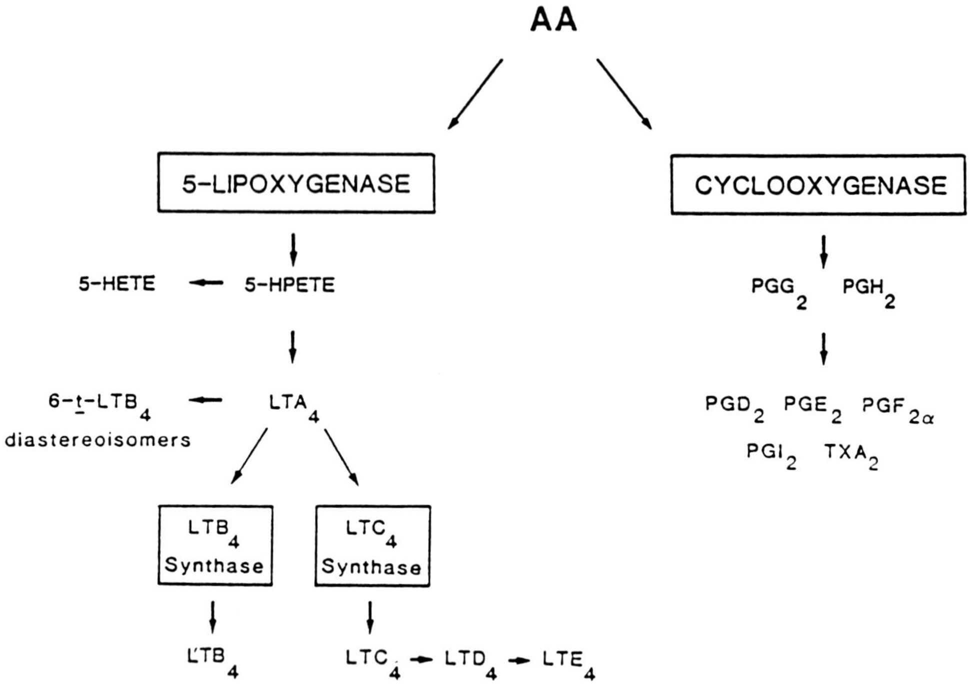

Figure 1 Metabolism of arachidonic acid (AA) by the 5-lipoxygenase and cyclooxygenase pathways. 5-HETE = 5-hydroxyeicosatetraenoic acid; 5-HPETE = 5-hydroperoxyeicosatetraenoic acid; 6-*t*-LTB_4 = 6-*trans*-LTB_4 diastereoisomers; LT = leukotriene; PG = prostaglandin.

zymatically to the unstable epoxide 5,6-oxido-7,9-*trans*-11,14-*cis*-eicosatetraenoic acid, leukotriene A_4 (LTA_4) (Borgeat and Samuelsson, 1979c). LTA_4 is metabolized by an epoxide hydrolase to 5*S*-12*R*-dihydroxy-6,14-*cis*-8, 10-*trans*-eicosatetraenoic acid, leukotriene B_4 (LTB_4) (Borgeat and Samuelsson, 1979c) or by glutathione-*S*-transferase termed leukotriene C_4 (LTC_4) synthase to 5*S*-hydroxy-6*R*-*S*-glutathionyl-7,9-*trans*-11,14-*cis*-eicosatetraenoic acid, leukotriene C_4 (LTC_4) (Murphy et al., 1979). LTC_4 is cleaved by gamma-glutamyltranspeptidase to 5*S*-hydroxy-6*R*-*S*-cysteinyl-glycyl-7, 9-*trans*-11,14-*cis*-eicosatetraenoic acid, leukotriene D_4 (LTD_4), which is cleaved by a dipeptidase to 5*S*-hydroxy-6*R*-*S*-cysteinyl-7,9-*trans* 11,14-*cis*-eicosatetraenoic acid, leukotriene E_4 (LTE_4) (Lewis et al., 1980a,b; Morris et al., 1980). LTA_4 also undergoes nonenzymatic hydrolysis to 5*S*,12*S*-dihydroxy-6,8,10-*trans*-14-*cis*-eicosatetraenoic acid diastereoisomers (5*S*,12*R*- and 5*S*,12*S*-dihydroxy-eicosatetraenoic acid diastereoisomers) (Borgeat and Samuelsson, 1979d).

B. Metabolism of Leukotrienes

The enzyme that metabolizes LTB_4, LTB_4–20 hydroxylase, is a member of the P-450 family and is located in neutrophils (Shak and Goldstein, 1984). LTB_4 is converted to 20-OH LTB_4 and by further oxidation to a biologically inactive molecule, 5*S*,12*R*-dihydroxy-20-aldehyde 2-6,14-*cis*-8,10-*trans*-eicosatetraenoic acid (20-CHO LTB_4). This is converted irreversibly to 5*S*,12*R*-dihydroxy,20-carboxy-6,14-*cis*-8,10-*trans*-eicosatetraenoic acid (20-COOH LTB_4) (Sutyak et al., 1989). An aldehyde reductase in microsomes converts 20-CHO LTB_4 back to 20-OH LTB_4.

Human neutrophils and eosinophils metabolize LTC_4, LTD_4, and LTE_4 via a peptidolytic or oxidative pathway as described above. The oxidative metabolism of LTC_4, LTD_4, and LTE_4 leads to generation of the respective sulfoxides and 6-*trans*-(C-12)-diastereoisomers of LTB_4 (Lee et al., 1982). LTE_4, can also be converted to *N*-acetyl-LTE_4 (Orning et al., 1985a).

C. Regulation of Leukotriene Synthesis

Arachidonic acid is released by the activation of phospholipase A_2 (Van Den Bosch, 1980) and in platelets by the activation of phospholipase C (Lapetina et al., 1981). The phospholipases are calcium dependent (Shukla, 1982), and their activity may be increased by many endogenous substances and mechanical stimuli (Van Den Bosch, 1980).

5-Lipoxygenase is associated with the cell membrane or free in the cytosol and may be activated by many stimuli (Dahlen et al., 1983; Voelkel et al., 1982; Armour et al., 1986; Bakhle et al., 1985). Rouzer et al. (1990) demonstrated that an additional component was necessary for cellular 5-lipoxygenase activity. Using a leukotriene synthesis inhibitor, Dixon et al. (1990) identified a membrane protein necessary for activating 5-lipoxygenase, which has been termed the 5-lipoxygenase-activating-protein (FLAP). When neutrophils are activated, there is translocation of 5-lipoxygenase by FLAP to the cell membrane, thereby bringing it in contact with arachidonic acid.

The LTA_4 hydrolase enzyme that converts LTA_4 to LTB_4 is widely distributed. LTA_4 may be converted by epoxide hydrolase in its cell of origin or in another cell to LTB_4 (Dahinden et al., 1985), converted by LTC_4 synthase to LTC_4 or undergo extracellular, nonenzymatic hydrolysis to 6-*trans*-LTB_4 and 12-epi-LTB_4 diastereoisomers. LTC_4 synthase is a glutathione-*S*-transferase and is widely distributed in tissues. The fact that LTC_4 synthase is membrane-bound suggests that LTC_4 may be formed at the membrane site.

D. Metabolism of Leukotrienes in Tissues

Using radiolabeled leukotrienes, Aharony et al. (1985) were able to demonstrate the conversion of LTA_4 to LTB_4, LTC_4, LTD_4, and LTE_4 in guinea pig lung

histamine compared to normal controls but were four- to fivefold more responsive to LTC_4 and LTD_4. Adelroth and co-workers studied the airway responsiveness to LTC_4 and LTD_4 and to methacholine in patients with asthma and compared these with normal controls. There was a correlation between the airway responsiveness to methacholine and the airway responsiveness to LTC_4 and LTD_4. There was also a correlation between airways responsiveness to methacholine and relative responsiveness to LTC_4 and LTD_4: subjects with the most responsive airways demonstrate the lowest relative responsiveness to LTC_4 and LTD_4 compared to methacholine (Adelroth et al., 1987). Thus, although LTC_4 and LTD_4 are potent bronchoconstrictor agonists when inhaled, the airways of asthmatic subjects were not as hyperresponsive to these agonists as they were to histamine or methacholine.

Using $\dot{V}_{30}$ as an index of airway bronchoconstriction, Davidson et al. (1987) demonstrated that LTE_4 is 39-fold more potent than histamine in normal and 14-fold more potent than histamine in asthmatic subjects. However, using airways-specific conductance as an index of bronchoconstriction, the relative potency of LTE_4 compared with histamine and methacholine was greater in asthmatic than in normal subjects (O'Hickey et al., 1988). There was also a correlation between the dose of LTE_4 causing a 35% fall in specific airways conductance (PD_{35} SG_{aw}) with the histamine PD_{35} SGaw and the methacholine PD_{35} SG_{aw}. More recently the potencies of histamine and methacholine were compared with those of LTC_4, LTD_4, and LTE_4 in normal and asthmatic subjects (Arm et al., 1990). The airways of asthmatic subjects were 14-fold, 15-fold, sixfold, ninefold, and 219-fold more responsive than the airways of normal subjects to histamine, methacholine, LTC_4, LTD_4, and LTE_4, respectively. Although LTC_4 and LTD_4 were 100- to 150-fold more potent than LTE_4 in constricting the airways of normal subjects, they were only four- to fivefold more potent than LTE_4 in asthmatic subjects. Thus the airways of asthmatic subjects demonstrated a selective and marked hyperresponsiveness to LTE_4.

The mechanism whereby leukotrienes produce a contractile response is unknown. The fact that prior administration of aspirin does not change leukotriene responsiveness suggests that secondary generation of cyclooxygenase products is not important (Weiss et al., 1983). The calcium channel blocker verapamil has been shown to inhibit LTD_4-induced bronchoconstriction in normal humans, suggesting that extracellular calcium entry is required for LTD_4-induced bronchoconstriction (Roberts et al., 1986a). In contrast, verapamil did not inhibit the response of asthmatic subjects to inhaled LTD_4, suggesting that there was a difference in the mechanism of action of LTD_4 in asthmatic subjects compared to normal subjects (Roberts et al., 1986b).

The site of leukotriene activity within the tracheobronchial tree is not clearly defined. Data from guinea pig studies suggest that leukotrienes are relatively selective peripheral airway agonists (Drazen et al., 1980). Holroyde et al. (1981) and Weiss et al. (1982b) suggested a predominantly peripheral site of action in normal subjects and noted that the inhalation of an aerosol of LTC_4 and LTD_4 had an effect on the $\dot{V}_{30}$ with little effect on the FEV_1. Weiss established that in normal subjects a 50-fold greater concentration of LTC_4 was required to achieve a 20% fall in FEV_1, compared to the concentration required to achieve a 30% fall in $\dot{V}_{30}$. However, in a number of studies where both SG_{aw} and $\dot{V}_{30}$ have been measured, inhalation of leukotriene has been shown to affect both indices. Thus Barnes et al. (1984b) compared the SG_{aw} and $\dot{V}_{30}$ following inhalation of LTC_4, LTD_4, and histamine in normal subjects and did not find a difference in response. In another study, Kern et al. (1986) observed the airway response to inhaled LTD_4 in normal subjects and found no difference.

Evidence from other studies suggests that the leukotrienes may have a response that is more marked in the central than the peripheral airways of asthmatic subjects. Bisgaard and co-workers (1985) reported that the airways of asthmatic subjects were more responsive than those of nonasthmatic subjects to LTD_4. The relative difference in potency between asthmatic and normal subjects was 100- to 1000-fold when measured in terms of FEV_1 but only 15-fold for differences in $\dot{V}_{30}$. Smith et al. (1985) found that a 30% fall in $\dot{V}_{30}$ in response to LTD_4 was accompanied by a 60% fall in asthmatic subjects but only a 30% fall in SG_{aw} in normal controls. Davidson et al. (1987) reported that a 30% fall in $\dot{V}_{30}$ induced by inhaled histamine was accompanied by a 10- and 13% fall in FEV_1 in asthmatic and normal subjects, respectively. When the same individuals inhaled LTE_4, a 30% fall in $\dot{V}_{30}$ was accompanied by a 17% fall in FEV_1 in asthmatic subjects and a 3% fall in FEV_1 in normal controls. More recently, Pichurko et al. (1989) compared the effects of inhalation of histamine or LTC_4 on maximal expiratory flow rate (V_{max}), while subjects breathed ambient air or 80% helium/20% oxygen and used both density dependence of V_{max} and the effects of a deep breath on expiratory flow rates as indices of the predominant site of response to LTC_4 or histamine aerosols. They found that there was a predominant central airway response to inhaled LTC_4 in asthmatic subjects, which was not seen with inhalation of histamine.

C. Leukotrienes and Airway Hyperresponsiveness

The in vitro observation that slow-reacting substance of anaphylaxis enhanced the contractile response of guinea pig ileum to histamine suggested that the sulfidopeptide leukotrienes might contribute to airway hyperresponsiveness (Brocklehurst, 1962). This was supported in a further study, where in the presence of calcium, LTE_4 but not LTC_4 or LTD_4 enhanced the contractile response to histamine in guinea pig tracheal spirals but not parenchymal strips (Lee et al., 1984a, 1985a). In addition, the contractile effect and effect on histamine responsiveness of LTE_4, LTE_4-sulfoxide, LTE_5, LTE_4 C-1 monoamine, LTE_4 *cis*-amide, and *N*-acetyl LTE_4 on guinea pig tracheal smooth muscle were studied. LTE_4 and its oxidative metabolite sulfoxide were able to induce an increase in airway hyperresponsiveness to histamine. This was dependent on the eicosanoid carboxyl group at C-1, the cysteine carboxyl group, and the free NH_2-terminal amino group of the cysteine in the structure of LTE_4. Although other analogs were able to produce bronchoconstriction, they did not elicit increased hyperrresponsiveness to histamine. The dissociation of the contractile response from enhancement of histamine response and requirement for structure suggested that the hyperresponsiveness was mediated via a receptor distinct from that which mediated contraction. The capacity of LTE_4 to enhance the response of guinea pig tracheal smooth muscle to histamine in vitro was inhibited by pretreatment with indomethacin, suggesting that the LTE_4 effect is mediated via the secondary generation of cyclooxygenase products (Lee et al., 1985a).

In normal subjects inhalation of a bronchoconstricting dose of LTD_4 did not significantly enhance the airway response to exercise (Bisgaard and Groth, 1987) or to isocapnic hyperventilation (Barnes et al., 1984a), although it increased the sensitivity of the airways to inhaled prostaglandin $F_{2\alpha}$ (Barnes et al., 1984c). Inhalation of a bronchoconstricting dose of LTD_4 in normal subjects produced an approximate twofold increase in airway methacholine responsiveness (Kern et al., 1986; Kaye and Smith, 1990). The inhalation of bronchconstricting doses of LTC_4 did not enhance airway response to inhalation of distilled water (Bianco et al., 1985). The in vitro finding that LTE_4 but not LTC_4 or LTD_4 augments histamine responsiveness of guinea pig tracheal smooth muscle (Lee et al., 1984a) led to further studies where the effect of LTE_4 on histamine hyperresponsiveness was tested in vivo (Arm et al., 1988b). Inhalation of LTE_4 up to 3 mM did not sensitize the airways of normal subjects to inhaled histamine, although LTE_4 produced a 35% fall in SG_{aw}. In contrast, preinhalation of a bronchoconstricting dose of LTE_4 in asthmatic subjects increased histamine responsiveness by approximately threefold. Methacholine inhalation, which led to a similar degree of decrease in SG_{aw} as LTE_4, did not elicit any change in histamine hyperresponsiveness, suggesting that the effect of LTE_4 was not related to the development of bronchoconstriction alone. Changes in airways histamine responsiveness were maximal at 4–7 hr after inhalation of LTE_4 and had returned to baseline values by 1 week.

D. Aspirin-Induced Asthma

A proportion of subjects with asthma are intolerant to aspirin. In these subjects ingestion of aspirin is followed within 1–2 hr by the onset of bronchospasm that may be accompanied by rhinitis and/or urticaria (Samter and Beers, 1968). The majority of subjects with aspirin-induced asthma (AIA) may be desensitized to

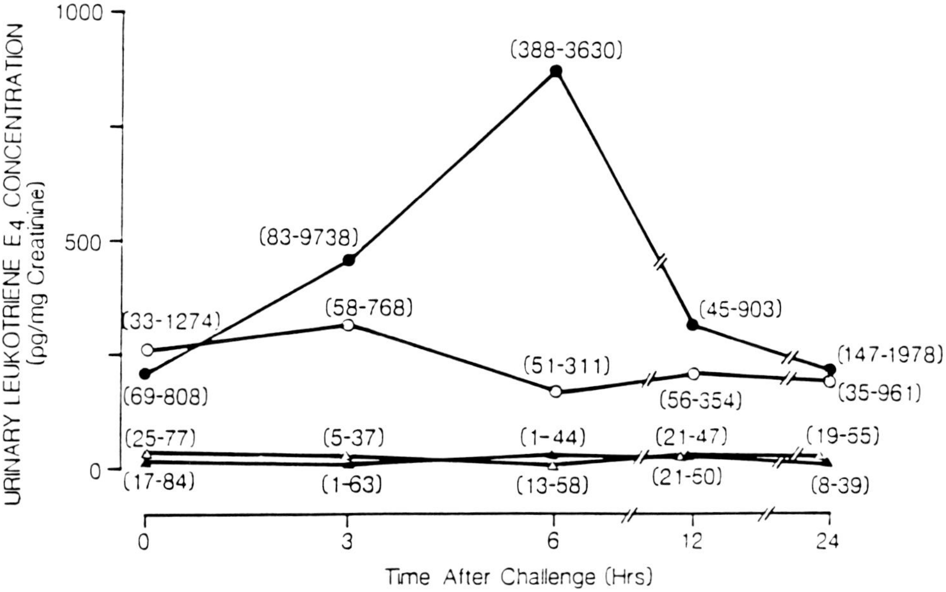

Figure 2 Urinary LTE_4 concentrations following aspirin (closed symbols) and placebo (open symbols) challenge in six aspirin-intolerant asthmatic subjects (●, ○) and in five asthmatic subjects who were tolerant to aspirin (▲, △). Each point is the geometrical mean (range). [From Christie et al., *Am. Rev. Respir. Dis.* (1991a).]

aspirin by the administration of incremental doses of aspirin orally (Pleskow et al., 1982), which may lead to an improvement in the severity of asthma and rhinitis (Stevenson et al., 1980). There is evidence that the leukotrienes may have a role in the pathogenesis of AIA. Arm et al. (1989a) compared airway responsiveness to histamine and LTE_4 in subjects with AIA and in a control group of subjects without AIA. LTE_4 was on average 145 times more potent than histamine in eliciting bronchoconstriction in subjects without AIA. In contrast, LTE_4 was 1870 times more potent than histamine in constricting the airways of subjects with AIA. Following oral desensitization to aspirin, there was a mean 20-fold decrease in the sensitivity to LTE_4 but no change in airway responsiveness to histamine. Release of LTC_4 into nasal secretions has been demonstrated following aspirin ingestion in subjects with AIA. LTC_4 was not released following ingestion of aspirin in subjects without AIA or in subjects with AIA following desensitization (Ferreri et al., 1988). Baseline urinary LTE_4 concentrations were raised in asthmatic subjects with aspirin intolerance compared to asthmatics who were aspirin tolerant (Christie et al., 1991a). In addition, following oral aspirin challenge there was an increase in urinary LTE_4 concentration, which

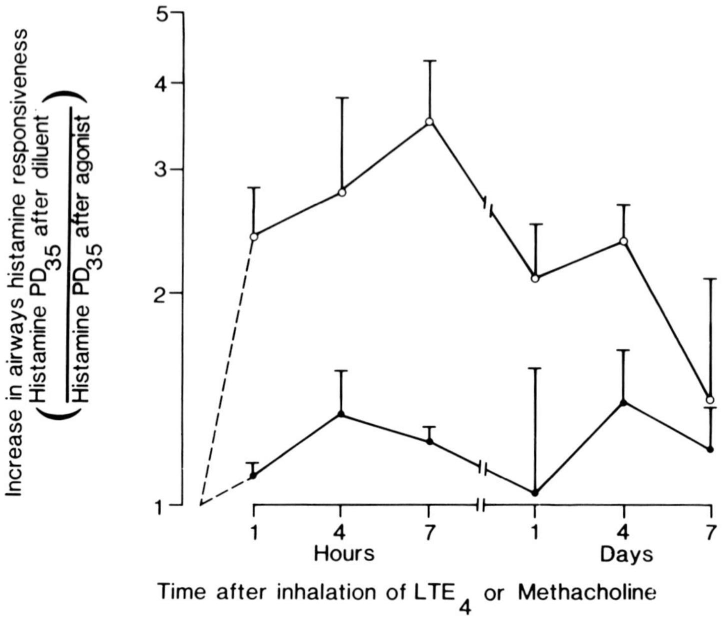

Figure 3 Time course of changes in airway histamine responsiveness after inhalation of bronchoconstricting doses of methacholine (●) and LTE_4 (○). Results are the GM ± SEM for four subjects with asthma and were calculated as the ratio of histamine PD_{35} after inhalation of diluent to histamine PD_{35} after inhalation of methacholine or of LTE_4. (From Arm et al., 1988b.)

was not observed following placebo challenge in the same subjects. The increase in LTE_4 was not a feature of bronchoconstriction alone as there was no increase in LTE_4 release following methacholine challenge in the aspirin-sensitive subjects. There was no change in urinary LTE_4 concentration in the non–aspirin-sensitive subjects following either aspirin or placebo challenge. The prior inhalation of a leukotriene receptor antagonist, SK&F 104353, inhibited aspirin-induced bronchoconstriction in five of six aspirin-sensitive subjects studied (Christie et al., 1991b), supporting the view that leukotrienes play a central role in AIA.

E. Release of Leukotrienes in Asthma

Automated reversed-phase high-performance liquid chromatography with radioimmunoassay can be used to analyze leukotrienes in complex biological fluids (Tagari et al., 1989). In humans, LTC_4 is converted enzymatically in blood to LTD_4 and LTE_4, which is excreted in the urine (Orning et al., 1985).

Measurement of urinary LTE_4 concentration may therefore act as a marker of systemic release of sulfidopeptide leukotrienes (Maltby et al., 1990). More direct evidence that leukotrienes are mediators of asthma comes from studies of their release. Thus Lam et al. (1988) analyzed the bronchoalveolar lavage (BAL) fluid of asthmatic subjects for LTC_4, LTD_4, and LTE_4 and compared these to normal controls. LTE_4 was the predominant leukotriene recovered from the BAL of asthmatic subjects and was not detected in the BAL of healthy subjects. Taylor et al. (1989) were able to demonstrate that urinary LTE_4 levels are raised during an acute severe attack of asthma and following antigen challenge in asthmatic subjects. Recently, Silber and co-workers demonstrated leukotriene release in the nasal lavage fluid of normal subjects following nasal hyperosmolar challenge (Silber et al., 1988). Smith and Lee were unable to demonstrate release of urinary leukotrienes following exercise-induced asthma in asthmatic subjects (Smith, C. M., and Lee, T. H., personal communication). Leukotrienes have been detected after the application of specific antigen to nasal airways of patients with allergic rhinitis (Creticos et al., 1989) and to conjunctiva of patients with allergic conjunctivitis (Proud et al., 1990). The release of leukotrienes following aspirin challenge has already been discussed.

F. Effects of Lipids

Fish oil diets are enriched in polyunsaturated acids, of which the two major types are eicosapentaenoic acid (EPA) and docosahexaenoic acid (DCHA). These fatty acids are incorporated into tissue phospholipids in mammals and competitively inhibit the conversion of arachidonic acid by the cyclooxygenase pathway to prostanoid metabolites (Corey et al., 1983). The endoperoxide and thromboxane A_3 derived from EPA are less active than the arachidonic acid–derived counterparts (Dyerberg et al., 1978; Whitaker et al., 1979). Docosahexaenoic acid is not metabolized to any cyclooxygenase product. EPA is converted via the lipoxygenase pathway to LTB_5, LTC_5, LTD_5, and LTE_5; DCHA is converted to the 7- and 4-hydroperoxy DCHA and their reduction products. LTB_5 is less active than LTB_4 in proinflammatory functions (Goldman et al., 1983; Lee et al., 1984b), but LTC_5 and LTC_4 are equiactive in constricting nonvascular smooth muscle (Dahlen et al., 1982). Incubation of PMN with EPA in vitro attenuates LTB_4 production with conversion to LTB_5 (Lee et al., 1984c). Monocyte monolayers treated with EPA demonstrate a decrease in PAF-acether generation following stimulation with calcium ionophore (Sperling et al., 1987). When murine mastocytoma cells grown in the peritoneal cavity of mice are treated with an EPA-enriched diet, 50% of phospholipid is replaced by EPA. If the cells are challenged with calcium ionophore, there is increased generation of LTB_5 with a reduction of LTB_4 and LTC_4 from membrane-derived arachidonic acid (Murphy et al., 1981). This has also been demonstrated in normal humans where an

EPA-enriched diet increases the content of EPA in PMN and monocytes, and on stimulation with ionophore in vitro, there is a decrease in release of arachidonic acid and its metabolites. Further, the adherence of PMN to endothelial cell monolayers pretreated with LTB_4 and the chemotactic response to LTB_4 are inhibited in response to an EPA-enriched diet (Lee et al., 1985b). The effect of a fish oil–supplemented diet in bronchial asthma has been evaluated in several studies. Although there was evidence of an attenuation of neutrophil function following 8 weeks dietary supplementation with fish oil, no effect on the severity of either mild to moderate or persistent severe asthma was noted (Arm et al., 1988c). However, 10 weeks of treatment with Max-EPA led to an attenuation of the late asthmatic response (Arm et al., 1989b). This is consistent with the capacity of EPA to modulate the inflammatory response. While fish oil supplements have had no effect on stable asthma, the results of studies in seasonal asthma are awaited.

G. Leukotriene Receptors

LTB_4

LTB_4 binds with high affinity and stereospecificity to human PMN (Goldman and Goetzl, 1982). Radiolabeled LTB_4 binding studies demonstrate the presence of two LTB_4 receptor populations: a high-affinity, low-density population mediating chemotaxis and a low-affinity, high-density population mediating lysozomal granule release (O'Flaherty et al., 1986).

Sulfidopeptide Leukotrienes

The differences of the rank order of relative contractile potencies for the sulfidopeptide leukotrienes in various tissues (Lewis et al., 1980b; Lee et al., 1984a), the difference in the time course of spasmogenic responses to the three compounds in the same tissue (Krilis et al., 1983), the distinct effect of LTE_4 in producing hyperresponsiveness (Lee et al., 1984a), as well as stereochemical requirements (Drazen et al., 1980) and radioligand binding studies (Krell et al., 1983; Aharony et al., 1989), suggest the involvement of two or more distinct receptor sites for the sulfidopeptide leukotrienes. Specific leukotriene receptor antagonists provide further evidence for leukotriene receptor heterogeneity (Drazen et al., 1980). The contractile activity of guinea pig lung parenchymal strips to low concentrations of LTD_4 was inhibited by the leukotriene antagonist FPL 55712, but the response of the same tissue to LTC_4 was not similarly inhibited. Subsequent studies on guinea pig pulmonary contractile tissues in the presence of L-serine borate complex and L-cysteine, which prevent the bioconversion of LTC_4 to LTD_4 and LTE_4, suggest the presence of distinct LTC_4 and LTD_4 receptors (Snyder and Krell, 1984; Weichman and Tucker, 1985).

Evidence to suggest a possible distinct LTE_4 receptor has been obtained for guinea pig trachea where incubation with LTE_4 but not with LTD_4 or LTC_4 results in an increase in histamine responsiveness (Lee et al., 1984a). Using binding and competition assays, Aharony et al. (1989) have suggested that LTE_4 binds to a subpopulation of LTD receptors. These reports are in contrast to studies conducted in the presence of bioconversion inhibitors on intralobar airways isolated from human subjects undergoing surgery for carcinoma of the bronchus, which did not reveal evidence for multiple leukotriene receptors (Buckner et al., 1986). Recent in vivo studies provide evidence that leukotriene receptor antagonists are able to inhibit antigen-induced bronchoconstriction (Eiser et al., 1989), AIA (Christie, P. E., 1991b), and exercise-induced asthma (Manning et al., 1990), suggesting a possible therapeutic role for these agents in asthma.

III. Conclusion

The sulfidopeptide leukotrienes have agonist activity on airways as well as an ability to induce airway hyperresponsiveness, which is a feature of asthma. Leukotriene B_4 has potent proinflammatory properties. The actions of leukotrienes in vitro and in vivo, the direct recovery of leukotrienes from biological fluids of asthmatic subjects, and the results of recent studies using newer, potent leukotriene receptor antagonists suggest that leukotrienes may play a role in the pathophysiology of bronchial asthma.

Discussion

Sullivan: How do your findings of increased LTE_4 basal excretion in aspirin (ASA) sensitivity relate to the recent report that ASA displaces lipid mediators from protein-binding sites? Could ASA cause LTE_4 release from binding sites?
Lee: The problems with reconciling that putative mechanism in ASA sensitivity are twofold: (1) The drugs that are firmly protein bound do not precipitate asthma in ASA sensitivity, although you cannot exclude different binding sites. (2) The postulated mechanism of PGF_2-alpha binding cannot explain target organ selectivity.
Kaliner: Kowalski in an abstract presented at the 1991 AAAI meeting (published in the *JACI* in March 1991) has shown that challenge of ASA-sensitive patients resulted in dramatic increases in LTC_4, PGD_2, and histamine in nasal washing at the time of rhinorrhea in response to oral ASA challenge.
Lee: You are suggesting that mast cells may be the source of released sulfidoleukotrienes in ASA sensitivity. There are additional studies to support that position.

Schleimer: Elevated levels of tryptase are found in the circulation after ASA challenge, adding more support to the role of mast cells in this disease.
Lee: John Oates's group has found increased histamine in the urine of patients with systemic mastocytosis who react adversely to ASA. These data also suggest that ASA can activate mast cells in selected patients.
Kaplan: Bradykinin contraction of the guinea pig ileum is more strongly augmented by leukotrienes than histamine, which you have studied. There may be a direct effect of leukotrienes on the contractile mechanism or the more complex suggestions you have raised.

References

Adelroth, E., Morris, M. M., Hargreave, F. E., and O'Byrne, P. (1987). Airway responsiveness and relative potency of leukotrienes C_4, D_4 and methacholine in asthmatics and normals. *N. Engl. J. Med.* 315:480–484.

Aharony, D., Dobson, P. T., and Krell, R. D. (1985). In vitro metabolism of (3H)-peptide leukotrienes in human and ferret lung: A comparison with the guinea pig. *Biochem. Biophys. Res. Commun.* 131:892–898.

Aharony, D., Catanese, C. A., and Falcone, R. (1989). Kinetic and pharmacologic analysis of [^{3}H] leukotriene E_4 binding to receptors on guinea pig lung membranes: Evidence for selective binding to a subset of leukotriene D_4 receptors. *J. Pharmacol. Exp. Ther.* 248:581–588.

Arm, J. P., Horton, C. E., House, F., Clark, T. J., Spur, B. W., and Lee, T. H. (1988a). Enhanced generation of leukotriene B_4 by neutrophils stimulated by unopsonized zymosan and by calcium ionophore after exercise-induced asthma. *Am. Rev. Respir. Dis.* 138(1):47–53.

Arm, J. P., Spur, B. W., and Lee, T. H. (1988b). The effects of inhaled leukotriene E_4 on the airway responsiveness to histamine in subjects with asthma and normal subjects. *J. Allergy Clin. Immunol.* 82:654–660.

Arm, J. P., Horton, C. E., Mencia-Huerta, J. M., House, F., Eiser, N. M., Clark, T. J. H., Spur, B. W., and Lee, T. H. (1988c). Effect of dietary supplementation with fish oil lipids on mild asthma. *Thorax* 43:84–92.

Arm, J. P., O'Hickey, S. P., Spur, B. W., and Lee, T. H. (1989a). Airway responsiveness to histamine and leukotriene E_4 in subjects with aspirin-induced asthma. *Am. Rev. Respir. Dis.* 140:148–153.

Arm, J. P., Horton, C. E., Spur, B. W., Mencia-Huerta, J. M., and Lee, T. H. (1989b). The effects of dietary supplementation with fish oil lipids on the airways response to inhaled allergen in bronchial asthma. *Am. Rev. Respir. Dis.* 139:1395–1400.

Arm, J. P., O'Hickey, S. P., Hawksworth, R. J., Fong, C. Y., Crea, A. E. G., Spur, B. W., and Lee, T. H. (1990). Asthmatic airways have a disproportionate hyperresponsiveness to LTE_4 as compared with normal airways, but not to LTC_4, LTD_4, methacholine, and histamine. *Am. Rev. Respir. Dis.* 42:1112–1118.

Armour, C. L., Black, J. L., Johnson, P. R., Vincenc, K. S., and Berend, N. (1986). Formyl peptide-induced contraction of human airways in vitro. *J. Appl. Physiol.* 60:141–146.

Bakhle, Y. S., Moncada, S., de Nucci, G., and Salmon, J. A. (1985). Differential release of eicosanoids by bradykinin, arachidonic acid and calcium ionophore A23187 in guinea-pig isolated perfused lung. *Br. J. Pharmacol.* 86:55–62.

Barnes, N., Watson, A., Piper, P. J., and Costello, J. F. (1984a). Action of inhaled leukotriene C and D on large and small airways. Effect of preinhalation of LTD on histamine dose response curve. *Am. Rev. Respir. Dis.* 129 (Suppl.):A1 (abstract).

Barnes, N. C., Piper, P. J., and Costello, J. F. (1984b). Effect of inhaled leukotrienes C_4 and D_4 in mild asthma. *Thorax* 39:697 (abstract).

Barnes, N., Watson, A., Kolouris, N., Piper, P. J., and Costello, J. (1984c). Effect of inhaled leukotriene D_4 on sensitivity to inhaled prostaglandin F_{2a}. *Thorax* 39:697 (abstract).

Bianco, S., Robuschi, M., Vaghi, A., Simone, P., Folco, G., Berti, F., and Pasargiklan, M. (1985). Effects of leukotriene C_4 on the bronchial response to an ultrasonic mist of distilled H_2O. *Prog. Respir. Res.* 19:82–86.

Bisgaard, H., and Groth, S. (1987). Bronchial effects of leukotriene D_4 inhalation in normal human lung. *Clin. Sci.* 72:585–592.

Bisgaard, H., Groth, S., and Madsen, F. (1985). Bronchial hyperreactivity to leukotriene D_4 and histamine in exogenous asthma. *Br. Med. J.* 290:1468–1471.

Borgeat, P., and Samuelsson, B. (1979a). Metabolism of arachidonic acid in polymorphonuclear leukocytes: Structural analysis of novel hydroxylated compounds. *J. Biol. Chem.* 245:7865–7868.

Borgeat, P., and Samuelsson, B. (1979b). Arachidonic acid metabolism in polymorphonuclear leukocytes: Unstable intermediate formation of dihydroxy acids. *Proc. Natl. Acad. Sci. USA* 76:3213–3217.

Borgeat, P., and Samuelsson, B. (1979c). Arachidonic acid metabolism in polymorphonuclear leukocytes: Effects of ionophore A23187. *Proc. Natl. Acad. Sci. USA* 76:2148–2152.

Borgeat, P., and Samuelsson, B. (1979d). Transformation of arachidonic acid by rabbit polymorphonuclear leukocytes. Formation of a novel dihydroxyeicosatetraenoic acid. *J. Biol. Chem.* 255:2643–2646.

Brocklehurst, W. E. (1962). Slow reacting substance and related compounds. *Prog. Allergy* 6:539–558.

Buckner, C. K., Krell, R. D., Lavaruso, R. B., Coursin, D. B., Bernstein, P. R., and Will, J. A. (1986). Pharmacological evidence that human intralobar airways do not contain different receptors that mediate contractions to leukotriene C_4 and D_4. *J. Pharmacol. Exp. Ther.* 237:558–562.

Camp, R. D. R., Coutts, A. A., Greaves, M. W., Kay, A. B., and Walport, M. J. (1983). Responses of human skin to intradermal injection of leukotrienes C_4, D_4 and B_4. *J. Pharmacol.* 80:497–502.

Christie, P. E., Tagari, P., Ford-Hutchinson, A. W., Charlesson, S., Chee, P., Arm, J. P., and Lee, T. H. (1991a). Urinary leukotriene E_4 concentrations increase after

Lapetina, E. G., Billah, M. M., and Cuatrecasas, P. (1981). The phosphatidylinositol cycle and the regulation of arachidonic acid production. *Nature* 292:367–369.

Laviolette, M., Coulombe, R., Picard, S., Braquet, P., and Borgeat, P. (1986). Decreased leukotriene B_4 synthesis in smokers'alveolar macrophages in vitro. *J. Clin. Invest.* 77:54–60.

Lee, C. W., Lewis, R. A., Corey, E. J., Barton, A., Oh, H., Tauber, A. I., and Austen, K. F. (1982). Oxidative inactivation of leukotriene C_4 by stimulated human polymorphonuclear leukocytes. *Proc. Natl. Acad. Sci. USA* 79:4166–70.

Lee, T. H., Austen, K. F., Corey, E. J., and Drazen, J. M. (1984a). LTE_4-induced airway hyperresponsiveness of guinea pig tracheal smooth muscle to histamine and evidence for 3 separate sulfidopeptide leukotriene receptors. *Proc. Natl. Acad. Sci. USA* 81:4922–4925.

Lee, T. H., Mencia-Huerta, J. M., Shih, C., Corey, E. J., Lewis, R. A., and Austen, K. F. (1984b). Characterization and biological properties of 5,12-dihydroxy derivatives of eicosapentaenoic acid including leukotriene B_5 and the double lipoxygenase product. *J. Biol. Chem.* 259:2383–2389.

Lee, T. H., Mencia-Huerta, J. M., Shih, C., Corey, E. J., Lewis, R. A., and Austen, K. F. (1984c). Effects of exogenous arachidonic, eicosapentaenoic, and docosahexaenoic acids on the generation of 5-lipoxygenase pathway products by ionophore-activated human neutrophils. *J. Clin. Invest.* 74:1922–1933.

Lee. T. H., Shore, S., Corey, E. J., Austen, K. F., and Drazen, J. M. (1985a). Leukotriene E_4 induced airway hyperresponsiveness to histamine. *J. Allergy. Clin. Immunol.* 75:140 (abstract).

Lee, T. H., Hoover, R. L., Williams, J. D., Sperling, R. I., Ravalese, J., Spur, B. W., Robinson, D. R., Corey, E. J., Lewis, R. A., and Austen, K. F. (1985b). Effect of dietary enrichment with eicosapentaenoic and docosahexaenoic acids on in vitro neutrophil and monocyte leukotriene generation and neutrophil function. *N. Engl. J. Med.* 312:1217–1224.

Leitch, A. G., Austen, K. F., and Drazen, J. M. (1983a). Effects of indomethacin on the guinea pig pulmonary response to intravenous leukotriene C_4 and D_4. *Clin. Sci.* 65:281–287.

Leitch, A. G., Corey, E. J., Austen, K. F., and Drazen, J. M. (1983b). Indomethacin potentiates the pulmonary response to aerosol. LTC_4 in the guinea pig. *Am. Rev. Respir. Dis.* 128:639–643.

Lewis, R. A., and Austen, K. F. (1982). Bronchoconstrictor effect of leukotriene C in humans. *Science* 216:196–198.

Lewis, R. A., Austen, K. F., Drazen, J. M., Clark, D. A., Marfat, A., and Corey, E. J. (1980a). Slow reacting substances of anaphylaxis: identification of leukotriene C-1 and D from human and rat sources. *Proc. Natl. Acad. Sci. USA* 77:3710–3714.

Lewis, R. A., Drazen, J. M., Austen, K. F., Clark, D. A., and Corey, E. J. (1980b). Identification of the C(6)-*S*-conjugate of leukotriene A with cysteine as a naturally occurring slow reacting substance of anaphylaxis (SRS-A). Importance of the 11-*cis* geometry. *Biochem. Biophys. Res. Commun.* 96:271–277.

Lewis, R. A., Goetzl, E. J., Drazen, J. M., Soter, N. A., Austen, K. F., and Corey, E. J. (1981). Functional characterisation of synthetic leukotriene B and its stereochemical isomers. *J. Exp. Med.* 154:1243–1248.

Maltby, N. H., Taylor, G. W., Ritter, J. M., Moore, K., Fuller, R. W., and Dollery, C. T. (1990). Leukotriene C_4 elimination and metabolism in man. *J. Allergy. Clin. Immunol.* 485:3–9.

Manning, P. J., Watson, R. M., Margolskee, D. J., Williams, V. C., Schwartz, J., and O'Byrne, P. M. (1990). Inhibition of exercise-induced bronchoconstriction by MK-571, a potent leukotriene D_4-receptor antagonist. *N. Engl. J. Med.* 323:1736–1739.

Mita, H., Yui, Y., Tanaguchi, N., Yasyeda, H., and Shida, T. (1985). Increased activity of 5-lipoxygenase in polymorphonuclear leukocytes from asthmatic patients. *Life Sci.* 37:907–914.

Morris, H. R., Taylor, G. W., Piper, P. J., and Tippins, J. R., (1980). Structure of slow reacting substance of anaphylaxis from guinea pig lung. *Nature* 285:104–105.

Murphy, R. C., Hammarstrom, S., and Samuelsson, B. (1979). Leukotriene C: A slow reacting substance from murine mastocytoma cells. *Proc. Natl. Acad. Sci. USA* 76:4275–4279.

Murphy, R. C., Pickett, W. C., Culp, B. R., and Lands, W. E. M. (1981). Tetraene and pentaene leukotrienes: Selective production from murine mastocytoma cells after dietary manipulation. *Prostaglandins* 22:613–622.

Nagy, L., Lee, T. H., Goetzl, E. J., Pickett, W., and Kay, A. B. (1982). Complement enhancement and chemotaxis of human neutrophils and eosinophils by leukotrienes and other lipoxygenase produces. *Clin. Exp. Immunol.* 47:541–547.

O'Byrne, P. M., Walters, E. H., Gold, B. D., Aizawa, H. A., Fabbri, I. M., Alpert, S. E., Nadel, J. A., and Holtzman, M. J. (1984). Neutrophil depletion inhibits airway hyperresponsiveness induced by ozone exposure. *Am. Rev. Respir. Dis.* 130:214–219.

O'Byrne, P. M., Leikauf, G. D., Aizawa, H., Betrel, R. A., Heki, J. F., Holtzman, M. J., and Nadel, J. A. (1986). Leukotriene B_4 induces airway hyperresponsiveness in dogs. *J. Appl. Physiol.* 59:1941–1946.

O'Flaherty, J., Kosfeld, S., and Nishihira, J. (1986). Binding and metabolism of leukotriene B_4 by neutrophils and their subcellular organelles. *J. Cell. Physiol.* 126:359–370.

O'Hickey, S. P., Arm, J. P., Rees, P. J., Spur, B. W., and Lee. T. H. (1988). The relative responsiveness to inhaled leukotriene E_4, methacholine and histamine in normal and asthmatic subjects. *Eur. Respir. J.* 1:913–917.

Orchard, M. A., Kagey-Sobotka, A., Proud, D., and Lichenstein, L. M. (1986). Basophil histamine release induced by a substance from stimulated human platelets. *J. Immunol.* 136:2240–2244.

Orning, L., Kaijser, L., and Hammarstrom, S. (1985). In vivo metabolism of leukotriene C_4 in man: Urinary excretion of leukotriene E_4. *Biochem. Biophys. Res. Commun.* 130:214–220.

Palmer, R. M. J., Stephney, R. J., Higgs, G. A., and Eakins, K. E. (1980). Chemokinetic activity of arachidonic and lipoxygenase products on leukocytes of different species. *Prostaglandins* 20:411–414.

Payan, D. G., and Goetzl, E. J. (1981). The dependence of human T lymphocyte migration on the 5-lipoxygenation of endogenous arachidonic acid. *J. Clin. Immunol.* 1:266–270.

Pichurko, B. M., Ingram. R. H., Jr., Sperling, R. I., Lafleur, J. E., Corey, E. J., Austen, K. F., and Drazen, J. M. (1989). Localization of the site of the bronchoconstrictor effects of leukotriene C_4 compared with that of histamine in asthmatic subjects. *Am. Rev. Respir. Dis.* 140:334–339.

Pleskow, W. W., Stevenson, D. D., Mathison, D. A., Simon, R. A., Schatz, M., and Zeiger, R. S. (1982). Aspirin desensitization in aspirin-sensitive asthmatic patients: Clinical manfestations and characterization of the refractory period. *J. Allergy. Clin. Immunol.* 69:11.

Proud, D., Sweet, J., Stein, Settipane, R. A., Kagey-Sobotka, A., Friedlaender, M. H., and Lichtenstein, L. M. (1990). Inflammatory mediator release on conjunctival provocation of allergic subjects with allergen. *J. Allergy. Clin. Immunol.* 85:896–905.

Roberts, S. A., Giembycz, M. A., Raeburn, D., Rodger, I. W., and Thomson, N. C. (1986a). In vitro and in vivo effect of verapamil on human airway responsiveness to leukotriene D_4. *Thorax* 41:12–16.

Roberts, J. A., Rodger, I. W., and Thomson, N. C. (1986b). Effect of verapamil and sodium cromoglycate on leukotriene D_4 induced bronchoconstriction in patients with asthma. *Thorax* 41:753–758.

Rouzer, C. A., Ford-Hutchinson, A. W., Morton, H. E., and Gillard, J. W. (1990). MK886, a potent and specific leukotriene biosynthesis inhibitor blocks and reverses the membrane association of 5-lipoxygenase in ionophore-challenged leukocytes. *J. Biol. Chem.* 265:1436–1442.

Samter, M., and Beers, R. F. (1968). Intolerance to aspirin: Clinical studies and consideration of its pathogenesis. *Ann. Intern. Med.* 6:975–983.

Samuelsson, B. (1983). Leukotrienes: Mediators of hypersensitivity reactions and inflammation. *Science* 220:568–575.

Shak, S., and Goldstein, I. M. (1984). Omega-oxidation is the major pathway for the catabolism of leukotriene B_4 in human polymorphonuclear leukocytes. *J. Biol. Chem.* 259:10181–10187.

Showell, H. J., Naccache, P. H., Borgeat, P., Picard, S., Vallerand, P., Becker, E. L., and Sha'afi, R. I. (1982). Characterisation of the secretory activity of leukotriene B_4 toward rabbit neutrophils. *J. Immunol.* 128:811–816.

Shukla, S. D. (1982). Phosphatidylinositol specific phospholipases C. *Life Sci.* 30:1323–1335.

Silber, G., Proud, D., Warner, J., Naclerio, R., Kagey-Sobotka, A., Lichtenstein, L., and Eggleston, P. (1988). In vivo release of inflammatory mediators by hyperosmolar solutions. *Am. Rev. Respir. Dis.* 137:606–612.

Sirois, P., Roy, S., and Borgeat, P. (1981). The lung parenchymal strip as a sensitive assay for leukotriene B_4. *Prostaglandins Leukotrienes Med.* 6:153–159.

Sirois, P., Brousseau, Y., Salari, H., and Borgeat, P. (1985). Correlation between the myotropic activity of leukotriene A_4 on guinea pig lung, trachea and ileum and its biotransformation in situ. *Prostaglandins* 30:21–36.

Smith, L. J., Greenberger, P. A., Patterson, R., Krell, R. D., and Bernstein, P. R. (1985). The effect of inhaled leukotriene D_4 in humans. *Am. Rev. Respir. Dis.* 131:368–372.

Snyder, D. W., and Krell, R. D. (1984). Pharmacological evidence for a distinct leukotriene C_4 receptor in guinea-pig trachea. *J. Pharmacol. Exp. Ther.* 231:616–611.

Sperling, R. I., Robin, J. L., Kylander, K. A., Lee, T. H., Lewis, R. A., and Austen, K. F. (1987). The effects of *N*-3 polyunsaturated fatty acids on the generation of platelet-activating factor-acether by human monocytes. *J. Immunol.* 12:4187–4191.

Stevenson, D. D., Simon, R. A., and Mathison, D. A. (1980). Aspirin-sensitive asthma: Tolerance to aspirin after positive oral aspirin challenges. *J. Allergy. Clin. Immunol.* 66:82–88.

Sutyak, J., Austen, K. F., and Soberman, R. J. (1989). Identification of an aldehyde dehydrogenase in the microsomes of human polymorphonuclear leukocytes that metabolizes 20-aldehyde leukotriene B_4. *J. Biol. Chem.* 264:14818–14823.

Tagari, P., Ethier, D., Carry, M., Korley, V., Charleson, S., Girard, Y., and Zamboni, R. (1989). Measurement of urinary leukotrienes by reversed-phase liquid chromatography and radioimmunoassay. *Clin. Chem.* 35:388–391.

Taniguchi, N., Mita, G., Saito, H., Yuo, Y., Kajita, T., and Shida, T. (1985). Increased generation of leukotriene C_4 from eosinophils in asthmatic patients. *Allergy* 40:571–573.

Taylor, G. W., Taylor, I., Black, P., Maltby, N. H., Turner, N., Fuller, R. W., and Dollery, C. T. (1989). Urinary leukotriene E_4 after antigen challenge and in acute asthma and allergic rhinitis. *Lancet* 1:584–588.

Van Den Bosch, H. (1980). Intracellular phospholipase A. *Biochim. Biophys. Acta* 604:191–246.

Voelkel, N., Reeves, S. T., Henson, P. M., and Murphy, R. C. (1982). Nonimmunological production of leukotrienes induced by platelet activating factor. *Science* 218:286–288.

Weichman, B. W., and Tucker, S. S. (1985). Differentiation of the mechanisms by which leukotrienes C_4 and D_4 elicit contraction of the guinea pig trachea. *Prostaglandins* 29:547–560.

Weiss, J. W., Drazen, J. M., Coles, N., McFadden, E. R., Weller, P. F., Corey, E. J., Lewis, R. A., and Austen, K. F. (1982a). Bronchoconstrictor effect of leukotriene C in humans. *Science* 216:196–198.

Weiss, J. W., Drazen, J. M., McFadden, E. R., Jr., Weller, P. F., Corey, E. J., Lewis, R. A., and Austen, K. F. (1982b). Comparative bronchoconstrictor effects of histamine, leukotriene C and leukotriene D in normal human volunteers. *Trans. Assoc. Am. Physicians* 95:30–35.

Weiss, J. W., Drazen, J. M., McFadden, E. R., Jr., Weller, P., Corey, E. J., Lewis, R. A., and Austen, K. F. (1983). Airway constriction in normal humans produced by inhalation of leukotriene D. Potency, time-course and effect of aspirin therapy. *JAMA* 249:2814–7.

Weller, P. F., Lee, C. W., Foster, D. W., Corey, E. J., Austen, K. F., and Lewis, R. A. (1983). Generation and metabolism of 5-lipoxygenase pathway leukotrienes by human eosinophils: Predominant production of leukotriene C_4. *Proc. Natl. Acad. Sci. USA* 80:7626–7630.

Whitaker, M. O., Wyche, A., Fitzpatrick, F., Sprecher, H., and Needleman, P. (1979). Triene prostaglandins: prostaglandin D_3 and eicosapentaenoic acid as potential antithrombotic substances. *Proc. Natl. Acad. Sci. USA* 76:5919–5923.

Zakrzewski, J. T., Sampson, A. P., Evans, J. M., Barnes, N. C., Piper, P. J., and Costello, J. F. (1989). The biotransformation in vitro of cysteinyl leukotrienes in blood of normal and asthmatic subjects. *Prostaglandins* 37(4):425–444.

15

Kinins and Mast Cell–Related Diseases

DAVID PROUD

The Johns Hopkins University School of Medicine
Baltimore, Maryland

I. Introduction

It is now over 40 years since Rocha e Silva and colleagues (1949) used the name "bradykinin" to describe a smooth muscle spasmogen that was liberated from plasma by the action of either trypsin or the venom of the snake *Bothrops jararaca*. In the years since these studies, major progress has been made in delineating the biochemical pathways by which bradykinin (Arg-Pro-Pro-Gly-Phe-Ser-Pro-Phe-Arg) and the closely related peptide lysylbradykinin are generated and metabolized physiologically in humans. Substantial advances have also been made in establishing the spectrum of pharmacological properties of these two biologically active peptides. In contrast, our understanding of the involvement of kinins in pathophysiological processes has developed much more slowly.

The concept that kinins may play a role in the pathogenesis of allergic events, for example, is not new. Within a year of its discovery, it was suggested that bradykinin may be generated during anaphylactic reactions (Beraldo, 1950). A decade later, when the pharmacological properties of pure bradykinin were first examined, it was again suggested that kinins could be important mediators of inflammatory diseases (Elliott et al., 1960). Despite this early interest in the

are derived from different genes and are biochemically and immunologically distinct from each other.

Plasma Kallikrein

Plasma kallikrein is synthesized in the liver and exists in the circulation as a zymogen, prekallikrein. This single-chain glycoprotein is a γ-globulin. In all plasmas tested, prekallikrein has been found in two major forms, with molecular weights of 85,000 and 88,000 (Mandle and Kaplan, 1977), but as many as seven different forms, with isoelectric points from 8.5 to 8.9, can be detected by isoelectric focusing because of heterogeneity of glycosylation (Hojima et al., 1985).

In vivo, activation of prekallikrein to kallikrein occurs principally as a result of the factor XII–dependent process, referred to as contact activation. This activation pathway involves the interaction of factor XII (Hageman factor), HMW kininogen, and prekallikrein with certain negatively charged surfaces. Of particular relevance to allergic diseases would be surfaces such as basement membranes and large anionic macromolecules such as mucus glycoproteins or proteoglycans, including mast cell heparin (Hojima et al., 1984). As mentioned above, plasma prekallikrein circulates as a complex with HMW kininogen (Mandle et al., 1976), and it has been shown that attachment of prekallikrein to the activating surface is facilitated by the HMW kininogen (Wiggins et al., 1977). Factor XII is not complexed with any other protein and attaches to the surface independently in a manner that results in a confirmational change that facilitates its activation (Griffin, 1978). Moreover, binding of these three proteins in close proximity on a surface results in high local concentrations that, presumably, enhance the rate of contact activation. Once surface attachment has occurred, the initial event is a relatively slow autoactivation of factor XII (Miller et al., 1980). In this process a single peptide bond is hydrolyzed to produce an active enzyme, factor XIIa, that can then convert prekallikrein to kallikrein. Once kallikrein is produced, it then activates the remainder of the factor XII in a reaction that is much more rapid than the initial autoactivation process (Dunn et al., 1982). HMW kininogen accelerates both the activation of prekallikrein by factor XIIa (Silverberg et al., 1980) and the feedback activation of factor XII by kallikrein (Griffin and Cochrane, 1976), although the mechanisms involved are not fully understood.

Prekallikrein is converted to kallikrein by the hydrolysis, within an internal disulfide bridge, of a single peptide bond, resulting in a heavy chain of 52,000 molecular weight connected to a light chain of either 33,000 or 38,000 molecular weight, depending on the form of prekallikrein (Mandle and Kaplan, 1977; Bouma et al., 1980). The enzymatic activity of the kallikrein is associated with the light chain (Mandle and Kaplan, 1977), while the binding sites for the surface and for HMW kininogen are on the heavy chain (Van der Graaf et al., 1982). Once activated, kallikrein can rapidly generate bradykinin from HMW-kininogen. Again, the proximity of these molecules on the surface could be expected to enhance the rate of this reaction. HMW-kininogen is the preferred substrate for plasma kallikrein (Pierce and Guimaraes, 1976). Indeed, in vivo, this enzyme does not liberate kinin from LMW kininogen.

Physiological regulation of the activity of plasma kallikrein and, indeed, of the contact activation process is achieved principally by means of two plasma protease inhibitors: C1-inactivator and α_2-macroglobulin. Not only are both these inhibitors capable of rapidly inactivating plasma kallikrein (McConnell, 1972), but C1-inactivator is also the principal inhibitor of activated factor XII (Forbes et al., 1970). Once plasma kallikrein is activated, therefore, it is the high affinity of this enzyme for HMW kininogen, together with their close proximity on the activating surface, that facilitates the release of bradykinin by kallikrein prior to its inactivation by the protease inhibitors. The lower affinity of LMW kininogen for plasma kallikrein, and the inability of this molecule to bind to surfaces, presumably explain why it is an ineffective substrate for this enzyme in vivo.

Tissue Kallikrein

Tissue kallikreins are single-chain, acidic glycoproteins with isoelectric points around pH 4.0 and reported molecular weights ranging from 25,000 to 43,000 (Nustad et al., 1978; Fiedler, 1979). Although it was originally believed that tissue kallikreins were derived only from the major exocrine organs, such as the pancreas, salivary glands, and the kidney, it is now apparent that these enzymes enjoy a much more widespread distribution that includes tissues such as the gut (Schachter et al., 1983), airways (Baumgarten et al., 1986b; Christiansen et al., 1987), and vessel walls (Nolly et al., 1985), as well as endocrine tissues, such as the pituitary gland (Powers and Nasjletti, 1983; Fuller et al., 1985). Immunoreactive tissue kallikrein has also been detected in plasma (Lawton et al., 1981; Shimamoto et al., 1984), but the majority of this material appears to represent biologically inactive enzyme that is cleared by the kidneys (Lawton et al., 1981).

In any given species, the tissue kallikreins from all organs are immunologically identical (Proud et al., 1977; Pisano, 1975). Moreover, in humans, sequence analysis of cDNA clones of pancreatic and renal kallikreins have shown the active enzyme from each tissue to have an identical sequence of 238 amino acids, and it is likely that a single gene codes for authentic tissue kallikrein (Baker and Shine, 1985; Fukushima et al., 1985). Although cloning studies show that kallikrein is synthesized, in all tissues examined to date, as a preproenzyme, conventional biochemical techniques show that in some tissues, such as the pancreas and kidney, kallikrein is present, and is released, primarily in the form of prokallikrein, while in other tissues, such as the salivary gland, only active kallikrein is detectable. The variable molecular weights reported for tissue kallikreins from different organs are most likely due to differential posttranslational glycosylation. Even from a single tissue source, isoelectric focusing reveals multiple forms of kallikrein, but removal of sialic acid by neuraminidase treatment abolishes this heterogeneity (Fiedler et al., 1970).

The factors that regulate kallikrein secretion from tissues are not fully understood, but studies performed to date have suggested that control mechanisms may vary from tissue to tissue. Mineralocorticoids appear to play a role in renal kallikrein secretion (Margolius et al., 1974), apparently stimulating secretion of the active enzyme more than that of the proenzyme (Lieberthal et al., 1983), while kallikrein secretion from the salivary glands is largely under sympathetic control (Barton et al., 1975). In contrast, secretion from intestinal goblet cells has been reported to be under cholinergic control (Schachter et al., 1983), and secretion of pancreatic kallikrein is enhanced by vagus nerve stimulation and by cholecystokinin (Farrell, 1960). Not only do we need to better understand the factors controlling kallikrein secretion, but, in those tissues in which prokallikrein is the principal form of the enzyme, studies on the mechanism of prokallikrein activation are necessary. While it is known that purified prokallikrein can be activated in vitro by enzymes such as trypsin or plasmin, the identity of the endogenous kallikrein-activating enzyme in tissues such as the kidney is unknown.

The interactions of tissue kallikrein with kininogens differs in three important ways from that of plasma kallikrein. First, while HMW kininogen is clearly the preferred substrate for plasma kallikrein, tissue kallikreins release kinin equally well from both HMW and LMW kininogens (Pierce and Guimaraes, 1976), providing them with a greater available pool of substrate. The second difference is that tissue kallikreins are unique among human enzymes in that they hydrolyze two dissimilar bonds within the kininogen moiety to release lysylbradykinin. The mechanisms involved in this interaction are not fully understood. The hydrolysis of an Arg-Ser bond at the C-terminal end of the kinin moiety is in keeping with the anticipated primary substrate specificity of kallikrein, and it has been suggested that this bond is hydrolyzed more rapidly than the Met-Lys bond at the amino terminal end of the kinin moiety (Fiedler, 1979). Studies with small peptides have confirmed the ability of kallikrein to hydrolyze methionyl bonds but indicate that this is highly dependent on the nature of the P2 and P3 amino acids. The bulky leucine residue at the P2 position in the peptide, Ser-Leu-Met-Lys-bradykinin, for example, is thought to be important for permitting the hydrolysis of the methionyl bond to release lysyslbradykinin (Iwanaga et al., 1977). It is presumed that the intact kininogen molecule provides an essential stereochemical confirmation to permit this bond to be hydrolyzed at high catalytic rates. The final difference between tissue and plasma kallikreins is that, while inhibition of plasma kallikrein by plasma protease inhibitors is very rapid, tissue kallikrein is resistant to inhibition. Indeed, in humans, only α_1-antiprotease shows any inhibitory capacity for tissue kallikrein, and even then inhibition occurs only over a period of many hours (Geiger et al., 1981). The combination of this resistance to inhibition and the ability to hydrolyze a larger available pool of substrate enhances the potential importance of tissue kallikrein in kinin generation during inflammatory disorders.

Mast Cell/Basophil Proteases

The central role of mast cells and basophils in allergic events has led several investigators to examine the possibility that kinin formation could occur as a direct result of the actions of enzymes released from these cells.

Antigen challenge of passively sensitized lung fragments was reported to result in the release of three enzymes with potential relevance to kinin formation: a kininogenase, an activator of plasma prekallikrein, and an enzyme capable of cleaving factor XII (Meier et al., 1979, 1983, 1986). The IgE dependence of the generation of these activities focused attention on the mast cell as a possible source of these enzymes. A factor XII–cleaving enzyme, apparently identical to neutrophil elastase, has been reported to be released from purified mast cells (Meier et al., 1989). Although this enzyme cleaves factor XII, however, it does not result in activation of this zymogen. Moreover, the presence of elastase in human mast cells has recently been disputed (Schechter et al., 1990). Prekallikrein activator activity has also been detected from stimulated mast cells (Newball et al., 1981), but relatively large numbers of mast cells are necessary to produce significant amounts of activity. Finally, highly purified human pulmonary mast cells have been shown to release a kininogenase (Proud et al., 1985). More recent studies have shown that this activity is due to mast cell tryptase (Proud et al., 1988b) but clearly indicate that, even under the unusual conditions (pH 5.5) required for optimal activity, this enzyme is a very weak kininogenase, displaying about 1% of the kinin-generating activity of tissue kallikrein. The properties of tryptase differ from those ascribed to the kininogenase from chopped lung and raise the possibility that this latter enzyme is not mast cell derived. It may represent a novel protease that remains to be characterized, or since it has now been shown that tissue kallikrein can be detected in bronchoalveolar lavage fluids (Christiansen et al., 1987), it is possible that the enzyme produced from chopped lung may represent tissue kallikrein that was released by an indirect mechanism.

Human basophils have also been reported to contain a kallikrein-like enzyme (Newball et al., 1979a,b). Human leukocytes containing basophils were shown to release arginine esterolytic activity, measured by its ability to hydrolyze the synthetic substrate *N*-α-*p*-tosyl-L-arginine methyl ester (TAME), upon IgE-mediated stimulation. Gel filtration of this activity suggested that it eluted with an apparent molecular weight of 1.2×10^6 and was associated with both kinin-generating and factor XII–cleaving activities. The presence of multiple functional activities and the unusually high molecular weight of this peak raise the possibility that several enzymes may actually have been present. The chromatographic separation was performed in low salt buffer and it is known, in the mast cell, that the interaction of several proteases with the cellular proteoglycan is only disrupted in high salt conditions. Moreover, in a limited number of recent studies using purified basophils (5–84%), the release of arginine esterase activity has been confirmed but no kinin-generating activity was detected (D. Proud, unpublished observations).

In summary, therefore, it is clear that kinin generation in allergic events occurs subsequent to mast cell or basophil activation. It has been conclusively shown, for example, that drugs that inhibit the release of mast cell mediators during the response to nasal provocation with allergen also decrease kinin generation (Naclerio et al., 1986; Pipkorn et al., 1987a). A major, direct role for mast cell or basophil enzymes in kinin generation, however, remains to be established. At this point, it is more likely that the major link between mast cell activation and kinin generation relates to the release of vasoactive mediators, such as histamine. These mediators increase vascular permeability and permit the influx of kininogens and the activation of plasma kallikrein. Thus antihistamines, such as azatadine and terfenadine, that both antagonize the actions of histamine at vascular H_1 receptors and inhibit histamine release in vivo are effective in reducing kinin generation during the immediate allergic response (Togias et al., 1986; Naclerio et al., 1990).

III. Kinin Generation During Mast Cell–Dependent Events

Although investigators have attempted to document kinin generation during allergic reactions for almost 40 years, early attempts focused on trying to demonstrate increases in systemic plasma kinins (Beraldo, 1950; Brocklehurst and Lahiri, 1962; Abe et al., 1967). These studies faced two major problems. First, it is now generally accepted that kinins are not systemic hormones. These peptides are rapidly destroyed in several vascular beds, and systemic levels of kinins are likely to increase dramatically only when extraordinary perturbations of the system occur. Second, while it may be argued that anaphylaxis could result in a sufficient stress to the body's control mechanisms that systemic kinins may be elevated, the technical difficulties of accurately measuring plasma kinins have only really been appreciated within the last decade, and the methods used in these earlier studies are now recognized as seriously flawed. Thus, by 1980, the best evidence to support the possible generation of kinins during allergic events was indirect, namely, that HMW kininogen was consumed during human anaphylaxis (Smith et al., 1980).

The first direct evidence that kinins could be generated during a local allergic reaction in humans was provided using a model of nasal provocation with allergen in which inflammatory mediators could be measured in secretions recovered by lavage (Proud et al., 1983). Insufflation of an appropriate allergen into the nasal cavity of an allergic individual resulted in the rapid manifestation of sneezing, nasal congestion, and rhinorrhea. Concomitant with this symptomatic response, markedly increased levels of kinins could be detected in recovered nasal lavages (Fig. 1). In this initial study of eight allergic and eight nonallergic subjects, allergen challenge resulted in striking increases in the levels of kinins in nasal lavages of allergic (5.6 ± 1.7 ng/ml; mean ± SE) but not nonallergic (0.04 ± 0.02 ng/ml) subjects. Typically, there were no increases in kinin levels following challenge with placebo, and the specificity of the response was further verified by demonstrating that challenge of allergic subjects with a nonrelevant allergen did not induce either a symptomatic response or the generation of kinins. The presence of kinins was highly correlated with the levels of histamine and of TAME-esterase activity and with the onset of symptoms ($p < 0.001$ in each case). In additional studies, it has also been shown that kinin generation correlates with the production of prostaglandin D_2 (PGD_2) and of sulfidopeptide leukotrienes (Pipkorn et al., 1987b). A major advantage of these studies was that, in contrast to the problems related with measuring plasma kinins, it was possible to rigorously validate the assay of kinins in nasal lavages and to definitively identify, by high-performance liquid chromatography (HPLC) analysis, the kinins generated as a mixture of both bradykinin and lysylbradykinin (Proud et al., 1983, and Fig. 2).

The nasal challenge model lent itself well to additional studies of the mechanisms of kinin formation, in part because the lavage procedure used apparently dilutes some of the enzyme-substrate interactions below K_m and essentially stops these reactions. It was shown that, during the allergic response, both HMW and LMW kininogens enter nasal secretions by transudation from plasma and, thereby, provide substrates for kinin-generating enzymes (Baumgarten et al., 1985). The presence of both bradykinin and lysylbradykinin during the allergic response suggested that two enzymes may be involved in kinin generation. Since plasma prekallikrein circulates as a complex with HMW kininogen, it was not surprising that immunoreactive plasma (pre)kallikrein could also be detected in nasal secretions during the allergic reaction. Biochemical studies revealed, however, that prekallikrein had been activated during the allergic reaction and had been subsequently bound to protease inhibitors (Baumgarten et al., 1986a). The presence of complexes of C1-inactivator with both kallikrein

kinin generation. Indeed, since nasal secretions also contain an aminopeptidase M–like enzyme that can convert lysylbradykinin to bradykinin (Proud et al., 1987), it is likely that the percentage of lysylbradykinin generated during the allergic response may initially be even higher than detected.

Following the initial demonstration of kinin formation during the immediate allergic response in the upper airways, analogous observations have been made in other target organs of the allergic response. Kinin levels were shown to be increased in bronchoalveolar lavages of asthmatic subjects responding to aerosolized allergen challenge compared to lavage samples from normal subjects (Christiansen et al., 1987). The increased levels of kinins correlated with levels of tissue kallikrein in lavage fluids. More recently, segmental allergen challenge has been used to demonstrate that allergen challenge of allergic asthmatic subjects results in increased kinin generation compared to saline challenge of the same subjects (Christiansen et al., 1989). Increased generation of both bradykinin and lysylbradykinin is also detected in recovered tear fluids from allergic subjects following conjunctival provocation with allergen (Proud et al., 1990). Finally, while it has proven technically more difficult to measure kinins directly in blister chamber fluids following allergen challenge of the skin, the presence of plasma kallikrein/C1-inactivator and factor XII/C1-inactivator complexes in these fluids provides strong indirect evidence that kinin generation occurs in the dermal allergic response (Atkins et al., 1987).

It is clear that the immediate response to allergen challenge does not adequately reflect chronic allergic disease, and several authors have suggested that the late-phase response may be a better model of the clinical entity. It was clearly of interest, therefore, to determine whether kinin generation also occurred during late allergic reactions. Studies in the upper airways have clearly demonstrated that kinins are produced during the late response, although at lower levels than observed during the immediate response to challenge (Naclerio et al., 1985). Kinin formation, again, correlates with the recurrence of symptoms and with the generation of histamine and TAME-esterase activity. In contrast to the early reaction, however, PGD_2 is not produced during the late response. It has been suggested that this reflects a role of basophils, rather than mast cells, in the late reaction, since, although both cell types produce histamine, the basophil, unlike the mast cell, does not produce PGD_2. Further support for this hypothesis has been provided by the demonstration that basophils can be detected in nasal secretions during the late response (Bascom et al., 1988). The mechanisms by which kinins are generated during the late-phase response in the upper airways have not been determined, but both bradykinin and lysylbradykinin are, again, produced (Fig. 2). Recent studies have shown that kinins are also present in high concentrations in bronchoalveolar lavage fluids obtained 19 hr after segmental lung challenge of allergic asthmatics with allergen. In contrast to the upper airways, kinin levels in bronchoalveolar lavages at this time are considerably higher than those collected 5 min after challenge (Liu et al., 1990). At this point, it is not possible to determine whether the differences between results in the upper and lower airways reflect different pathologies or variations in methodologies. In the skin, it also seems likely that kinin generation can occur during the late-phase response, since formation of plasma kallikrein/C1-inactivator and factor XII/C1-inactivator complexes did not peak until several hours after challenge (Atkins et al., 1987). Moreover, tissue kallikrein has been detected in late-phase skin blister fluids (Dorsch et al., 1982).

Finally, kinin formation has also been documented in a condition in which mast cell activation apparently occurs by an antigen-independent mechanism. Some individuals report a history of symptoms of rhinitis upon exposure to cold, windy environments. It has proven possible to reproduce symptoms in such subjects by nasal provocation with cold, dry air. In 12 such subjects, provocation with cold, dry air, but not with warm, moist air, led to a significant increase in the levels of kinins in recovered nasal lavages (2.9 ± 0.07 ng/ml), while no such response was observed in subjects without a history of sensitivity to cold environments (Togias et al., 1985). In the symptomatic subjects, increases in kinins correlated with increases in histamine and TAME-esterase activity ($p < 0.001$) and with symptom scores ($p < 0.05$). The increase in histamine in nasal lavages during this reaction has been presumed to reflect mast cell activation. One hypothesis to explain such an activation is that the provocation procedure results in evaporative water loss that increases the osmolarity of the nasal mucosa (Togias et al., 1988). This increased osmolarity may then lead to mast cell histamine release, since mast cells can be activated in vitro when placed in hyperosmolar environments (Eggleston et al., 1983). Regardless of the mechanism involved, these studies clearly demonstrate that kinin generation is associated with several types of mast cell–dependent inflammatory reactions.

IV. Kinins in the Pathophysiology of Allergic Events

The studies listed above provide solid evidence that kinin formation occurs during mast cell–dependent reactions, but they do not address the issue of whether kinin generation plays a role in the pathogenesis of such reactions. Some insight into the potential importance of kinins in disease processes can be gained from a general consideration of their pharmacological properties and by evaluating the effects of exogenously administered bradykinin on relevant target organs.

In general, the pharmacological properties of kinins suggest that they are ideal mediators of inflammatory reactions. Both bradykinin and lysylbradykinin display the same range of properties, although some minor differences in their relative potencies have been reported in some tissues, probably reflecting differential rates of metabolism by peptidases. In addition to their abilities to contract many types of smooth muscle and to act as peripheral vasodilators, kinins are approximately 100-fold more potent than histamine in inducing vascular permeability, and as a direct consequence of this, they are extremely effective inducers of edema (Garcia-Leme, 1978). Kinins are also capable of stimulating epithelial ion transport (Musch et al., 1983; Leikauf et al., 1985; Widdicombe et al., 1985) and can stimulate sensory Aδ and C-fibers to cause pain and hyperalgesia (Kaufman et al., 1980; Taiwo and Levine, 1988; Haley et al., 1989). Moreover, they are clearly capable of inducing the release of biologically active lipids, including platelet-activating factor and prostaglandins, from a variety of cell types (Hong and Levine, 1976; McIntyre et al., 1985; Churchill et al., 1989). With this broad spectrum of properties in mind, it must be realized that the potential role of kinins in mast cell–dependent events will be a reflection, in the organ in question, of the specific types of target cells that display kinin receptors and are, therefore, susceptible to stimulation. Thus, although studies of the effects of exogenously applied kinins demonstrate variations in the types of responses induced in different target tissues, it is clear that these peptides induce a symptomatic response that is relevant, in each case, to that observed during allergic events in the tissue in question.

In the lower airways of humans, for example, several investigators have shown that aerosolized bradykinin is a potent bronchoconstrictor in asthmatic, but not in normal, subjects (Herxheimer and Stresemann, 1961; Varonier and Panzani, 1968; Simonsson et al., 1973; Fuller et al., 1987). Bradykinin can cause constriction in vitro of bronchial smooth muscle from several animal species, but it has been reported to be, at best, a weak constrictor of isolated human airway tissue samples (Bhoola et al., 1962; Simonsson et al., 1973; Newball et al., 1976), although Simonnson and colleagues (1973) reported that tissues from subjects with chronic airflow obstruction tended to be more sensitive than those from subjects with normal airflow. The lack of a pronounced direct effect of bradykinin on smooth muscle, together with the ability of bradykinin to induce cough in all subjects, has led to the suggestion that this peptide exerts its effects, in part, by stimulation of afferent C-fibers (Fuller et al., 1987). The ability of bradykinin to stimulate such fibers has been demonstrated in dogs (Kaufman et al., 1980).

There is also evidence that kinins may increase the volume of airway secretions during asthmatic reactions. Lysylbradykinin has been shown to increase production of respiratory mucus macromolecules in canine tracheal explants (Baker et al., 1977), and bradykinin has been shown to be able to increase secretion from canine tracheal glands by a reflex mechanism after stimulation of bronchial C-fibers (Davis et al., 1982). Moreover, since bradykinin can stimulate chloride secretion across respiratory epithelium (Leikauf et al., 1985; Widdicombe et al., 1985), transepithelial water transport could also contribute to increased airway secretions. Although it may be expected that bradykinin could also stimulate secretions as a result of increased vascular permeability and transudation of plasma, there have been no studies in vivo in humans confirming that this occurs.

The final physiological response that could occur upon bradykinin generation during allergic events in the lower airways is an alteration of ciliary beat frequency, since bradykinin has been reported to increase ciliary beat frequency via a prostaglandin-dependent pathway (Tamaoki et al., 1989).

In the upper airways, it has been shown that administration of bradykinin to the human nasal mucosa results in a dose-dependent induction of symptoms of rhinitis, regardless of the atopic status of the subject (Proud et al., 1988a). Although some individual variations were noted in the pattern of symptoms recorded following unilateral provocation, the principal symptoms reported were nasal obstruction on the challenged side, rhinorrhea, and sore throat. Bradykinin did not induce sneezing, suggesting that, in contrast to the lower airways, this peptide does not stimulate afferent sensory fibers. Anterior rhinomanometry demonstrated objectively that both the magnitude and duration of the induced unilateral nasal obstruction were dose-dependent. The ability of bradykinin to induce obstruction and rhinorrhea has recently been confirmed by others (Holmberg et al., 1990). Clearly, the nasal vasculature is a major target for the actions of bradykinin. Nasal provocation results in a striking dose-dependent increase in the levels of albumin and TAME-esterase activity in recovered nasal secretions (Proud et al., 1988a; Fig. 3), indicating a marked increase in vascular permeability. This observation is consistent with the autoradiographic demonstration that vascular smooth muscle was a major binding site for radiolabeled bradykinin in human turbinate nasal mucosa (Baraniuk et al., 1990). The increased vascular permeability induced by bradykinin would not only contribute to the rhinorrhea associated with kinin challenge, but the associated edema could play a role in increasing nasal obstruction. The ability of bradykinin to induce respiratory glycoconjugate release from the nasal mucosa (Baraniuk et al., 1990) could also contribute to rhinorrhea, as could transepithelial water transport associated with bradykinin-evoked chloride secretion (Leikauf et al., 1985; Widdicombe et al., 1985). Although it has been reported that bradykinin can release histamine from rodent mast cells (Johnson and Erdoe, 1973; Ishizaka et al., 1985), the ability of bradykinin to induce symptoms of rhinitis does not appear to be due to mast cell activation, since histamine levels in nasal secretions did not increase following kinin challenge (Proud et al., 1988a; Fig. 3). This is consistent with the observation that bradykinin is not a secretagogue for human mast cells or basophils in vitro (Lawrence et al., 1989).

In the skin, the effects of bradykinin, again, appear to be directed principally toward vascular tissues. In contrast to substance P, which causes a marked wheal-and-flare response, bradykinin causes a wheal and localized erythema but very little flare. Antihistamines markedly attenuate the substance P–induced flare

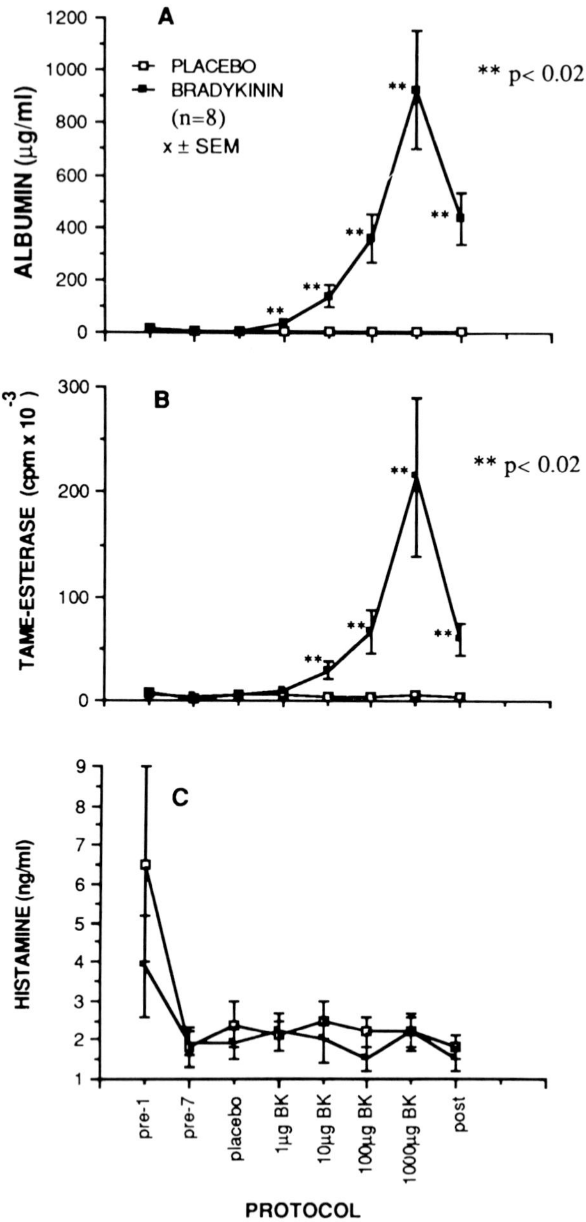

Figure 3 Protein and mediator levels in nasal lavages after provocation with bradykinin. Values are those in the lavages performed 10 min after administration of the material indicated in the protocol. (Reproduced with permission from Proud et al., 1988a.)

but have little effect on the response to bradykinin (Crossman and Fuller, 1988). These observations are, again, consistent with the inability of bradykinin to induce histamine release from human skin mast cells (Lawrence et al., 1989) and suggest that the response to intradermal bradykinin is largely a result of local increased vascular permeability.

V. Pharmacological Intervention Studies

Definitive proof for a role of kinins in allergic events can only be provided by demonstrating that blocking the actions of these peptides during such reactions leads to symptomatic relief. Studies in this regard are in their early stages and have been of two types: those studies that have attempted to determine if kinins may act indirectly in a manner susceptible to existing pharmacological agents, and those studies that have tried to interfere directly with the interactions of kinins with their specific receptors.

Kinins are known to stimulate the release of prostaglandins from several cell types, including epithelial (Churchill et al., 1989) and endothelial cells (McIntyre et al., 1985). Moreover, prostaglandins have been shown to enhance the ability of kinins to increase vascular permeability in some models (Williams and Peck, 1977), and in some tissues, actions of kinins have been shown to be mediated via prostanoids. It is not surprising, therefore, that the ability of cyclooxygenase inhibitors to modulate the proinflammatory effects of kinins have been evaluated in several target tissues of the allergic response. Despite the ability of prostanoids to enhance bradykinin-evoked increases in vascular permeability in rabbit skin (Williams and Peck, 1977), cyclooxygenase inhibition has proven ineffective in reducing the effects of intradermally administered bradykinin in humans (Crossman and Fuller, 1988). Prostaglandins also do not appear to play a part in the ability of angiotensin-converting enzyme inhibitors to potentiate the effects of kinins (McAlpine and Thomson, 1989). In the guinea pig lung, bronchoconstriction evoked by bradykinin can be inhibited by pretreatment with cyclooxygenase inhibitors (Collier et al., 1960). In humans, however, oral administration of 1 g of aspirin did not reduce bradykinin-induced bronchoconstriction in asthmatics (Fuller et al., 1987). The effects of aspirin on vascular permeability in the lower airways have not bee evaluated. In the upper airways, however, a 2-day pretreatment with aspirin had no effect on the symptoms of rhinitis induced by bradykinin provocation and failed to significantly reduce increased vascular permeability, although a slight inhibitory trend was noticed (Proud et al., unpublished observations). Since cyclooxygenase inhibitors are not effective as antiallergic drugs, the demonstration that this class of drug is also ineffective in blocking the effects of exogenously administered kinins is important if the hypothesis that kinins may play a role in allergic events is to remain tenable.

In the lung, the ability of bradykinin to induce bronchoconstriction has been inhibited by sodium cromoglycate, nedocromil sodium, and ipratroprium bromide (Fuller et al., 1987; Dixon and Barnes, 1989). These observations have been interpreted as supporting the concept that this action of bradykinin is mediated, at least in part, by neural reflexes. Unfortunately, this is not a specific effect for bradykinin, so these agents cannot be used to accurately delineate the importance of this peptide in allergic events in the lower airways.

Clearly, the most direct way to interfere with the actions of kinins is to prevent them from occupying their specific receptors. Considerable excitement was generated, therefore, when the first generation of kinin receptor antagonists was recently developed (Vavrek and Stewart, 1985). One such compound, [$DArg^0$, Hyp^3, $DPhe^7$]-bradykinin, was selected for evaluation as a potentially useful therapeutic agent. The compound was able to antagonize the effects of bradykinin on contraction of isolated intestinal and uterine smooth muscle preparations with a pA_2 of approximately 6, but, like bradykinin, the antagonist has a short half-life in vivo.

In vivo studies of allergic sheep showed that inhalation of this antagonist 30 min before provocation with aerosolized bradykinin led to a significant reduction of the bradykinin-evoked bronchoconstriction (Soler et al., 1990), a surprising observation in light of the presumed short half-life of the antagonist. In the same study, this compound had no effect on the immediate response to allergen challenge but was capable of inhibiting both the influx of neutrophils and the hyperreactivity to methacholine that is usually observed 2 hr after antigen challenge in this model.

Unfortunately, studies using this same compound in the upper airways in humans have proven less encouraging. In the first placebo-controlled, double-blind study of a kinin antagonist in humans, a 500-μg dose of [$DArg^0$, Hyp^3, $DPhe^7$]-bradykinin was administered 5 min prior to challenge with 20 μg of bradykinin, after it was shown that doses of the antagonist up to 2 mg had no partial agonist activity. By using a 25-fold excess of antagonist and by pre-administering the drug to favor receptor occupancy, it was hoped that conditions would enhance the possibility of a positive drug effect. Under these conditions, however, the antagonist had no effect on the symptomatic response to bradykinin provocation, nor did it reduce bradykinin-induced increases in vascular permeability, as assessed by the levels of albumin in recovered lavage fluids (Pongracic et al., 1991). This lack of antagonism was not due to clearance or metabolism of the compound in the 5 min prior to bradykinin challenge, since in a second double-blind study, in which the antagonist and bradykinin were administered simultaneously, the compound was still ineffective. The failure of this compound to inhibit the response to provocation with bradykinin in humans could reflect an inability of the compound to gain access to the appropriate receptor, or it could be that the effects of bradykinin are mediated via a subtype of receptor for which this compound is not an antagonist. Perhaps, the most likely possibility, however, is that the compound is simply not sufficiently potent to be effective. Regardless of the reason, it is clear that this particular antagonist is not an appropriate compound to delineate the role of kinins in allergic events in humans.

Although the results with [DArg^0, Hyp^3, DPhe^7]-bradykinin in humans have been disappointing, the work performed with antagonists to date has provided an impetus for several laboratories and pharmaceutical companies to focus on developing improved compounds. Antagonists with enhanced potency and improved stability have already been produced, and the next few years seem certain to provide exciting new opportunities for better understanding the mechanisms of kinin action and for definitively delineating the role of kinins in allergic and inflammatory diseases.

Acknowledgments

I acknowledge support from Grant Number HL 32272 from the National Institutes of Health. This is Publication Number 075 from the Johns Hopkins Asthma and Allergy Center.

References

Abe, K., Watanabe, N., Kumagai, N., Mouri, T., and Yoshinaga, K. (1967). Circulating plasma kinin in patients with bronchial asthma. *Experientia* 23:626–627.

Atkins, P. C., Miragliotta, G., Talbot, S. F., Zweiman, B., and Kaplan, A. P. (1987). Activation of plasma Hageman factor and kallikrein in ongoing allergic reactions in the skin. *J. Immunol.* 139:2744–2748.

Baker, A. P., Hillegass, L. M., Holden, D. A., and Smith, W. J. (1977). Effect of kallidin, substance P, and other basic polypeptides on the production of respiratory macromolecules. *Am. Rev. Respir. Dis.* 115:811–817.

Baker, A. R., and Shine, J. (1985). Human kidney kallikrein: cDNA cloning and sequence analysis. *DNA* 4:445–450.

Baraniuk, J. N., Lundgren, J. D., Mizoguchi, H., Peden, H., Gawin, A., Merida, M., Shelhamer, J. H., and Kaliner, M. A. (1990). Bradykinin and respiratory mucous membranes. Analysis of bradykinin binding site distribution and secretory responses in vitro and in vivo. *Am. Rev. Respir. Dis.* 141:706–714.

Barton, S., Sanders, E. J., Schachter, M., and Uddin, M. (1975). Autonomic nerve stimulation, kallikrein content and acinar cell granules of the cat's submandibular gland. *J. Physiol.* 251:363–369.

Bascom, R., Wachs, M., Naclerio, R. M., Pipkorn, U., Galli, S. J., and Lichtenstein, L. M. (1988). Basophil influx occurs after nasal antigen challenge: effects of topical corticosteroid pretreatment. *J. Allergy Clin. Immunol.* 81:580–589.

Baumgarten, C. R., Togias, A. G., Naclerio, R. M., Lichtenstein, L. M., Norman, P. S., and Proud, D. (1985). Influx of kininogens into nasal secretions after antigen challenge of allergic individuals. *J. Clin. Invest.* 76:191–197.

Baumgarten, C. R., Nichols, R. C., Naclerio, R. M., Lichtenstein, L. M., Norman, P. S., and Proud, D. (1986a). Plasma kallikrein during experimentally-induced allergic rhinitis: Role in kinin formation and contribution to TAME-esterase activity in nasal secretions. *J. Immunol.* 137:977–982.

Baumgarten, C. R., Nichols, R. C., Naclerio, R. M., and Proud, D. (1986b). Concentrations of glandular kallikrein in human nasal secretions increase during experimentally-induced allergic rhinitis. *J. Immunol.* 137:1323–1328.

Beraldo, W. T. (1950). Formation of bradykinin in anaphylactic and peptone shock. *Am. J. Physiol.* 163:283–289.

Bhoola, K. D., Collier, H. O. J., Schachter, M., and Shorley, P. G. (1962). Actions of some peptides on bronchial muscle. *Br. J. Pharmacol.* 19:190–197.

Bouma, B. N., Miles, L. A., Barretta, G., and Griffin, J. H. (1980). Human plasma prekallikrein. Studies of its activation by activated factor XII and of its inactivation by diisopropyl phosphofluoridate. *Biochemistry* 19:1151–1160.

Brocklehurst, W. E., and Lahiri, S. C. (1962). The production of bradykinin in anaphylaxis. *J. Physiol.* 160:15P–16P.

Christiansen, S. C., Proud, D., and Cochrane, C. G. (1987). Detection of tissue kallikrein in the bronchoalveolar lavage fluids of asthmatic subjects. *J. Clin. Invest.* 79:188–197.

Christiansen, S. C., Proud, D., Sarnoff, R. B., Cochrane, C. G., and Zuraw, B. L. (1989). Human bronchial kallikrein (HBK) in bronchoalveolar lavage (BAL) fluid following local allergen challenge. *J. Allergy Clin. Immunol.* 83:285 (Abstr.).

Churchill, L., Chilton, F. H., Resau, J. H., Bascom, R., Hubbard, W. C., and Proud, D. (1989). Cyclooxygenase metabolism of endogenous arachidonic acid by cultured human tracheal epithelial cells. *Am. Rev. Respir. Dis.* 140:449–459.

Collier, H. O. J., Holgate, J. A., Schachter, M., and Shorley, P. G. (1960). The broncoconstrictor action of bradykinin in the guinea pig. *Br. J. Pharmacol.* 15:290–297.

Crossman, D. C., and Fuller, R. W. (1988). Bradykinin-induced wheal and flare is not mediated by histamine release or cyclooxygenase products. *Br. J. Clin. Pharmacol.* 26:113–115.

Davis, B., Roberts, A. M., Coleridge, H. M., and Coleridge, J. C. G. (1982). Reflex tracheal gland secretion evoked by stimulation of bronchial C-fibers in dogs. *J. Appl. Physiol.* 53:985–991.

Dixon, C. M. S., and Barnes, P. J. (1989). Bradykinin-induced bronchoconstriction: Inhibition by nedocromil sodium and sodium cromoglycate. *Br. J. Clin. Pharmacol.* 27:831–836.

Dolovich, J., Back, N., and Arbesman, C. E. (1970). Kinin-like activity in nasal secretions of allergic patients. *Int. Arch. Allergy* 38:337–344.

Dorsch, W., Ring, J., Reimann, H. J., and Geiger, R. (1982). Mediator studies in skin blister fluid from patients with dual reactions after intradermal allergen injection. *J. Allergy Clin. Immunol.* 70:236–242.

Dunn, J. T., Silverberg, M., and Kaplan, A. P. (1982). The cleavage and formation of activated Hageman factor by autodigestion and by kallikrein. *J. Biol. Chem.* 275:1779–1784.

Eggleston, P. A., Kagey-Sobotka, A., Schleimer, R. P., and Lichtenstein, L. M. (1983). Interaction between hyperosmolar and IgE-mediated histamine release from basophils and mast cells. *Am. Rev. Respir. Dis.* 130:86–91.

Elliott, D. F., Horton, E. W., and Lewis, G. P. (1960). Actions of pure bradykinin. *J. Physiol.* 153:473–480.

Farrell, M. M. (1960). Pancreatic kallikrein in physiological and pathological conditions. In *Polypeptides Which Affect Smooth Muscles and Blood Vessels*. Edited by M. Schachter. Oxford, Pergamon Press, pp. 247–252.

Fiedler, F. (1979). Enzymology of glandular kallikreins. In *Handbook of Experimental Pharmacology: Bradykinin, Kallidin and Kallikrein*. Vol. 25 (Suppl.). Edited by E. G. Erdos. Berlin, Springer-Verlag, pp. 103–161.

Fiedler, F., Hirschauer, C., and Werle, E. (1970). Anreicherung von prakallikrein B aus schweinepankreas und eigerschafter verschiederer former des pankreaskallikreins. *Hoppe-Seyler's Z. Physiol. Chem.* 351:225–238.

Forbes, C. O., Pensky, J., and Ratnoff, O. D. (1970). Inhibition of activated Hageman factor and activated plasma thromboplastin antecedent by purified C1 inactivator. *J. Lab. Clin. Med.* 76:809–815.

Fukushima, D., Kitamura, N., and Nakanishi, S. (1985). Nucleotide sequence of cloned cDNA for human pancreatic kallikrein. *Biochemistry* 24:8037–8043.

Fuller, P. F., Clements, J. A., Whitfield, P. F., and Funder, J. W. (1985). Kallikrein gene expression in the rat anterior pituitary. *Mol. Cell. Endocrinol.* 39:99–105.

Fuller, R. W., Dixon, C. M. S., Cuss, F. M. C., and Barnes, P. J. (1987). Bradykinin-induced bronchoconstriction in humans. Mode of action. *Am. Rev. Respir. Dis.* 135:176–180.

Garcia-Leme, J. (1978). Bradykinin system. In *Handbook of Experimental Pharmacology, Vol. 50, Inflammation*. Edited by J. R. Vane, and S. H. Ferreira. Berlin, Springer-Verlag, pp. 464–522.

Geiger, R., Stuckstedte, U., Clausnitzer, B., and Fritz, H. (1981). Progressive inhibition of human glandular (urinary) kallikrein by human serum and identification of the progressive antikallikrein as α_1-antitrypsin (α_1-protease inhibitor). *Hoppe-Seyler's Z. Physiol. Chem.* 362:317–325.

Griffin, J. H. (1978). Role of surface in surface-dependent activation of Hageman factor (blood coagulation factor XII). *Proc. Natl. Acad. Sci. USA* 75:1998–2002.

Griffin, J. H., and Cochrane, C. G. (1976). Mechanisms for the involvement of high molecular weight kininogen in surface-dependent reactions of Hageman factor. *Proc. Natl. Acad. Sci. USA* 73:2554–2558.

Gustafson, E. J., Schmaier, A. H., Wachtfogel, Y. T., Kaufman, N., Kuchich, U., and Colman, R. W. (1989). Human neutrophils contain and bind high molecular weight kininogen. *J. Clin. Invest.* 84:28–35.

Haley, J. E., Dickenson, A. H., and Schachter, M. (1989). Electrophysiological evidence for a role of bradykinin in chemical nociception in the rat. *Neurosci. Lett.* 97:198–202.

Herxheimer, H., and Stresemann, E. (1961). The effect of bradykinin aerosol in guinea pigs and man. *J. Physiol.* 158:38–39.

Hojima, Y., Cochrane, C. G., Wiggins, R. C., Austen, K. F., and Stevens, R. L. (1984). In vitro activation of the contact (Hageman factor) system of plasma by heparin and chondroitin sulfate E. *Blood* 63:1453–1459.

Hojima, Y., Pierce, J. V., and Pisano, J. J. (1985). Purification and characterization of multiple forms of human plasma prekallikrein. *J. Biol. Chem.* 260:400–406.

Holmberg, K., Bake, B., and Pipkorn, U. (1990). Vascular effects of topically applied bradykinin on the human nasal mucosa. *Eur. J. Pharmacol.* 175:35–41.

Hong, S. L., and Levine, L. (1976). Stimulation of prostaglandin biosynthesis by bradykinin and thrombin and their mechanisms of action on MC5-5 fibroblasts. *J. Biol. Chem.* 251:5814–5816.

Ishizaka, T., Iwata, M., and Ishizaka, K. (1985). Release of histamine and arachidonate from mouse mast cells induced by glycosylation-enhancing factor and bradykinin. *J. Immunol.* 134:1880–1887.

Iwanaga, S., Han, Y. N., Kato, H., and Suzuki, T. (1977). Actions of various kallikreins on HMW kininogen and its derivatives. In *Kininogenases 4. Physiological Properties and Pharmacological Rationale*. Edited by G. L. Haberland, J. W. Roher, and T. Suzuki. Stuttgart/New York, Schattauer Verlag, pp. 79–90.

Johnson, A. R., and Erdos, E. G. (1973). Release of histamine from mast cells by vasoactive peptides. *Proc. Soc. Exp. Biol. Med.* 142:1251–1256.

Kaplan, A. P., and Silverberg, M. (1987). The coagulation-kinin pathway of human plasma. *Blood* 70:1–15.

Kaufman, M. P., Coleridge, H. M., Coleridge, J. C. G., and Baker, D. G. (1980). Bradykinin stimulates afferent vagal C-fibers in intrapulmonary airways of dogs. *J. Appl. Physiol.* 48:511–517.

Kitamura, N., Kitagawa, H., Fukushima, D., Takagaki, Y., Miyata, T., and Nakanishi, S. (1985). Structural organization of the human kininogen gene and a model for its evolution. *J. Biol. Chem.* 260:8610–8617.

Lawrence, I. D., Warner, J. A., Cohan, V. L., Lichtenstein, L. M., Kagey-Sobotka, A., Vavrek, R. J., Stewart, J. M., and Proud, D. (1989). Induction of histamine release from human skin mast cells by bradykinin analogs. *Biochem. Pharmacol.* 38:227–233.

Lawton, W. J., Proud, D., Frech, M. E., Pierce, J. V., Keiser, H. R., and Pisano, J. J. (1981). Characterization and origin of immunoreactive glandular kallikrein in rat plasma. *Biochem. Pharmacol.* 30:1731–1737.

Leikauf, G. D., Ueki, I. F., Nadel, J. A., and Widdicombe, J. H. (1985). Bradykinin stimulates Cl secretion and prostaglandin E_2 release by canine tracheal epithelium. *Am. J. Physiol.* 248:F48–F55.

Lieberthal, W., Oza, N. B., Arbeit, L., Bernard, D. B., and Levinsky, N. G. (1983). Effects of alterations in sodium and water metabolism on urinary excretion of active and inactive kallikrein in man. *J. Clin. Endocrinol. Metab.* 56:513–519.

Liu, M. C., Hubbard, W. C., Proud, D., Stealey, B., Galli, S., Kagey-Sobotka, A., Bleecker, E. R., and Lichtenstein, L. M. (1990). Late inflammation following antigen challenge of the airways in allergic asthmatics. *J. Allergy Clin. Immunol.* 85:263 (abstract).

Mandle, R. J., Jr., and Kaplan, A. P. (1977). Hageman factor substrates. Human plasma prekallikrein. Mechanism of activation by Hageman factor and participation in Hageman factor–dependent fibrinolysis. *J. Biol. Chem.* 252:6097–6104.

Mandle, R. J., Jr., Colman, R. W., and Kaplan, A. P. (1976). Identification of prekallikrein and HMW-kininogen as a circulating complex in human plasma. *Proc. Natl. Acad. Sci. USA* 73:4179–4183.

Margolius, H. S., Horwitz, D., Geller, R. G., Alexander, R. W., Gill, J. R., Pisano, J. J., and Keiser, H. R. (1974). Urinary kallikrein excretion in normal man. Relationships to sodium intake and sodium-retaining steroids. *Circ. Res.* 35:812–819.

McAlpine, L. G., and Thomson, N. C. (1989). The effect of indomethacin and enalapril on the cutaneous response to bradykinin. *Br. J. Clin. Pharmacol.* 27:870–872.

McConnell, D. J. (1972). Inhibitors of kallikrein in human plasma. *J. Clin. Invest.* 51:1611–1623.

McIntyre, T. M., Zimmerman, G. A., Satoh, K., and Prescott, S. M. (1985). Cultured endothelial cells synthesize both platelet activating factor and prostacyclin in response to histamine, bradykinin and adenosine-triphosphate. *J. Clin. Invest.* 76:271–280.

Meier, H. L., Newball, H. H., Berninger, R. W., Talamo, R. C., and Lichtenstein, L. M. (1979). Purification of lung kallikrein of anaphylaxis. *J. Allergy Clin. Immunol.* 63:191 (Abstr.).

Meier, H. L., Kaplan, A. P., Lichtenstein, L. M., Revak, S., Cochrane, C. G., and Newball, H. H. (1983). Anaphylactic release of a prekallikrein activator from human lung in vitro. *J. Clin. Invest.* 72:574–582.

Meier, H. L., Flowers, B., Silverberg, M., Kaplan, A. P., and Newball, H. H. (1986). The IgE-dependent release of a Hageman factor cleaving factor from human lung. *Am. J. Pathol.* 123:146–154.

Meier, H. L., Schulman, E. S., Heck, L. W., MacGlashan, D., Newball, H. H., and Kaplan, A. P. (1989). Release of elastase from purified human lung mast cells and basophils. Identification as a Hageman factor cleaving enzyme. *Inflammation* 13:295–308.

Miller, G., Silverberg, M., and Kaplan, A. P. (1980). Autoactivatability of human Hageman factor (factor XII). *Biochem. Biophys. Res. Commun.* 92:803–810.

Muller-Esterl, W., Fritz, H., Machleidt, W., Ritonja, A., Brzin, J., Kotnik, M., Turk, V., Kellermann, J., and Lottspeich, F. (1985). Human plasma kininogens are identical with α_2-thiol proteinase inhibitors. Evidence from immunological, enzymological and sequence data. *FEBS Lett.* 182:310–314.

Musch, M. W., Kachur, J. F., Miller, R. J., Field, M., and Stoff, J. S. (1983). Bradykinin-stimulated electrolyte secretion in rabbit and guinea pig intestine. Involvement of arachidonic acid metabolites. *J. Clin. Invest.* 71:1073–1083.

Naclerio, R. M., Proud, D., Togias, A. G., Adkinson, N. F., Jr., Meyers, D. A., Kagey-Sobotka, A., Plaut, M., Norman, P. S., and Lichtenstein, L. M. (1985). Inflammatory mediators in late antigen-induced rhinitis. *N. Engl. J. Med.* 313:65–70.

Naclerio, R. M., Bartenfelder, D., Proud, D., Togias, A. G., Meyers, D. A., Kagey-Sobotka, A., Norman, P. S., and Lichtenstein, L. M. (1986). Theophylline reduces histamine release during pollen-induced rhinitis. *J. Allergy Clin. Immunol.* 78:874–876.

Naclerio, R. M., Kagey-Sobotka, A., Lichtenstein, L. M., Freidhoff, L., and Proud, D. (1990). Terfenadine, an H_1 antihistamine, inhibits histamine release in the human. *Am. Rev. Respir. Dis.* 142:167–171.

Newball, H. H., Keiser, H. R., Webster, M. E., and Pisano, J. J. (1976). Effects of bradykinin on human airways. In *Chemistry and Biology of the Kallikrein-Kinin System in Health and Disease*. Edited by J. J. Pisano and K. F. Austen. Washington, D.C., DHEW Publ. No. (NIH) 76–791, pp. 505–511.

Newball, H. H., Berninger, R. W., Talamo, R. C., and Lichtenstein, L. M. (1979a). Anaphylactic release of a basophil kallikrein-like activity. I. Purification and characterization. *J. Clin. Invest.* 64:457–465.

Newball, H. H., Talamo, R. C., and Lichtenstein, L. M. (1979b). Anaphylactic release of a basophil kallikrein-like activity. II. A mediator of immediate hypersensitivity reactions. *J. Clin. Invest.* 64:466–475.

Newball, H. H., Meier, H. L., Kaplan, A. P., Revak, S. D., Cochrane, C. G., and Lichtenstein, L. M. (1981). Activation of Hageman factor by proteases released during antigen challenge of human lung. *Trans. Assoc. Am. Physicians* 94:126–134.

Nolly, H., Scicli, A. G., Scicli, G., and Carretero, O. A. (1985). Characterization of a kininogenase from rat vascular tissue resembling tissue kallikrein. *Circ. Res.* 56:816–821.

Nustad, K., Orstavik, T. B., Gautvik, K. M., and Pierce, J. V. (1978). Glandular kallikreins. *Gen. Pharmacol.* 9:1–9.

Ohkubo, I., Kurachi, K., Takasawa, T., Shiokawa, H., and Sasaki, M. (1984). Isolation of a human cDNA for α_2-thiol proteinase inhibitor and its identity with low molecular weight kininogen. *Biochemistry* 23:5691–5697.

Pierce, J. V., and Guimaraes, J. A. (1976). Further characterization of highly purified human plasma kininogens. In *Chemistry and Biology of the Kallikrein-Kinin System in Health and Disease*. Edited by J. J. Pisano and K. F. Austen. Washington, D.C., DHEW Publ. No. (NIH) 76-791, pp. 121–127.

Pipkorn, U., Proud, D., Lichtenstein, L. M., Kagey-Sobotka, A., Norman, P. S., and Naclerio, R. M. (1987a). Inhibition of mediator release in allergic rhinitis by pretreatment with topical glucocorticosteroids. *N. Engl. J. Med.* 316:1506–1510.

Pipkorn, U., Proud, D., Lichtenstein, L. M., Schleimer, R. P., Peters, S. P., Adkinson, N. F., Jr., Kagey-Sobotka, A., Norman, P. S., and Naclerio, R. M. (1987b). Effect of short-term systemic glucocorticoid treatment on human nasal mediator release after antigen challenge. *J. Clin. Invest.* 80:957–961.

Pisano, J. J. (1975). Chemistry and biology of the kallikrein-kinin system. In *Proteases and Biological Control*. Edited by E. Reich, D. B. Rifkin, and E. Shaw. Cold Spring Harbor, NY, Cold Spring Harbor Lab., pp. 199–222.

Pongracic, J. A., Naclerio, R. M., Reynolds, C. J., and Proud, D. (1991). A competitive kinin receptor antagonist, [DArg^0, Hyp^3, DPhe^7]-bradykinin, does not affect the response to nasal provocation with bradykinin. *Br. J. Clin. Pharmacol.* 31:287–294.

Powers, C. A., and Nasjletti, A. (1983). A kininogenase resembling glandular kallikrein in the rat pituitary pars intermedia. *Endocrinology* 112:1194–1200.

Proud, D., and Kaplan, A. P. (1988). Kinin formation: Mechanisms and role in inflammatory disorders. *Annu. Rev. Immunol.* 6:49–83.

Proud, D., Bailey, G. S., Nustad, K., and Gautvik, K. M. (1977). The immunological similarity of rat glandular kallikreins. *Biochem. J.* 167:835–838.

Proud, D., Pierce, J. V., and Pisano, J. J. (1980). Radioimmunoassay of human high molecular weight kininogen in normal and deficient plasmas. *J. Lab. Clin. Med.* 95:563–574.

Proud, D., Perkins, M., Pierce, J. V., Yates, K. N., Highet, P. F., Herring, P. L., Mangkornkanok/Mark, M., Bahu, R., Carone, F., and Pisano, J. J. (1981). Characterization and localization of human renal kininogen. *J. Biol. Chem.* 256:16034–16039.

Proud, D., Togias, A., Naclerio, R. M., Crush, S. A., Norman, P. S., and Lichtenstein, L. M. (1983). Kinins are generated in vivo following nasal airway challenge of allergic individuals with allergen. *J. Clin. Invest.* 72:1678–1685.

Proud, D., Nakamura, S., Carone, F. A., Herring, P. L., Kawamura, M., Inagami, T., and Pisano, J. J. (1984). The kallikrein-kinin and renin-angiotensin system in rat renal lymph. *Kidney Int.* 25:880–885.

Proud, D., MacGlashan, D. W., Jr., Newball, H. H., Schulman, E. S., and Lichtenstein, L. M. (1985). Immunoglobulin E–mediated release of a kininogenase from purified human lung mast cells. *Am. Rev. Respir. Dis.* 132:405–408.

Proud, D., Baumgarten, C. R., Naclerio, R. M., and Ward, P. E. (1987). Kinin metabolism in nasal secretions during experimentally induced allergic rhinitis. *J. Immunol.* 138:428–434.

Proud, D., Reynolds, C. J., LaCapra, S., Kagey-Sobotka, A., Lichtenstein, L. M., and Naclerio, R. M. (1988a). Nasal provocation with bradykinin induces symptoms of rhinitis and a sore throat. *Am. Rev. Respir. Dis.* 137:613–616.

Proud, D., Siekierski, E. S., and Bailey, G. S. (1988b). Identification of human lung mast cell kininogenase as tryptase and relevance of tryptase kininogenase activity. *Biochem. Pharmacol.* 37:1473–1480.

Proud, D., Sweet, J., Stein, P., Settipane, R. A., Kagey-Sobotka, A., Friedlaender, M. H., and Lichtenstein, L. M. (1990). Inflammatory mediator release on conjunctival provocation of allergic subjects with allergen. *J. Allergy Clin. Immunol.* 85:896–905.

Rocha e Silva, M., Beraldo, W. T., and Rosenfeld, G. (1949). Bradykinin, a hypotensive and smooth muscle stimulating factor released from plasma globulin by snake venoms and by trypsin. *Am. J. Physiol.* 156:261–273.

Salvesen, G., Parkes, C., Abrahamson, M., Grubb, A., and Barrett, A. J. (1986). Human low molecular weight kininogen contains three copies of a cystatin sequence that are divergent in structure and in inhibitory activity for cysteine proteinases. *Biochem. J.* 234:429–434.

Schachter, M., Peret, M. W., Billing, A. G., and Wheeler, G. D. (1983). Immunolocalization of the protease kallikrein in the colon. *J. Histochem. Cytochem.* 31:1255–1260.

Schechter, N. M., Irani, A-M. A., Sprows, J. L., Abernethy, J., Wintroub, B., and Schwartz, L. B. (1990). Identification of a cathepsin G–like proteinase in the MC_{TC} type of human mast cell. *J. Immunol.* 145:2652–2661.

Schmaier, A. H., Zuckerberg, A., Silverman, C., Kuchobhotla, J., Tuszynski, G. P.,

16

Mast Cell Cytokines

JOHN J. COSTA

Beth Israel Hospital and
Harvard Medical School
Boston, Massachusetts

PARRIS R. BURD
DEAN D. METCALFE

National Institute of Allergy and
Infectious Diseases
National Institutes of Health
Bethesda, Maryland

I. Background

Until recently, the mechanisms invoked to explain the participation of mast cells in physiological and pathological processes were limited to groups of molecules termed preformed (histamine, proteoglycans, proteolytic enzymes) and newly generated (leukotrienes, prostaglandins, platelet activating factor) mast cell mediators. It is now appreciated that an additional class of mediators known as cytokines are synthesized and released by mast cells, and that mast cell cytokines may also play an important role in the pathophysiology of allergic and immunological diseases.

Cytokines are protein or glycoprotein molecules synthesized and secreted by cells. The interleukins, interferons, and colony-stimulating factors were the first categories of cytokines discovered and have since been extensively studied. In general, induction of cytokine genes occurs in response to cellular injury or activation, although there are also examples of constitutive cytokine production. Table 1 provides a list of the cell types for which cytokine synthesis has been demonstrated to date. As can be seen, an extensive and broad diversity of cell types are included. In addition, these cells are widely distributed throughout the organism, underscoring their important role in modulating cellular responses.

Table 1 Spectrum of Cells Producing Cytokines

Mast cells	Endothelial cells
T cells	Epithelial cells
B cells	Keratinocytes
Neutrophils	Fibroblasts
Eosinophils	Astrocytes
Monocytes	Microglial cells
Macrophages	Hepatocytes
Platelets	Renal cells
Megakaryocytes	Mesangial cells
NK cells	Smooth muscle cells
Osteoblasts	Pancreatic β cells
Synoviocytes	Endometrial stromal cells
Bone marrow stromal cells	

Table 2 Spectrum of Cytokine Functions

Stem cell colony-stimulating factors
Lineage-specific cell growth and/or differentiation
Induction of MHC antigens
Cellular activation
Initiation of the acute-phase response
Enhancement of endothelial/leukocyte/lymphocyte adhesion
Promotion of chemotaxis
Modulation of cellular biological activities
Transcriptional induction
Arachidonic acid metabolism
Protein phosphorylation
Cytotoxic/tumoricidal activity
Antiviral activity
Induction of other cytokines and/or cytokine receptors

Cytokines exert their biological effects by interaction with specific cytokine receptor molecules located on the surface of target cells. As a group, cytokines possess a broad spectrum of bioactivities and have been found to play a part in cell growth, repair, inflammation, and the immune response. Table 2 provides a summary of the spectrum of functions attributable to cytokines. Detailed descriptions of individual cytokine functions have been the subject of several recent reviews (Strober and James, 1988; Mizel, 1989; Paetkau and Mills, 1989; Wolpe and Cerami, 1989). One important feature of cytokines not apparent from a summary list is that cytokine molecules are both pleiotrophic, with each having multiple functions, and redundant, with more than one cytokine possessing a given bioactivity (Paul, 1989). In addition, in vivo these molecules do not exist in isolation, but rather as a network in which the expression of one cytokine may be influenced both by other cytokines and by noncytokine mediators (Akira et al., 1990).

II. Effects of Cytokines on Mast Cells

Not surprisingly, the biology of mast cells themselves is influenced by cytokines. As has been described, several cytokines have been demonstrated to either stimulate or inhibit the growth or differentiation of mast cells. The ability of interleukin (IL)-3 to promote the outgrowth of mast cells in bone marrow cultures of both murine (Schrader et al., 1981; Tertian et al., 1981; Razin et al., 1981, 1984; Ihle et al., 1983) and human (Kirshenbaum et al., 1989; Bressler et al., 1990) origins, and to support the survival and proliferation of long-term in vitro–derived murine mast cell lines (Nagao et al., 1981; Pluznik et al., 1982) is well established. In addition, IL-4 (Mosmann et al., 1986; Smith and Rennick, 1986), IL-9 (Hultner et al., 1989a, 1990; Renauld et al., 1990), and IL-10 (Thompson-Snipes et al., 1990) have been demonstrated to act synergistically with IL-3 to enhance the proliferation of cultured IL-3-dependent murine mast cells. The combination of IL-3 and IL-4 also has been shown to trigger the proliferation of purified mouse peritoneal connective tissue–type mast cells grown in methylcellulose (Tsuji et al., 1990). Under similar conditions, neither cytokine alone was able to induce extensive colony formation, although IL-3 alone could support the survival of these cells and proliferation could be induced by $Fc_{\epsilon}RI$ crosslinking followed by culture in the presence of IL-3 (Takagi et al., 1989).

Recently, a new substance termed mast cell growth factor (Boswell et al., 1990) or stem cell factor (Zsebo et al., 1990a) has been found to support the growth of several mast cell lines as well as to augment mast cell proliferation in response to IL-3 and/or IL-4. This new factor has been shown to be encoded by the *Sl* locus (Copeland et al., 1990; Zsebo et al., 1990b; Huang et al., 1990), and to be the ligand for the c-*kit* protooncogene (Williams et al., 1990; Zsebo et al., 1990b).

In contrast to these cytokines that promote mast cell growth, there are now several examples of cytokines that have an inhibitory influence on mast cell proliferation. Addition of granulocyte/macrophage colony-stimulating factor (GM-CSF) to murine bone marrow cultures resulted in a decrease from 95% mast cells to less than 1% mast cells after 2–3 weeks of culture in the presence of IL-3 (Bressler et al., 1989). In a separate study, transforming growth factor (TGF)-β_1

was found to cause a dose-dependent, reversible inhibition of murine bone marrow–derived cultured mast cells (BMCMC) proliferation as assessed by tritiated thymidine incorporation (Broide et al., 1989). Prolonged exposure of BMCMC to TGF-β_1 did not affect cell viability, histamine content, or staining properties, nor was any influence on either antigen or calcium ionophore-induced β-hexosaminidase release or leukotriene C4 generation observed. Interferon (IFN)-γ also appears to have an inhibitory influence on mast cell proliferation. One group of investigators has demonstrated a dose-dependent, reversible suppression of colony formation by mouse peritoneal connective tissue–type mast cells cultured in IL-3 after antigen mediated $Fc_\epsilon RI$ crosslinking, or in response to culture in the presence of IL-3 and IL-4 (Takagi et al., 1990). Other workers have shown that addition of IFN-γ to cultures of murine bone marrow grown in the presence of IL-3 at either the time of seeding or after 7 days results in a marked decrease in the number of mast cells observed (Nafziger et al., 1990). However, there was no apparent effect of IFN-γ on the growth of 3-week BMCMC, suggesting that the inhibitory effect of this cytokine was restricted to the mast cell precursors.

In addition to its antiproliferative effect, IFN-γ also has been shown to reduce mast cell natural cytotoxicity for WEHI-164 target cells by 50% in a dose- and time-dependent fashion (Bissonnette and Befus, 1990). This inhibition was associated with a decreased release of tumor necrosis factor (TNF)α into the culture supernatants, although spontaneous histamine release was unaffected and remained less than 10% for both control and IFNγ-treated cultures. IFN-α/β was found to have similar effects, although somewhat higher doses were required to obtain an equivalent degree of inhibition. Preincubation of the mast cells with actinomycin D or cycloheximide to inhibit RNA and protein synthesis, respectively, also was sufficient to cause a 50% decrease in mast cell–mediated cytotoxicity, and in the presence of these drugs, neither class of interferon had any additional inhibitory effect, suggesting that new protein synthesis was required for interferon to influence the cell. In an earlier study, this group demonstrated that a 24-hr preincubation with IFN-α/β resulted in a dose-dependent inhibition of histamine release following antigen-mediated crosslinking of $Fc_\epsilon RI$ in rat peritoneal mast cells (Swieter et al., 1989). In contrast, IFN-α/β had no effect on histamine release induced in response to substance P or compound 48/80.

Several other effects of cytokines on mast cells have been documented. IL-3 has been shown to stimulate chemotaxis of mouse peritoneal mast cells, with an additional minor chemokinetic component (Matsuura and Zetter, 1989). No chemotactic activity was observed in response to IL-4, nor was any synergistic effect noted with the combination of IL-3 and IL-4. Mast cells have recently been found to possess functional laminin receptors that mediate the adhesion and spreading of these cells on a laminin-coated surface in response to $Fc_\epsilon RI$ crosslinking (Thompson et al., 1989). Both IL-3 and TGF-β_1 (Thompson et al.,

1990) have been shown to enhance mast cell adhesion to laminin. Finally, preincubation of purified human lung mast cells with IL-1α followed by antigen-mediated $Fc_{\epsilon}RI$ crosslinking resulted in enhanced leukotriene C4 and prostaglandin D2 release compared with cells that had not been exposed to IL-1 (Salari and Chan-Yeung, 1989). This effect of IL-1 was both time- and dose-dependent. It is likely that future studies will reveal a multitude of additional influences of cytokines on mast cells. The challenge will be to correlate and integrate these primarily in vitro observations with physiological mast cell functions and responses in vivo.

It is appropriate to sound a note of caution regarding the need to reproduce the animal data in humans, as there can be significant differences in the observed responses. Perhaps the best example to illustrate this point is the different results observed in the aforementioned investigations on the culture of human or mouse bone marrow in IL-3. While murine bone marrow grown in the presence of mouse IL-3 yields a nearly pure population of mast cells after 3 weeks, analogous experiments with human bone marrow cultures supplemented with human IL-3 produce a culture of mixed cellularity with 25–35% basophils and only 1–5% mast cells.

It should also be noted that the effect(s) of cytokines on mast cells and basophils sometimes appear to be markedly different, and it cannot be assumed that responses observed in one cell type can then be generalized to the other. For example, there is now a considerable body of evidence indicating that IL-3, GM-CSF, IL-1, and IL-5 can influence histamine release from basophils, either by causing direct release or by enhancing the histamine release observed in response to other stimuli (Haak-Frendscho et al., 1988a,b; Hirai et al., 1988, 1990; Valent et al., 1989; Alam et al., 1989; MacDonald et al., 1989; Schleimer et al., 1989; Massey et al., 1989; Bischoff et al., 1990). Similarly, exposure of purified human adenoidal mast cells to human IL-1 was reported to cause a direct release of histamine, although the magnitude of the response was small (less than 10%) (Subramanian and Bray, 1987). In contrast to these studies, recombinant human GM-CSF, IL-1, TNF, and gibbon IL-3 did not cause any histamine release from murine BMCMC (Broide et al., 1990), nor was any histamine release observed after exposure of purified mouse peritoneal mast cells to recombinant human IL-1α, IL-1β, or mouse IL-1α (Coleman, 1990). Similarly, purified human lung mast cells also did not release histamine in response to recombinant human IL-3 (Valent et al., 1990).

III. Production of Cytokines by Mast Cells

The focus of the first paper demonstrating mast cell cytokine production was not the mast cell at all, but rather the ability of a retrovirus carrying the v-*abl* oncogene to produce cell lines capable of growth in the absence of exogenously added growth factors. Using the Abelson murine leukemia virus to transform murine multilineage hematopoietic colonies, Chung et al. (1986) obtained transformed mast cell lines. Several of these lines were found to contain messenger RNA (mRNA) for GM-CSF and to release bioactive GM-CSF, as shown by the ability of culture supernatants from these transformed cells to support the growth of FDC-P1 cells in the presence of excess neutralizing anti-IL-3 antibody. These authors looked for, but were unable to find, IL-3 message or bioactivity in these cell lines.

The following year, the presence of IL-4 message and bioactivity was demonstrated in fetal liver-derived mast cell lines that had also been transformed by infection with the Abelson murine leukemia virus (Brown et al., 1987). In addition, these investigators detected IL-4 mRNA in the original CFTL mast cell lines from which the transformed cell lines were derived, thus providing one of the first clues that nontransformed mast cells might be capable of cytokine synthesis. However, IL-4 bioactivity was not detected in culture supernatants from the nontransformed mast cell lines. Of the transformed cell lines examined, one (MMC34) was found to contain mRNA for IL-3 and GM-CSF, as well as IL-4. This ability of mast cells to transcribe multiple cytokine genes was confirmed in a subsequent study in which several subclones of the transformed mast cells used by Chung were further characterized (Humphries et al., 1988). In addition to GM-CSF and IL-3 mRNA expression and bioactivities, IL-6 bioactivity and another substance with growth factor activity for pre-B cells were also detected in the supernatants of these mast cell cultures. The levels of mRNA for IL-3 and the protooncogene c-*myc* were observed to be higher in the log phase of cell growth, compared to the plateau phase when the cells had reached maximum density. In contrast, the levels of GM-CSF mRNA appeared to be similar in both the log and plateau phases of growth. The drawback to these studies, however, was that they left open to question the influence of the virally-induced transformed phenotype on the transcription and translation of cytokines in mast cells.

At about this same time, several laboratories were actively pursuing the production by mast cells of another cytokine, TNFα. The impetus for these investigations was the observation that purified murine peritoneal mast cells were cytotoxic for certain specific target cells (Farram and Nelson, 1980). Using IL-3-dependent BMCMC and mouse peritoneal mast cells, subsequent investigators defined the specificity of mast cell–mediated killing as being consistent with a natural cytotoxic, as opposed to natural killer, bioactivity based on the ability of these cells to lyse WEHI-164 but not YAC-1 target cells (Ghiara et al., 1985; Ernst et al., 1985). Other workers confirmed this selectivity of killing and additionally demonstrated that mast cell natural cytotoxicity could be augmented by bridging of their surface IgE receptors (Okuno et al., 1986). It was soon appreciated that mast cell–mediated cytotoxicity and that of TNFα displayed similar target cell specificity and kinetics of killing (Jadus et al., 1986).

These investigators also demonstrated that anti-TNFα antibodies could partially block bone marrow–derived mast cell cytotoxicity, and that new protein synthesis was not required for expression of this cytotoxicity. Based on these observations, the authors suggested that mast cell natural cytotoxicity was mediated through a TNFα-like molecule that was preformed and stored in the cytoplasmic granules.

This hypothesis has now been independently confirmed by several groups. Cytotoxic activity has been demonstrated in both lysates and supernatants of mast cells from a variety of sources, and this activity is inhibited by anti-TNFα antibodies (Young et al., 1987; Kasper and Tharp, 1987; Richards et al., 1988; Bissonnette and Befus, 1990; Tharp et al., 1989). In addition, Young and co-workers utilized subcellular fractionation to show that the cytotoxic activity was localized, at least partially, to the mast cell cytoplasmic granules. Using immunoblot analysis and affinity purification with anti-TNFα antibodies, these workers demonstrated a single protein band of 50 kDa. However, this observation did not completely resolve the controversy surrounding the actual identity of this cytotoxic substance, as purified TNFα had been shown to have a molecular weight of 17–20 kDa.

Recent work has provided the definitive proof that this cytotoxic activity was actually TNFα. Several independent groups have demonstrated the presence of TNFα mRNA in several different long-term mast cell lines, BMCMC, mast-like cells cultured from normal human bone marrow, as well as in an in vivo population of mast cells, purified mouse peritoneal mast cells (Steffen et al., 1989; Ohno et al., 1990a,b; Gordon and Galli, 1990; Gurish et al., 1991). The very low, but detectable, levels of TNFα message constitutively transcribed in unstimulated mast cells have been found to increase dramatically within 30–60 min after $Fc_{\epsilon}RI$ crosslinking. The $Fc_{\epsilon}RI$-mediated induction of TNFα mRNA was associated with an increase in the amount of cytotoxic activity present in both culture supernatants and cell lysates, and this cytotoxicity could be almost completely inhibited by anti-TNF antiserum. Using Western blot analysis, Ohno and co-workers demonstrated that material released into RBL-2H3 cell supernatants after IgE receptor crosslinking comigrated with recombinant murine TNFα, with a molecular weight of 17 kDa. In the study by Gordon and Galli, it was shown that inhibition of new mRNA synthesis by pretreatment of highly purified mouse peritoneal mast cells with actinomycin D did not significantly alter the quantity of TNFα present in the cell lysates of unstimulated cells, thus firmly establishing that mast cells can store significant quantities of preformed TNFα in vivo. However, taken together, these studies reveal that there is considerable heterogeneity both in the amounts of granule-associated, preformed TNFα present and in the quantity of TNFα synthesized de novo after $Fc_{\epsilon}RI$ crosslinking among the various mast cells so far examined.

As previously mentioned, earlier studies with the Abelson murine leukemia virus–transformed cell lines suggested that mast cells could produce multiple cytokines. The confirmation that nontransformed mast cells could also serve as a source of multiple, biologically active cytokines was based on a series of observations that demonstrated that activation of several different subclones of the nontransformed, IL-3-dependent CFTL murine mast cell line by antigen-mediated $Fc_{\epsilon}RI$ crosslinking or by calcium ionophores resulted in acquisition of the ability to survive and proliferate in culture in the absence of an exogenous source of IL-3 (Plaut et al., 1989). This response could be prevented by pretreatment of the cultures with the immunosuppressive drug cyclosporin A, a potent inhibitor of lymphokine synthesis in T cells. These results suggested that the stimulated mast cells were supporting their own growth by autocrine cytokine synthesis and secretion. Further investigation revealed that these antigen- or calcium ionophore–stimulated mast cells contained mRNA for multiple cytokines, including IL-2, IL-3, IL-4, IL-5, IL-6, and γ-IFN. More important, the supernatants of these cultures were demonstrated to contain IL-3, IL-4, and IL-6 bioactivities. Addition of blocking antibodies for IL-3 and IL-4 to the antigen-stimulated mast cell cultures abrogated the autocrine proliferative response.

Since this initial observation, several studies have confirmed that in vitro stimulation of murine mast cells with ionophores, phorbol esters (such as the protein kinase C agonist phorbol 12-myristate 13-acetate (PMA), or by antigen-mediated $Fc_{\epsilon}RI$ crosslinking results in the transcription of a broad spectrum of cytokine genes. In one study that examined cytokine transcription and translation in several different IL-3 dependent and independent long-term mast cell lines, mRNA for IL-1, IL-3, IL-5, IL-6, GM-CSF, γ-IFN, MIP-1α, MIP-1β, TCA3, and JE, as well as IL-1, IL-4, and IL-6 bioactivity, was documented (Burd et al., 1989). To date, murine mast cells are the only cell type that has been found to contain transcripts for all four members of the murine MIP-1 family of cytokines (MIP-1α, MIP-1β, TCA3, and JE). A fifth member of this family, RANTES, has been described in humans but not yet in mice. The genes encoding the MIP-1 group of cytokines are chromosomally linked, and their protein products share significant structural similarities (Wolpe and Cerami, 1989). Their biological activities include prostaglandin-independent pyrogenic activity (Davatelis et al., 1989) and induction of an oxidative burst and selective degranulation of neutrophils (Wolpe et al., 1988). MIP-1α and MIP-1β (Wolpe et al., 1988) and JE, also referred to as MCAF or monocyte chemoattractant protein-1 (Yoshimura and Leonard, 1990), have been shown to be chemotactic for granulocytes and monocytes, respectively. Injection of MIP-1α and MIP-1β (Wolpe et al., 1988) or TCA3 (Wilson et al., 1990) into the footpads of mice induced a rapid, localized inflammatory reaction characterized by swelling and an accumulation of neutrophils. MIP-1α has also been found to inhibit hematopoietic stem cell proliferation (Graham et al., 1990). Although translation of these mRNAs into bioactive protein has yet to be demonstrated in mast cells, the potent proinflammatory properties of this group of cytokines suggest they may play a central role in allergic inflammatory disease. Further studies are needed to determine their involvement in mast cell–mediated responses.

Based on the data from the aforementioned studies, it now appears clear that although the aggregate spectrum of cytokines transcribed by activated mast cells is quite broad, the response of an individual cell line is a subset of this aggregate that varies from one cell line to the next. This suggests a clonal basis for the different patterns of cytokine gene induction seen in response to IgE receptor–mediated or chemical stimulation in the cell lines examined so far.

Other investigators have shown that elaboration of multiple cytokines in response to $Fc_{\epsilon}RI$ crosslinking or chemical activation is not limited to long-term mast cell lines. In the first of these studies, both IgE receptor–mediated and chemical stimulation of primary mouse BMCMC was found to result in the induction of mRNA for IL-3 and GM-CSF, and the subsequent release of the corresponding bioactivities into the culture media (Wodnar-Filipowicz et al., 1989). Both primary mouse BMCMC and permanent IL-3-dependent mucosal mast cell lines derived from these cultures have been shown to constitutively produce IL-6 and to contain IL-6 mRNA (Hultner et al., 1989b). A more recent investigation using 6-week mouse BMCMCs has demonstrated that nearly all the cytokine mRNAs previously detected in one or another of the mast cell lines in response to $Fc_{\epsilon}RI$ crosslinking or chemical stimulation also can be induced in these primary mast cell cultures (Costa et al., 1990). This observation is probably attributable to the fact that these bone marrow–derived mast cell cultures are actually comprised of a heterogeneous population of mast cells derived from multiple progenitors, as opposed to an individual cloned cell line. Several recent studies support this hypothesis. In situ hybridization analysis of BMCMC 1 hr after antigen-mediated $Fc_{\epsilon}RI$ crosslinking revealed that only 50% of the cells contained detectable amounts of IL-6 mRNA (Gurish et al., 1991). In addition, in both the unstimulated and antigen-activated cultures, the authors reported considerable variation in the amount of IL-6 mRNA observed between individual cells, as indicated by differences in the number of silver grains located over the cells. Another group of investigators who examined cytokine mRNA expression in single BMCMC using the polymerase chain reaction, observed significant differences in the levels of the IL-3-specific products in each individual cell, with some cells being entirely negative-(Razin et al., 1991). Inasmuch as the mast cells distributed throughout the tissues of animals and humans also represent a heterogeneous population of cells, the information derived from experimental investigation of primary bone marrow–derived mast cell cultures may more closely reflect the spectrum of responses one could expect to elicit after IgE receptor–mediated activation of mast cells present within the intact organism. Table 3 summarizes the spectrum of cytokine genes demonstrated to be transcribed and/or translated in mast cell lines or primary mast cell cultures. Note that

Table 3 Cytokine Production by Mast Cells

I. Constitutively transcribed cytokines[a]
TNFα[b]
TGFβ
IL-4
IL-6[b]
JE
II. Cytokines transcribed in activated cells
A. Proinflammatory type[c]
IL-6[b]
TNFα[b]
MIP-1α
MIP-1β
TCA[3]
JE
B. Growth factor type
IL-1[b]
IL-2
IL-3[b]
IL-4[b]
IL-5
GM-CSF
C. Others
IFN-γ

[a]Observed in some but not all of the mast cells examined so far.
[b]Both mRNA and bioactivity have been detected.
[c]This categorization is based on the cytokine mRNA expression pattern observed in primary mouse BMCMC (Costa et al., 1990).

despite the large number of cytokines for which mRNA has been detected, bioactivities corresponding to TNFα and IL-6 have been found in unstimulated mast cells, while IL-1, IL-3, IL-4, IL-6, GM-CSF, and TNFα bioactivities have been found in the supernatants of stimulated mast cell cultures.

Several studies have revealed that the temporal appearance and relative amounts of cytokine mRNA observed in response to $Fc_{\epsilon}RI$ crosslinking or calcium ionophore stimulation are not uniform (Burd et al., 1989; Wershil et al., 1990; Gurish et al., 1991). It now appears that $Fc_{\epsilon}RI$-mediated cytokine gene induction falls into one of two major response patterns (Costa et al., 1990); the first is characterized by rapid and relatively high-level mRNA induction. Included in this group are all four members of the murine MIP-1 family, as well as TNFα and IL-6, whose mRNAs can be detected within 30 min after $Fc_{\epsilon}RI$

crosslinking. Interestingly, the cytokines within this group also share functional bioactivities, possessing (but not limited to) predominantly proinflammatory properties. Pretreatment of BMCMC with cycloheximide did not inhibit the induction of any of these genes, indicating that new protein synthesis is not required for their expression. In contrast, pretreatment with cyclosporin A completely blocked the induction of MIP-1α, MIP-1β, and TCA3. The second group of cytokine genes induced in BMCMC after $Fc_{\epsilon}RI$ crosslinking includes IL-1, IL-3, IL-5, and GM-CSF. In contrast in the proinflammatory group, the appearance of these messages is temporally delayed and of lesser magnitude. Message for these cytokines could not be detected until 1–2 hr after $Fc_{\epsilon}RI$ crosslinking, and induction of these genes was inhibited by both cyclosporin A and cycloheximide. This group of cytokines also shares functional characteristics, with predominantly, although again not limited to, growth-promoting properties. The possibility that under physiological conditions either one or the other of these groups may be expressed exclusively would add specificity to what is now a generalized cytokine induction response, and future studies will need to address this issue. In this regard, mRNA analysis of single cells has revealed that coculture of both BMCMC and purified peritoneal mast cells with 3T3 fibroblasts results in an increased percentage of cells containing IL-3 message, thus demonstrating that other physiological conditions may have important influences on mast cell cytokine production (Razin et al., 1991).

In addition to the variability observed with regard to the appearance of cytokine mRNAs after $Fc_{\epsilon}RI$ crosslinking, several studies have demonstrated that there are also differences in the duration of cytokine message expression (Gordon and Galli, 1990; Ohno et al., 1990b; Gurish et al., 1991). In mouse BMCMC, induction of TNFα mRNA occurs within 30 min after IgE receptor aggregation, reaches peak levels at 30–60 min, and then decreases rapidly such that by 4 hr after activation, levels are similar to those seen in unstimulated cells. While the expression of IL-6 mRNA was similar to TNF, message for GM-CSF could only be detected at 1 and 2 hr after $Fc_{\epsilon}RI$ crosslinking. In the IL-3-independent C1.MC/C57.1 mast cell line, activation of the cells with the calcium ionophore ionomycin resulted in progressively increasing levels of IL-3 message over the subsequent 24 hr whereas IL-4 expression was greatest at 4 hr and had significantly diminished by 24 hr poststimulation (Wershil et al., 1990). The study by Gurish also demonstrated that the induction of cytokine genes was not accompanied by any alteration in the steady-state levels of message for the alpha subunit of the high-affinity IgE receptor or two other mast cell mediators, including carboxypeptidase A and a generic chymotryptic serine protease. The mRNA encoding the proteoglycan peptide core was found to increase slightly.

Another important finding is that the pattern of cytokine gene induction varies depending on the type of stimulus used to activate the cells (Plaut et al., 1989; Burd et al., 1989, 1990). Thus, while both $Fc_{\epsilon}RI$ crosslinking and calcium ionophore similarly cause rapid mast cell histamine release, they result in the induction of different patterns of cytokine genes, with further differences both in the kinetics of message expression and in the ability of drugs such as cyclosporin A or the protein synthesis inhibitor cycloheximide to prevent the appearance of these cytokine mRNAs. Three hours after activation of 6-week BMCMC with 1 μM calcium ionophore A23187, mRNA for IL-3, IL-5, and GM-CSF could be detected but, in contrast to the response seen with IgE and antigen, not for IL-1 (Burd et al., 1990). In addition, ionophore-mediated induction of these growth-promoting cytokines was not inhibited by cycloheximide, representing another difference from Fc_ϵRI-mediated induction. In contrast, however, calcium ionophore produced a high-level induction of the proinflammatory cytokines, with the appearance of message for MIP-1α, MIP-1β, TCA3, and TNFα inhibited by cyclosporin A but not cycloheximide, thus closely mimicking (although not identical to) the response observed after Fc_ϵRI crosslinking. These authors also showed that exposure of BMCMC to the protein kinase C agonist PMA yielded yet another distinct pattern of cytokine gene induction. Although the entire group of proinflammatory cytokine genes could be detected after cellular activation with this agent, induction of MIP-1α, MIP-1β, and TCA3 was unaffected by pretreatment with cyclosporin A and inhibited by cycloheximide. Of the group of growth-promoting cytokines, PMA was only able to induce mRNA for IL-1, and this was also inhibited by cycloheximide and not cyclosporin. Taken together, these data indicate that mast cells possess several distinct signaling pathways, each of which results in the induction of multiple cytokine genes. However, the relationship between the transcription and translation of cytokine genes in mast cells is not completely clear at this time. The observation of IL-2 mRNA in the absence of any detectable IL-2 bioactivity in response to calcium ionophore stimulation indicates that mRNA induction may not always be accompanied by synthesis and release of a bioactive protein (Plaut et al., 1989).

Another unique aspect of PMA-mediated cytokine gene induction is that it was not accompanied by detectable histamine release (Burd et al., 1990). Thus, the limitation of PMA-induced cytokine gene expression to the proinflammatory group of molecules and IL-1, which is also a potent proinflammatory molecule, is intriguing because it raises the possibility that mast cells may be capable of responding to as yet unidentified non–Fc_ϵRI-mediated stimuli by synthesis of proinflammatory cytokines, without concomitant production and release of the mediators associated with the immediate hypersensitivity response. In this regard, a recent preliminary communication has reported that substance P, thrombin, and nerve growth factor (NGF) are able to transiently induce the appearance of message for MIP-1α in BMCMC (Costa et al., 1991). Of note was the observation that expression of MIP-1α message in response to either substance P or NGF was not accompanied by histamine release, thus suggesting that physiological stimuli other than Fc_ϵRI crosslinking may influence mast cell participation in pathological and physiological processes via induction of cytokine genes.

Currently, very little information is available regarding the mechanism(s) of cytokine gene induction in mast cells. A requirement for prolonged receptor crosslinkage and extracellular calcium has been demonstrated, based on the ability of the monovalent hapten DNP-lysine and the calcium chelator EDTA to block antigen-induced IL-3 and IL-4 production (Plaut et al., 1990). In another study that examined IL-3 and GM-CSF expression in the IL-3-dependent PB-3c cell line, it was demonstrated that depletion of protein kinase C by long-term PMA exposure did not inhibit induction of either IL-3 or GM-CSF in response to the calcium ionophore A23187 (Wodnar-Filipowicz and Moroni, 1990). In addition, although neither of these mRNAs could be detected by Northern analysis in unstimulated cells, nuclear run on assays revealed that both the IL-3 and GM-CSF genes were being constitutively transcribed. Furthermore, the marked induction of IL-3 seen in response to calcium ionophore was felt not to be due to a significant increase in IL-3 gene transcription, although ionophore did have a weak stimulatory effect on the transcriptional induction of the GM-CSF gene. Rather, these authors demonstrated that exposure to calcium ionophore stabilized both IL-3 and GM-CSF messages, with no sign of mRNA decay for up to 3 hr after the addition of actinomycin D. GM-CSF message could also be stabilized by PMA. These results indicate that in PB-3c cells, expression of IL-3 and GM-CSF is influenced by calcium ions, with a major component of the inductional response being posttranscriptional message stabilization. However, it should be noted that PB-3c cells have previously been shown to constitutively express high levels of c-*fos* mRNA (Conscience et al., 1986). In contrast, unstimulated 6-week BMCMC did not contain c-*fos* message, although c-*fos* transcripts were rapidly induced after $Fc_\epsilon RI$ crosslinking (Burd and Costa, unpublished observations). Finally, one study has reported the half-life of IL-3, IL-5, and TNFα messages after $Fc_\epsilon RI$ crosslinking to be similar, with a value of approximately 30 min (Gordon, and Galli, 1990).

IV. Potential Physiological Influences of Mast Cell–Derived Cytokines

The discovery that mast cells respond to immunological stimulation by induction of a broad panel of cytokine genes and secretion of bioactive cytokine molecules suggests that in vivo, mast cells may serve as a source for a wide variety of multifunctional cytokines. The constitutive production demonstrated for several of these molecules raises the possibility that resident mast cells may influence their local microenvironment by producing cytokines in the absence of $Fc_\epsilon RI$-mediated cellular activation. Moreover, it seems reasonable to consider that, in addition to the preformed and newly generated mediators traditionally associated with mast cell activation, mast cell–derived cytokines must also be regarded as having potential influences on the pathophysiology of diseases when there is evidence of mast cell activation. Furthermore, given that mast cell degranulation results in the local release of proteoglycans that have the ability to bind a variety of growth factors (reviewed in Ruoslahti and Yamaguchi, 1991), $Fc_{\epsilon}RI$-mediated cytokine production may provide a means by which the function, concentration, and spatial distribution of these molecules can be controlled within the tissue microenvironment.

In this regard, a recent study has shown that the appearance of granulocytes at sites where IgE-mediated mast cell degranulation occurred 6 hr earlier is markedly diminished in mast cell–deficient mice, and local injection of anti-TNFα antiserum causes a 50% decrease in neutrophil influx in similarly treated normal mice (Wershil et al., 1991).

There have also been several reports of in vivo IgE-dependent cytokine production, although the cellular source of these cytokines was not determined. Treatment of organ cultures of normal human skin with a variety of agents known to cause mast cell degranulation (e.g., anti-IgE, morphine sulfate, compound 48/80, and calcium ionophore A23187) resulted in the rapid appearance of the endothelial adhesion molecule ELAM-1 in the adjacent microvasculature (Klein et al., 1989). This response could be blocked by pretreatment of the cultures with the mast cell–stabilizing drug cromolyn sodium, as well as with antibodies to TNFα. These findings are consistent with a model in which IgE-mediated release of mast cell–derived TNFα activates the dermal endothelium with the resultant expression of an antigen that is important for endothelial-leukocyte interactions. Increased ICAM-1 expression on vascular endothelium has also been demonstrated in human skin biopsies taken 6 hr after antigen challenge (Kyan-Aung et al., 1991).

Antigen challenge of atopic subjects using skin blister chambers has demonstrated the appearance of IL-1β, IL-3, GM-CSF, and IL-6 in blister fluid within the first 12 hr after challenge (Charlesworth et al., 1990; Massey et al., 1991; Lee et al., 1991). IL-6 mRNA has also been detected by Northern blot analysis of tissue from sites of passive cutaneous anaphylaxis in mice (Mican et al., 1991). Increased numbers of cells expressing mRNA for IL-3, IL-4, IL-5, and GM-CSF have also been identified by in situ hybridization at allergen-challenged skin sites in atopic human subjects (Hamid et al., 1991). Although the mast cell has not been proven to be the source of these cytokines, either direct or indirect mast cell participation is likely, since the cutaneous late-phase response is known to be generated by triggering of cutaneous mast cells via IgE-dependent mechanisms. However, even in IgE-dependent reactions, recent data indicate that mast cells are not the only cellular source of cytokines. In situ hybridization of lymphocytes in bronchoalveolar lavage (BAL) fluid from allergen-challenged atopic individuals revealed a dramatic increase in the percentage of cells containing IL-2 and IL-4 message (Dishuck et al., 1991), and

BAL lymphocytes from atopic asthmatics showed increased expression of IL-2, -3, -4, -5, and GM-CSF compared with nonatopic, nonasthmatic controls (Robinson et al., 1991). In addition, human peripheral blood mononuclear phagocytes from atopic donors have been demonstrated to produce IL-1β and TNFα in response to IgE/anti-IgE immune complexes (Borish et al., 1991).

Recently, a population of non-B, non-T cells that contain high-affinity IgE receptors and that produce significant quantities of IL-3 and IL-4 in response to $Fc_{\epsilon}RI$ crosslinking has been identified in mice (Ben-Sasson et al., 1990). Infection with *Nippostrongylus brasiliensis* markedly enhances this IgE receptor-mediated IL-4 production (Conrad et al., 1990). Although the identity of these cells is uncertain, the existence of yet another population of cells that respond to IgE receptor crosslinking with production of cytokines strengthens the concept that this is probably an important mechanism by which immune and inflammatory responses can be modulated.

The discovery that mast cells produce cytokines has expanded the role of this cell beyond that of a simple effector cell to include possible functions as a regulatory and modulatory element of both inflammatory and immune responses. However, it must be emphasized that to date, virtually all the studies describing cytokine production by mast cells have utilized murine or rodent mast cell lines or primary mast cell cultures. The extent to which human mast cells are also capable of cytokine synthesis and secretion is yet to be fully determined. This being said, it should also be noted that models of inflammation in murine systems have proven to be remarkably accurate predictors of the analogous human biological processes.

It is not unreasonable to speculate that many or all of the cell types participating in allergic and inflammatory diseases will eventually be found to produce one or more cytokines. The challenge will be to elucidate the circumstances under which these molecules are produced in vivo, and to understand the way in which each cell type uses cytokines to influence other resident and recruited cells. The study of the effects of cytokine production by mast cells and other cells on allergic inflammatory disease is only in its infancy. This is an exciting and rapidly progressing era in biomedical research, and it is likely that future studies in this area will finally provide long-awaited answers regarding the role of the mast cell in both health and disease.

Discussion

Sullivan: Recent studies have suggested that in vitro gene expression may not occur if physiological levels of corticosteroids are present. Are mast cell cytokine genes suppressed by corticosteroids? Do these responses occur in the presence of physiological levels of corticosteroids?
Costa: To my knowledge, there are no published studies that address this issue,

although the finding of inhibition of IL-6 induction in certain cell lines cultured in the presence of physiological concentrations of glucocorticoids highlights the importance of this question.

Lichtenstein: I have long felt that IgE receptor occupancy up-regulates the mast cell. You showed that in one cell line IgE alone increased cytokine message. Is this reproducible?

Costa: We have consistently observed the induction of selected cytokine messenger RNAs in response to the addition of IgE in the absence of any crosslinking antigen, suggesting that IgE binding to its receptor generates a signal that results in cytokine induction.

Bienenstock: Please elaborate on the non-B, non-T cell as described by Paul and co-workers.

Costa: The work of Ben-Sasson, Conrad, and Paul has revealed the existence of a population of non-B, non-T cells from mouse spleen, which can be stimulated to secrete high levels of IL-4 in response to plate-bound IgE or IgG. Recent investigation of the morphology and ultrastructure of these cells has revealed two populations, one of which resembles basophils and the other, immature cells. Which of these is the source of the IL-4 is not clear at this time.

Lichtenstein: What is the relationship of the pattern of mast cell cytokine mRNA expression to the TH_2 pattern of cytokines?

Costa: The initial studies of mast cell cytokine production suggested mast cells were more like TH_2 cells than TH_1 cells because of the detection of IL-3, IL-4, and IL-6. As the literature on mast cell cytokines has grown, it has become clear that although the spectrum of mast cell cytokines may overlap with that of TH_2 cells, it is not identical to it.

Lee: Are growth factor cytokines synchronously produced?

Costa: In our study, the growth-promoting group of cytokines (IL-1, IL-3, IL-5, and GM-CSF) were not detected at 30 min after IgE-receptor crosslinking but all were present 2 hr postactivation, suggesting synchronous induction. Gordon and Galli have also recently reported that IL-3 and IL-5 message both peaked 2 hr after IgE receptor crosslinking.

Stevens: We have found that activated mast cells contain mRNA for a number of cytokines, but that certain transcripts are preferentially induced (e.g., IL-6 mRNA is 100–1000-fold higher than IL-3 mRNA). Have you found preferential inductions of any of these 12 cytokine transcripts?

Costa: Our observations support those you are describing. We observed significant differences in the relative levels of mRNA for various cytokines after IgE receptor crosslinking. IL-6, TNFα, and the MIP-1 family of cytokines demonstrate a strong induction response, whereas message for the growth-promoting cytokines (IL-1, IL-3, IL-5, and GM-CSF) are present at relatively much lower levels. Of course, the levels of mRNA cannot be used to make inferences regarding the subsequent levels of bioactive protein released.

Galli: I would like to make two points. The first is that Costa and Sullivan are correct in emphasizing the importance of determining which cytokines are expressed by physiologically relevant mast cell populations in vivo; these may differ from those produced by mast cells generated in vitro. Of course, it will also be critical to examine patterns of mast cell cytokines produced at sites of disease processes or immunological responses, and to test whether such mast cell–derived cytokines importantly contribute to the expression of biological responses in vivo. The second point is offered only partly in jest. Ehrlich named the mast cell "mastzellen," or "well-fed," cell to indicate that it may have a role in regulating the nutrition of the connective tissue and to emphasize that its cytoplasm is packed with granules. The recognition that the already long list of mast cell–associated mediators apparently includes multiple cytokines whose effects can importantly influence many biological processes prompts the suggestion that "mast cell" can now be reserved as the short form of the more appropriate term "master cell."
Costa: Galli's comments are correct. In general, because there are so many cells that are capable of cytokine synthesis, we must be careful about implicating the mast cell without clear evidence that this is the cell from which the cytokine in question is coming.

References

Akira, S., Hirano, T., Taga, T., and Kishimoto, T. (1990). Biology of multifunctional cytokines: IL 6 and related molecules (IL 1 and TNF). *FASEB J.* 4:2860–2867.

Alam, R., Welter, J. B., Forsythe, P. A., Lett-Brown, M. A., and Grant, J. A. (1989). Comparative effect of recombinant IL-1, -2, -3, -4, and -6, IFN-γ, granulocyte-macrophage–colony-stimulating factor, tumor necrosis factor-α, and histamine releasing factors on the secretion of histamine from basophils. *J. Immunol.* 142:3431–3435.

Ben-Sasson, S. Z., Le Gros, G., Conrad, D. H., Finkelman, F. D., and Paul, W. E. (1990). Cross-linking Fc receptors stimulate splenic non-B, non-T cells to secrete interleukin 4 and other lymphokines. *Proc. Natl. Acad. Sci. USA* 87:1421–1425.

Bischoff, S. C., de Weck, A. L., and Dahinden, C. A. (1990). Interleukin 3 and granulocyte-macrophage-colony-stimulating factor render human basophils responsive to low concentrations of complement component C3a. *Proc. Natl. Acad. Sci. USA* 87:6813–6817.

Bissonnette, E. Y., and Befus, A. D. (1990). Inhibition of mast cell-mediated cytotoxicity by IFN-α/β and -γ. *J. Immunol.* 145:3385–3390.

Borish, L., Mascali, J. J., and Rosenwasser, L. J. (1991). IgE-dependent cytokine production by human peripheral blood mononuclear phagocytes. *J. Immunol.* 146:63–67.

Boswell, H. S., Mochizuki, D. Y., Burgess, G. S., Gillis, S., Walker, E. B., Anderson, D., and Williams, D. E. (1990). A novel mast cell growth factor (MCGF-3)

Hirai, K., Yamaguchi, M., Misaki, Y., Takaishi, T., Ohta, K., Morita, Y., Ito, K., and Miyamoto, T. (1990). Enhancement of human basophil histamine release by interleukin 5. *J. Exp. Med.* 172:1525–1528.

Huang, E., Nocka, K., Beler, D. R., Chu, T-Y., Buck, J., Lahm, H-W., Wellner, D., Leder, P., and Besmer, P. (1990). The hematopoietic growth factor KL is encoded by the *Sl* locus and is the ligand of the c-*kit* receptor, the gene product of the *W* locus. *Cell* 63:225–233.

Hultner, L., Moeller, J., Schmitt, E., Jager, G., Reisbach, G., Ring, J., and Dormer, P. (1989a). Thiol-sensitive mast cell lines derived from mouse bone marrow respond to a mast cell growth-enhancing activity different from both IL-3 and IL-4. *J. Immunol.* 142:3440–3446.

Hultner, L., Szots, H., Welle, M., Van Snick, J., Moeller, J., and Dormer, P. (1989b). Mouse bone marrow-derived IL-3-dependent mast cells and autonomous sublines produce IL-6. *Immunology* 67:408–413.

Hultner, L., Druez, C., Moeller, J., Schmitt, E., Uyttenhove, C., Rude, E., Dormer, P., and Van Snick, J. (1990). Mast cell growth enhancing activity (MEA) is structurally related and functionally identical to the novel mouse T cell growth factor P40/TCGF III. *Eur. J. Immunol.* 20:1413–1416.

Humphries, R. K., Abraham, S., Krystal, G., Lansdorp, P., Lemoine, F., and Eaves, C. J. (1988). Activation of multiple hemopoietic growth factor genes in Abelson virus–transformed myeloid cells. *Exp. Hematol.* 16:774–781.

Ihle, J. N., Keller, J., Oroszlan, S., Henderson, L. E., Copeland, T. D., Fitch, F., Prystowsky M. B., Goldwasser, E., Schrader, J. W., Palaszynski, E., Dy, M., and Lebel, B. (1983). Biological properties of homogeneous interleukin 3. I. Demonstration of WEHI-3 growth factor activity, P cell-stimulating factor activity, colony-stimulating factor activity, and histamine-producing cell-stimulating factor activity. *J. Immunol.* 131:282–287.

Jadus, M. R., Schmunk, G., Djeu, J. Y., and Parkman, R. (1986). Morphology and lytic mechanisms of interleukin 3–dependent natural cytotoxic cells: tumor necrosis factor as a possible mediator. *J. Immunol.* 137:2774–2783.

Kasper, C., and Tharp, M. (1987). Mast cells are cytotoxic against TNF-sensitive and TNF-resistant targets. *Fed. Proc. Fed. Am. Soc. Exp. Biol.* 46:1225 (abstract).

Kirshenbaum, A. S., Goff, J. P., Dreskin, S. C., Irani, A-M., Schwartz, L. B., and Metcalfe, D. D. (1989). IL-3-dependent growth of basophil-like cells and mastlike cells from human bone marrow. *J. Immunol.* 142:2424–2429.

Klein, L. M., Lavker, R. M., Matis, W. L., and Murphy, G. F. (1989). Degranulation of human mast cells induces an endothelial antigen central to leukocyte adhesion. *Proc. Natl. Acad. Sci. USA* 86:8972–8976.

Kyan-Aung, U., Haskard, D. O., Poston, R. N., Thornhill, M. H., and Lee, T. H. (1991). Endothelial leukocyte adhesion molecule-1 and intercellular adhesion molecule-1 mediate the adhesion of eosinophils to endothelial cells in vitro and are expressed by endothelium in allergic cutaneous inflammation in vivo. *J. Immunol.* 146:521–528.

Lee, C. E., Dixon, P. S., and Charlesworth, E. N. (1991). Interleukin-6 is released in the cutaneous late phase response to antigen challenge. *J. Allergy Clin. Immunol.* 87:208 (abstract).

MacDonald, S. M., Schleimer, R. P., Kagey-Sobotka, A., Gillis, S., and Lichtenstein, L. M. (1989). Recombinant IL-3 induces histamine release from human basophils. *J. Immunol.* 142:3527–3532.

Massey, W. A., Randall, T. C., Kagey-Sobotka, A., Warner, J. A., MacDonald, S. M., Gillis, S., Allison, A. C., and Lichtenstein, L. M. (1989). Recombinant human IL-1α and -1β potentiate IgE-mediated histamine release from human basophils. *J. Immunol.* 143:1875–1880.

Massey, W., Friedman, B., Kato, M., Lichtenstein, L. M., Liu, M., and Schleimer, R. (1991). Allergen-induced late-phase reaction (LPR) sites contain IL-3 and GM-CSF activity. *J. Allergy Clin. Immunol.* 87:207 (abstract).

Matsuura, N., and Zetter, B. R. (1989). Stimulation of mast cell chemotaxis by interleukin 3. *J. Exp. Med.* 170:1421–1426.

Mican, J. M., Burd, P. R., and Metcalfe, D. D. (1991). Demonstration of IL-6 mRNA in mouse skin after IgE mediated mast cell degranulation. *J. Allergy Clin. Immunol.* 87:206 (abstract).

Mizel, S. B. (1989). The interleukins. *FASEB J.* 3:2379–2388.

Mosmann, T. R., Bond, M. W., Coffman, R. L., Ohara, J., and Paul, W. E. (1986). T-cell and mast cell lines respond to B-cell stimulatory factor 1. *Proc. Natl. Acad. Sci. USA* 83:5654–5658.

Nafziger, J., Arock, M., Guillosson, J-J., and Wietzerbin, J. (1990). Specific high affinity receptors for interferon-γ on mouse bone marrow-derived mast cells: inhibitory effect of interferon-γ on mast cell precursors. *Eur. J. Immunol.* 20:113–117.

Nagao, K., Yokoro, K., and Aaronson, S. A. (1981). Continuous lines of basophil/mast cells derived from normal mouse bone marrow. *Science* 212:333–335.

Ohno, I., Tanno, Y., Yamauchi, K., Takishima, T. (1990a). Production of tumour necrosis factor by mastocytoma P815 cells. *Immunology* 69:312–315.

Ohno, I., Tanno, Y., Yamauchi, K., and Takishima, T. (1990b). Gene expression and production of tumour necrosis factor by a rat basophilic leukaemia cell line (RBL-2H3) with IgE receptor triggering. *Immunology* 70:88–93.

Okuno, T., Takagaki, Y., Pluznik, D. H., and Djeu, J. Y. (1986). Natural cytotoxic (NC) cell activity in basophilic cells: Release of NC-specific cytotoxic factor by IgE receptor triggering. *J. Immunol.* 136:4652–4658.

Paetkau, V., and Mills, G. B. (1989). Cytokines and mechanisms of lymphocyte activation. *Immunol. Allergy Clin. North Am.* 9:21–43.

Paul, W. E. (1989). Pleiotropy and redundancy: T cell-derived lymphokines in the immune response. *Cell* 57:521–524.

Plaut, M., Pierce, J. H., Watson, C. J., Hanley-Hyde, J., Nordan, R. P., and Paul, W. E. (1989). Mast cell lines produce lymphokines in response to cross-linkage of $Fc_{\epsilon}RI$ or to calcium ionophores. *Nature* 339:64–67.

Plaut, M., Kagey-Sobotka, A., Niv, Y., Pierce, J. H., and Paul, W. E. (1990). Regulation of mast cell lymphokine production. *FASEB J.* 4:A1705 (abstract).

Pluznik, D. H., Tare, N. S., Zatz, M. M., and Goldstein, A. L. (1982). A mast/basophil cell line dependent on colony stimulating factor. *Exp. Hematol.* 10(Suppl.):211–218.

Razin, E., Cordon-Cardo, C., and Good, R. A. (1981). Growth of a pure population of

mouse mast cells in vitro with conditioned medium derived from concanavalin A-stimulated splenocytes. *Proc. Natl. Acad. Sci. USA* 78:2559–2561.
Razin, E., Ihle, J. N., Seldin, D., Mencia-Huerta, J-M., Katz, H. R., Leblanc, P. A., Hein, A., Caulfield, J. P., Austen, K. F., and Stevens, R. L. (1984). Interleukin 3: A differentiation and growth factor for the mouse mast cell that contains chondroitin sulfate E proteoglycan. *J. Immunol.* 132:1479–1486.
Razin, E., Leslie, K. B., and Schrader, J. W. (1991). Connective tissue mast cells in contact with fibroblasts express IL-3 mRNA. Analysis of single cells by polymerase chain reaction. *J. Immunol.* 146:981–987.
Renauld, J-C., Goethals, A., Houssiau, F., Merz, H., Van Roost, E., and Van Snick, J. (1990). Human P40/IL-9. Expression in activated $CD4^+$ T cells, genomic organization, and comparison with the mouse gene. *J. Immunol.* 144:4235–4241.
Richards, A. L., Okuno, T., Takagaki, Y., and Djeu, J. Y. (1988). Natural cytotoxic cell-specific cytolytic factor produced by IL-3-dependent basophilic/mast cells. Relationship to TNF. *J. Immunol.* 141:3061–3066.
Robinson, D. S., Hamid, Q., Ying, S., Bentley, A. M., Durham, S. R., and Kay, A. B. (1991). Cytokine mRNA profile and T-cell activation in bronchoalveolar lavage (BAL) cells from atopic asthmatics and controls. *J. Allergy Clin. Immunol.* 87:208 (abstract).
Ruoslahti, E., and Yamaguchi, Y. (1991). Proteoglycans as modulators of growth factor activities. *Cell* 64:867–869.
Salari, H., and Chan-Yeung, M. (1989). Interleukin-1 potentiates antigen-mediated arachidonic acid metabolite formation in mast cells. *Clin. Exp. Allergy* 19:637–642.
Schleimer, R. P., Derse, C. P., Friedman, B., Gillis, S., Plaut, M., Lichtenstein, L. M., and MacGlashan, Jr., D. W. (1989). Regulation of human basophil mediator release by cytokines. I. Interaction with antiinflammatory steroids. *J. Immunol.* 143:1310–1317.
Schrader, J. W., Lewis, S. J., Clark-Lewis, I., and Culvenor, J. G. (1981). The persisting (P) cell: histamine content, regulation by a T cell–derived factor, origin from a bone marrow precursor, and relationship to mast cells. *Proc. Natl. Acad. Sci. USA* 78:323–327.
Smith, C. A., and Rennick, D. M. (1986). Characterization of a murine lymphokine distinct from interleukin 2 and interleukin 3 (IL-3) possessing a T-cell growth factor activity and a mast-cell growth factor activity that synergizes with IL-3. *Proc. Natl. Acad. Sci. USA* 83:1857–1861.
Steffen, M., Abboud, M., Potter, G. K., Yung, Y. P., and Moore, M. A. S. (1989). Presence of tumour necrosis factor or a related factor in human basophil/mast cells. *Immunology* 66:445–450.
Strober, W., and James, S. P. (1988). The interleukins. *Pediatr. Res.* 24:549–557.
Subramanian, N., and Bray, M. A. (1987). Interleukin 1 releases histamine from human basophils and mast cells in vitro. *J. Immunol.* 138:271–275.
Swieter, M., Ghali, W. A., Rimmer, C., and Befus, A. D. (1989). Interferon-α/β inhibits IgE-dependent histamine release from rat mast cells. *Immunology* 66:606–610.
Takagi, M., Nakahata, T., Koike, K., Kobayashi, T., Tsuji, K., Kojima, S., Hirano, T.,

Miyajima, A., Arai, K-I., and Akabane, T. (1989). Stimulation of connective tissue–type mast cell proliferation by crosslinking of cell-bound IgE. *J. Exp. Med.* 170:233–244.
Takagi, M., Koike, K., and Nakahata, T. (1990). Anti-proliferative effect of IFN-α on proliferation of mouse connective tissue–type mast cells. *J. Immunol.* 145:1880–1884.
Tertian, G., Yung, Y-P., Guy-Grand, D., and Moore, M. A. S. (1981). Long-term in vitro culture of murine mast cells. I. Description of a growth factor-dependent culture technique. *J. Immunol.* 127:788–799.
Tharp, M. D., Kasper, C., Thiele, D., Charley, M. R., Kennerly, D. A., and Sullivan, T. J. (1989). Studies of connective tissue mast cell–mediated cytotoxicity. *J. Invest. Dermatol.* 93:423–428.
Thompson, H. L., Burbelo, P. D., Segui-Real, B., Yamada, Y., and Metcalfe, D. D. (1989). Laminin promotes mast cell attachment. *J. Immunol.* 143:4188–4192.
Thompson, H. L., Burbelo, P. D., and Metcalfe, D. D. (1990). Regulation of adhesion of mouse bone marrow–derived mast cells to laminin. *J. Immunol.* 145:3425–3431.
Thompson-Snipes, L., Dhar, V., O'Garra, A., Moore, K., Bond, M., and Rennick, D. (1990). Cytokine synthesis inhibitory factor is a potent co-factor for mast cell growth. *FASEB J.* 4:A1705 (abstract).
Tsuji, K., Nakahata, T., Takagi, M., Kobayashi, T., Ishiguro, A., Kikuchi, T., Naganuma, K., Koike, K., Miyajima, A., Arai, K-I., and Akabane, T. (1990). Effects of interleukin-3 and interleukin-4 on the development of "connective tissue–type" mast cells: Interleukin-3 supports their survival and interleukin-4 triggers and supports their proliferation synergistically with interleukin-3. *Blood* 75:421–427.
Valent, P., Besemer, J., Muhm, M., Majdic, O., Lechner, K., and Bettelheim, P. (1989). Interleukin 3 activates human blood basophils via high affinity binding sites. *Proc. Natl. Acad. Sci. USA* 86:5542–5546.
Valent, P., Besemer, J., Sillaber, C., Butterfield, J. H., Eher, R., Majdic, O., Kishi, K., Klepetko, W., Eckersberger, F., Lechner, K., and Bettelheim, P. (1990). Failure to detect IL-3-binding sites on human mast cells. *J. Immunol.* 145:3432–3437.
Wershil, B. K., Levine, A. D., Nauert, J. P., Gordon, J. R., and Galli, S. J. (1990). Ionomycin stimulation of a growth factor-independent mouse mast cell line induces differential IL-3 and IL-4 gene expression and release of product. *FASEB J.* 4:A1943 (abstract).
Wershil, B. K., Wang, Z-S., Gordon, J. R., and Galli, S. J. (1991). The recruitment of neutrophils during IgE-dependent cytaneous late phase reactions in the mouse is mast cell–dependent: Partial inhibition of the reaction with antiserum against tumor necrosis factor alpha. *J. Clin. Invest.* (in press).
Williams, D. E., Eisenman, J., Baird, A., Rauch, C., Van Ness, K., March, C. J., Park, L. S., Martin, U., Mochizuki, D. Y., Boswell, H. S., Burgess, G. S., Cosman, D., and Lyman, S. D. (1990). Identification of a ligand for the c-*kit* proto-oncogene. *Cell* 63:167–174.
Wilson, S. D., Kuchroo, V. K., Israel, D. I., and Dorf, M. E. (1990). Expression and characterization of TCA3: A murine inflammatory protein. *J. Immunol.* 145:2745–2750.
Wodnar-Filipowicz, A., and Moroni, C. (1990). Regulation of interleukin 3 mRNA

xpression in mast cells occurs at the posttranscriptional level and is mediated by calcium ions. *Proc. Natl. Acad. Sci. USA* 87:777–781.

Wodnar-Filipowicz, A., Heusser, C. H., and Moroni, C. (1989). Production of the haemopoietic growth factors GM-CSF and interleukin-3 by mast cells in response to IgE receptor-mediated activation. *Nature* 339:150–152.

Wolpe, S. D., and Cerami, A. (1989). Macrophage inflammatory proteins 1 and 2: members of a novel superfamily of cytokines. *FASEB J.* 3:2565–2573.

Wolpe, S. D., Davatelis, G., Sherry, B., Beutler, B., Hesse, D. G., Nguyen, H. T., Moldawer, L. L., Nathan, C. F., Lowry, S. F., and Cerami, A. (1988). Macrophages secrete a novel heparin-binding protein with inflammatory and neutrophil chemokinetic properties. *J. Exp. Med.* 167:570–581.

Yoshimura, T., and Leonard, E. J. (1990). Secretion by human fibroblasts of monocyte chemoattractant protein-1, the product of gene JE. *J. Immunol.* 144:2377–2383.

Young, J. D-E., Liu, C-C., Butler, G., Cohn, Z. A., and Galli, S. J. (1987). Identification, purification, and characterization of a mast cell–associated cytolytic factor related to tumor necrosis factor. *Proc. Natl. Acad. Sci. USA* 84:9175–9179.

Zsebo, K. M., Wypych, J., McNiece, I. K., Lu, H. S., Smith, K. A., Karkare, S. B., Sachdev, R. K., Yuschenkoff, V. N., Birkett, N. C., Williams, L. R., Satyagai, V. N., Tung, W., Bosselman, R. A., Mendiaz, E. A., and Langley, K. E. (1990a). Identification, purification, and biological characterization of hematopoietic stem cell factor from buffalo rat liver–conditioned medium. *Cell* 63:195–201.

Zsebo, K. M., Williams, D. A., Geissler, E. N., Broudy, V. C., Martin, F. C., Atkins, H. L., Hsu, R-Y., Birkett, N. C., Okino, K. H., Murdock, D. C., Jacobsen, F. W., Langley, K. E., Smith, K. A., Takeishi, T., Cattanach, B. M., Galli, S. J., and Suggs, S. V. (1990b). Stem cell factor is encoded at the *Sl* locus of the mouse and is the ligand for the c-*kit* tyrosine kinase receptor. *Cell* 63:213–224.

17

Lessons to Be Learned from Sodium Cromoglycate and Related Drugs

RATKO DJUKANOVIĆ and STEPHEN T. HOLGATE

University of Southampton
Southampton, England

I. Introduction

The association of mast cell mediators with allergic disease dates back to the observation of Dale and Laidlaw of histamine reproducing the acute bronchoconstriction observed in clinical asthma (Dale and Laidlaw, 1910). The cellular localization of histamine to mast cells by Riley and West (1953) firmly established this cell as a source of mediators for allergic tissue responses. Over the last 20 years, a large number of preformed and newly generated mediators with biological actions pertinent to allergic tissue responses have been ascribed to the mast cell, providing opportunities for the pharmaceutical industry to develop inhibitory drugs targeted toward this cell type and its mediators. The success of H_1-histamine antagonists, in particular the recent, more potent and selective drugs, testifies to the success of this strategy. However, although antihistamines have been shown to have proven efficacy in allergic rhinitis and urticaria, their application to the treatment of other allergic disorders, particularly of a more chronic nature, such as asthma and atopic ezcema, has been disappointing. Thus, a relentless effort has been expended to discover drugs capable of inhibiting the release of all mediators from activated mast cells, and it is within this context that sodium cromoglycate is most frequently associated.

Before reviewing the mechanisms of action of this drug and its cogeners, it is worth highlighting the evidence for mast cell involvement in asthma and allied disorders.

II. Evidence for Mast Cell Involvement in Asthma

While it has long been hypothesized that mast cells are implicated in the pathogenesis of human asthma, largely on the basis of in vitro and animal studies, definitive proof of this has been long awaited. Over 35 years ago an acute bronchoconstriction provoked by inhaled allergen in atopic asthmatics had been described (reviewed by Pepys, 1973), and because its time course was similar to that of the allergen-induced skin wheal reaction, mast cells were thought to be responsible. The application of sensitive and specific assays for mast cell–dependent products has now clearly shown that the early asthmatic response is accompanied by an increase in histamine (Casale et al., 1987a; Chan-Yeung et al., 1989; Wenzel et al., 1990), prostaglandin (PG) D_2 (Wenzel et al., 1990), leukotrienes (LT) C_4 (Wenzel et al., 1990) and E_4 (Chan-Yeung et al., 1989), and tryptase (Wenzel et al., 1988) in bronchoalveolar lavage fluid, which is paralleled by an increase in circulating concentrations of histamine (Howarth et al., 1987) (Fig. 1) and the urinary excretion of the τ-methyl metabolite of histamine (De Monchy et al., 1986).

Evidence for mast cell involvement in day-to-day asthma has been more difficult to obtain. As long ago as 1949 Herxheimer noticed that H_1-histamine antagonists, when administered intravenously to patients with asthma, resulted in bronchodilatation (Herxheimer, 1949), an observation that has subsequently been confirmed with oral and inhaled administration of more selective and potent antagonists (Rafferty and Holgate, 1987; Kemp et al., 1987). Studies in atopic asthma have demonstrated increased releasability of lavage mast cells (Wardlaw et al., 1988) in keeping with ultrastructural evidence of loss of mast cell granular content in endobronchial biopsies by electron microscopy (Beasley et al., 1989; Djukanović et al., 1990) (Fig. 2). When taken with the observation of increased baseline concentrations of histamine (Casale et al., 1987b), PGD_2 (Liu et al., 1990), and tryptase (Wenzel et al., 1988) in lavage fluid of asthmatics, these studies and others demonstrating a bronchodilator effect of H_1 antagonists can be explained on the basis of persistent mast cell mediator release, imparting an increase in bronchial tone.

In addition to allergen, the mast cell may also be involved in other forms of provoked bronchoconstriction. One example is the effect of inhaled adenosine or adenosine 5'-monophosphate (AMP), which in patients with extrinsic or intrinsic asthma produces a rapid onset of bronchoconstriction that is exquisitely sensitive to inhibition by H_1-histamine antagonists (Rafferty et al., 1987) (Fig.

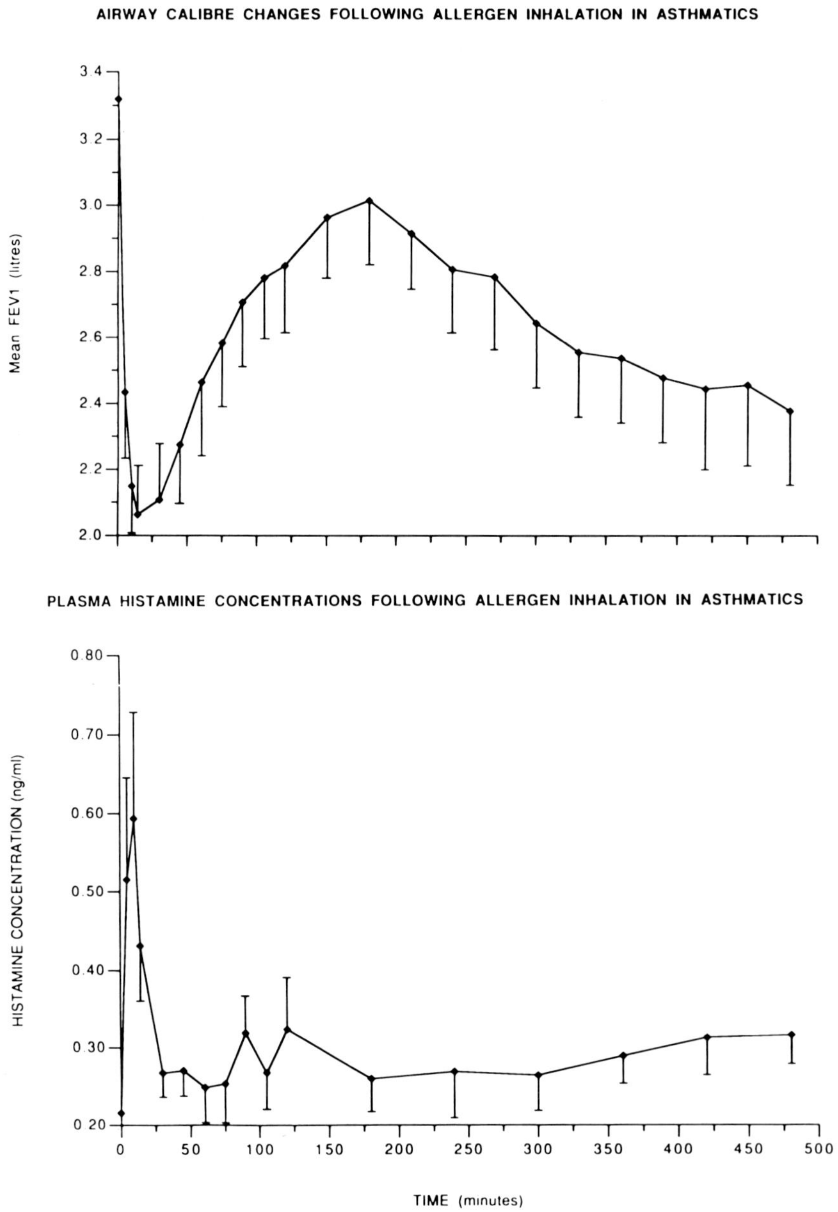

Figure 1 Changes in plasma histamine concentration measured by radioimmunoassay (bottom panel) following allergen bronchial challenge that induced an early and late asthmatic response (top panel) in a group of atopic asthmatic subjects.

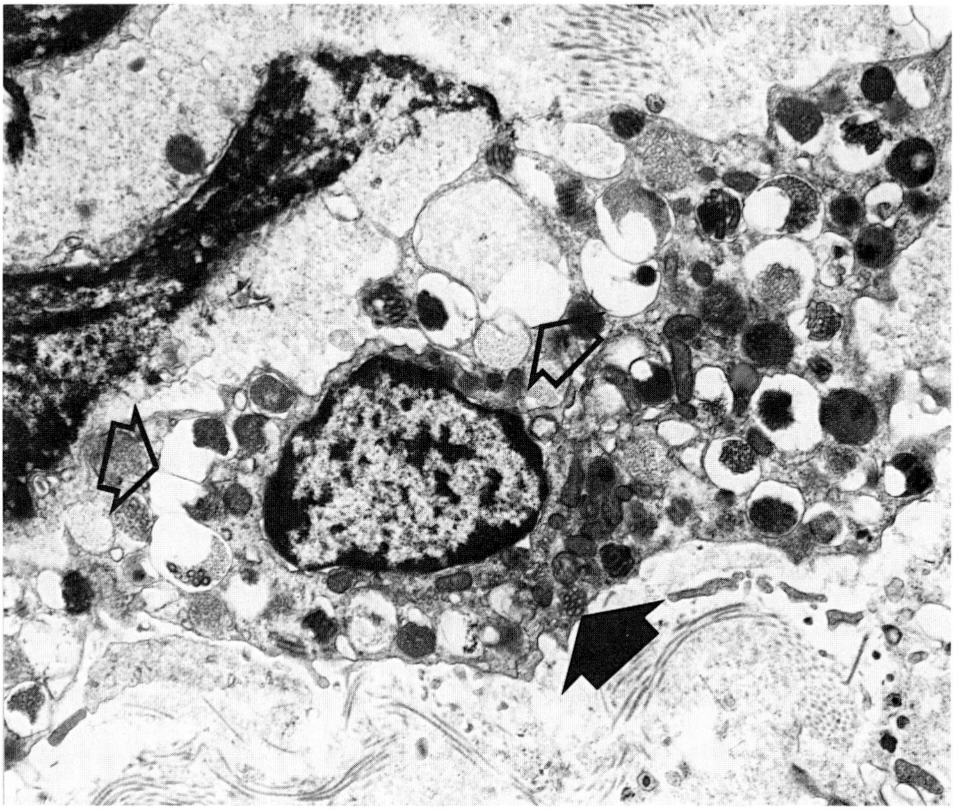

Figure 2 Mast cell in the submucosa of a subject with atopic asthma. Note the characteristic scroll appearance of intact granules (filled arrow) and varying degrees of loss of granular content as a sign of degranulation with the formation of degranulation channels (open arrow). Uranyl acetate–lead citrate stain; transmission electron microscopy, magnification × 12,000.

3). This response is mediated through an interaction of adenosine with A_2-purinoreceptors on the surface of mast cells with augmentation of degranulation (Phillips et al., 1989). The rapid development of tachyphylaxis with repeated AMP challenge is supported by the in vitro observation of receptor down-regulation on exposure to adenosine and related analogs (Daxun et al., 1989).

Although there still exists considerable controversy over the mechanisms of exercise-induced asthma (EIA), one view that is receiving increasing support is the hyperosmolar release of mediators from primed mast cells consequent upon hyperventilation and water loss from the airway surface to meet the increased

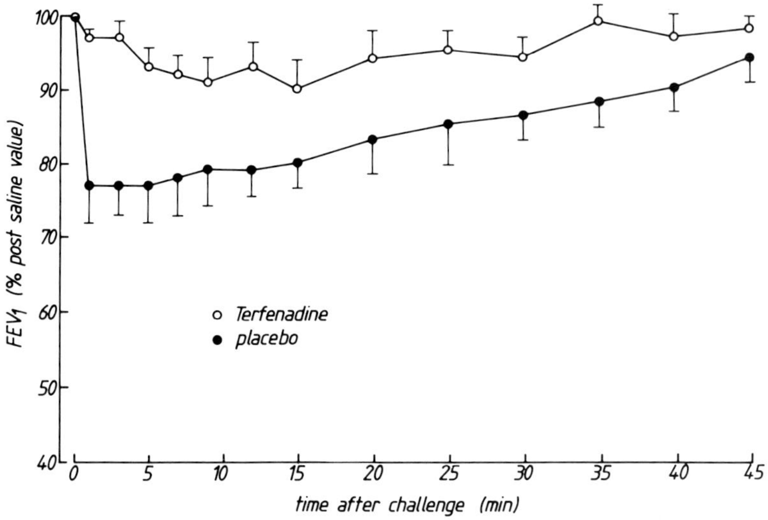

Figure 3 Effect of a potent H_1-histamine antagonist, terfenadine (180 mg), on adenosine 5'-monophosphate–induced bronchoconstriction.

requirement to humidify the inspired air (Anderson et al., 1985). Careful study has shown that the bronchoconstriction produced by exercise in asthma can be reproduced by isocapnic hyperventilation (ICH) (Howarth et al., 1984), cold air (Gilbert et al., 1988) or hypertonic saline challenge (Kivity et al., 1986). The capacity of H_1-histamine antagonists such as oral terfenadine to ablate the response to ICH (Finnerty et al., 1990) and hypertonic saline (Finnerty et al., 1989) supports an important role for mast cell activation in these events. The situation with EIA is not quite so straightforward in that H_1-histamine antagonists, administered either orally or by inhalation, attenuate the response at best by a mean of approximately 30% less than that achieved with either hypertonic saline or ICH (Finnerty and Holgate, 1990). The recent demonstration that LTD_4 antagonists and inhibitors of the 5-lipoxygenase pathway of arachidonic acid metabolism also exert a suppressive effect on EIA (Manning et al., 1990; Israel et al., 1990) indicates an important contribution from this class of lipid mediators. The ability of H_1-histamine antagonists to attenuate EIA achieves a maximum within the first 5–10 min of the response, with diminishing effect thereafter (Finnerty and Holgate, 1990), whereas the reverse is true of the LTD_4 antagonists, with their maximum effect being observed over the latter two-thirds of the response (Manning et al., 1990). Both these observations are in

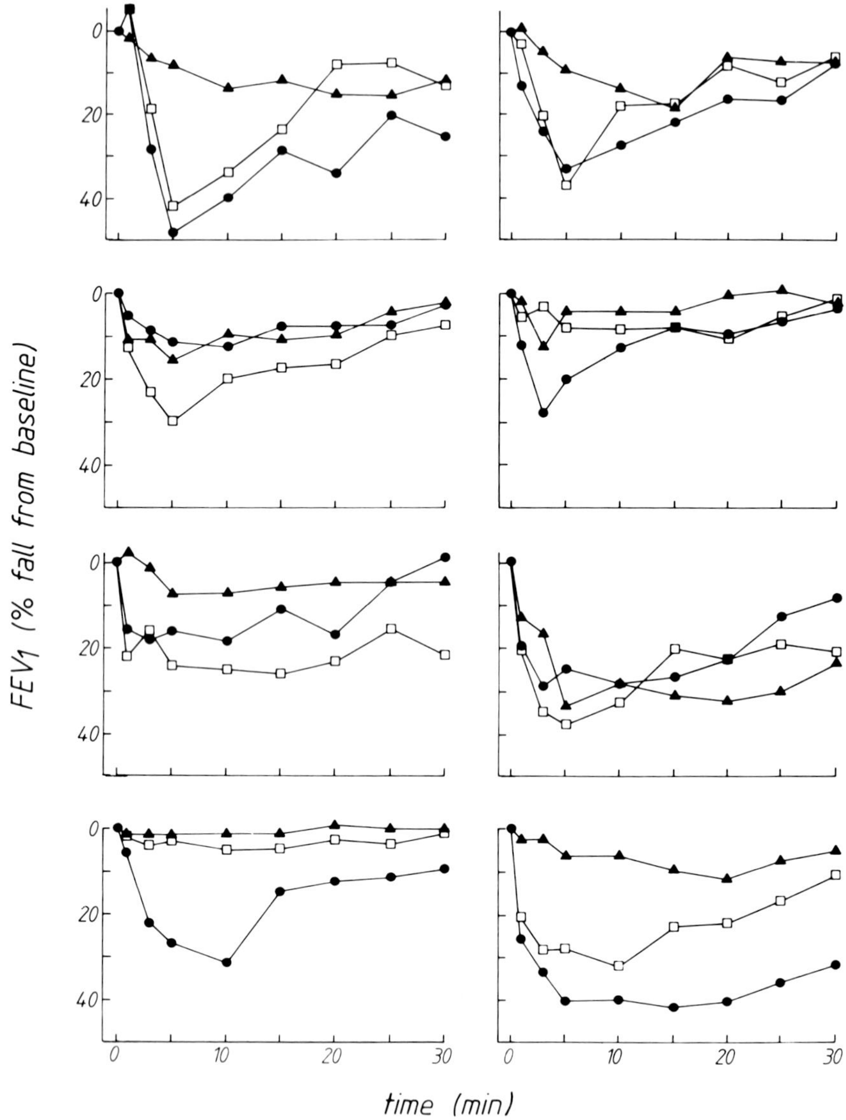

Figure 4 Effect of pretreatment with a histamine H_1-antagonist (terfenadine, 180 mg, ▲), a cyclooxygenase inhibitor (flurbiprofen, 100 mg, □), and placebo (●) on the immediate fall in FEV_1 produced by isocapnic hyperventilation in eight asthmatic subjects.

keeping with the known time course of action of histamine and cysteinyl leukotrienes as contractile agonists. Measurement of mediators in bronchial lavage fluid has shown that hypertonic saline challenge causes an increase in histamine and PGD_2 (Gravelyn et al., 1988), although at the time of writing similar changes with exercise have not been recorded (Broide et al., 1990). One possibility is that these stimuli cause a rapid burst of mediator release, with constrictor effects that persist long after the mediator has been cleared, as occurs with a single administration of either one or a mixture of mediators. An additional possibility is the involvement of non–mast cell mechanisms such as stimulation of airway reflexes and rebound vascular engorgement.

There are other good examples of agonists causing indirect bronchoconstriction not involving mast cells, including platelet-activating factor (PAF) (Cuss et al., 1986), bradykinin (Simonsson et al., 1973), and sulfur dioxide (Jackson-Myers et al., 1986), all of which are stimulants of airway sensory nerves to activate both local and central constrictor reflexes.

III. Studies with Mast Cell–Stabilizing Agents

Sodium cromoglycate was first introduced as a prophylactic agent for treating asthma by Howell and Altounyan in 1967 on the basis of its proven efficacy in treating patients with this disease. This observation was followed by the clear demonstration of an inhibitory activity of the drug on acute bronchoconstriction provoked by inhaled allergen (Altounyan, 1987) and exercise (Davies, 1968), providing what was thought at that time to be convenient human test systems to evaluate this class of drug. The recognition that the early asthmatic response to inhaled allergen involves mast cell activation and the clear demonstration by Cox (1967) that sodium cromoglycate could inhibit IgE-dependent histamine secretion from rat peritoneal mast cells led to the labelling of this drug as a mast cell–stabilizing agent. Subsequent studies have amply proven the inhibitory effect of sodium cromoglycate on mediator release from mast cells isolated from the lungs of a large number of species, including humans (Flint et al., 1985; Assem and Mongar, 1970). However, although it is active against connective tissue–type mast cells in rodents (Garland, 1973), sodium cromoglycate proved to be inactive against mast cells isolated from human skin (Lowman et al., 1988), in contrast to those obtained from mucosal sites (Church and Hiroi, 1987). The difference in potency of cromoglycate-like drugs on lung mast cell function at different sites was capitalized upon the introduction of nedocromil sodium, a more potent inhibitor of mast cell mediator secretion. In *Ascaris*-sensitized monkeys, this drug was effective only on mucosal mast cells, which introduced both increased potency and selectivity (Wells et al., 1986).

The ability of both sodium cromoglycate and nedocromil sodium to inhibit

increases in the total number of mast cells when mucosal biopsies from atopic asthmatics have been compared with normal controls, some patients show very high mast cell counts, both in the epithelium and in the submucosa (Djukanović et al., 1990). This could suggest that these are the asthmatic patients who might best respond to sodium cromoglycate and related drugs and raises the interesting possibility that it is the mast cells' role in this disease that may contribute more to therapeutic efficacy of this group of drugs than is currently accepted.

V. Concluding Comments

While the precise mechanisms of action of sodium cromoglycate and related drugs have yet to be fully elucidated, the use of these compounds in dissecting the pathophysiology of asthma has proven invaluable. While their inhibitory effects on mast cells undoubtedly account for some of their therapeutic efficacy, particularly in the challenge situation, other activities, especially inhibition of neural pathways and late-phase leukocyte recruitment, are also of considerable importance and probably relevant to their clinical efficacy. With the rapidly increasing knowledge of mast cell ontogeny and biochemistry, the mechanism of action of this class of drugs in inhibiting mediator release is within the reach of scientists. However, it is a salatory thought that the discovery of sodium cromoglycate stemmed from careful clinical observation by Roger Altounyan and that despite 25 years of research the mechanism of action of the drug is still not known. Thus, although our knowledge about the pathogenesis of asthma continually increases, there are still many features of this disease about which we are still totally ignorant.

Discussion

Casale: Since increased BAL fluid histamine levels are found in a number of inflammatory lung diseases, wouldn't you expect increased mast cell degranulation in intrinsic asthma, which is also possibly an inflammatory disease?
Djukanović: Yes, I agree entirely. There is no reason why histamine and tryptase may not be elevated in intrinsic asthma as well, which is also viewed as an inflammatory disease.
Schwartz: Tryptase levels in BAL fluid from intrinsic asthmatics appeared not to be normally distributed. Only two subjects had markedly elevated levels, which raised the mean of the entire population. Do you think that atopy could have been missed in these subjects?
Djukanović: We were able to identify some intrinsic asthmatics who had elevated tryptase levels in their BAL fluid, suggesting mast cell release of this mediator in this type of asthma as well as in atopic asthma. I am not surprised by this as I feel

that what we call intrinsic asthma may have an allergic component as well and we may not be able to identify the allergen that causes it. Our difficulty with studying intrinsic asthmatics has been that most of these patients have to be treated with inhaled and/or oral steroids, and this affects our BAL findings.

Dvorak: I would like to compliment you on your ultrastructural demonstration of piecemeal degranulation and anaphylactic degranulation of mast cells in asthma tissue biopsies. I agree with your interpretation of these images exactly. We have found similar images (piecemeal degranulation > anaphylactic degranulation) in approximately 70% of biopsies we have studied taken from ileostomies of inflammatory bowel disease patients when all active disease had been removed prior to biopsy.

Djukanović: Thank you. There is now clear evidence of mast cell degranulation occurring in asthma in ways similar to those observed in vitro, i.e., via piecemeal degranulation and, less frequently, anaphylactic mechanism. There is little evidence in our biopsy of asthmatic airways for basophil involvement.

Platts-Mills: You described mast cells in the lung that were anaphylactically degranulating "without antigen challenge." However, I suspect what you really did was to study patients who had spent the previous night at home in a house with high levels of allergen.

Djukanović: I agree that it is possible that the anaphylactic type of degranulation we have seen was due to prior allergen exposure, possibly during the night before the investigation. What I said was that it was interesting to see anaphylactic degranulation occurring in vivo without bronchial challenge with allergen either by aerosol or by local instillation.

Galli: What is the current understanding of the mechanisms by which cromolyn affects the mast cell and other effector cells?

Djukanović: There is enough evidence to suggest that, as far as the mast cell in concerned, phosphorylation of a 78-kDa protein and inhibition of protein kinase C are two ways whereby cromolyn sodium may inhibit mast cell mediator release. This may theoretically affect cytokine release, but there is nothing to prove that. Another way whereby SCG may modulate inflammatory responses is by its action on neural reflexes and other inflammatory cells such as eosinophils, macrophages, and platelets.

References

Altounyan, R. E. C. (1987). Inhibition of experimental asthma by a new compound—Disodium cromoglycate, "Intal." *Acta Allergol.* 22:487.

Altounyan, R. E. C., Cole, M., and Lee, T. B. (1986). Inhibition of sulphur dioxide induced bronchoconstriction by nedocromil sodium and sodium cromoglycate in non-asthmatic atopic subjects. *Eur. J. Respir. Dis.* 69(Suppl. 147):274–276.

Anderson, S. D. (1989). Exercise-induced asthma, in: *Allergy: Principles and Practice*.

Edited by E. Middleton, C. E. Ree, E. F. Ellis, N. F. Adkinson, and J. W. Yunginger. St. Louis, Washington, D.C., Toronto, Mosby, pp. 1156–1175.

Anderson, S. D., Schoeffer, R. E., Black, J. L., and Daviskas, E. (1985). Airway cooling as the stimulus to exercise-induced asthma—A re-avaluation. *Eur. J. Respir. Dis.* 67:20–30.

Assem, E. S. K., and Mongar, J. L. (1970). Inhibition of allergic reactions in man and other species by cromoglycate. *Int. Arch. Allergy Appl. Immunol.* 38:68–77.

Beasley, R., Roche, W. R., Roberts, J. A., and Holgate, S. T. (1989). Cellular events in the bronchi in mild asthma and after bronchial provocation. *Am. Rev. Respir. Dis.* 139:806–817.

Broide, D. H., Eisman, S., Ramsdell, J. W., Ferguson, P., Schwartz, L. B., and Wasserman, S. I. (1990). Airway levels of mast-cell-derived mediators in exercise-induced asthma. *Am. Rev. Respir. Dis.* 141:563–568.

Cartier, A., Thomson, N. C., Frith, P. A., Roberts, R., and Hargreave, F. E. (1982). Allergen-induced increase in bronchial responsiveness to histamine: relationship to the late asthmatic response and change in airway calibre. *J. Allergy Clin. Immunol.* 70:170–177.

Casale, T. B., Wood, D., Richerson, H. B., Trapp, S., Metzger, W. J., Zavala, D., and Hunninghake, G. W. (1987a). Elevated bronchoalveolar lavage fluid histamine levels in allergic asthmatics are associated with methacholine bronchial responsiveness. *J. Clin. Invest.* 79:1197–1203.

Casale, T. B., Wood, D., Richerson, H. B., Zehr, B., Zavala, D., and Hunninghake, G. W. (1987b). Direct evidence of a role for mast cells in the pathogenesis of antigen-induced bronchoconstriction. *J. Clin. Invest.* 80:1507–1511.

Chan-Yeung, M., Chan, H., Tse, K. S., Salari, H., and Lam, S. (1989). Histamine and leukotrienes release in bronchoalveolar fluid during plicatic acid-induced bronchoconstriction. *J. Allergy Clin. Immunol.* 84:762–768.

Chilvers, E. R., Dixon, C. M. S., and Ind, P. W. (1987). Mechanism of metabisulphate-induced bronchoconstriction in atopic non-asthmatic subjects. *Thorax* 42: 745–746.

Church, M. K., and Hiroi, J. (1987). Inhibition of IgE-dependent histamine release from human dispersed lung mast cells by anti-allergic drugs and salbutamol. *Br. J. Pharmacol.* 90:421–429.

Correia, L., and Theoharides, T. C. (1991). Inhibition of mast cell secretion is associated with phosphorylation of a major protein kinase C substrate. *FASEB J.* 5:3704 (abstract).

Cox, J. S. G. (1967). Disodium cromoglycate (FPL 670, Intal): A specific inhibitor of reaginic antibody-antigen mechanisms. *Nature (Lond.)* 216:1328–1329.

Crimi, N., Palermo, F., Oliveri, R., Cacopardo, B., Vancheri, C., and Mistretta, A. (1986). Adenosine-induced bronchoconstriction: Comparison between nedocromil and sodium cromoglycate. *Eur. J. Respir. Dis.* 69(Suppl. 147):258–262.

Cuss, F. M., Dixon, C. M. S., and Barnes, P. J. (1986). Effects of inhaled platelet-activating factor on pulmonary function and bronchial responsiveness in man. *Lancet* 2:189–192.

Dale, H. H., and Laidlaw, P. P. (1910). The physiological action of beta-imidazolylethylamine. *J. Physiol. (Lond.)* 41:318–344.

Davies, S. E. (1968) Effect of disodium cromoglycate on exercise induced asthma. *Br. Med. J.* 3:593–594.

Daxun, Z., Rafferty, P., Richards, R., Summerell, S., and Holgate, S. T. (1989). Airway refractoriness to adenosine 5'-monophosphate after repeated inhalation by atopic-nonasthmatic subjects. *J. Allergy. Clin. Immunol.* 83:152–158.

De Monchy, J. G., Keyzer, J. J., and Kauffman, H. F. (1986). Histamine in late asthmatic reactions following house dust mite inhalation. Histamine in late asthmatic reactions following house dust mite inhalation. *Agents Actions* 16:252–255.

Dixon, C. M. S., and Barnes, P. J. (1988). Bradykinin induced bronchoconstriction: Inhibition by nedocromil and cromoglycate. *Thorax* 43:225 (abstract).

Djukanović, R., Wilson, J. W., Britten, K. M., Wilson, S. J., Walls, A. F., Howarth, P. H., and Holgate, S. T. (1990). Quantitation of mast cells and eosinophils in the bronchial mucosa of symptomatic atopic asthmatics and healthy controls using immunohistochemistry. *Am. Rev. Respir. Dis.* 142:863–871.

Djukanović, R., Polosa, R., Mann, M., and Holgate, S. T. (1991). The effect of allergen bronchial challenge on methacholine and bradykinin airway responsiveness (1991). *Eur. Respir. J.* (in press).

Finnerty, J. P., and Holgate, S. T. (1990). Evidence for the roles of prostaglandins as mediators of exercise-induced asthma: inhibitory effect of terfenadine and flurbiprofen alone and in combination. *Eur. Respir. J.* 3:540–547.

Finnerty, J. P., Wilmot, J., and Holgate, S. T. (1989). Inhibition of hypertonic saline-induced bronchoconstriction by terfenadine and flurbiprofen: evidence for the predominant role of histamine. *Am. Rev. Respir. Dis.* 140:593–597.

Finnerty, J. P., Harvey, A., and Holgate, S. T. (1990). The effect of terfenadine and flurbiprofen on isocapnic hyperventilation-induced asthma. *Am. Rev. Respir. Dis.* 141:172 (abstract).

Flint, K. C., Leung, K. B. P., Pearce, F. L., Hudspith, B. N., Brostoff, J., and Johnson, N. M. (1985). Human mast cells recovered by bronchoalveolar lavage: their morphology, histamine release and the effects of sodium cromoglycate. *Clin. Sci.* 68:427–432.

Garland, L. G. (1973). Effect of cromoglycate on anaphylactic histamine release from rat peritoneal mast cells. *Br. J. Pharmacol.* 49:128–130.

Gilbert, I. A., Fouke, J. M., and McFadden, E. R. (1988). Intra-airway thermodynamics during exercise and hyperventilation in asthmatics. *J. Appl. Physiol.* 64:2167–2174.

Gravelyn, T. R., Pan, P. M., and Eschenbacher, W. L. (1988). Mediator release in an isolated airway segment in subjects with asthma. *Am. Rev. Respir. Dis.* 137:641–646.

Herxheimer, H. (1949). Antihistamines in bronchial asthma. *Br. Med. J.* 2:901–905.

Hoag, J. E., and McFadden, E. R. (1991). Long-term effect of cromolyn sodium on nonspecific bronchial hyperresponsiveness: A review. *Ann. Allergy* 66:53–63.

Howarth, P. H., Pao, G. J-K., Church, M. K., and Holgate, S. T. (1984). Exercise and isocapnic hyperventilation-induced bronchoconstriction in asthma: Relevance of circulating basophils to measurements of plasma histamine. *J. Allergy Clin. Immunol.* 73:391–399.

Howarth, P. H., Durham, S. R., Kay, A. B., and Holgate, S. T. (1987). The relationship between mast cell mediator release and bronchial reactivity in allergic asthma. *J. Allergy Clin. Immunol.* 80:703–711.

Howell, J. B. L., and Altounyan, R. E. C. (1967). Double-blind trial of disodium cromoglycate in the treatment of allergic bronchial asthma. *Lancet* 2:539–542.

Israel, E., Dermarkarian, R., Rosenberg, M., Sperling, R., Taylor, G., Rubin, P., and Drazen, J. M. (1990). The effects of a 5-lipoxygenase inhibitor on asthma induced by cold dry air. *N. Engl. J. Med.* 323:1740–1744.

Jackson-Myers, D., Bigby, B. G., Calvayrac, P., Shepard, D., and Boushey, H. A. (1986). Interaction of cromolyn and a muscarinic antagonist in inhibiting bronchial reactivity to sulphur dioxide and to isocapnic hyperpnoea alone. *Am. Rev. Respir. Dis.* 133:1154–1158.

Joos, G. F., Pauwels, R. A., and Van Der Straeten, M. E. (1989). The effect of nedocromil sodium on the bronchoconstrictor effect of neurokinin A in subjects with asthma. *J. Allergy Clin. Immunol.* 83:663–668.

Kay, A. B. (1991). Lymphocytes in asthma. *Respir. Med.* 85:87–90.

Kemp, J. P., Meltzer, E. O., Orgel, H. A., Welch, M. J., Bucholtz, G. A., Middleton, E., Spector, S. L., Newton, J. J., and Perhach, J. L. (1987). A dose-response study of the bronchodilator action of azelastine in asthma. *J. Allergy Clin. Immunol.* 79:893–899.

Kivity, S., Greif, J., Reisner, B., Fireman, E., and Topilsky, M. (1986). Bronchial inhalation challenge with ultrasonically nebulised saline: comparison to exercise-induced asthma. *Ann. Allergy* 57:355–358.

Leung, K. B. P., Flint, K. C., Brostoff, J., Hudspith, B. N., Johnson, N. M., and Pearce, F. L. (1986). A comparison of nedocromil sodium and sodium cromoglycate on human lung mast cells obtained by bronchoalveolar lavage and by dispersion of lung fragments. *Eur. J. Respir. Dis.* 147(Suppl.):223–226.

Liu, M. C., Bleecker, E. R., Lichtenstein, L. M., Kagey-Sobotka, A., Niv, Y., Mclemore, T. L., Permutt, S., Proud, D., and Hubbard, W. C. (1990). Evidence for elevated levels of histamine, prostaglandin D_2, and other bronchoconstricting prostaglandins in the airways of subjects with mild asthma. *Am. Rev. Respir. Dis.* 142:126–132.

Lowhagen, O., and Rak, S. (1985). Modification of bronchial hyperreactivity after treatment with sodium cromoglycate during the pollen season. *J. Allergy Clin. Immunol.* 75:460–467.

Lowman, M. A., Benyon, R. C., and Church, M. K. (1988). Human skin mast cells: Effects of salbutamol and sodium cromoglycate on histamine release induced by anti-IgE and substance P. *Skin Pharmacol.* 1:63–64.

Manning, P. J., Watson, R. M., Margolskee, D. J., Williams, V. C., Schwartz, J. I., and O'Byrne, P. M. (1990). Inhibition of exercise-induced bronchoconstriction by MK-571, a potent leukotriene D_4-receptor antagonist. *N. Engl. J. Med.* 323:1736–1739.

Moqbel, R., Walsh, G. M., and Kay, A. B. (1986a). Inhibition of human granulocyte activation by nedocromil sodium. *Eur. J. Respir. Dis.* 69(Suppl. 147):227–229.

Moqbel, R., Walsh, G. M., MacDonald, A. J., and Kay, A. B. (1986b). Effect of disodium cromoglycate on activation of human eosinophils and neutrophils following reversed (anti-IgE) anaphylaxis. *Clin. Allergy* 16:73–83.

Pepys, J. (1973). Immunopathology of allergic disease. *Clin. Allergy* 3:1–22.

Phillips, G. D., Bagga, P. K., Djukanovic, R., and Holgate, S. T. (1989). The influence of refractoriness to adenosine 5'-monophosphate on allergen-provoked bronchoconstriction in asthma. *Am. Rev. Respir. Dis.* 140:321–326.

Rafferty, P., and Holgate, S. T. (1987). Terfenadine (Seldane^R) is a potent and selective histamine H_1 receptor antagonist in asthmatic airways. *Am. Rev. Respir. Dis.* 135:181–184.

Rafferty, P., Beasley, C. R. W., and Holgate, S. T. (1987). The contribution of histamine to immediate bronchoconstriction provoked by inhaled allergen and adenosine 5'-monophosphate in atopic asthma. *Am. Rev. Respir. Dis.* 136:369–373.

Riley, J. F., and West, G. B. (1953). Presence of histamine in tissue mast cells. *J. Physiol. (Lond.)* 120:528–537.

Silverman, M., Connolly, N. M., Balfour-Lynn, L., and Godfrey, S. (1972). Long-term trial of disodium cromoglycate and isporenaline in children with asthma. *Br. Med. J.* 3:378–381.

Simonsson, B., Skoogh, B. E., Bergh, N. P., Andersson, R., and Svedmyr, N. (1973). In vivo and in vitro effect of bradykinin on bronchial motor tone in normal subjects and patients with airways obstruction. *Respiration* 30:378–388.

Theoharides, T. C., Seighart, W., Greengard, P., and Douglas, W. W. (1980). Antiallergic drug cromolyn may inhibit secretion by phosphorylation of a mast cell protein. *Science* 207:80–82.

Thorel, T., Ameisen, J. C., Joseph, M., Vorng, H., Tonnel, A. B., Marquette, C. H., and Capron, A. (1987). Preventative effect of nedocromil sodium on the abnormal response to aspirin of platelets from aspirin-sensitive asthmatics. *Am. Rev. Respir. Dis.* 135:398 (abstract).

Thorel, T., Joseph, M., Tsicipoulos, A., Tonnel, A. B., and Capron, A. (1988). Inhibition by nedocromil sodium of IgE-mediated activation of human mononuclear phagocytes and platelets in allergy. *Int. Arch. Allergy Appl. Immunol.* 85:232–237.

Wardlaw, A. J., Dunnette, S., Gleich, G. J., Collins, J. V., and Kay, A. B. (1988). Eosinophils and mast cells in bronchoalveolar lavage in subjects with mild asthma. Relationship to bronchial hyperreactivity. *Am. Rev. Respir. Dis.* 137:62–69.

Wells, E., Jackson, C. G., Harper, S. T., Mann, J., and Eady, R. P. (1986). Characterization of primate bronchoalveolar mast cells. II. Inhibition of histamine, LTC_4, and PGD_2 release from primate bronchoalveolar mast cells and comparison with rat peritoneal mast cells. *J. Immunol.* 127:3941–3945.

Wenzel, S. E., Fowler, A. A., and Schwartz, L. B. (1988). Activation of pulmonary mast cells by bronchoalveolar lavage allergen challenge. In vivo release of histamine and tryptase in atopic subjects with and without asthma. *Am. Rev. Respir. Dis.* 137:1002–1008.

Wenzel, S. E., Larsen, G. L., Johnston, K., Voelkel, N. F., and Westcott, J. Y. (1990). Elevated levels of leukotriene C_4 in bronchoalveolar lavage fluid from atopic asthmatics after endobronchial allergen challenge. *Am. Rev. Respir. Dis.* 142:112–119.

18

The Effects of Anti-inflammatory Steroids on Mast Cells

ROBERT P. SCHLEIMER

Johns Hopkins Asthma and Allergy Center
The Johns Hopkins University School of Medicine
Baltimore, Maryland

I. Introduction

This chapter will consider the information available on the effects of glucocorticoids ("steroids") on mast cells and has been divided into three major parts. Discussion will first focus on the effects of in vivo treatment with steroids on numbers and distribution of mast cells. In the next section the effects of steroids on mast cell function in experimental inflammatory reactions and diseases that are associated with mast cell activation will be considered. The final major section will analyze in vitro studies of steroid action on mast cell proliferation, mast cell function, and the biochemical mechanisms of mast cell activation. For all three sections it has been necessary to pull together data from studies employing several different species, including rodent, rabbit, dog, sheep, and human. In many cases there are clear species differences, and where such differences are of interest in application of results to humans, these differences have been highlighted. The effects of steroids on mast cells and basophils have been reviewed previously (Schleimer, 1989). This review represents an extension of this previous review, focusing only on the mast cell and bringing to the discussion relevant new information.

release in the rat. Norn (1965, 1967, 1968) demonstrated that in vivo treatment of rats with hydrocortisone, methylprednisolone, betamethasone, and other steroids caused no change in the total number of peritoneal mast cells, but inhibited subsequent antigen-mediated histamine release tested in vitro. In contrast, this steroid treatment did not inhibit the mast cell mediator release stimulated with 48/80, alpha-chymotrypsin, polymyxin B, or phospholipase (Norn, 1967). Marquardt and Wasserman (1983) showed that a 5-day treatment with dexamethasone in vivo in rats inhibited both antigen and ionophore A23187-induced mediator release from rat peritoneal mast cells in vitro. Infection of rats with *Nippostrongylus brasiliensis* or other parasites induces a large increase in mucosal mast cell numbers in the gut and elsewhere. Olson and Schiller (1978) demonstrated that cortisone treatment decreased both the primary and secondary worm expulsion, which are thought to be mast cell dependent. Cortisone also reduced the number of mast cells in the gut and blocked the increase in mast cells seen following infection (Olson and Schiller, 1978; Barrett et al., 1988). King et al. (1985) extended these studies with some elegant experiments in which the effects of steroids on mucosal mast cell numbers and intestinal anaphylaxis were determined. These investigators measured the rat mast cell protease-II (RMCP-II) as an indicator of mucosal mast cell number (see Fig. 2). As expected, infection of rats with *Nippostrongylus* caused a large increase in mast cells and RMCP-II in gut. Challenge of these animals with i.v. *Nippostrongylus* antigen produced systemic anaphylaxis in which the gut was the primary shock organ. Treatment of rats for 24 or 48 hr with methylprednisolone depleted the mucosal mast cell numbers and RMCP-II levels in the gut and other tissues, without having effects on IgE levels or connective tissue mast cell numbers in the ear. Furthermore, the steroid treatment blocked the systemic anaphylactic reaction and the increase in RMCP-II found in the blood following antigen, presumably by depletion of the MMC in the treated rats (King et al., 1985).

Soda and colleagues (1991) recently followed up these studies and provided morphological evidence of a mechanism for this effect of steroids. When *N. brasiliensis*–infected rats were treated with dexamethasone, Soda et al. (1991) observed engulfment of mast cells by tissue macrophages within 4–7 hr (Fig. 3). Greater than 90% of the intestinal mucosal mast cells were destroyed by macrophages, and as in the studies by King et al. (1985), these investigators found no evidence for release of the mast cell mediators, histamine, or RMCP-II.

Although corticosteroid treatment has been shown to delay or slightly shift the dose response of antigen required for anaphylaxis in guinea pigs, steroids are relatively ineffective in blocking the acute anaphylactic response in the guinea pig (Goadby and Smith, 1964; Forsberg and Sorenby, 1981; Forsberg et al., 1982) (see Section III.A). In vivo treatment of guinea pigs with steroid followed by removal of lung tissue and challenge in vitro has been shown to inhibit the leukotriene or SRS release while not inhibiting histamine release (Goadby and

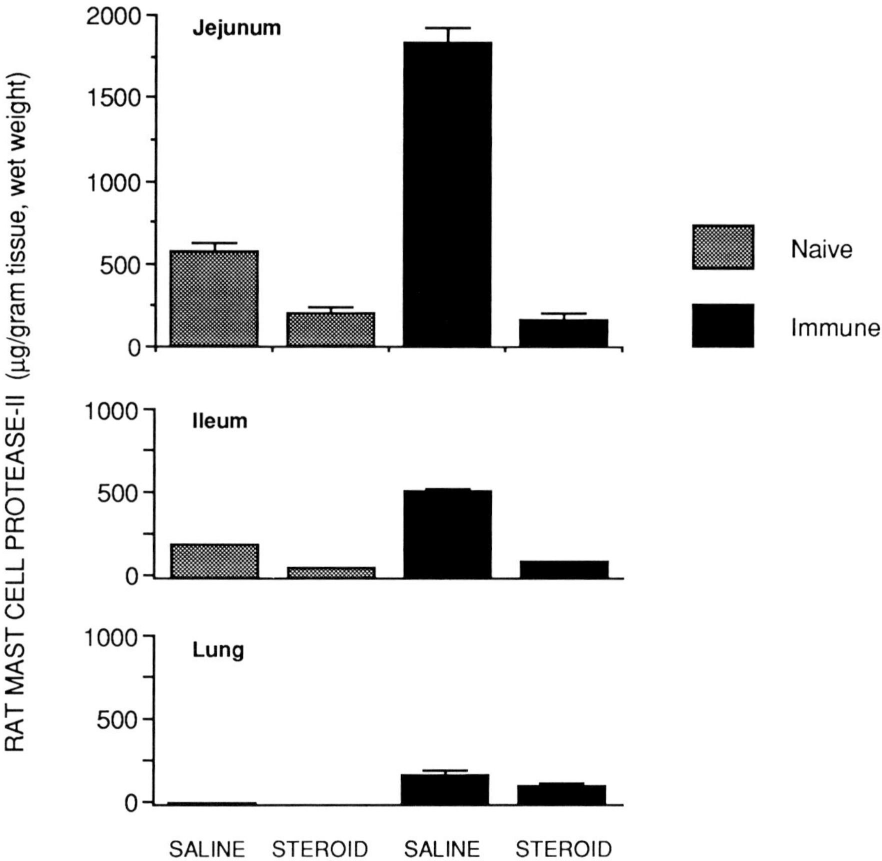

Figure 2 The effects of immunization and corticosteroid treatment on distribution of RMCP-II in rat tissues. [Adapted from King et al. (1985).]

Smith, 1964; Forsberg and Sorenby, 1981; Forsberg et al., 1982; Andersson et al., 1985). Andersson and collaborators (1982a,b, 1985) have analyzed steroid effects in detail in guinea pigs and have observed that the immunization protocol is critical as a determinant of the subsequent steroid effects. When antigen is given with aluminum hydroxide ($A1OH_3$) as an adjuvant, guinea pigs produce an IgE and IgG response to antigen. When antigen is given alone without the adjuvant, only an IgG response is produced. Since, in the guinea pig, both IgG_1 and IgE antibodies can sensitize mast cells, the isotype of antibody can be critical in such experiments. Andersson et al. (1982a,b) found that the release of histamine in vitro and the bronchospasm in vivo following challenge with recruiting leukocytes to the challenge site; these recruited leukocytes are felt to be responsible for releasing the mediators that induce the late-phase response (Atkins et al., 1977; Metzger et al., 1985; Bochner et al., 1990b). The effects of oral corticosteroid therapy on the acute response to experimental allergen challenge in humans are controversial. Herxheimer (1954) reported a reduction of the acute response to antigen challenge by steroids. Similarly, Martin et al. (1980) demonstrated an increase in the quantity of antigen required to cause a standard reduction in airflow in antigen-sensitive patients. Inhibition of the response to antigen was associated with reduced peak levels of neutrophil chemotactic activity following antigen challenge (Martin et al., 1980). In contrast to the work of Martin et al. and Herxheimer, several groups have demonstrated that parenteral steroid treatment causes a selective decrease in the late-phase response with little or no effect on the acute, mast cell–dependent response (McCarthy and Pepys, 1971; Booij-Noord et al., 1972; Pepys et al., 1974; Nakazawa et al., 1976). This pattern of steroid effect, i.e., selective inhibition of the late-phase response, is also seen in the upper airways and in skin in humans (see Sections III.C and III.E). The advent of effective topically active steroids that are rapidly metabolized and thus produce relatively few systemic side effects has led to a resurgence of the use of steroids in the treatment of asthma. Studies in the airways as well as in nasal challenge (see Section III.C) have shown that topical steroid treatment, but not oral steroid administration, clearly reduces the acute response to antigen challenge in the upper and lower airways (Dahl and Johansson, 1982; Burge, 1982). Such treatment requires several weeks for optimal effect (Dahl and Johansson, 1982). Firm evidence has been obtained in the nasal challenge model that this effect of topical steroids is associated with reduced appearance of mast cell mediators (see Section III.C). Oral steroid treatment has been shown to block both acute and late-phase allergic responses in the airways of rats and sheep (Church et al., 1972; Church and Miller, 1978; Abraham et al., 1983; Delehunt et al., 1984).

C. Hayfever

As in the case of asthma, there is good evidence for a role of the mast cell in the etiology of allergic rhinitis or hayfever. Antigen challenge of allergic subjects produces symptoms such as sneezing and nasal airway narrowing, along with an increased appearance of mast cell mediators such as histamine, prostaglandin D_2, leukotrienes, and others in nasal lavage (Naclerio et al., 1983). As in the lower airways, a late-phase response is seen in nasal antigen challenge of allergic subjects, and the profile of mediators released during the late response suggests that basophils may be involved (Naclerio et al., 1985). In subjects who experience nasal stuffiness and rhinitis upon exposure to cold air during the winter months, nasal challenge with cold, dry air produces release of mast cell mediators. Similar challenge of control subjects does not cause mediator release (Togias et al., 1985). Basophils as well as both formalin-sensitive and -resistant mast cells have been demonstrated in the human nose (Otsuka et al., 1985). The efficacy of topical steroids such as hydrocortisone, dexamethasone, or prednisolone in hayfever has been demonstrated by many different groups (Schwartz, 1954; Herxheimer and McAllen, 1956; Godfrey et al., 1957; Norman et al., 1966). Steroids such as these produce considerable systemic effects at concentrations that are required for activity and have been recently replaced by a new group of steroids such as budesonide, beclomethasone dipropionate, flunisolide, and others, which are rapidly metabolized and therefore cause relatively fewer systemic side effects (Mygind, 1973; Pipkorn, 1982a). The ability of topical steroid treatment to reduce epithelial mast cell numbers in the nose has been discussed earlier. As is the case with the study of lower airways responses to experimental allergen challenge, there is general agreement that steroid treatment both orally and topically blocks the late-phase response in the nose (Pelikan and DeVries, 1974; Vilsvik et al., 1975; Mygind et al., 1977; Pelikan, 1984). Also, as is the case in lower airways, topical steroid treatment is much more effective in reducing the acute response to antigen challenge than is oral steroid treatment (Pelikan and DeVries, 1974; Okuda et al., 1983; Mygind, 1973; Mygind et al., 1977; Pipkorn, 1982a,b; Pipkorn et al., 1987a,b). With regard to mast cell mediators, 2- or 3-day oral steroid treatment fails to inhibit the release of (probably mast cell–derived) histamine and prostaglandin D_2 in the acute response to antigen challenge in humans while blocking the late-phase appearance of (possibly basophil-derived) histamine (Pipkorn et al., 1987b). In contrast, topical treatment for 1 week with flunisolide substantially reduced the appearance of mast cell mediators following antigen challenge of allergic subjects (Pipkorn et al., 1987a).

D. Cold Urticaria

Idiopathic cold urticaria is a syndrome in which patients experience local skin urticaria upon exposure to cold. When skin biopsies of patients who suffer from cold urticaria are challenged by cooling in vitro, mast cells in the tissue degranulate, releasing histamine (Kaplan et al., 1981). Biopsy following ice challenge reveals mast cell degranulation in the skin of cold urticaria patients (Juhlin and Shelley, 1961). Whether cold challenge of basophils from patients with cold urticaria causes degranulation is controversial (Kaplan et al., 1981; Juhlin and Shelley, 1961). Combined treatment with ACTH and triamcinolone failed to inhibit the acute response to cold challenge (Juhlin and Shelley, 1961). Keahey and Greaves (1980) reported that prednisone treatment (20 mg prednisone/day for 3–5 days) inhibited the appearance of histamine in the venous circulation of the arm following cold challenge in two patients and enhanced it in a third. It has been the experience of Kaplan (personal communication) that prednisone treatment (40–60 mg/day for 1 week) has no effect on the response to cold challenge in cold urticaria patients.

E. Skin Reactions

Whereas the critical role of mast cells in cold urticaria seems clear, in other skin reactions following antigen challenge the importance of mast cells is less certain. Allergic responses in the skin with an IgE-dependent etiology are most likely to be among those that depend on mast cell activation. As in other challenged sites, challenge of the skin with allergen in a sensitive subject yields an acute reaction, which subsides and is replaced by the late-phase reaction (Gleich, 1982). Serum from a sensitive individual can passively sensitize the skin of a nonallergic subject to express the acute and late-phase responses (Solley et al., 1976). Transfer of the ability to express an acute and late-phase reaction is blocked if the serum is heated at 56°C for 4 hr, which inactivates IgE but not IgG, or if the serum is passed over an IgE immunoabsorbant. Furthermore, addition of high concentrations of IgE myeloma, which compete with antigen-specific IgE for the limited number of mast cell IgE Fc receptors, also prevent the sensitization (Solley et al., 1976). While it seems likely that the acute response to antigen challenge in the skin is a mast cell–mediated response, the role of mast cells in elicitation of the late-phase response is not clear (see Section III.F).

It was appreciated early that oral cortisone and ACTH do not inhibit the immediate skin reaction, or reaginic response, to intradermal challenge with allergen in allergic subjects (Cooke et al., 1951; Feinberg et al., 1951; Stollerman et al., 1951; Mancini et al., 1961). These studies were extended to show that oral steroid treatment clearly inhibits the late-phase response but does not inhibit the immediate wheal-and-flare response to 48/80 or histamine or antigen (Slott and Zweiman, 1974; Poothullil et al., 1976; Gronneberg et al., 1981). Recent studies using a cutaneous blister chamber model confirmed that oral steroid treatment for up to 3 days fails to inhibit the release of mast cell mediators (histamine and tryptase) during the acute response to antigen challenge (Atkins et al., 1990; Charlesworth et al., 1990). As discussed earlier, in the nose and the lower airways, prolonged (i.e., greater than 1 week) treatment with topical steroids leads to an inhibition of the acute airways response to antigen. Pipkorn et al. (1989) have shown that topical steroid treatment of skin for 1–2 weeks inhibits the immediate skin reaction following challenge with both antigen and histamine, being more effective against the former. Similarly, Ståhle and Hägermark (1984) showed that clobetasol-17-propionate inhibited 48/80-induced cutaneous flare responses better than histamine-induced flare responses. Thus, in the skin, as in the nose, topical steroid treatment has efficacy in inhibiting acute antigen responses. While this appears to be the result of a reduction of epithelial mast cells in the nose rather than inhibition of mast cell degranulation, the mechanism in the skin has not been determined, although the 1–2-week treatment used by Pipkorn et al. (1989) was not of sufficient duration to reduce total skin histamine (Lavker and Schechter, 1985—see Fig. 1). While most studies suggest no effect of oral steroids on the acute mast cell response following challenge, a study by Olson et al. (1990) demonstrates that subjects receiving prolonged oral steroid therapy (in most cases daily or alternate-day steroids for at least a year) had a diminished wheal response to the mast cell activator codeine but not to histamine.

F. The Role of Mast Cells in the Late-Phase Response

The common, though as yet unproved, view is that the late-phase accumulation of leukocytes (especially neutrophils and eosinophils) results from the direct action of mast cell mediators in recruiting leukocytes from the blood. Certainly the size of the late-phase reaction correlates in intensity with the size of the acute (mast cell–mediated) reaction (DeShazo et al., 1979; Gleich, 1982). Administration of codeine into the skin of normal subjects yields mast cell degranulation and a wheal-and-flare response that is not followed by a late-phase response, however, leading to the conclusion that mast cell degranulation may not be sufficient for induction of a late-phase response (Dolovich et al., 1983). Since some stimuli are incomplete (e.g., can cause histamine release in the absence of formation of leukotrienes), it is premature to conclude that, at least under some circumstances, mast cell activation *per se* is not sufficient to produce late-phase responses. In rats, injection of purified rat mast cell granules or a 1400-molecular-weight factor further purified from the granules, termed IFA (inflammatory factor of anaphylaxis), has been reported to induce a late-phase reaction in the skin as measured by leukocyte infiltration (Oertel and Kaliner, 1981a,b).

Recently, several laboratories have demonstrated that rodent mast cells are capable of releasing cytokines following IgE-mediated activation (Plaut et al., 1989; Gordon and Galli, 1990). Among these cytokines are IL-1 and TNF, two cytokines that could theoretically participate in the LPR in several ways (Bochner et al., 1990a). These cytokines can stimulate a variety of leukocytes and can increase vascular permeability, two proinflammatory actions of theoretical relevance to the LPR. Most relevant to the recruitment of leukocytes in the LPR is the activation of endothelial cells to express adhesion molecules, including ELAM-1, ICAM-1, and VCAM-1, after exposure to IL-1 or TNF. These adhesion molecules can induce leukocyte adhesion and transendothelial migration, two key events in LPR leukocyte recruitment (Leung et al., 1991; Schleimer et al., 1991a). Interestingly, VCAM-1 has selectivity for lymphocytes, eosinophils, and basophils versus neutrophils (Bochner et al., 1991). Induction of VCAM-1 by IL-4 would be expected to recruit a spectrum of leukocytes (eosinophils, lymphocytes, and basophils) similar to that observed in the LPR (Schleimer et al., 1991b). Whether these cytokines (especially IL-1, TNF, and IL-4) are produced by human mast cells in vivo following antigen exposure has not yet been established. Evidence suggestive (some of which is circumstantial) that they are includes the following: (1) Purified human mast cells have been reported to produce TNF in vitro after challenge with antigen or morphine (Gordon et al., 1991; Walsh et al., 1991); (2) antigen challenge in vivo results in endothelial activation, adhesion molecule expression, and IL-1 production (Leung et al., 1991; Kyan-Aung et al., 1991; Benenati et al., 1991; Bochner et al., 1990a); and (3) activation of mast cells in human lung or skin organ culture results in endothelial activation (Klein et al., 1989; Matis et al., 1990). Although it is attractive to suggest that antigen stimulation results in mast cell cytokine release, followed by endothelial activation and recruitment of the leukocytes responsible for the LPR, considerable gaps in our knowledge exist and such a model would be, at this time, premature. Accepting, for the moment, that this hypothesis has some merit, then the ability of glucocorticoids to inhibit the LPR leukocyte recruitment must be explained in the context of the model. Although human mast cells have proven to be resistant to glucocorticoids when degranulation has been studied in vitro (see Section IV), mast cell cytokine release may be distinguished from preformed mediator release in this regard. Although steroids are potent inhibitors of cytokine release in a number of cell types, the effects of steroids on mast cell cytokine release have yet to be tested. Fitting all the available data, the most reasonable model for steroid action in the LPR is that they inhibit the release of the factors (both chemoattractants and endothelial activators) that recruit leukocytes in the LPR (Schleimer et al., 1989b; Schleimer, 1990; Bochner et al., 1987). If mast cells are responsible for LPR leukocyte recruitment via the release of endothelial-activating cytokines, then we anticipate that such mast cell cytokine release is inhibited by glucocorticoids.

IV. In Vitro Studies with Steroids on Mast Cells

Great strides have been made in the understanding of the molecular biology of glucocorticoid actions. Steroids bind to specific receptors, and the steroid-receptor complex, in turn, binds to glucocorticoid response elements (GRE) in the promoter regions of relevant genes and induces their transcription. Steroids also alter gene translation and posttranslational modifications (LaPointe et al., 1989; Miesfeld, 1990). A suitable explanation of the mechanism by which steroids suppress the expression of some genes (e.g., cytokines) has yet to emerge. However, recently, the ability of steroids to inhibit the expression of the collagenase gene has been shown to result from an interaction between the steroid-receptor complex and a factor (AP-1 or c-*Jun*/c-*fos*) that is an endogenous activator of transcription for that gene (Yang-Yen et al., 1990; Schüle et al., 1990). By binding AP-1, the steroid-receptor complex prevents it from activating expression of the collagenase gene. This important observation suggests that steroids may have some direct actions in the cytoplasm and that some of the other inhibitory effects of steroids (e.g., on cytokine production) may result from similar molecular mechanisms. The identities of the genes whose expression is altered by steroids during the modification of mast cell functions have not been established.

A. Effects on Proliferation

Ginsburg et al. (1981) grew mast cells from mouse lymph node cultures. In these cultures, no mast cells arose if the lymph node cells were first depleted of T cells. If supernatants from activated T cells were added to the lymph node cultures depleted of T cells, mast cells did arise (Ginsburg et al., 1981). Subsequently, many groups have successfully grown T-cell-factor–dependent mast cells from bone marrow, fetal liver, and other tissues from several species (Nagao et al., 1981; Nabel et al., 1981; Razin et al., 1981, among others). The factor from T lymphocytes responsible for promoting the growth of mast cells is interleukin-3 or multi-colony-stimulating factor (multi-CSF) (Ihle et al., 1983). Subsequently, other mast cell growth-promoting factors have been discovered and cells other than T cells (e.g., epidermal cells) have been shown to produce IL-3 (Rennick et al., 1985; Luger et al., 1985; Lee et al., 1986). Recently c-*kit* and the c-*kit* ligand (also known as stem cell factor or mast cell growth factor) have been shown to represent the receptors and ligand, respectively, responsible for the propagation and differentiation of formalin-resistant (sometimes referred to as "connective tissue") rodent mast cells (see Witte, 1990, for review). The effects of steroids on this system are of great relevance but are at this time unknown.

The effects of glucocorticoids on IL-3-dependent mast cells from mouse bone marrow have been analyzed by Robin et al. (1985) and Benhamou et al. (1986). Their results will be discussed in more detail in the following sections; with regard to proliferation, 1 μM dexamethasone had a relatively minor effect on bone marrow mast cell proliferation during a 96-hr culture period (70 $\pm$ 18% of baseline in seven experiments). Culpepper and Lee (1985) found that corticosteroids inhibit the production of the mast cell growth factor interleukin-3 in cloned mouse T-helper lymphocytes. Thus, although the direct antiproliferative effects of steroids on bone marrow–derived mast cells are modest, by inhibiting the production of IL-3 and other mast cell growth factors they may significantly suppress the numbers of mast cells that are dependent, in the short term, on growth factors.

As discussed earlier, steroid treatment of rats infected with *N. brasiliensis* causes near-total depletion of the large number of mast cells that reside in the

dependent histamine release selectively is a straightforward one in which steroid-induced lipocortin is inhibiting phospholipase activation. Another steroid-induced anti-inflammatory protein, "vasocortin," has been shown to inhibit degranulation of rat mast cells induced by dextran and concanavalin A (Carnuccio et al., 1989).

Two different groups (Robin et al., 1985; Benhamou et al. 1986) have studied the effects of steroids on bone marrow–derived, mucosal mast cell mediator release processes. Both these groups have demonstrated that 24-hr steroid incubation causes inhibition of the release of granule-contained mediators such as β-hexoseaminidase and histamine, as well as inflammatory metabolites of phospholipid metabolism such as LTB_4, LTC_4, and PAF (Robin et al., 1985; Benhamou et al., 1986). Interestingly, prostaglandin D_2 production was increased by the steroid treatment, apparently as a result of increased levels of prostaglandin D_2–synthesizing enzymes in the steroid-treated cells (Robin et al., 1985). In the bone marrow–derived mast cells, treatment with steroids led to a reduction in IgE Fc receptors, in contrast to the findings in human basophils and in mature murine peritoneal mast cells (Robin et al., 1985; Benhamou et al., 1986; Schleimer et al., 1982; Daeron et al., 1982). While it seems possible that the reduction in IgE Fc receptors on bone marrow mast cells by steroid treatment may play a role in the inhibitory effect of steroids on the mast cell mediator release process, it is unlikely that this is the only explanation (Benhamou et al., 1986). Studies by Collado-Escobar (1990a,b) have shown that inhibition of activation of intracellular biochemical processes (PI hydrolysis, calcium elevations, arachidonate release) and secretion of serotonin in RBL-2H3 cells (a tumor analog of the rat mucosal mast cell) are lost in permeabilized cells, suggesting a rapidly reversible action, possibly mediated by a relatively low-molecular-weight factor. These authors also concluded that steroids act at an early (receptor and/or G protein) biochemical step. As mentioned previously, the ability of steroids to inhibit mediator release from mouse, rat, and guinea pig mast cells contrasts with the lack of inhibition of mediator release by steroids in human mast cells from lung parenchyma, lung airway, and gut (Daeron et al., 1982; Heiman and Crews, 1984a,b; Schleimer et al., 1983, 1986). Thus, whatever the mechanism of inhibition in rodent cells (indeed, at this time it must be considered to be unknown), these findings reveal a basic difference between human and rodent mast cells.

V. Summary and Conclusions

Anti-inflammatory steroids are effective against a host of inflammatory diseases that arise from diverse pathological processes. Some of these diseases, especially the IgE-mediated allergic diseases, are felt to involve the activation of mast cells.

The major effects of anti-inflammatory steroids on mast cells are as follows (Schleimer, 1989):

A. Distribution and Numbers

Steroids clearly reduce the numbers of mucosal mast cells in normal, allergic, and parasite-infected hosts. The connective tissue mast cell subtype seems much less sensitive to this effect of glucocorticoids (although prolonged topical application is effective), and studies on the effects of steroids on the c-*kit*/c-*kit* ligand system should be revealing. Glucocorticoids achieve reduction of mucosal mast cell numbers most likely by inhibiting the production of IL-3 or other mast cell growth factors; some direct effects on mast cell proliferation, production of mast cell precursors, or migration may also occur. In rats, the loss of mucosal mast cells (during a parasite infestation) induced by steroids appears to involve engulfment of the mast cells by macrophages. Since, especially during an ongoing parasite infestation, gut mucosal mast cells may require ongoing release of growth factors by lymphocytes (and/or other cells) to maintain elevated numbers, inhibition of growth factor release by steroids may also be an initiating event for this phagocytosis. Steroids may, alternatively, directly induce a mast cell "apoptosis" or programmed cell death, although it seems less likely, since steroid antiproliferative or cytotoxic effects on mast cells in vitro are modest.

B. Inhibition of Mast Cell Functions

In the rat, mouse, guinea pig, and perhaps other species, glucocorticoids inhibit degranulation of mast cells. In humans, although glucocorticoids can reduce the number of epithelial mucosal mast cells, thus reducing the appearance of mediators following antigen challenge in vivo at a mucosal surface such as the nose, there is no direct evidence that steroids can directly inhibit production and release of preformed and newly generated inflammatory mediators by mast cells. This conclusion is supported by both in vitro and in vivo findings. The failure of oral glucocorticoids to inhibit the acute-phase allergic response in the skin, the nose, and the airways as well as mast cell–dependent responses such as cold challenge, in cold urticaria patients supports this conclusion. The ability of topical steroids to reduce the response to antigen challenge in the airways and in the skin most likely results from a localized reduction in mast cells numbers and/or decreased access of antigen to mast cells in the tissue, as well as a decreased response of the various tissues to mast cell mediators that are released.

A new concept of the role of the mast cell in allergic reactions has evolved recently in which mast cell–derived cytokines may play a prominent role. Mast cell–derived cytokines may contribute to the recruitment and activation of leukocytes at allergic reaction sites. Although no data are available at present, it seems likely that glucocorticoids will inhibit the release of cytokines from mast cells since inhibition of cytokine release is a well-established glucocorticoid effect.

Acknowledgments

I would like to express gratitude to Dr. John Bienenstock for providing the electron micrograph and to Ms. Bonnie Hebden for excellent secretarial assistance in the preparation of the manuscript.

Discussion

Metcalfe: Can you comment on the sensitivity of mast cells to steroids? In our studies, mast cells (and lymphocytes) die at concentrations of steroids that have no effect on such cells as fibroblasts.

Schleimer: Both lymphocytes and mast cells of certain species are very sensitive to corticosteroids. In humans there is a suggestion that T-cell-dependent mast cells (mucosal mast cells containing the enzyme tryptase) are depleted more easily by steroids than are connective tissue mast cells. This might be due to their greater dependence on T-cell-derived factors.

Dvorak: In inflammatory bowel disease (IBD), there is no mast cell injury in the gut, and gut mast cells are increased whether the patients are taking steroids or not.

Schleimer: It is possible that steroid-resistant T cells in the gut of IBD patients are producing mast cell growth-promoting factors that can overcome the effects of steroids. It is not uncommon for cytokines and steroids to exhibit opposing effects.

Claman: What is the current status of lipocortin?

Schleimer: The concept that the anti-inflammatory action of steroids acted by influencing the enzyme PLA2 had substantial appeal. Inhibition of PLA2 should reduce the inflammatory effects of both cyclooxygenase and lipoxygenase enzymes by reducing the availability of substrate. Several studies have led to the diminishment of this enthusiasm: (1) Steroids may exhibit anti-inflammatory effects without reducing arachidonate production in vivo. (2) Many studies have shown that steroids may effect eicosanoid release without inducing lipocortin generation and by mechanisms that do not involve effects on PLA2. (3) The suggestion that lipocortin might act as a mediator of steroid action became less likely when the molecule was cloned and a signal peptide was missing. These data suggest that lipocortin would only be released by dead and dying cells, rather than be a secreted product. However, recombinant lipocortin has been found to have some anti-inflammatory actions and is being studied further.

Kennerly: Work by Ed Dennis suggests that lipocortin acts by substrate deple-

tion, through binding of phospholipases. The presence of lipocortin is not in sufficiently high concentrations to reduce phospholipase concentrations, suggesting that lipocortin would not be active in vivo.
Schleimer: It is interesting that the purification of lipocortin involved an affinity chromatography step in which lipocortin bound to insolubilized PLA2. These data suggest that lipocortin must bind, either specifically or nonspecifically, to PLA2.

References

Abraham, W. M., Delehunt, J. C., Yerger, L., and Marchette, B. (1983). Characterization of a late phase pulmonary response after antigen challenge in allergic sheep. *Am. Rev. Respir. Dis.* 128:839–844.

Ädelroth, E., Rosenhall, L., Johansson, S., Linden, M., and Venge P. (1990). Inflammatory cells and eosinophils activity in asthmatics investigated by bronchoalveolar lavage. *Am. Rev. Respir. Dis.* 142:91–99.

Andersson, P., and Brattsand, R. (1982a). Protective effects of the glucocorticoid, budesonide, on lung anaphylaxis in actively sensitized guinea pigs: inhibition of IgE-but not IgG-mediated anaphylaxis. *Br. J. Pharmacol.* 76:139–147.

Andersson, P., Brattsand, R., Brange, C., Kallstrom, L., and Stahre, G. (1982b). Protective effects of budesonide on lung anaphylaxis in actively sensitized guinea pigs. Inhibition of "IgE"-mediated anaphylaxis. *Eur. J. Respir. Dis.* 122 (Suppl.): 260–262.

Andersson, P., Chignard, M., Brange, C., Nilsson, T., Juhlin, M., and Le-Covedic, J. P. (1985). Effect of glucocorticosteroid treatment on antigen-induced mediator release from sensitized guinea-pig lungs. In *Glucocorticosteroids, Inflammation, and Bronchial Hyperreactivity*. Edited by J. C. Hogg, R. Ellul-Micallef, and R. Brattsand. Amsterdam, Excerpta Medica, pp. 132–135.

Asboe-Hansen, G. (1950). Effect of the adrenocorticotropic hormone of the pituitary on mesenchymal tissues. *Scand J. Clin. Lab Invest.* 2:271–275.

Asboe-Hansen, G. (1952). The mast cell. Cortisone action on connective tissues. *Proc. Soc. Exp. Biol. Med.* 80:677–679.

Atkins, P. C., Norman, M., Weiner, H., and Zweiman, B. (1977). Release of neutrophil chemotactic activity during immediate hypersensitivity reactions in humans. *Ann. Intern. Med.* 86:415–418.

Atkins, P. C., Schwartz, L. B., Adkinson, N. F., von Allmen, C., Valenzamo, M., and Zweiman, B. (1990). In vivo antigen-induced cutaneous mediator release: Simultaneous comparisons of histamine, tryptase, and prostaglandin D_2 release and the effect of oral corticosteroid administration. *J. Allergy Clin. Immunol.* 86:360–370.

Baker, B. L. (1952). Mast cells of the omentum in relation to states of adrenocortical deficiency and excess. *Ann. NY Acad. Sci.* 56:684–690.

Barrett, K. E., Neva, F. A., Gam, A. A., Cicmanec, J., London, W. T., Phillips, J. M., and Metcalfe, D. D. (1988). The immune response to nematode parasites: Modulation of mast cell numbers and function during *Strongyloides stercoralis* infections in nonhuman primates. *Am. J. Trop. Med. Hyg.* 38:574–581.

Benenati, S., Bochner, B., Horn, T., Farmer, E., and Schleimer, R. (1991). Endothelial-leukocyte adhesion molecule-1 (ELAM-1) expression following cutaneous allergen challenge. *J. Allergy Clin. Immunol.* 87:304 (abstract).

Benhamou, M., Ninio, E., and Salem, P. (1986). Decrease in IgE Fc receptor expression on mouse bone marrow–derived mast cells and inhibition of PAF-acether formation and of β-hexosaminidase release by dexamethasone. *J. Immunol.* 136:1385–1392.

Bochner, B. S., Rutledge, B. K., and Schleimer, R. P. (1987). Interleukin 1 production by human lung tissue. II. Inhibition by antiinflammatory steroids. *J. Immunol.* 139:2303–2307.

Bochner, B. S., Charlesworth, E. N., Lichtenstein, L. M., Gillis, S., Dinarello, C. A., Derse, C. P., and Schleimer, R. P. (1990a). Interleukin-1 is released at sites of human cutaneous allergic reactions. In *J. Allergy Clin. Immunol.* 86:830–839.

Bochner, B. S., Lamas, A. M., Benenati, S. V., and Schleimer, R. P. (1990b). On the central role of vascular endothelium in allergic reactions. *Late Phase Allergic Reactions*. Edited by R. Dorsch. Boca Raton, FL, CRC Press, pp. 221–235.

Bochner, B. S., Luscinskas, F. W., Gimbrone, M. A., Newman, W., Sterbinsky, S. A., Derse-Anthony, C., Klunk, D., and Schleimer, R. P. (1991). Adhesion of human basophils, eosinophils, and neutrophils to IL-1-activated human vascular endothelial cells: contributions of endothelial cell adhesion molecules. *J. Exp. Med.* 173:1553–1556.

Booij-Noord, H., deVries, K., Sluiter, H. J., and Orie, N. G. M. (1972). Late bronchial obstructive reaction to experimental inhalation of house dust extract. *Clin. Allergy* 2:43–61.

Brocklehurst, W. E. (1960). The release of histamine and formation of a slow reacting substance (SRS-A) during anaphylactic shock. *J. Physiol.* 151:416–423.

Burge, P. S. (1982). The effects of corticosteroids on the immediate asthmatic reaction. *Eur. J. Respir. Dis.* 122(Suppl.):163–166.

Carnuccio, R., Di Rosa, M., Ialenti, A., Iuvone, T., andSautebin, L. (1989). Selective inhibition by vasocortin of histamine release induced by dextran and concanavalin-A from rat peritoneal cells. *Br. J. Pharmacol.* 98:32–34.

Cavallero, C., and Braccini, C. (1951). Effect of cortisone on the mast cells of the rat. *Proc. Soc. Exp. Biol. Med.* 78:141–143.

Charlesworth, E. N., Kagey-Sobotka, A., Schleimer, R. P., Norman, P. S., and Lichtenstein, L. M. (1990). Prednisone inhibits the appearance of inflammatory mediators and the influx of eosinophils and basophils associated with the cutaneous late-phase response to antigen. *J. Immunol.* 146:671–676.

Church, M. K., and Miller, P. (1978). Time courses of the anti-anaphylactic and anti-inflammatory effects of dexamethasone in the rat and mouse. *Br. J. Pharmacol.* 62:481–486.

Church, M. K., Collier, H. O. J., and James, G. W. L. (1972). The inhibition by dexamethasone and disodium cromoglycate of anaphylactic bronchoconstriction in the rat. *Br. J. Pharmacol.* 46:56–65.

Cohan, V. L., Undem, B. J., Fox, C. C., Adkinson, N. F., Jr., Lichtenstein, L. M., and Schleimer, R. P. (1989). Dexamethasone does not inhibit the release of mediators from human mast cells residing in airway, intestine or skin. *Am. Rev. Respir. Dis.* 140:951–954.

Collado-Escobar, D., Ali, H., and Beaven, M. A. (1990a). On the mechanism of action of dexamethasone in a rat mast cell line (RBL-2H3 cells). *J. Immunol.* 144:3449–3457.

Collado-Escobar, D., Cunha-Melo, J. R., and Beaven, M. A. (1990b). Treatment with dexamethasone down-regulates IgE-receptor-mediated signals and up-regulates adrenosine-receptor-mediated signals in a rat mast cell (RBL-2H3) line. *J. Immunol.* 144:244–250.

Cooke, R. A., Sherman, W. B., Menzel, A. E. O., et al. (1951). ACTH and cortisone in allergic diseases. *J. Allergy* 22:211–236.

Csaba, B., and Kassay, L. (1966). Effect of cortisone on anaphylactic shock in the guinea pig. *Acta Physiol. Acad. Sci. Hung.* 30:91–97.

Culpepper, J. A., and Lee, F. (1985). Regulation of IL-3 expression by glucocorticoids in cloned murine T-lymphocytes. *J. Immunol.* 135:3191–3197.

Daeron, M., Sterk, A. R., Hirata, F., and Ishizaka, T. (1982). Biochemical analysis of glucocorticoid-induced inhibition of IgE-mediated histamine release from mouse mast cells. *J. Immunol.* 129:1212–1218.

Dahl, R., and Johansson, S. A. (1982). Importance of duration of treatment with inhaled budesonide on the immediate and late bronchial reaction. *Eur. J. Respir. Dis.* 122(Suppl.):167–175.

Delehunt, J. C., Yerger, L., Ahmed, T., and Abraham, W. M. (1984). Inhibition of antigen-induced bronchoconstriction by methylprednisolone succinate. *J. Allergy Clin. Immunol.* 73:479–483.

Dembinska-Kiec, A., Grodzinska, L., Panczenko, B., and Gryglewski, R. J. (1978). Effect of corticosteroids on the release of histamine and prostaglandins from fragments of mesentery of immunized guinea pigs. *Pharmacol. Res. Commun.* 10:153–160.

DeShazo, R., Levinson, A. I., Dvorak, H. F., and Davis, R. W. (1979). The late phase skin reaction: evidence for activation of the coagulation system in an IgE-dependent reaction in man. *J. Immunol.* 122:692–698.

Devitt, J. E., Pirozynski, W. J., and Samuels, P. B. (1953). Mast cell resistance to hormonal influence. *Proc. Soc. Exp. Biol. Med.* 83:335–337.

Doherty, G. B., Moorthi, D. S., Shah, T., et al. (1981). The effect of methylprednisolone and indomethacin on hypoxia mediated histamine release. *Ann. Allergy* 46:241–245.

Dolovich, J., Denberg, J., Kwee, Y. N., Belda, T., Blajchman, J., and Hargreave, F. E. (1983). Does nonimmunologic mast cell mediator release/activation elicit a late cutaneous response? *Ann. Allergy* 50:241–244.

Enerbäck, L., Pipkorn, U., and Granerus, G. (1986). Intraepithelial migration of nasal mucosal mast cells in hay fever. *Int. Arch. Allergy Appl. Immunol.* 80:44–51.

Feinberg, S. M., Dannenberg, T. B., and Malkiel, S. (1951). ACTH and cortisone in allergic manifestations. *J. Allergy* 22:195–210.

Forsberg, K., and Sorenby, L. (1981). The influence of a new corticosteroid, budesonide, on anaphylactic bronchoconstriction and SRS-A release in the guinea pig. *Agents Actions* 11:391–395.

Forsberg, K., Ryrfeldt, A., and Sorenby, L. (1982). Protective effects of budesonide on

leukocyte adhesion molecule-1 in elicited late phase allergic reactions. *J. Clin. Invest.* 87:1805–1809.

Lewis, G. P., and Whittle, B. J. R. (1977). The inhibition of histamine release from rat peritoneal mast cells by nonsteroid anti-inflammatory drugs and its reversal by calcium. *Br. J. Pharmacol.* 61:229–235.

Luger, T. A., Wirth, U., and Kock, A. (1985). Epidermal cells synthesize a cytokine with interleukin 3-like properties. *J. Immunol.* 134:915–919.

Malbon, C. C. (1989). Physiological regulation of transmembrane signaling elements. *Am. J. Respir. Cell Mol. Biol.* 1:449–450.

Malkiel, S. (1951). The influence of ACTH and cortisone on histamine and anaphylactic shock in the guinea pig. *J. Immunol.* 66:379–384.

Malone, D. G., Wilder, R. L., Saavedra-Delgado, A. M., and Metcalfe, D. D. (1987). Mast cell numbers in rheumatoid synovial tissues. *Arthritis Rheumatism* 30:130–137.

Mancini, R. E., Colombi, P. A., Galli, H., and Orcivoli, L. (1961). Effect of glucocorticoid hormones on experimentally induced allergic reactions on human skin. *J. Allergy* 32:471–482.

Marquardt, D. L., and Wasserman, S. I. (1983). Modulation of rat serosal mast cell biochemistry by in vivo dexamethasone administration. *J. Immunol.* 131:934–939.

Martin, G. L., Atkins, P. C., Dunsky, E. H., and Zweiman, B. (1980). Effects of theophyline, terbutaline, and prednisone on antigen-induced bronchospasm and mediator release. *J. Allergy Clin. Immunol.* 66:204–212.

Matis, W. L., Lavker, R. M., and Murphy, G. F. (1990). Substance P induces the expression of an endothelial-leukocyte adhesion molecule by microvascular endothelium. *J. Invest. Dermatol.* 94:492–495.

McCarthy, D. S., and Pepys, J. (1971). Allergic broncho-pulmonary aspergillosis. *Clin. Allergy* 1:415–432.

Metzger, W. J., Hunninghake, G. W., and Richerson, H. B. (1985). Late asthmatic responses: Inquiry into mechanisms and significance. *Clin. Rev. Allergy* 3:145–165.

Michell, R. H. (1975). Inositol phospholipids and cell surface receptor function. *Biochim. Biophys. Acta* 415:81–147.

Miesfeld, R. L. (1990). Molecular genetics of corticosteroid action. *Am. Rev. Respir. Dis.* 141:S11–S17.

Mygind, N. (1973). Local effect of intranasal beclomethasone dipropionate aerosol in hay fever. *Br. Med. J.* 4:464–466.

Mygind, N., Johnsen, N. J., and Thomsen, J. (1977). Intranasal allergen challenge during corticosteroid treatment. *Clin. Allergy* 7:69–74.

Nabel, G., Galli, S. J., Dvorak, A. M., Dvorak, H. F., and Cantor, H. (1981). Induced T-lymphocytes synthesize a factor that stimulates proliferation of cloned mast cells. *Nature* 291:332–334.

Naclerio, R. M., Meier, H. C., Adkinson, N. F., Kagey-Sobotka, A., Meyers, D. A., Norman, P. S., and Lichtenstein, L. M. (1983). In vivo demonstration of inflammatory mediator release following nasal challenge with antigen. *Eur. J. Respir. Dis.* 128(Suppl.):26–32.

Naclerio, R. M., Proud, D., Togias, A. G., Adkinson, N. F., Jr., Meyers, D. A.,

Kagey-Sobotka, A., Plaut, M., Norman, P. S., and Lichtenstein, L. M. (1985). Inflammatory mediators in late antigen-induced rhinitis. *N. Engl. J. Med.* 313:65–70.

Nagao, K., Yokoro, K., and Aaronson, S. A. (1981). Continuous lines of basophil mast cells derived from normal mouse bone marrow. *Science* 212:333–335.

Nakazawa, T., Yoyoda, T., Furukawa, M., Taya, T., and Kobayashi, S. (1976). Inhibitory effects of various drugs on dual asthmatic responses in wheat flour-sensitive subjects. *J. Allergy Clin. Immunol.* 58:1–9.

Nelson, C. T., Fox, C. L., and Freeman, E. B. (1950). Inhibitory effect of cortisone on anaphylaxis in the mouse. *Proc. Soc. Exp. Biol. Med.* 75:181–183.

Nishizuka, Y. (1984). The role of protein kinase C in cell surface signal transduction and tumour promotion. *Nature* 308:693–698.

Norman, P. S., Winkenwerder, W. C., Murgatroyd, G. W., and Parsons, J. W. (1966). Evidence for the local action of intranasal dexamethasone aerosols in the suppression of hay fever symptoms. *J. Allergy* 38:93–99.

Norn, S. (1965). Influence of anti-rheumatic agents on the release of histamine from rat peritoneal mast cells after an antigen-antibody reaction. *Acta. Pharmacol. Toxicol.* 22:369–378.

Norn, S. (1967). Effect of histamine liberators on rat peritoneal mast cells and influence of antirheumatic agents. *Acta. Pharmacol. Toxicol* 25:281–289.

Norn, S. (1968). Influence of anti-rheumatic agents on the release of histamine from sensitized rat peritoneal mast cells. *Acta Pharmacol Toxicol.* 26:470–474.

Oertel, H. L., and Kaliner, M. (1981a). The biologic activity of mast cell granules. III. Purification of inflammatory factors of anaphylaxis (IF-A) responsible for causing late-phase reactions. *J. Immunol.* 127:1398–1402.

Oertel, H., and Kaliner, M. (1981b). The biologic activity of mast cell granules in rat skin: effects of adrenocorticosteroids on late-phase inflammatory responses induced by mast cell granules. *J. Allergy Clin. Immunol.* 68:238–245.

Okuda, M., Sakaguchi, K., and Ohtsuka, H. (1983). Intranasal beclomethasone: Mode of action in nasal allergy. *Ann. Allergy* 50:116–120.

Olson, C. E., and Schiller, E. L. (1978). *Strongyloides ratti* infections in rats. II. Effects of cortisone treatment. *Am. J. Trop. Med. Hyg.* 27:527–531.

Olson, R., Karpink, M. H., Shelanski, S., Atkins, P. C., and Zweiman, B. (1990). Skin reactivity to codeine and histamine during prolonged corticosteroid therapy. *J. Allergy Clin. Immunol.* 86:153–159.

Otsuka, H., Denburg, J., Dolovich, J. et al. (1985). Heterogeneity of metachromatic cells in human nose: Significance of mucosal mast cells. *J. Allergy Clin. Immunol.* 76:695–702.

Otsuka, H., Denburg, J. A., Befus, A. D., Hitch, D., Lapp, P., Rajan, R. S., Bienenstock, J., and Dolovich, J. (1986). Effect of beclomethasone dipropionate on nasal metachromatic cell sub-populations. *Clin. Allergy* 16:589–595.

Peachell, P. T., and Schleimer, R. P. (1991). Functional desensitization of beta agonist responses in human lung mast cells (HLMC). *FASEB J.* 5:A1007.

Pelikan, Z., and DeVries, K. (1974). Effects of some drugs applied topically to the nasal mucosa before nasal provocation tests with allergen. *Acta Allerg.* 29:337–353.

Pepys, J., Davies, R. J., Breslin, A. B. X., Hendrick, D. J., and Hutchcroft, B. J.

(1974). The effects of inhaled beclomethasone dipropionate (Becotide) and sodium cromoglycate on asthmatic reactions to provocation tests. *Clin. Allergy* 4:13–24.

Pipkorn, U. (1982a). Budesonide and nasal mucosal histamine content and anti IgE induced histamine release. *Allergy* 37:591–595.

Pipkorn, U. (1982b). The effect of budesonide on the immediate reaction to allergen challenge—A rhinomanometric study. *Eur. J. Respir. Dis.* 122(Suppl.):185–191.

Pipkorn, U. (1983). Effect of topical glucocorticoid treatment on nasal mucosal mast cells in allergic rhinitis. *Allergy* 38:125–129.

Pipkorn, U., Proud, D., Lichtenstein, L. M., Kagey-Sobotka, A., Norman, P. S., and Naclerio, R. M. (1987a). Inhibition of mediator release in allergic rhinitis by pretreatment with topical glucocorticosteroids. *N. Engl. J. Med.* 316:1506–1510.

Pipkorn, U., Proud, D., Lichtenstein, L. M., Schleimer, R. P., Peters, S. T., Adkinson, N. F., Jr., Kagey-Sobotka, A., Norman, P. S., and Naclerio, R. M. (1987b). Effect of short-term systemic glucocorticoid treatment on human nasal mediator release after antigen challenge. *J. Clin. Invest.* 80:957–961.

Pipkorn, U., Hammarlund, A., and Enerbäck, L. (1989). Prolonged treatment with topical glucocorticoids results in an inhibition of the allergen-induced weal-and-flare response and a reduction in skin mast cell numbers and histamine content. *Clin. Exp. Allergy* 19:19–25.

Plaut, M., Pierce, J. H., Watson, C. J., Hanley-Hyde, J., Nordan, R. P., and Paul, W. E. (1989). Mast cell lines produce lymphokines in response to cross-linkage of $FC_{\epsilon}RI$ or to calcium ionophores. *Nature* 339:64–67.

Poothullil, J., Umemoto, L., Dolovich, J., Hargreave, F. E., and Day, R. P. (1976). Inhibition by prednisone of late cutaneous allergic responses induced by antiserum to human IgE. *J. Allergy Clin. Immunol.* 57:164–167.

Razin, E., Rifkind, A. B., Cardo, C. C., and Good, R. A. (1981). Selective growth of a population of human basophil cells in vitro. *Proc. Natl. Acad. Sci. USA* 78:5793–5796.

Rennick, D. M., Lee, F. D., Yokota, T., Arai, K. I., Cantor, H., and Nabel, G. J. (1985). A cloned MCGF cDNA encodes a multilineage hematopoietic growth factor: multiple activities of interleukin-3. *J. Immunol.* 134:910–914.

Rich, A. R., Berthrong, M., and Bennett, I. L. (1950). The effect of cortisone upon the experimental cardiovascular and renal lesions produced by anaphylactic hypersensitivity. *Bull. Johns Hopkins Hosp.* 87:549–564.

Robin, J. L., Seldin, D. C., Austen, K. F., and Lewis, R. A. (1985). Regulation of mediator release from mouse bone marrow–derived mast cells by glucocorticoids. *J. Immunol.* 135:2719–2726.

Salvato, G. (1959). Mast cells in bronchial connective tissue of man. Importance of such cells in allergic tissue injury. *Exper.* 15:308–309.

Saunders, F. J. (1951). Studies on the role of the adrenal in anaphylaxis and histamine shock. *Endocrinology* 49:185–188.

Schild, H. O. (1939). Histamine release in anaphylactic shock from various tissues of the guinea pig. *J. Physiol.* 95:394–408.

Schleimer, R. P. (1988). Glucocorticosteroids: Their mechanisms of action and use in allergic diseases. In *Allergy: Principles and Practice*. Edited by E. Middleton, Jr.,

C. E. Reed, E. F. Ellis, N. F. Adkinson, Jr., and J. W. Yunginger. St. Louis, Mosby, pp. 739–765.

Schleimer, R. P. (1989). The effects of glucocorticoids on mast cells and basophils. In *Anti-inflammatory Steroid Action. Basic and Clinical Aspects.* Edited by R. P. Schleimer, H. N. Claman, and A. Oronsky. San Diego, Academic Press, pp. 226–258.

Schleimer, R. P. (1990). Effects of glucocorticoids on inflammatory cells relevant to their therapeutic applications in asthma. *Am. Rev. Respir. Dis.* 141:S59–S69.

Schleimer, R. P., Lichtenstein, L. M., and Gillespie, E. (1981). Inhibition of basophil histamine release by anti-inflammatory steroids. *Nature* 292:454–455.

Schleimer, R. P., MacGlashan, D. W., Gillespie, E., and Lichtenstein, L. M. (1982). Inhibition of basophil histamine release by antiinflammatory steroids II. Studies on the mechanism of action. *J. Immunol.* 129:1632–1636.

Schleimer, R. P., Schulman, E. S., MacGlashan, D. W., Jr., Peters, S. P., Adams, G. K. III, Lichtenstein, L. M., and Adkinson, N. F., Jr. (1983). Effects of dexamethasone on mediator release from human lung fragments and purified human lung mast cells. *J. Clin. Invest.* 71:1830–1835.

Schleimer, R. P., Davidson, D. A., Peters, S. P., and Lichtenstein, L. M. (1985). Inhibition of basophil leukotriene release by antiinflammatory steroids. *Int. Arch. Allergy Appl. Immunol.* 77:241–243.

Schleimer, R. P., Davidson, D. A., Lichtenstein, L. M., and Adkinson, N. F., Jr. (1986). Selective inhibition of arachidonic acid metabolite release from human lung tissue by antiinflammatory steroids. *J. Immunol.* 136:3006–3011.

Schleimer, R. P., Undem, B. J., Meeker, S., Bollinger, M. E., Adkinson, N. F., Jr., Lichtenstein, L. M., and Adams, G. K., III. (1987). Dexamethasone inhibits the antigen-induced contractile activity and release of inflammatory mediators in isolated guinea pig lung tissue. *Am. Rev. Respir. Dis.* 135:562–566.

Schleimer, R. P., Claman, H. N., and Oronsky, A., (1989a). *Anti-inflammatory Steroid Action. Basic and Clinical Aspects.* San Diego, Academic Press.

Schleimer, R. P., Freeland, H. S., Peters, S. P., Brown, K. E., and Derse, C. P. (1989b). An assessment of the effects of glucocorticoids on degranulation, chemotaxis, binding to vascular endothelial cells and formation of leukotriene B4 by purified human neutrophils. *J. Pharmacol. Exp. Ther.* 250:598–605.

Schleimer, R. P., Benenati, S. V., Friedman, B., and Bochner, B. S. (1991a). Do cytokines play a role in leukocyte recruitment and activation in the lungs? *Am. Rev. Respir. Dis.* 143:1169–1174.

Schleimer, R. P., Sterbinsky, S. A., Kaiser, J., Bickel, C. A., Klunk, D. A., Tomioka, K., Newman, W., Luscinskas, F. W., Gimbrone, M. A., Jr., McIntyre, B. W., and Bochner B. S. (1991b). Interleukin-4 induces adherence of human eosinophils and basophils but not neutrophils to endothelium: Association with expression of VCAM-1. *J. Immunol.* 148:1086–1092.

Schoch, E. P., and Glick, D. (1952). The effect of cold stress, ACTH, cortisone, pyrogen, and nitrogen mustard on tissue mast cells in the skin and subcutaneous tissues of the rat. *J. Invest. Dermatol.* 18:119–132.

Schüle, R., Rangarajan, P., Kliewer, S., Ransone, L. J., Bolado, J., Yang, N., Verma,

I. M., and Evans, R. M. (1990). Functional antagonism between oncoprotein c-Jun and the glucocorticoid receptor. *Cell* 62:1217–1226.

Schwartz, E. (1954). Oral hydrocortisone therapy in bronchial asthma and hay fever. *J. Allergy* 25:112–119.

Seale, J. P. (1983). Effect of corticosteroids in asthma is not due to suppression of leukotriene release. *N. Engl. J. Med.* 308:846.

Segal, D. M., Taurog, J. D., and Metzger, H. (1977). Dimeric immunoglobulin E serves as a unit signal for mast cell degranulation. *Proc. Natl. Acad. Sci. USA* 74:2993–2997.

Siraganian, R. P. (1983). Histamine secretion from mast cells and basophils. *Trends Pharm. Sci.* 4:432–437.

Slott, R. I., and Zweiman, B. (1974). A controlled study of the effect of corticosteroids on immediate skin test reactivity. *J. Allergy Clin. Immunol.* 54:229–234.

Smith, D. E., and Lewis, Y. S. (1954). Influence of hypophysis and adrenal cortex upon tissue mast cell of the rat. *Proc. Soc. Exp. Biol. Med.* 87:515–518.

Soda, K., Kawabori, S., Perdue, M. H., and Bienenstock, J. (1991). Macrophage engulfment of mucosal mast cells in rats treated with dexamethasone. *Gastroenterology* 100:929–937.

Solley, G. O., Gleich, G. J., Jordan, R. E., and Schroeter, A. L. (1976). The late phase of the immediate wheal and flare skin reaction. Its dependence upon IgE antibodies. *J. Clin. Invest.* 58:408–420.

Solotorovsky, M., and Winsten, S. (1954). Inhibition of fatal anaphylactic shock in the mouse with cortisone. *J. Immunol.* 72:177–178.

Spector, S. L., English, G., and Jones, L. (1980). Clinical and nasal biopsy response to treatment of perennial rhinitis. *J. Allergy Clin. Immunol.* 66:129–137.

Ståhle, M., and Hägermark, Ö. (1984). Effects of topically applied clobetasol-17-propionate on histamine release in human skin. *Acta. Dermatol. Venereol.* 64:239–242.

Stollerman, G. H., Rubin, S. J., and Plotz, C. M. (1951). Effect of cortisone on passively induced skin hypersensitivity in man. *Proc. Soc. Exp. Biol. Med.* 76:261–265.

Togias, A. G., Naclerio, R. M., Proud, D., et al. (1985). Nasal challenge with cold, dry air results in release of inflammatory mediators. Possible mast cell involvement. *J. Clin. Invest.* 76:1375–1381.

Tolone, G., Bonasera, L., and Tolone, C. (1978). Influence of hydrocortisone on the modulation of the inflammatory response. *Br. J. Exp. Pathol.* 59:366–372.

Turner, C. R., and Spannhake, E. W. (1990). Acute topical steroid administration blocks mast cell increase and the late asthmatic response of the canine peripheral airways. *Am. Rev. Respir. Dis.* 141:421–427.

Walsh, L. J., Trinchieri, G., Waldorf, H. A., Whitaker, D., and Murphy, G. F. (1991). Human dermal mast cell contain and release tumor necrosis factor a, which induces endothelial leukocyte adhesion molecule 1. *Proc. Natl. Acad. Sci. USA* 88:4220–4224.

Wegelius, D., and Asboe-Hansen, G. (1956). Hormonal effects on mast cells. Studies on living connective tissue in the hamster cheek pouch. *Acta Endocrinol.* 22:157–165.

Witte, O. N. (1990). Steel locus defines new multipotent growth factor. *Cell* 63:5–6.

Yang-Yen, H.-F., Chambard, J.-C., Sun, Y.-L., Smeal, T., Schmidt, T. J., Drouin, J., and Karin, M. (1990). Transcriptional interference between c-*Jun* and the glucocorticoid receptor: Mutual inhibition of DNA binding due to direct protein-protein interaction. *Cell* 62:1205–1215.

Zachariae, L., and Moltke, E. (1954). Influence of hydrocortisone on mast cells of normal skin and healing wounds in the rabbit. *Acta Endocrinol.* 16:300–304.

to provide evidence for a causal relationship between exposure and the disease; second, to establish protocols for environmental control that are appropriate for routine treatment of allergic patients. Our objective is to outline the evidence for a relationship between sensitivity to allergens and asthma and then to describe briefly the evidence for threshold levels above which the risk of disease increases. These thresholds are important, because they establish a background for evaluating the relationship between changes achieved in avoidance regimes and evidence for clinical improvement. Finally, the evidence about avoidance measures will be considered before we discuss the procedures currently being recommended.

II. Sensitivity and Disease

A. Asthma

Reports of immediate skin sensitivity among patients with asthma were made as early as 1921 (Kern, 1921). However, the allergen source used most often in those reports was a very poorly defined "house dust" extract, which makes it difficult to evaluate their significance. In 1964, Spieksma and Voorhorst demonstrated that dust mites were the major source of house dust allergens in Europe and also developed techniques for growing *Dermatophagoides pteronyssinus* (Voorhorst et al., 1967). Using extracts of this mite and the closely related *D. farinae*, it rapidly became clear that sensitivity to dust mites was very common among patients with asthma and that this sensitivity was characterized by skin-sensitizing IgE antibodies. Initial studies were of clinic populations, but these were followed by population surveys and case-control studies that established unequivocally the association between mite sensitivity and disease (Smith et al., 1969; Miyamoto et al., 1968). Most recently, two prospective studies—one in England (Sporik et al., 1990) and the other in New Zealand (Sears et al., 1989)—have confirmed a very strong association between the development of mite sensitivity and asthma. In each of these studies dust mite sensitivity appeared to be the major factor, with cat sensitivity as an additional factor (Sporik et al., 1990; Sears et al., 1989). In neither of the studies did sensitivity to pollens play an important role. Thus, increasingly the epidemiological evidence about development of asthma in childhood has focused on mite sensitivity and mite exposure (Platts-Mills and de Weck, 1989). However, it is important to recognize that many other allergens, both indoors and outdoors, can be associated with asthma.

Recently, we analyzed the prevalence of sensitivity among adults and children presenting to two different emergency rooms in the United States. These case-control studies confirm the association between sensitivity and asthma and focused attention on three different sources of indoor allergens: dust mites, cats, and cockroaches (Pollart et al., 1989; Gelber et al., 1990). The significance of sensitivity was found to be stronger among "uninsured" and nonwhite populations, suggesting that indoor allergen sensitivity (and possibly exposure) may be very important among that population with the highest prevalence, morbidity, and mortality from asthma (Gelber et al., 1990). Those studies, however, also identify a significant number of patients with asthma who have low serum IgE and no evidence of sensitivity. In those individuals it seems unlikely that allergen exposure (or environmental control) plays a significant role. With improvements in the definition of sensitivity to the major inhalants, it has become easier to define nonatopic or intrinsic asthma. Patients with intrinsic asthma are not necessarily "nonallergic" since some of them have skin sensitivity and serum IgE antibodies to allergens such as *Trichophyton*, *Aspergillus*, or yeasts such as *Candida albicans* (Ward et al., 1989). In addition, some of these patients improve with prolonged use of specific antifungal therapy (Platts-Mills et al., 1986). We now recognize three classifications of adult asthmatics: (1) extrinsic asthmatics with sensitivity to a well-defined inhaled allergen, where there are good reasons for considering that that allergen (or allergens) is contributing to the disease; (2) asthmatics who lack inhalant sensitivity but have positive skin tests to a noninhaled allergen such as *Trichophyton* or foods that might play a role in their disease; (3) patients who have low total IgE, negative serum assays for IgE antibodies, and negative skin tests to a range of allergens.

Defining patients accurately is very important before considering environmental control. It is perhaps worth remembering Rackemann's final criterion for intrinsic asthma—that these patients "do not improve in hospital" (Rackemann, 1947). That is, he already recognized that those asthmatics without skin sensitivity to inhalants did not improve when they were removed from their home environment. Studies of environmental control need to focus on patients who have the potential to benefit.

B. Atopic Dermatitis

Patients with AD have higher levels of total IgE, more positive skin tests, and higher levels of serum IgE antibodies than any other patient group (Juhlin et al., 1969; Barnetson et al., 1981; Chapman et al., 1983). Despite the overwhelming evidence that most of the patients are indeed "atopic," there is still major confusion about whether allergens are an important cause of the skin disease. Among young children, food sensitivity is extremely common, and Sampson and his colleagues have demonstrated that double-blind food challenge can exacerbate skin disease in children with specific IgE antibodies (Sampson, 1983). They also showed that prolonged avoidance of foods to which these patients have specific sensitivity will not only produce clinical improvement, but also lead to progressive reductions in spontaneous release of mediators from circulating basophils (Sampson, 1988). However, food sensitivity is less obvious as a cause of disease among older children or adults. Indeed, over the age of 7 years, children with AD usually become sensitive to inhalants (Chapman et al., 1983; Tuft, 1949). In addition to demonstrating wheal-and-flare skin sensitivity, application of allergen to the skin of older patients with AD will produce a response that is macroscopically and histologically eczema (Mitchell et al., 1982). Thus, there is excellent evidence that many older children and adults with AD are sensitive to inhalants, and there is good evidence that exposure to these allergens experimentally can produce eczema. As with asthma, environmental control studies have two objectives: to gain further evidence for a role of allergen exposure in the disease *and* to develop practical protocols that can be recommended as part of routine treatment of those patients who have inhalant sensitivity.

III. Relationship of Exposure to Disease

Given that some individuals become sensitized to common inhalant allergens and that this sensitization increases the risk of developing asthma, there must be some level of exposure that can produce these changes. In all areas of air pollution, the policy has been to define a threshold level of exposure that carries a certain risk. However, before we discuss thresholds, it is important to recognize that these allergens are not toxic to nonallergic or genetically nonresponsive individuals. At present, we cannot accurately define the individuals who are genetically prone to develop allergic disease. The first statement of a risk level was made for dust mites by Spieksma, who suggested that 500 mites/g of dust was associated with asthma among mite-allergic individuals (Voorhorst et al., 1967). Subsequently, several studies demonstrated that patients living in houses with $\geq$100 mites/g of dust were more likely to present with asthma associated with mite sensitivity (Korsgaard, 1983a; Peat et al., 1989). Counting mites requires skill, is very time consuming, and gives only a partial estimate of the allergen content of dust since much of the allergen is fecal and mite bodies do not become airborne (Platts-Mills and Chapman, 1987; Tovey et al., 1981). Between 1980 and 1986, a series of assays were developed to measure specific mite allergens initially with polyclonal antisera and radioactive antigen and then with monoclonal antibodies and ELIZA technique (Chapman et al., 1987; Luczynska et al., 1989). During these studies it became clear that 500 mites/g was approximately equivalent to 10 μg *Der p* I (or *Der f* I)/g of dust (and that 100 mites/g is equivalent to 2 μg *Der p* I/g of dust). More recently, these two allergens have been referred to as dust mite group I allergens (Platts-Mills and Chapman, 1987; Platts-Mills and de Weck, 1989). Assays of this kind have now been applied to confirm the relationship between levels of exposure and asthma. Thus, in Berlin and Marseilles mite-allergic asthmatics were significantly more likely to have lived in a house with ≥2 μg group I allergen/g of dust (Charpin et al., 1990; Lau et al., 1989). These data do not distinguish between the level necessary to induce *sensitization* and the level that will give rise to *symptoms of asthma*.

Inherent in the concept of these thresholds is the view that high levels of exposure will increase the number of individuals who develop asthma. There are now three studies that suggest that high levels of exposure to dust mites can increase the number of patients who develop asthma. First, in Papua New Guinea introduction of blankets was associated with an increase in the prevalence of asthma from ~0.7% to 7%; all the wheezing individuals (predominantly adult males) in that "epidemic" were skin test positive to mites, and the mean level of exposure was ~1400 mites/g of blanket dust (Dowse et al., 1985). Second, comparing the town of Briancon (2000 meters high) with Marseilles, Vervloet and his colleagues found lower mean levels of mites at high altitude, as well as a significantly lower prevalence of both mite sensitivity and asthma (Charpin et al., 1990). Third, our recent prospective study on children in the south of England suggested that at-risk children who spent early childhood in a house with ≥10 μg group I mite allergen/g of dust were almost five times more likely to have symptoms of asthma at the age of 11 years than those whose houses had less than this level (Sporik et al., 1990).

In relating these studies to avoidance regimes, two different phases of the disease now need to be considered. First, avoidance could be recommended during the early years to prevent patients becoming allergic. Second, avoidance measures should be recommended to any symptomatic allergic patient. At present, there is very little controlled data that demonstrates what level of reduction of exposure is effective for either of these objectives. However, we do know that children raised in houses with less than 2 μg group I allergen/g of dust do not often develop sensitivity. We also know that when chronic mite-allergic asthmatics were taken from houses with ~13.5 μg group I mite allergen/g to a hospital room with ~0.2 μg/g, they showed dramatic improvement in symptoms and highly significant reductions in nonspecific bronchial reactivity (Platts-Mills et al., 1982). These studies can be seen as providing a target level of reductions that might be effective, but there is still only limited data on changes in allergen exposure in houses that are actually associated with improvement in either asthma or AD.

Most of the epidemiological data and the measurements of exposure relate to mite allergens; this reflects the high prevalence of mite sensitivity among asthmatics in many parts of the world. However, there is preliminary data about some other allergens, and approaches to reducing exposure have been proposed. For cat allergens, a level of 8 μg *Fel d* I has been proposed as a level above which most cat-allergic patients will have symptoms (Gelber et al., 1990). However, cat allergen can be passively transferred on clothing; many houses without cats will have levels between 8 and 1 μg, and it is not clear whether this is a level that can give rise to symptoms or sensitization. For cockroach allergen, published exposure levels have been in units, which cannot as yet be compared with the levels for other allergens. For the fungi exposure, levels can only be given as spore counts or viable units. The relationship between the concentration of fungal spores and either the quantity of allergen or symptoms is not clear. Thus, at present it is not possible to propose threshold levels for exposure to any of the fungi or to attempt to define the changes that need to be achieved to improve symptoms.

IV. Avoidance Measures

A. Dust Mite

Methods for reducing dust mite exposure can be divided into physical measures and chemical measures (Table 1). Each measure can, in theory, be evaluated by

Table 1 Avoidance Measures for Dust Mites

Physical measures
Covering mattresses and pillows[a]
Hot washing bedding every week or 2 weeks[a]
Removing carpets and upholstered furniture from bedroom[a]
Vacuum cleaning once per week, using a cleaner with good filters and mask for patient[a]
Reducing humidity of house *either* by opening windows or by air conditioning, depending on climate
Establishing polished flooring (wood or vinyl) throughout the house
Chemical measures for carpets and/or sofas
Acaricides
Benzyl benzoate
Pyrethroids
Pirimiphos methyl
Fungicide
Natamycin
Denaturing agents
Tannic acid
Physical killing of mites
Liquid nitrogen[b]
Steam cleaning[c]

[a]Priority measures that should be recommended in all cases.
[b]Pirimiphos methyl is not currently marketed for household use, and a practical technique for using liquid nitrogen has not been established.
[c]Steam cleaning is effective only at "industrial strength", many methods of steam cleaning will simply apply warmth, wet the carpet, and increase mite growth.

its effectiveness either in controlling mite allergens *or* in reducing symptoms. In practice, none of these measures carried out on its own will have a major impact on symptoms, and successful trials of avoidance have always used a combination of measures. Most successful studies have used a regime applied to most of the house (Platts-Mills and Chapman, 1987; Walshaw and Evans, 1986; Dorward et al., 1988). Surprisingly, two controlled studies that reported successful results focused only on the patients' bedrooms (Murray and Ferguson, 1983; Lau-Schadendorf et al., 1991). In each case mattresses and pillows were covered, bedding was washed in hot water, clutter was removed, and carpets were either removed or treated with a chemical compound. Both studies reported a significant improvement in symptoms and nonspecific bronchial hyperreactivity (BHR). Reduction in BHR related to reduced exposure to dust mite allergens has been reported in children moved to high-altitude sanatoria (Kerrebijn, 1970; Vervloet et al., 1982), in adults kept in an allergen-free unit in London (Platts-Mills et al., 1982), and among patients whose bedrooms were "cleaned" (Murray et al., 1983; Lau-Schadendorf et al., 1991). Because of the importance of this conclusion, it is worth pointing out that there are other possible explanations of these results. In most cases, following effective avoidance measures the patients had less symptoms and therefore used less treatment, particularly less inhaled beta$_2$-adrenergic agonists. Thus, it is possible that reduced nonspecific BHR was actually related to reduced use of these bronchodilators, which have been suspected of increasing BHR. In addition, as the patients improve they take more exercise, which may also have contributed to reductions in BHR.

Reducing humidity is a logical measure to reduce mite growth and in some areas is the simplest approach. Thus, in northern areas of the United States or in Denmark, where indoor humidity has risen because the houses are tightly sealed, simply opening a window may reduce the humidity below 7 g/kg and thus discourage mite growth (Korsgaard, 1983b). By contrast, in many areas of the world outdoor humidity is very high and therefore opening windows will not be effective. Typical examples are Brazil and the Gulf Coast of the United States (Arruda et al., 1991). Thus, although there are situations where increasing ventilation is an important measure, this is not a universal solution. The real conclusion is that it is very unhealthy to live with fitted carpets and upholstered sofas if the house is both warm and humid. The problem can be solved by removing the furnishings, controlling the humidity, or keeping the temperature down. Obviously, different situations will demand different solutions.

The use of chemicals to control mite growth in carpets is not simple. Although many different chemicals will kill mites in culture, it is difficult to apply these chemicals so that they will penetrate through to the bottom of the carpet. Carpets not only consist of multiple layers of material, but become filled with debris from the house. These layers create a refuge for mites, which cannot easily be penetrated. Thus, a recent International Workshop concluded that further work was needed in developing both preparations to clean carpets and methods of applying them so that they reach the live mites (Platts-Mills et al., 1991). At present, two preparations are marketed in the United States: a powder form of benzyl benzoate and tannic acid solution. Tannic acid denatures mite allergens rapidly but has no effect on live mites; thus the effect can only be short lived: ~1 month to 6 weeks. Benzyl benzoate powder presents a difficult problem of assessment because the powder applied to the carpet (i.e., 75 g/m^2) will increase the quantity of "dust" recovered for several weeks after application. Thus, results have to be expressed as total allergen recovered rather than as a concentration. Furthermore, the powder is thought to act as a cleaning agent by removing allergen from the carpet; if so, the presence of allergen on the recovered dust may represent allergen removed from the carpet rather than persistent growth of mites (Hayden et al., 1991). Overall, it appears that total recovery of group II mite allergen may be the best guide to acaricidal activity, and that allergen levels are decreased when treatment with benzyl benzoate is vigorous. However, it is difficult to say what change is enough, and perhaps more important, there are no studies that show what effect treatment with acaricides has on airborne mite allergen during disturbance.

The best documented measures are covering mattresses and pillows; a recent study showed that vapor-permeable cases can reduce mite allergen in dust off a mattress from ~20 μg/g to <1 μg/g (Owen et al., 1990). This is almost certainly a sufficient reduction to produce clinical benefit, and there can be no reason for not advising covering mattresses and pillows for all asthmatic patients who are shown to be allergic to mites.

B. Cat Allergens

Until recently, the only widely recommended avoidance measure for cat allergens was removing the cat permanently. However, this advice is often ignored by patients even when they have severe symptoms. Indeed, it has been estimated that 2 million patients in the United States are allergic to cats and have a cat in the house. The major cat allergen is a protein of molecular weight 34,000 named *Felis domesticus* I (*Fel d* I) first defined by Ohman and his colleagues (Ohman et al., 1974). Recently, Chapman et al. reported the use of monoclonal antibodies to *Fel d* I, both to purify the allergen and to develop very sensitive two-site immunoassays (Chapman et al., 1988). Using these assays, it was possible to monitor changes in airborne cat allergen in response to different measures and to design a protocol to reduce airborne cat allergen with the cat still in the house (Luczynska et al., 1990; De Blay et al., 1991). This protocol (Table 2) appears to have the potential for reducing airborne cat allergen by ~90%, but has not yet been used in clinical trials.

Although many other allergens are relevant to asthma, there are only very scattered pieces of data on methods of avoidance. In most cases the procedures

Table 2 Proposed Procedure for Reducing Airborne Cat Allergen Levels

A.	Either remove cat completely or keep outdoors
B.	Use polished flooring, no carpeting
	Minimize upholstered furniture
	Vacuum-clean with high-efficiency filter
	Use air filtration
	Wash cat weekly

recommended have not been evaluated because there are no available assays suitable for monitoring changes in exposure. As discussed previously, for the fungi, without a simple assay it is difficult to monitor changes occurring during avoidance or to define a target reduction in exposure. Thus, although there are obvious measures (such as removing a guinea pig or killing cockroaches) and measures that seem reasonable (such as the regularly recommended protocols for reducing exposure to fungi), it is difficult to provide evidence that such measures actually reduced exposure *or* symptoms. It is important to remember that many measures that seemed reasonable, such as vacuum-cleaning carpets more often for mites or using a room air filter to reduce airborne cat allergen, may actually increase exposure unless they are part of a full plan of avoidance.

C. Avoidance Measures for Atopic Dermatitis

It has been well known for many years that most patients with severe atopic dermatitis improve when they are admitted to hospital. One explanation of this phenomenon is that they improve because of reduced exposure to dust mite and other indoor allergens (Platts-Mills et al., 1983; Tuft, 1949). Korsgaard and his colleagues have carried out avoidance studies on patients with AD and reported encouraging results (Beck and Korsgaard, 1989). Similarly, we have had good experience suggesting that if avoidance measures are carried out aggressively, many patients improve dramatically (Platts-Mills et al., 1983). One of the problems is to document improvement. Recently we developed an assay for human IgG in skin scales on the patient's sheet (Deuell et al., 1991). This assay is, in effect, monitoring the quantity of serum coming through the skin and being scratched off with skin scales. It appears to be an excellent guide to the severity of disease. In preliminary studies patients not only improved when they were admitted to hospital unit, but also continued their improvement when they returned home to a modified environment. These results support the view originally proposed by Tuft that measures to reduce exposure to house dust allergens can be an important part of the management of eczema (Tuft, 1949). However, controlled trials of avoidance are urgently needed to establish this form of treatment.

V. Conclusions

Over the last 10 years evidence has come from many areas that the management of asthma is not satisfactory. Rising admission rates for children and rapidly increasing quantities of medicine prescribed are matched by increasing mortality rates. There are two major explanations: either that some important cause (or causes) of the disease has increased, or that pharmaceutical treatments that appear beneficial have harmful side effects. There is evidence for both these possibilities; however, the conclusion in either case is that we should focus on identifying and reducing the causes of asthma. Over the same period, accurate evaluation of indoor allergen avoidance has become possible. It is now possible to measure indoor levels of mite, cat, and cockroach allergens and begin to make statements about the quantitative changes necessary to achieve significant improvement in symptoms. Within the next few years, it should be possible to define specific regimes that will achieve, for example, a 90% reduction is exposure to mite or cat allergens in the treated room or rooms. It will also be possible to advise patients with some confidence what improvement can be expected (and what percent of patients may expect such an improvement). At present, it is clear that certain mite avoidance measures (e.g., covering mattresses and pillows) should be recommended to all mite allergic individuals. Within the next few years, diagnosis of sensitivity and the recommendation of specific appropriate avoidance regimes should become a first line of treatment that is considered for all asthmatics.

Opinions about the role that allergens play in asthma have swung from one extreme to the other over the last 70 years. Several developments have helped to rationalize the situation over the last 20 years. Our scientific understanding of allergens and allergen exposure has increased dramatically so that it is possible to make quantitative statements and compare results from many parts of the world. Understanding of the role that allergens play has changed completely so that the major perennial allergens are now considered as a dominant *cause* of BHR rather than as a "trigger factor" (Platts-Mills et al., 1990). Thus, allergen avoidance regimens, like other therapeutic regimens, are increasingly judged by their ability to produce reductions in BHR. Indeed, the best evidence that allergen exposure is causally related to asthma has come from studies showing either that reduced exposure can lead to a reduction in BHR *or* that exposure to high levels of allergen is associated with the development of BHR. Overall, the analysis of asthma has become much clearer, and it is possible to state with confidence that a large proportion of asthma among children over 2 years old and young adults is related to allergen exposure. This makes it possible to focus avoidance measures much more specifically on patients who would be expected to benefit. Finally, it is important to recognize that the indoor environment is quantitatively the dominant source of inhaled proteins and that specific measurements of indoor exposure are essential in designing avoidance regimes and in the management of allergic asthmatics.

Acknowledgment

This work was supported by NIH Grant AI-20565.

Discussion

Kennerly: Have the effects of benzyl benzoates or other chemicals been tested for their effect on airborne allergens?
Platts-Mills: No, the studies to date have been on reservoir dust, and they need to be extended to airborne dust.
Casale: What factors do you think are contributing to the increase in morbidity from asthma in people over 45 years old?
Platts-Mills: While it is possible that there are more environmental factors that have not been identified, I don't think that is the explanation of the increase in asthma in people over 45. I suspect that most of these cases are indeed intrinsic, including such antigens as *Trichophyton*; however, that would not explain why it is getting worse.
Metcalfe: Does liquid nitrogen work, and what is the effect of "hot water" vacuum cleaners?
Platts-Mills: Mat Colloff, in Glasgow, has demonstrated the feasibility of using liquid nitrogen to kill mites. It is very effective on sofas, but it is not clear that it will become widely used. Most hot water vacuum cleaners do not kill mites effectively because the hot water doesn't get down far enough. Furthermore, they often increase mite growth presumably because they increase humidity.
Hanifin: You have suggested an association between dust mites and eczema. Is there evidence about roaches and asthma?
Platts-Mills: It has been reported that many of the children with eczema in the Dermatology Clinic at Grady Hospital in Atlanta are allergic to roaches.
Goldstein: If dust mite allergens are not airborne, how do they work to induce asthma?
Platts-Mills: Dust mite allergens are usually undetectable in an undisturbed room. However, they become airborne during disturbance. When airborne, they are mainly on particles $> 10\ \mu m$ in diameter. We believe that about 10% of these particles enter the lung and give rise to local foci of inflammation, which cumulatively cause bronchial reactivity.
Casale: Is there data on the role of stuffed animals in mite allergy?

Platts-Mills: We published results showing very high levels of dust mite allergens in soft toys. We have also speculated that stuffed animals that are not washed regularly act as a reservoir of live mites to reinfect bedding.

References

Arruda, K., Rizzo, M. C., Chapman, M. D., Fernandez-Caldas, E., Baggio, D., Platts-Mills, T. A. E., and Naspitz, C. K. (1991). Exposure and sensitization to dust mite allergens among asthmatic children in Sao Paulo, Brazil. *Clin. Exp. Allergy* 21:433–439.

Barnetson, R. S., Merrett, T. G., and Ferguson, A. (1981). Studies on hyperimmunoglobulinaemia E in atopic diseases with particular reference to food allergens. *Clin. Exp. Immunol.* 46:54–60.

Beck, H-I., and Korsgaard, J. (1989). Atopic dermatitis and house dust mites. *Br. J. Dermatol.* 120:245–251.

Chapman, M. D., Rowntree, S., Mitchell, E. B., Di Prisco de Fuenmajor, M. C., and Platts-Mills, T. A. E. (1983). Quantitative assessments of IgG and IgE antibodies to inhalant allergens in patients with atopic dermatitis. *J. Allergy Clin. Immunol.* 72:27–33.

Chapman, M. D., Heymann, P. W., Wilkins, S. R., Brown, M. J., and Platts-Mills, T. A. E. (1987). Monoclonal immunoassays for the major dust mite *(Dermatophagoides)* allergens, *Der p* I and *Der f* I, and quantitative analysis of the allergen content of mite and house dust extracts. *J. Allergy Clin. Immunol.* 80:184–194.

Chapman, M. D., Aalberse, R. C., Brown, M. J., and Platts-Mills, T. A. E. (1988). Monoclonal antibodies to the major feline allergen *Fel d* I. II. Single step affinity purification of *Fel d* I, N-terminal sequence analysis, and development of a sensitive two-site immunoassay to assess *Fel d* I exposure. *J. Immunol.* 140:812–818.

Charpin, D., Birnbaum, J., Haddi, E., Genard, G., Toumi, M., and Vervloet, D. (1990). Attitude and allergy to house dust mites: An epidemiological study in primary school children. *J. Allergy Clin. Immunol.* 85:185.

De Blay, F., Chapman, M. D., and Platts-Mills, T. A. E. (1991). Airborne cat allergen (*Fel d* I): Environmental control with the cat in situ. *Am. Rev. Respir. Dis.* 143:1334–1339.

Deuell, B., et al. (1991). Atopic dermatitis (AD): The role of dust mite allergy and monitoring of disease activity by assay of IgG in skin scales. *J. Allergy Clin. Immunol.* 87:237.

Dorward, A. J., Colloff, M. J., MacKay, N. S., McSharry, C., and Thomson, N. C. (1988). Effect of house dust mite avoidance measures on adult atopic asthma. *Thorax* 43:98–105.

Dowse, G. K., Turner, K. J., Stewart, G. A., Alpers, M. P., and Woolcock, A. J. (1985). The association between Dermatophagoides mites and the increasing prevalence of asthma in village communities within the Papua New Guinea highlands. *J. Allergy Clin. Immunol.* 75:75–83.

Gelber, L., Pollart, S., Chapman, M. D., and Platts-Mills, T. A. E. (1990). Serum IgE antibodies and allergen exposure as a risk factor for acute asthma. *J. Allergy Clin. Immunol.* (abstract). 85:193.

Hayden, M. L., Rose, G., Diduch, K. B., Domson, P., Chapman, M. D., Heymann, P. W., and Platts-Mills, T. A. E. (1992). Reduction of dust mite allergens in carpets using Benzyl benzoate in the form of a wet powder. *J. All. Clin. Immunol.* (in press).

Ishizaka, K., Ishizaka, T., and Hornbrook, M. M. (1967). Allergen-binding activity of gamma-E, gamma-G and gamma-A antibodies in sera from atopic patients. In vitro measurements of reaginic antibody. *J. Immunol.* 98:490–501.

Juhlin, L., Johansson, G. O., Bennich, H., Högman, C., and Thyresson, N. (1969). Immunoglobulin E in dermatoses. Levels in atopic dermatitis and urticaria. *Arch. Dermatol.* 100:12–16.

Kern, R. A. (1921). Dust sensitization in bronchial asthma. *Med. Clin. North Am.* 5:751–758.

Kerrebijn, K. F. (1970). Endogenous factors in childhood CNSLD: Methodological aspects in population studies. In *Bronchitis III*. Edited by N. G. M. Orie and R. van der Lende. The Netherlands, Royal Vangorcum Assen, pp. 38–48.

Korsgaard, J. (1983a). House dust mites and absolute indoor humidity. *Allergy* 38:85–92.

Korsgaard, J. (1983b). Mite asthma and residency. A case-control study on the impact of exposure to house-dust mites in dwellings. *Am. Rev. Respir. Dis.* 128:231–235.

Lau, S., Falkenhorst, G., Weber, A., Werthman, I., Lind, P., Bucttner-Goetz, P., and Wahn, U. (1989). High mite-allergen exposure increases the risk of sensitization in atopic children and young adults. *J. Allergy Clin. Immunol.* 84:718–725.

Lau-Schadendorf, S., Ehnert, B., and Wahn, U. (1991). Reduction of mite allergen exposure and bronchial hyperreactivity. 2nd International Workshop. University Childrens Hospital, Berlin.

Luczynska, C. M., Arruda, L. K., Platts-Mills, T. A. E., Miller, J. D., Lopez, M., and Chapman, M. D. (1989). A two-site monoclonal antibody Eliza for the quantitation of the major *Dermatophagoides* spp. allergens, *Der p* I and *Der f* I. *J. Immunol. Meth.* 118:227–235.

Luczynska, C. M., Li, Y., Chapman, M. D., and Platts-Mills, T. A. E. (1990). Airborne concentrations and particle size distribution of allergen derived from domestic cats *(Felis domesticus)*: Measurements using cascade impactor, liquid impinger and a two site monoclonal antibody assay for *Fel d* I. *Am. Rev. Respir. Dis.* 141:361–367.

Mitchell, E. B., Crow, J., Chapman, M. D., Jouhal, S. S., Pope, F. M., and Platts-Mills, T. A. E. (1982). Basophils in allergen-induced patch test sites in atopic dermatitis. *Lancet* 1:127–130.

Miyamoto, T., Oshima, S., Ishizaka, T., and Sato, S. (1968). Allergic identity between the common floor mite (*Dermatophagoides farinae*, Hughes 1961) and house dust as a causative agent in bronchial asthma. *J. Allergy* 42:14–28.

Murray, A. B., and Ferguson, A. C. (1983). Dust-free bedrooms in the treatment of asthmatic children with house dust or house dust mite allergy: A controlled trial. *Pediatrics* 71:418–422.

Murray, A. B., Ferguson, A. C., and Morrison, B. J. (1983). Diagnosis of house dust mite allergy in asthmatic children: what constitutes a positive history? *J. Allergy Clin. Immunol.* 71:21–28.

Norman, P. S., Lichtenstein, L. M., and Ishizaka, K. (1973). Diagnostic tests in ragweed hay fever. A comparison of direct skin tests, IgE antibody measurements, and basophil histamine release. *J. Allergy Clin. Immunol.* 52:210–224.

Ohman, J. L., Jr., Lowell, F. C., and Bloch, K. J. (1974). Allergens of mammalian origin. III. Properties of a major feline allergen. *J. Immunol.* 113:1668–1677.

Owen, S., Morgenstern, J., Hepworth, J., and Woolcock, A. (1990). Control of house dust mite antigen in bedding. *Lancet* 335:396–397.

Peat, J. K., Salome, C. M., Sedgwick, C. J., Kerrebijn, J., and Woolcock, A. J. (1989). A prospective study of bronchial hyperresponsiveness and respiratory symptoms in a population of Australian school children. *Clin. Exp. Allergy* 19:299–306.

Platts-Mills, T. A. E., and Chapman, M. D. (1987). Dust mites: Immunology, allergic disease, and environmental control [published erratum appears in *J. Allergy Clin. Immunol.* 1988; 82(5 Pt 1):841]. *J. Allergy Clin. Immunol.* 80:755–775. (review).

Platts-Mills, T. A. E., and de Weck, A. L. (1989). Dust mite allergens and asthma—A world wide problem. *J. Allergy Clin. Immunol.* 83:416–427.

Platts-Mills, T. A. E., Tovey, E. R., Mitchell, E. B., Moszoro, H., Nock, P., and Wilkins, S. R. (1982). Reduction of bronchial hyperreactivity during prolonged allergen avoidance. *Lancet* 2:675–678.

Platts-Mills, T. A. E., Mitchell, E. B., Rowntree, S., Chapman, M. D., and Wilkins, S. R. (1983). The role of dust mite allergens in atopic dermatitis. *Clin. Exp. Dermatol.* 8:233–247.

Platts-Mills, T. A., Fiocco, G. P., Pollart, S., Hayden, M. L., Jackson, S., and Wilkins, S. R. (1986). *Trichophyton* allergy in a 24-year-old man with "intrinsic" asthma. *Ann. Allergy* 56:454–455.

Platts-Mills, T. A. E., et al. (1990). Role of allergens in asthma and airway hyperresponsiveness: Relevance to immunotherapy and allergen avoidance. In *Asthma: Its Pathology and Treatment*. Edited by M. A. Kaliner, P. J. Barnes, and C. G. A. Persson. New York, Marcel Dekker, pp. 595–631.

Platts-Mills, T. A. E., Thomas, W. R., Aalberse, R. C., Vervloet, D., and Chapman, M. D. (1992). Dust mite allergens and asthma: Report of a second international workshop. *J. All. Clin. Immunol.* (in press).

Pollart, S. M., Chapman, M. D., Fiocco, G. P., Rose, G., and Platts-Mills, T. A. (1989). Epidemiology of acute asthma: IgE antibodies to common inhalant allergens as a risk factor for emergency room visits. *J. Allergy Clin. Immunol.* 83:875–882.

Rackemann, F. M. (1947). A working classification of asthma. *Am. J. Med.* 3:601–609.

Sampson, H. A. (1983). Role of immediate food hypersensitivity in the pathogenesis of atopic dermatitis. *J. Allergy Clin. Immunol.* 71:473–480.

Sampson, H. A. (1988). The role of food allergy and mediator release in atopic dermatitis. *J. Allergy Clin. Immunol.* 81:635–645.

Sears, M. R., Hervison, G. P., Holdaway, M. D., Hewitt, C. J., Flannery, E. M., and Silva, P. A. (1989). The relative risks of sensitivity to grass pollen, house dust mite, and cat dander in the development of childhood asthma. *Clin. Exp. Allergy* 19:419–424.

Smith, J. M., Disney, M. E., Williams, J. D., and Goels, Z. A. (1969). Clinical significance of skin reactions to mite extracts in children with asthma. *Br. Med. J.* 1:723–726.

Sporik, R., Holgate, S. T., Platts-Mills, T. A. E., and Cogswell, J. (1990). Exposure to house dust mite allergen (*Der p* I) and the development of asthma in childhood: A prospective study. *N. Engl. J. Med.* 323:502–507.

Tovey, E. R., Chapman, M. D., Wells, C. W., and Platts-Mills, T. A. E. (1981). The distribution of dust mite allergen in the houses of patients with asthma. *Am. Rev. Respir. Dis.* 124:630–635.

Tuft, L. A. (1949). Importance of inhalant allergen in atopic dermatitis. *J. Invest. Dermatol.* 12:211–219.

Vervloet, D., Penaud, A., Razzouk, H., Senft, M., Arnaud, A., Boutin, C., and Charpin, J. (1982). Altitude and house dust mites. *J. Allergy Clin. Immunol.* 69:290–296.

Voorhorst, R., Spieksma, F. Th. M., Varekamp, H., Leupen, M. J., and Lyklema, A. W. (1967). The house dust mite *(Dermatophagoides pteronyssinus)* and the allergens it produces: Identity with the house dust allergen. *J. Allergy* 39:325–339.

Walshaw, M. J., and Evans, C. C. (1986). Allergen avoidance in house dust mite sensitive adult asthma. *Q. J. Med.* 58:199–215.

Ward, G. W., Jr., Karlsson, G., Rose, G., and Platts-Mills, T. A. E. (1989). *Trichophyton* asthma: Sensitization of bronchi and upper airways to dermatophyte antigen. *Lancet* 1:859–862.

20

Anaphylaxis

TIMOTHY J. SULLIVAN

University of Texas Southwestern Medical Center
Dallas, Texas

> In 1895, one year after the introduction of serotherapy, a two year old asthmatic boy was given an equine antiserum for prophylaxis against diphtheria. Anaphylaxis occurred and the child was dead within ten minutes (Lamson, 1924).

Anaphylaxis is an acute, severe, systemic reaction to antigens or other stimuli that is widely thought to be mediated by the sudden release of overwhelming amounts of mast cell mediators (Sullivan, 1988a). The purposes of this chapter are to review the basis for the theory that mast cells and their mediators play critical roles in human anaphylaxis, and to relate those concepts to current approaches to the diagnosis and management of anaphylaxis.

I. Historical Perspective

The case noted above was one of many instances of anaphylaxis that had been observed in humans and in experimental animals before 1902 (Lamson, 1924; May, 1985). Even though the patient was the child of Professor Langerhans, the mechanism of his death was not understood, and despite intense consideration, his death did not generate any new studies or insight into the nature of anaphylaxis. The development of a model of experimental anaphylaxis and the recognition of the existence of immunopathology by Paul Portier and Charles Richet in 1902 (May, 1985) however, led to a rapid expansion in knowledge of anaphylaxis and hypersensitivity (Table 1). A Nobel Prize was awarded to Richet in 1913 for these studies.

By 1907 passive transfer of specific anaphylactic sensitivity from a sensitized animal to a naïve animal had been discovered (Otto, 1907; Friedmann, 1908). In 1921, Prausnitz and Kustner demonstrated local passive transfer of human IgE-mediated sensitivity to human skin. Using the P-K method for assessment of specific reactivity after physicochemical treatments of serum containing IgE to ragweed antigens, the Ishizakas (1967) isolated and characterized human IgE in 1967. This accomplishment, coupled with the discovery of IgE myelomas (Johansson and Bennich, 1967), led to many new insights, including the development of assays for specific IgE, the isolation and characterization of the IgE Fc receptors expressed on mast cells and other cell types, and identification and study of the heavy-chain epsilon gene.

Table 1 Critical Events in Leading to Our Current Understanding of Anaphylaxis

IgE and anaphylaxis	
1902	Discovery of experimental anaphylaxis (May, 1985)
1907	Passive transfer of experimental anaphylaxis (Otto, 1907; Friedmann, 1908)
1921	Passive transfer of specific human IgE to human skin (Prausnitz and Kustner, 1921)
1967	Isolation and characterization of human IgE (Ishizaka and Ishizaka, 1967)
Antigens and anaphylaxis	
1902	Discovery of protein antigen–induced anaphylaxis (May, 1985)
1924	Hapten-induced anaphylaxis (Landsteiner, 1924)
1936	Experimental anaphylaxis induced and elicited by a free drug (arsphenamine) (Landsteiner and Jacobs, 1936)
1960	Demonstration of requirement for two or more IgE-binding sites on a single molecule to initiate human IgE-mediated inflammation (Farah et al., 1960)
Mast cells and anaphylaxis	
1902	Discovery of in vivo anaphylaxis (May, 1985)
1910	Discovery of in vitro tissue responses to antigen (Schultz, 1910)
1913	Recognition of similarity of in vitro anaphylaxis to effects of histamine (Dale, 1913)
1953	Recognition of association of tissue histamine with mast cells (Riley and West, 1953)
1958	Development of isolated mast cell experimental systems (Uvnas, 1958)
1987	Demonstration of elevated mast cell tryptase levels during human anaphylaxis (Schwartz et al., 1987)

The discovery of protein antigen–induced anaphylaxis (May, 1985) also led to detailed studies of the basis for the specificity of the reactions. Landsteiner and associates (1924, 1936, 1938, 1944) introduced the concept of haptenation, covalent attachment of a low-molecular-weight molecule to a larger carrier molecule, and studied precipitin and anaphylactic reactions induced by haptens. Systematic studies beginning in 1924 demonstrated that anaphylaxis could be mediated by hapten-specific antibodies: haptens could be presented on any carrier (Landsteiner, 1924). Indeed, anaphylaxis could be elicited without a carrier protein, if the hapten was presented in a multivalent form (Landsteiner, 1938). Landsteiner (1924) showed that univalent hapten did not cause anaphylaxis. Univalent hapten could prevent anaphylaxis to multivalent hapten carrier conjugates, providing more evidence in support of the concept that antibody binding to more than one site on an antigen was an essential aspect of the induction of anaphylaxis (Landsteiner, 1924). Landsteiner and Jacobs (1936) were the first to develop an in vivo experimental model of anaphylaxis induced and elicited by the administration of a low-molecular-weight drug, arsphenamine. Eisen and co-workers demonstrated the ability of carriers substituted with two or more hapten groups to activate human mast cells through IgE and the ability of univalent haptens to inhibit (Farah et al., 1960). These principles led to a clearer understanding of how IgE activates mast cells and the development of skin tests to detect IgE to penicillin (Sullivan et al., 1981) and several other drug-derived haptens.

Evidence that mast cells play a critical role in anaphylaxis also can be traced directly from the same initial experiments of Portier and Richet (May, 1985). In 1910, Schultz recognized the ability of antigen to cause responses in vitro in smooth muscle preparations from anaphylactically sensitized animals. Dale recognized the close similarity of these responses to antigen to responses by the same tissues to the addition of histamine (Dale, 1913). These observations and hypotheses were presented in 1913. In 1953, Riley and West demonstrated that tissue histamine is located predominantly in mast cells and generated the hypothesis that mast cells were of central importance in anaphylaxis. Studies of the role of mast cells and their mediators in anaphylaxis began in earnest when experimental systems using isolated mast cells were introduced in 1958 by Uvnas. These studies led to confirmation of the presence of histamine in mast cells and the release of histamine from sensitized cells by antigen. The first unambiguous biochemical data linking mast cells to human anaphylaxis, however, were presented in 1987 when Schwartz and co-workers detected increased levels of mast cell tryptase in the serum of patients experiencing anaphylaxis.

Studies of mediators released from antigen-stimulated tissues and from mast cells have strengthened the evidence that mediators of anaphylaxis are released from mast cells (Wasserman and Marquardt, 1988). Mediators released from mast cells that are capable of causing tissue responses seen in anaphylaxis include histamine, sulfidopeptide leukotrienes, prostaglandin D_2, and platelet-activating factor (PAF). Activation of mast cells also can lead to the release of preformed tumor necrosis factor (TNF) and the activation and expression of genes for TNF and IL-6 (Gordon et al., 1990). TNF also can mediate many of the vascular and cardiac disorders seen in anaphylaxis, with IL-6 in some manner playing a permissive role in the TNF actions (Starnes et al., 1988, 1990; Pober and Cotran, 1990). In addition to antigen-IgE mechanisms, mast cells can be activated by complement anaphylatoxins, diverse chemicals and drugs, and mast cell–activating cytokines (Sullivan, 1988a; Wasserman and Marquardt, 1988).

Taking these classical lines of evidence as a whole, there is considerable support for the concept that the release of mediators from mast cells is the central event in anaphylaxis. In experimental IgE-mediated anaphylaxis, a multisystem reaction results from a sudden, massive release of mast cell mediators. In clinical anaphylaxis, the acute, life-endangering reaction is associated with mast cell mediator release.

How well does this theory account for the clinical phenomena of anaphylaxis and the responses to therapy?

II. Clinical Anaphylaxis

The stimuli known to cause anaphylaxis can be stratified according to the scheme outlined in Table 2 (Sullivan, 1988a). In addition to antigen-IgE activation, anaphylaxis can be elicited by agents that directly activate mast cells, such as opiates, vancomycin, and polymyxin B. Anaphylatoxins can cause anaphylaxis after generation by immunological reactions to blood products or direct activation by aggregated antibodies in heterologous antiserum preparations. Anaphylaxis also can occur in rare individuals during exercise, after cold exposure, during exposure to endogenous or exogenous changes in steroid hormone levels,

Table 2 Classification of Causes of Systemic Anaphylaxis

IgE-mediated anaphylaxis
Haptens
Complete antigens
Direct activation of mast cells
Anaphylaxis mediated by anaphylatoxins
Anaphylaxis of unknown mechanisms
Physical factors
Mastocytosis
Idiopathic

Table 3 Clinical Manifestations of Anaphylaxis

System	Manifestation
Skin	Generalized, perineal, or vaginal pruritus; angioedema; urticaria and other pruritic rashes
Eye	Pruritus, conjuctival suffusion, lacrimation
Nose	Pruritus, congestion, sneezing, rhinorrhea
Mouth	Metallic taste
Upper airway	Sensation of narrowing airway, hoarseness, stridor, oropharyngeal or laryngeal edema, complete obstruction
Lower airway	Dyspnea, tachypnea, wheezing, use of accessory muscles of respiration, cyanosis, respiratory arrest
Cardiovascular	Tachycardia, hypotension, ventricular and supraventricular rhythm disturbances, cardiac arrest
Gastrointestinal	Nausea, vomiting, cramping abdominal pain, diarrhea, bloody diarrhea
Neurological	Fear of impending death, weakness, dizziness, syncope, seizure

in patients with mastocytosis, and during treatment with some recombinant immunoregulatory molecules. Some patients experience recurrent episodes of anaphylaxis with no known exogenous or endogenous stimulus. Clearly, clinical anaphylaxis can be initiated by several mechanisms independent of IgE.

The symptoms and signs of anaphylaxis (Table 3) are typical of IgE-mediated allergic reactions (Sullivan, 1988a). None is pathognomonic of anaphylaxis. A metallic taste in the mouth is noted when the plasma histamine exceeds 4 ng/ml (Kaliner, 1982) and is highly suggestive of anaphylaxis if characteristic acute respiratory or cardiovascular manifestations also are present.

Biphasic or protracted anaphylaxis occurs in approximately half of patients with life-endangering reactions (Stark and Sullivan, 1986). Initial response to therapy can be followed by asymptomatic intervals of up to 8 hr, with recurrence of anaphylaxis in the same organ systems involved in the early response. In some severe reactions, conventional therapy is unable to fully reverse the respiratory or cardiovascular dysfunction for a period of hours to days, rarely for more than a week. In some instances anaphylaxis is rapidly fatal, and in others progression to a fatal outcome is more gradual over hours to days.

III. IgE and Anaphylaxis

The relationship between the presence of IgE to penicillin or to Hymenoptera venoms and risk of anaphylaxis has been determined in prospective trials (Sullivan, 1988b; Reisman, 1988). A patient with no IgE to either antigen has virtually no risk of anaphylaxis to either antigen. The presence of IgE indicates a risk of an acute reaction in 43–67% of patients exposed to the antigen. The IgE is not sufficient, however, to assure a clinical reaction to an antigen. These and related data strongly indicate that IgE can mediate anaphylaxis in humans (Wasserman and Marquardt, 1988; Sullivan, 1988b; Reisman, 1988).

IV. Mast Cells and Anaphylaxis

The clinical manifestations of anaphylaxis include reactions in diverse organs typical of IgE-mediated allergic diseases that are closely linked to mast cell activation. H_1 antihistamines are associated with relief from some of the manifestations of anaphylaxis, providing additional evidence consistent with the notion that mast cells are contributing to or mediating the reactions.

The strongest evidence of a role for mast cells in anaphylaxis comes from assessments of serum tryptase during anaphylaxis (Schwartz et al., 1987, 1989). Anaphylaxis stimulated by penicillin, insect venom, exercise, food, heteroantiserum, and nonsteroidal anti-inflammatory drugs has been associated with marked increases in serum tryptase. This molecule is expressed in mast cells and at very low levels in basophils. Serum levels reflect mast cell tryptase release since the amount that could arise from basophils is so low it would not be detected in this assay. Serum levels peak 1–2 hr after the onset of anaphylaxis and then decline with a half-clearance value of approximately 2 hr (Schwartz et al., 1989).

There are, however, instances of apparent antigen-induced or idiopathic anaphylaxis that are not accompanied by increased serum tryptase levels (T. Sullivan and L. Schwartz, unpublished data), raising serious concern about the accuracy of the mast cell hypothesis for all forms of anaphylaxis. Mast cell–deficient mice do not display evidence of anaphylaxis when stimulated through IgE (Martin et al., 1989). But these animals do express a reaction resembling anaphylaxis when actively sensitized mast cell-deficient animals are challenged with antigen. While much remains to be done to characterize the nature of these reactions, the data raise the possibility that antigen can cause acute reactions in the virtual absence of mast cells. Alternatively, mast cells may be able to secrete histamine and other mediators under some circumstances without releasing tryptase and other granule core materials. Still another possibility is that mast cells can selectively release TNF or IL-6, resulting in vascular and other responses (Starnes et al., 1988, 1990; Pober and Cotran, 1990) in a manner distinctly different from conventional granule and lipid mediator release.

Similar considerations apply to the phenomena of biphasic and protracted anaphylaxis. Antigen-induced mast cell secretion of histamine-containing granules and of lipid mediators ceases within less than an hour in all experimental systems studied to date. The nature of the recurrent and sustained reactions is not known, but deserves careful study. The release of TNF, IL-6, or other cytokines after activation of mast cells genes (Gordon et al., 1990) could account for these reactions (Starnes et al., 1988, 1990; Pober and Cotran, 1990) but the roles of these mediators in the vascular and other responses in anaphylaxis have not been studied.

Tryptase-negative anaphylaxis, antigen-induced "anaphylaxis" in mast cell–deficient mice, and biphasic and protracted anaphylaxis present challenges to the concept that anaphylaxis is entirely the result of the release of mediators from mast cells. Since no other cell type has been shown to account for these apparent discrepancies, and no evidence for or against the other possibilities noted has been presented, these issues are currently unresolved.

V. Roles of Specific Mediators in Anaphylaxis

The pathophysiological changes that result in clinical anaphylaxis are primarily the result of the effects of mediators on blood vessels, cardiac muscle, and airway smooth muscle. Vascular caliber is increased by histamine acting on both H_1 and H_2 receptors, PGD_2, PAF, and leukotrienes (Wasserman and Marquardt, 1988; Kaliner et al., 1982). Histamine, and to a lesser degree the other mediators, also increase the permeability of postcapillary venules. These same mediators also are thought to cause the pulmonary responses seen in anaphylaxis (Wasserman and Marquardt, 1988).

The multiple acute actions of mediators of anaphylaxis on the heart (Wasserman and Marquardt, 1988; Kaliner et al., 1982; Del Balzo et al., 1985, 1988, 1990; Graver et al., 1986; Hattori and Levi, 1986; Robertson et al., 1987; Wolff and Levi, 1988) are summarized in Table 4. The usual alterations in cardiac function are decreased force of contraction, decreased coronary artery

Table 4 Cardiac Anaphylaxis

Dysfunction	Probable mediators
Tachycardia	Histamine H_2
Bradycardia	Histamine H_1
V. rhythm disorders	Histamine
Negative inotropism	H_1, LT, PAF
Positive inotropism	H_2, PGD_2
Coronary constriction	PGD_2, TXA_2, PAF

Denburg: Could you comment on the role of mast cell mediators in radiocontrast media reactions?

Sullivan: In the small number of patients we have studied, all patients with hypotension or respiratory symptoms have been tryptase positive.

Galli: There clearly may be differences in the pathogenesis of immunological responses in human and mouse. However, some models of active anaphylaxis that in normal mice are associated with extensive mast cell degranulation, pulmonary mechanical changes, and death also induce similar pulmonary mechanical changes and death rates in genetically mast cell–deficient mice. This finding indicates that the mast cell degranulation associated with these experimental models of active anaphylaxis is not essential for some of the clinically important aspects of the responses. I wouldn't want to suggest that mast cells don't have an important role in many forms of active anaphylaxis in humans; several lines of evidence you have summarized indicate that they almost certainly do have such a role in many instances. However, do you think that examples of human anaphylaxis exist in which effector mechanisms other than the mast cell may be important?

Sullivan: There may very well be contributions by FcϵRII (CD 23)-bearing cells, but no data are available to permit our assessment of their contributions. Mast cell mediators may induce other cell types to become activated even if they cannot be activated by antigen in a direct manner.

Schwartz: Tryptase levels are not elevated in serum during serum sickness and immune complex–mediated diseases, despite hypotension. Thus, I suspect that complement-derived anaphylatoxins act directly on the vasculature rather than on mast cells and that this clinical event should not be called anaphylaxis. Protracted or biphesic anaphylaxis could reflect a dual mechanism with anaphylaxis early, complement activation late. Levels of tryptase and C3a or C5a should provide precise diagnostic markers to sort this out.

Sullivan: There may be syndromes that resemble anaphylaxis that do not involve mast cells. Some patients with "idiopathic anaphylaxis" are tryptase negative and therefore may have non–mast cell origins.

Kaplan: During anaphylaxis, other plasma cascades are affected and can contribute to the syndrome. We collaborated with Larry Lichtenstein in studies of immunotherapy in insect sting allergy and obtained data on controls who had severe reactions. The had depletion of their kininogen and presumed formation of bradykinin, and autoanticoagulated. This was not due to circulating heparin from mast cells but to consumption of coagulation factors. Their factor V, for example, dropped to zero. Thus, when there is massive activation, many proteolytic processes are set in motion that can contribute to symptoms.

Sullivan: Those are very interesting observations. Perhaps the increased vascular permeability dilutes the contact system factors, initiating coagulation cascades that extend back into the vessels in affected tissues.

References

Besredka, A. (1908). Du mechanisme de l'anaphylaxie. *Ann. Inst. Pasteur (Paris)* 22:446–508.

Bussolino, F., Camussi, G., and Baglioni, C. (1988). Synthesis and release of platelet-activating factor by human vascular endothelial cells treated with tumor necrosis factor or Interleukin 1a. *J. Biol. Chem.* 263:11856–11861.

Dale, H. H. (1913). An anaphylactic reaction of plain muscle in the guinea pig. *J. Pharmacol. Exp. Ther.* 4:167.

Del Balzo, U. H., Levi, R., and Polley, M. J. (1985). Cardiac dysfunction caused by purified human C3a anaphylatoxin. *Proc. Natl. Acad. Sci. USA* 82:886–890.

Del Balzo, U., Polley, M. J., and Levi, R. (1988). Activation of the third complement component (C3) and C3a generation in cardiac anaphylaxis: Histamine release and associated inotropic and chronotropic effects. *J. Pharmacol. Exp. Ther.* 246:911–916.

Del Balzo, U., Sakuma, I., and Levi, R. (1990). Cardiac dysfunction caused by recombinant human C5A anaphylatoxin: Mediation by histamine, adenosine and cyclooxygenase arachidonate metabolites. *J. Pharmacol. Exp. Ther.* 253:171–179.

De Weck, A. L., and Girard, J. P. (1972). Specific inhibition of allergic reactions to penicillin in man by a monovalent hapten. II. Clinical studies. *Int. Arch. Allergy Appl. Immunol.* 42:798–815.

Farah, F. S., Kern, M., and Eisen, H. N. (1960). Specific inhibition of wheal and erythema responses with univalent haptens and univalent antibody fragments. *J. Exp. Med.* 112:1211–1126.

Friedmann, U. (1908). Ueber passive ueberempfindlichkeit. *Munchen Med. Wochenschr.* 54:2414.

Gordon, J. R., Burd, P. R., and Galli, S. J. (1990). Mast cells as a source of multifunctional cytokines. *Immunol. Today* 11:458–464.

Graver, L. M., Robertson, D. A., Levi, R., Becker, C. G., Weksler, B. B., and Gay, W. A. (1986). IgE-mediated hypersensitivity in human heart tissue: Histamine release and functional changes. *J. Allergy Clin. Immunol.* 77:709–714.

Hattori, Y., and Levi, R. (1986). Effect of PGD_2 on cardiac contractility: A negative inotropism secondary to coronary vasoconstriction conceals a primary positive inotropic action. *J. Pharmacol. Exp. Ther.* 237:719–724.

Ishizaka, K., and Ishizaka, T. (1967). Identification of gamma E antibodies as a carrier of reagenic activity. *J. Immunol.* 99:1187–1198.

Johansson, S. G. O., and Bennich, H. (1967). Immunochemical studies of an atypical (myeloma) immunoglobulin. *Immunology* 73:381–394.

Kaliner, M., Shelhamer, J. H., and Ottesen, E. A. (1982). Effects of infused histamine: Correlation of plasma histamine levels and symptoms. *J. Allergy Clin. Immunol.* 69:283–289.

Kawakami, M., Ishibashi, S., Ogawa, H., Murase, T., Takaku, F., and Shibata, S. (1986). Cachectin/TNF as well as interleukin-1 induces prostacyclin synthesis in cultured vascular endothelial cells. *Biochem. Biophys. Res. Commun.* 141:482–487.

Kilbourn, R. G., Gross, S. S., Jubran, A., Adams, J., Griffith, O. W., Levi, R., and

Lodato, R. F. (1990). N^G-Methyl-L-arginine inhibits tumor necrosis factor-induced hypotension: Implications for the involvement of nitric oxide. *Proc. Natl. Acad. Sci. USA* 87:3629–3632.
Lamson, R. W. (1924). Sudden death associated with the injection of foreign substances. *JAMA* 82:1091–1098.
Landsteiner, K. (1924). Experiments on anaphylaxis to azoproteins. *J. Exp. Med.* 39:631–637.
Landsteiner, K. (1938). Anaphylactic shock by azodyes. II. *J. Exp. Med.* 67:79–87.
Landsteiner, K. (1944). Bibliography. *J. Immunol.* 48:1–16.
Landsteiner, K., and Jacobs, J. (1936). Studies on the sensitization of animals with simple chemical compounds. III. Anaphylaxis induced by arsphenamine. *J. Exp. Med.* 64:717–721.
Martin, T. R., Galli, S. J., Katona, I. M., and Drazen, M. (1989). Role of mast cells in anaphylaxis. Evidence for the importance of mast cells in the cardiopulmonary alterations and death induced by anti-IgE in mice. *J. Clin. Invest.* 83:1375–1383.
May, C. D. (1985). The ancestry of allergy: Being an account of the original experimental induction of hypersensitivity recognizing the contribution of Paul Portier. *J. Allergy Clin. Immunol.* 75:485–495.
Otto, R. (1907). Zur Frage der serum-ueberembindlichkeit. *Munchen Med. Wochenschr.* 54:1665–1670.
Prausnitz, C., and Kustner, H. (1921). Studien ueber die Ueberempfindlichkeit. *Z. Bakt.* 86:160–169.
Pober, J. S., and Cotran, R. S. (1990). Cytokines and endothelial cell biology. *Physiol. Rev.* 70:427–451.
Reisman, R. E. (1988). Insect allergy. In *Allergy, Principles and Practice*. Edited by E. Middleton, Jr., C. E. Reed, E. F. Ellis, N. F. Adkinson, and J. W. Yunginger. St. Louis, Mosby, pp. 11345–1364.
Riley, J. F., and West, J. B. (1953). The presence of histamine in tissue mast cells. *J. Physiol.* (Lond.) 120:528–537.
Robertson, D. A., Genovese, A., and Levi, R. (1987). Negative inotropic effect of platelet-activating factor on human myocardium: A pharmacological study. *J. Pharmacol. Exp. Ther.* 243:834–839.
Schultz, W. H. (1910). Physiological studies in anaphylaxis. I. *J. Pharmacol. Exp. Ther.* 1:549–567.
Schwartz, L. B., Metcalfe, D. D., Miller, J. S., Earl, H., and Sullivan, T. J. (1987). Tryptase levels as an indicator of mast-cell activation in systemic anaphylaxis and mastocytosis. *N. Engl. J. Med.* 316:1622–1626.
Schwartz, L. B., Yunginger, J. W., Miller, J., Bokhari, R., and Dull, D. (1989). Time course of appearance and disappearance of human mast cell typtase in the circulation after anaphylaxis. *J. Clin. Invest.* 83:1551–1555.
Stark, B. J., and Sullivan, T. J. (1986). Biphasic and protracted anaphylaxis. *J. Allergy Clin. Immunol.* 78:76–83.
Starnes, H. F., Jr., Warren, R. S., Jeevanandam, M., Gabrilove, J. L., Larchian, W., Oettgen, H. F., and Brennan, M. F. (1988). Tumor necrosis factor and the acute metabolic response to tissue injury in man. *J. Clin. Invest.* 82:1321–1325.
Starnes, H. F., Pearce, M. K., Tewari, A., Yim, J. H., Zou, J., and Abrams, J. S.

(1990). Anti-IL6 monoclonal antibodies protect against lethal *Escherichia coli* infection and lethal tumor necrosis factor-α challenge in mice. *J. Immunol.* 145:4185–4191.

Stuehr, D. J., Fasehun, O. A., Kwon, N. S., Gross, S. S., Gonzalez, J. A., Levi, R., and Nathan, C. F. (1991). Inhibition of macrophage and endothelial cell nitric oxide synthase by diphenyleneiodonium and its analogs. *FASEB J.* 5:98–103.

Sullivan, T. J. (1988a). Systemic anaphylaxis. In *Current Therapy in Allergy, Immunology and Rheumatology-3*. Edited by L. M. Lichtenstein, and A. S. Fauci. Philadelphia, B. C. Decker, pp. 91–98.

Sullivan, T. J. (1988b). Drug allergy. In *Allergy, Principles and Practice*. Edited by E. Middleton, Jr., C. E. Reed, E. F. Ellis, N. F. Adkinson, and J. W. Yunginger. St. Louis, Mosby, pp. 1523–1536.

Sullivan, T. J., Wedner, H. J., Shatz, G. S., Yecies, L. D., and Parker, C. W. (1981). Skin testing to detect penicillin allergy. *J. Allergy Clin. Immunol.* 68:171–180.

Uvnas, B. (1958). The mechanism of histamine liberation. *J. Pharm. Pharmacol.* 10:1–13.

Wasserman, S. I., and Marquardt, D. L. (1988). Anaphylaxis. In *Allergy, Principles and Practice*. Edited by E. Middleton, Jr., C. E. Reed, E. F. Ellis, N. F. Adkinson, and J. W. Yunginger. St. Louis, Mosby, pp. 1365–1376.

Wolff, A. A., and Levi, R. (1988). Ventricular arrhythmias parallel cardiac histamine efflux after coronary artery occlusion in the dog. *Agents Actions* 25:296–306.

21

The Pathophysiology of Allergic Rhinitis and Its Implications for Management

ALKIS G. TOGIAS and LAWRENCE M. LICHTENSTEIN

The Johns Hopkins University School of Medicine
Baltimore, Maryland

I. Introduction

Allergic rhinitis affects between 15 and 20% of the U.S. population, which translates to approximately 30 million people (Ricketti, 1985). It is one of the most common chronic illnesses in the Western world, the most common in those under 18 years, and the third most common in the 18–44-year age group in the United States (Collins, 1988). It is not clear whether its prevalence is steadily rising; however, as the population of the industrialized world tends to spend progressively longer periods in poorly ventilated indoor environments (Samet et al., 1987), the exposure to potent indoor aeroallergens increases. More and more evidence is accumulating that relates indoor allergenic exposure to sensitization and to the development of airway symptomatology (Sporik et al., 1990; Price et al., 1990).

Despite the availability of potent therapeutic regimens, a large number of individuals with allergic rhinitis do not obtain adequate relief. This is, to some extent, due to the anatomical relationships of the nasal cavities to the narrow drainage orifices of the paranasal sinuses and of the eustachian tube, which allow for frequent inflammatory/infectious complications of the sinuses and the middle ear. However, .it may also be secondary to the fact that a very important pathophysiological concept—that mucosal inflammation is a consistently underlying phenomenon in this condition—has still not found its way into clinical practice. In the past decade, significant steps in establishing this concept and understanding its relationship to the clinical features of allergic rhinitis have been taken. These steps were largely facilitated by the accessibility of the human nasal mucosa to experimental manipulations. This has turned allergic rhinitis into an excellent model for the investigation of allergic diseases. It was, for example, in a model of nasal provocation that the first confirmation of mast cell mediator production and release upon mucosal contact with antigen was obtained in the human respiratory tract (Naclerio et al., 1983), and it was during the nasal late-phase reaction to antigen that a potential role for the basophil leukocyte in this phase of the allergic response was first suggested (Naclerio et al., 1985).

In this review we present the most recent achievements in our understanding of the mechanisms of allergic rhinitis and attempt to relate them to the clinical presentation of the disease. To do so, we will first briefly discuss some of the clinical features of this condition and will later reappraise these features, after exploring their pathophysiological aspects.

II. Clinical Features of Allergic Rhinitis

In the minds of many physicians, allergic rhinitis is perceived as an illness comprised of multiple, independent, acute episodes of localized, nasal mucosal anaphylaxis. This picture derives from the fact that patients tend to primarily describe their acute symptomatology, which involves nasal and conjunctival pruritus associated with bouts of sneezing and lacrimation, rhinorrhea, and, to a lesser degree, nasal congestion. In the majority of cases, the patients can clearly relate these symptoms to specific antigenic exposure. However, this clinical presentation is only a snapshot in the course of the disease. More extensive questioning reveals a different picture: patients are almost continuously symptomatic, but the chronic symptomatology is characterized by moderate to severe congestion, postnasal drainage, sinus pressure, and headaches, instead of itching and sneezing or profuse rhinorrhea. Patients have difficulty identifying any relationship between these symptoms and exposure to offending allergens. This picture is more evident in individuals with perennial allergic rhinitis, who seem to be the majority of allergy sufferers (Turkeltaub and Gergen, 1988), but such a history can be elicited from patients with simple seasonal disease, within the time frame of their pollen season. In attempting to explain this presentation, one can generate several hypotheses. A quantitative relationship between symptoms and allergen exposure may be present, with high allergen doses resulting in the acute presentation and lower doses leading to low-grade symptomatology. However, this hypothesis does not explain the above-described qualitative differences in the symptoms. A more attractive hypothesis is that the reaction that follows an encounter with a large amount of antigen does not end with the easily recognizable acute symptoms, but results in mucosal inflammation, which leads to the development of the more chronic clinical presentation. This hypothesis introduces the concept of late-phase reactions, which have been described in the skin (Dolovich et al., 1973; Solley et al., 1976) and in the upper and lower airways (Pelican, 1978; Booij-Nord et al., 1971; Robertson et al., 1974) following experimental antigen provocation.

A second interesting feature is that patients with allergic rhinitis, especially those with perennial disease, frequently pinpoint nonspecific irritants as well as sudden weather changes as triggers of acute nasal symptoms. Since no evidence exists that any of these irritants, such as cigarette smoke, perfumes, and other strong odors, are immunological sensitizers, it is reasonable to believe that the reported symptoms are the result of increased nonspecific irritability of the nasal mucosa, similar to the hyperreactivity of the lower airways in asthmatic individuals.

In patients with seasonal pollinosis, the symptomatology closely correlates with the pollen counts. However, it has been consistently reported that, when the pollen counts begin to drop, a lag time occurs before the symptoms decrease (Norman and Lichtenstein, 1988). This "hysteresis" may be attributed to the introduction of other allergens (such as mold spores) or to a buildup of pollen levels in the indoor environment, but it may equally well represent increased sensitivity to the pollen, a phenomenon that was described in the 1960s by Connell as "priming" (Connell, 1968, 1969).

The above characteristics of the natural history of allergic rhinitis point away from the concept of sporadic contact with antigen leading to episodes of acute symptomatology, unrelated to each other, and suggest a complex pathophysiology in which an underlying alteration of mucosal function dominates. The recognition that allergic rhinitis is a chronic inflammatory condition may help reconciliate the main features of the clinical presentation.

III. Advances in Our Understanding of the Pathophysiology of Allergic Rhinitis

A. Antigen Challenge

The study of allergic diseases is simplified because the etiological factors are easily identifiable through epicutaneous or intradermal skin testing or through the detection of specific IgE antibodies against these factors in the patient's serum (Norman and Lichtenstein, 1988). Furthermore, because of their rather localized nature, allergic reactions can be safely induced experimentally in the human nose, lung, or skin. This greatly facilitates the development of human models to study the pathophysiology of these conditions. Antigen provocations are, therefore, central to the development of models to study airway dysfunction. An additional advantage is that, since the basic allergic reaction involves the same mechanism, regardless of the target organ, observations in one organ, such as the skin, can be extrapolated to the airways, and vice versa. In the skin and the lower airways, rather invasive approaches are required to establish models to study the immunological, biochemical, and cellular events that follow the introduction of antigen. In contrast, the nasal mucosa provides a readily accessible part of the airway that can be sampled sequentially without traumatic effect. Thus, the development of a nasal antigen challenge model by Naclerio and his associates in the early 1980s (Naclerio et al., 1983) has offered significant information on the pathophysiology of allergic rhinitis and has helped generate more complete hypotheses to explain the clinical picture of this condition. This model has also allowed comparisons with other, mostly lower airway models. From these comparisons the concept was developed that not only the basic antigen-IgE-mediated acute allergic reactions, but also the late inflammatory phenomena observed in the upper airways of individuals with allergic rhinitis after antigen provocation, are almost identical to those in the lower airways of asthmatic patients.

In 1873 Blackley, afflicted with allergic rhinitis, was the first to introduce grass pollen in his own nasal cavities and experience an acute allergic reaction (Blackley, 1873). Since then nasal antigen challenge has been extensively used for both experimental and clinical evaluation of patients with allergic rhinitis (Salvaggio et al., 1964; Connell, 1967, Bernstein and Safferman, 1973; McLean et al., 1976). In the early studies the end-points were either antigen-induced symptoms or nasal airway resistance. Histamine was established in the beginning of the century as a mediator of allergic symptomatology (Dale and Laidlaw, 1910, 1919), but elucidation of the basic allergic reaction as the result of the interaction of antigen with basophil and mast cell–bound specific IgE antibodies occurred much later (Ishizaka and Ishizaka, 1967, 1975). As more inflammatory mediators were recognized as products of the antigen-induced mast cell and basophil activation in in vitro systems and in animal models of anaphylaxis, some attempts were made to demonstrate the release of these substances at the specific site of an allergic reaction in humans. Owing to the poor sensitivities of the initially available detection methods, the early results were rather equivocal (Dolovich et al., 1970; Okazaki et al., 1977; Eggleston et al., 1978; Okuda and Otsuka, 1977).

With the advent of more sensitive assays and the development of a nasal antigen challenge model in which secretions are collected before and after challenge by lavaging the nasal cavities with normal saline, the release of preformed and newly generated mast cell mediators such as histamine and prostaglandin (PG) D_2 was confirmed (Naclerio et al., 1983). Subsequent studies by many investigators have reproduced these findings and have widened the spectrum of inflammatory mediators that can be recovered in increased quantities following nasal antigen provocation (Proud et al., 1983; Creticos et al., 1984; Baumgarten et al., 1985; Brown et al., 1987; Freeland et al., 1989; Miadonna et al., 1987, 1989; Tonnesen et al., 1988; Krayenbuhl et al., 1989; Volovitz et al., 1988; Castells and Schwartz, 1988; Ophir et al., 1988; Shaw et al., 1985; Nagakura et al., 1988; Chan-Yeung et al., 1988). In addition to the measurement of inflammatory mediators, the technique of nasal lavage allows for simultaneous quantitation and differentiation of the cellular contents of nasal secretions (Bascom et al., 1988a, b). It is, therefore, possible to correlate the presence of inflammatory cells with the mediators that they release and to comment on their state of activation (Bascom et al., 1988a, 1989).

B. The Early Inflammatory Events

Symptoms

The reaction occurring within seconds after antigen is insufflated into the nasal cavities closely mimics the bouts of acute symptomatology reported by patients as part of the natural history of the disease. Sneezing, unquestionably the most prominent symptom, correlates well with the elevations in mediators recovered in lavage fluids 10 min after challenge (Naclerio et al., 1983).

Mast Cell Activation

The pattern of mediators—histamine, PGD_2, and mast cell tryptase—indicates mast cell activation (Schwartz and Austen, 1988). In addition, there is good evidence of mast cell degranulation in nasal mucosal biopsies after antigen challenge (Kawabori et al., 1983; Kawabori and Unno, 1983; Gomez et al., 1986). Histamine may be also derived from basophils, but although the metachromatic cells in nasal secretions of symptomatic patients with allergic rhinitis are largely basophils (Okuda et al., 1978; Hastie et al., 1979), it is not clear whether these cells are present in the secretions of allergic individuals when they are asymptomatic, out of the pollen season. Sulfidopeptide leukotrienes are also released in nasal secretions (Creticos et al., 1984; Shaw et al., 1985), but their source is unclear: the mast cells in the human nasal mucosa have not been characterized with regard to their capability of producing these arachidonic acid metabolites. The mast cells from human lung tissue produce equal amounts of LTC_4 and PGD_2 (Peters et al., 1984), but those collected through bronchoalveolar lavage from asthmatics generate largely PGD_2 (Cohan et al., 1989). Under electron microscopy, the mast cells of the nasal mucosa appear to have crystalline and reticular components of their secretory granules almost identical to lung mast cells, but the morphological sequence of antigen-induced degranulation is not the same (Friedman and Kaliner, 1985). Okuda and Otsuka (1987) report that the majority of metachromatic cells within the epithelium share many characteristics with the "mucosal mast cells" described by Enerback (1981) in the rat intestine. According to the same investigators, only these cells are found degranulated following the application of antigen to the nasal mucosa; the mast cells of the deeper layers (lamina propria), which morphologically appear to be related to the "connective tissue mast cells" of rat peritoneum (Bienenstock et al., 1982), do not show evidence of degranulation after antigen challenge (Okuda et al., 1985).

Are Other Cells Involved?

Some of the inflammatory mediators detected during the acute nasal reaction to antigen cannot be totally attributed to mast cell activation. For example, it appears that human mast cells release a small amount of platelet-activating factor (PAF) in their environment, after antigen provocation (Triggiani et al., 1990), compared to other inflammatory cells. Miadonna et al. (1989) published evidence of activation of the PAF metabolic pathway in the nose following antigen challenge. We have only detected high levels of lyso-PAF in nasal lavage fluids, with the use of gas chromatography, mass spectrometry (unpublished observations). We have also detected significant elevations of major basic protein (MBP), the sole proteinaceous constituent of the eosinophil granule core, in post–antigen challenge lavages (Bascom et al., 1989). Although basophils contain some MBP, the quantity is less than 3% of the MBP content of eosinophils (Ackerman et al., 1983). Based on these findings, the possibility exists that, in addition to the mast cells, other cell types may be activated in the early reaction to antigen in vivo. The eosinophil is a logical candidate: it has been claimed that this cell bears low-affinity receptors for IgE (Capron et al., 1984), but it is clear that it releases not only MBP, but LTC_4 and PAF as well (Silberstein et al., 1986; Lee et al., 1984). There is, however, no definitive evidence that antigen can activate eosinophils in an in vivo model of anaphylaxis. It is possible that some unknown mast cell factor induces eosinophil activation in the course of the acute reaction to antigen. The concept of eosinophil activation during the acute reaction is rendered less tenable by the fact that very few eosinophils are present in the nasal mucosa of individuals who are asymptomatic and out of the pollen season. As part of this discussion, it is worth noting that monocytes and macrophages have also been said to possess low-affinity IgE receptors (Capron et al., 1983) and could, theoretically, carry IgE molecules and be activated by antigen. These cells can also produce PAF and leukotrienes upon stimulation (Arnoux et al., 1980; Williams et al., 1984; Rankin et al., 1982).

Acute Effects of Mast Cell Mediators

Mast cell mediators are clearly capable of inducing the symptoms of the acute nasal allergic response. Knowledge of the actions of these autacoids derives from animal experimentation, from ex vivo studies on human tissues, and, most important, from direct in vivo challenge of humans. The effects of several of these mediators have been examined in the nose (Togias et al., 1987; Secher et al., 1982; Miadonna et al., 1987; Bisgaard et al., 1984; Karim et al., 1978; Pipkorn et al., 1984; Proud et al., 1988; Mezawa et al., 1989; Doyle et al., 1989). Among them, histamine appears to be the one that most closely mimics the symptoms of acute allergic rhinitis. Sneezing, pruritus, rhinorrhea, and nasal congestion are hallmarks of the clinical response to nasal histamine challenge (Togias et al., 1987). In addition, histamine induces marked vascular permeability manifested by increases in albumin in returned lavage fluids (Togias et al., 1987) and by the generation of kinins, by allowing kininogen and plasma kallikrein to flood the extravascular tissues (Baumgarten et al., 1986). Most of these responses are totally blocked by H_1 receptor antagonists (Togias et al., 1987); however, inhibition of histamine-induced nasal congestion requires the addition of H_2 antagonists, presumably because the nasal vasculature carries both H_1 and H_2 receptors (Secher et al., 1982). Other mast cell–derived mediators can only partially reproduce the acute rhinitic symptoms, when introduced in the human nose. PGD_2 causes rhinorrhea and nasal congestion in the hands of some investigators (Doyle et al., 1989), but has no effects in the hands of others (Mezawa et al., 1989). LTD_4 results in nasal congestion and increased nasal blood flow (Miadonna et al., 1987; Bisgaard et al., 1984), as well as in some rhinorrhea (Mezawa et al., 1989). The role of mast cell tryptase is unknown, since it has not yet been used to stimulate the human nose. This enzyme may contribute to kinin formation (Baumgarten et al., 1986) and may lead to the generation of C3a anaphylatoxin (Schwartz et al., 1983), but neither effect is likely to be of physiological importance. Recently, tryptase has been shown to potentiate histamine-induced contractility of isolated dog bronchial smooth muscle (Sekizawa et al., 1989).

As noted, histamine and other mast cell mediators may also lead to the generation of additional inflammatory substances, by interacting with blood vessels and promoting vascular permeability. Bradykinin and lysyl-bradykinin are present in large quantities in the nasal fluids immediately following provocation with antigen (Proud et al., 1983). The role of these mediators in allergic rhinitis may be significant. When bradykinin is used to challenge the human nose, it leads to some nasal congestion and rhinorrhea and induces impressive vascular leakage, as shown by the presence of albumin in nasal lavage fluids (Proud et al., 1988). The vascular effects of bradykinin have been well

recovered in later stages, between 2 and 12 hr: sulfidopeptide leukotrienes (Pipkorn et al., 1987a) and kinins (Naclerio et al., 1985), which are, however, not as abundant as in the early phase. When samples are analyzed with HPLC, LTE_4 is recovered from late lavages in larger amounts than in the early response (Pipkorn et al., 1987a). This implies that metabolism of LTC_4 to E_4 may be occurring during late inflammation and that this may not be readily appreciated because the immunoassay used in these measurements detects primarily LTC_4 and has only 10% cross-reactivity with LTE_4.

Two eosinophil products, major basic protein and eosinophil-derived neurotoxin, found in high levels in late lavages, are only present in low levels in the lavages performed immediately after antigen challenge (Bascom et al., 1989). Both correlate with the number of eosinophils in lavage fluids, suggesting that these cells not only infiltrate the nasal mucosal surface, but are also activated in the course of antigen-induced inflammation.

The Role of the Basophil Leukocyte in Late Inflammation

If, based on the above findings, one accepts the notion that mast cells do not produce mediators during late inflammation, the obvious next question concerns the source of histamine and other mediators in late lavages. All the evidence we have accumulated points toward the basophil leukocyte. Cell pellets from nasal lavages can be evaluated by relatively simple handling (Bascom et al., 1988b). Staining with alcian blue identifies the metachromatic granules contained in mast cells and basophils (Gilbert and Ornstein, 1975). Our studies have demonstrated a 12-fold increase in the number of alcian blue–positive cells in late nasal lavage fluids (Bascom et al., 1988a). In the same study, the correlation between histamine levels and these cells was highly significant ($r = 0.72$, $p < 0.0001$), implying that they were the source of histamine in the nasal fluids. At least 68% of the alcian blue–positive-staining cells were identified as basophils by standard light microscopy criteria (Galli et al., 1984). During the same study we evaluated the effects of a 7-day nasal treatment with topical steroids on the mediators and the infiltrating cells of the late phase (Bascom et al., 1988a; Pipkorn et al., 1987b). Among the several effects of topical steroids, we found inhibition of histamine release in late lavages and a significant suppresion of the alcian blue–positive cell influx.

Since alcian blue–staining cells represent only 2% of the total cell population in late lavage fluids, electron microscopy to confirm their identity is not feasible. However, we have managed to isolate these cells and study their functional characteristics ex vivo (Iliopoulos et al., 1989). The average histamine content per alcian blue–staining cell (~1 pg) was similar to that reported for peripheral blood basophils and less than that contained in human mast cells. When the nasal cells were challenged with anti-IgE, their response was similar to that of peripheral blood basophils: both populations released histamine optimally at the same dose (0.1 μg/ml), which is 100-fold less than the optimal dose for mast cells. In addition, the cells in the nasal fluid were sensitive to f-Met-Leu-Phe (2×10^{-6} M), a secretagogue for basophils and not for human lung mast cells (Siraganian and Hook, 1977; Cohan et al., 1989). Dimaprit, an agonist for the H_2 histamine receptor, inhibited the anti-IgE-induced response of the nasal histamine-containing cells in a dose-dependent manner, suggesting that these cells possess an H_2 receptor through which histamine exerts a negative feedback on its own release. This is, again, a characteristic of human basophils and not mast cells (Lichtenstein and Gillespie, 1975). We also performed dual-color immunofluorescence and flow cytometric analysis of the cells in nasal lavages during the late inflammatory stages. The vast majority of IgE-bearing cells coexpressed CD18 and other leukocyte markers not present on mast cells (unpublished observations). All these approaches demonstrate clearly that basophil leukocytes are recruited in nasal secretions following antigen challenge and are activated to release histamine, thus participating in the late antigen-induced inflammation. The significance of this phenomenon is, at this point, not totally clear, because we do not know to what extent the late symptoms, which are different from those in the early reaction, are mediated by histamine and other basophil mediators.

The finding of basophils during the late after-antigen-challenge inflammation is consistent with previous work that found these cells in nasal secretions and on the superficial layers of the epithelium during the naturally occurring disease (Okuda et al., 1978; Hastie et al., 1979). This emphasizes the importance of late inflammation as more representative of allergic rhinitis. In addition, it is worth noting that in our recent studies of late antigen-induced inflammation in the lower airways of asthmatic patients, BAL fluids, 20 hr after subsegmental antigen provocation, contained 30-fold more basophils than the baseline lavage, while mast cell numbers were not changed (Guo et al., 1990). Finally, in a versatile model of allergic skin reactions in which blisters are raised, unroofed, and replaced with a chamber where antigen is injected and samples are removed hourly, a high correlation was observed between late histamine release, the size of the skin late-phase reaction, and the influx of basophils during hours 6–12 after antigen challenge (Charlesworth et al., 1989).

Nasal Priming to Antigen

As initially described by Connell, the nasal mucosa becomes more sensitive to antigen as a result of a previous antigen exposure. He found that his subjects, who were exposed to natural antigen on daily basis, noted a progressive increase in their symptomatology despite the stable pollen counts. In other studies, he was able to reproduce this effect with repetitive intranasal antigen provocations

(Connell, 1968, 1969). The phenomenon was later confirmed by other investigators who monitored clinical or physiological end-points such as symptoms, nasal airway resistance, or eustachian tube function (Bacon et al., 1981; Juliusson and Bende, 1988; Skoner et al., 1989). These studies did not address the mechanism of priming, and it was not clear, therefore, whether priming was a specific phenomenon related to the acute immunological response to antigen challenge or was due to the development of nonspecific hyperirritability of the mucosa, secondary to inflammation.

In 1989, Wachs and colleagues published their observations on the pathogenesis of nasal priming. Ten subjects with seasonal allergic rhinitis were challenged while asymptomatic with ragweed pollen on four separate occasions: days 1, 15, 16, and 17. During each of these challenges they received the same number of pollen grains in a stepwise increasing protocol. The nasal response was monitored not only by symptom scores, but also with nasal lavages, the returned fluids of which were assayed for several inflammatory mediators. The cellular contents of the lavage fluids, prior to each provocation, were also examined. These investigators showed that the clinical response to antigen on day 16 was significantly stronger than those on days 1 and 15, which were reproducible. Furthermore, the response on day 17 was even greater than that on day 16. The dose-response curves for the generation of mast cell–derived mediators such as histamine and PGD_2 were shifted to the left every day additional antigen was administered to the nasal cavity. Similar findings were reported for LTC_4 and TAME esterase activity. On days 16 and 17, the eosinophils and neutrophils in nasal lavage fluids were significantly elevated over the previous 2 days. This study offered significant insight into the mechanism of priming by implicating increased mast cell mediator release (Wachs et al., 1989). It remained unclear, however, whether this was the result of the increased number of mast cells in the nasal mucosal epithelium, or whether the preexisting cells were driven to a state of hyperreleasability by the infiltrating eosinophils and neutrophils or other aspects of the inflammatory process.

In other studies, the lowest dose of an initial, increasing dose antigen challenge protocol was readministered 12 hr after the first provocation, resulting in a markedly increased response (Pipkorn et al., 1987b). The pattern of priming with regard to mediators was somewhat different at 12 hr in that only histamine and the secondary mediators, such as the kinins, were elevated, compared to the initial challenge, suggesting that, at this stage of nasal inflammation, the potentiation may have been secondary to the influx of basophils in the nasal mucosa. This would lead only to higher histamine release in response to antigen, but not to higher PGD_2, since the contribution of the mast cells was unchanged. It is worth noting that both systemic and local steroids totally abolished the primed response at 12 hr, suggesting that this was related to the antigen-induced mucosal inflammation (Pipkorn et al., 1987a,b).

The relationship between priming and the late-phase reaction does not seem to be necessarily causal. In a large study of 55 consecutive ragweed hayfever patients, Iliopoulos et al. (1990) found that 47% of these subjects demonstrated a late-phase reaction, arbitrarily defined as a threefold increase over baseline in two mediators in nasal lavage fluids. These subjects were also rechallenged with antigen 10 hr after the initial provocation, and 41% had mediator levels greater than those of the early reaction. However, among the 21 subjects who demonstrated a priming response, 11 developed a late reaction and 10 did not. It appears that the antigen-induced inflammation can manifest itself with different phenomena in different individuals, thus increasing the complexity of the natural disease.

Nasal Nonspecific Hyperreactivity

Our interest in studying nonspecific hyperreactivity in the nose comes from the observations in the lower airways of asthmatics, where this phenomenon, manifested as an increased physiological response to histamine, cholinergic agonists, such as methacholine, and physical challenges, such as dry air hyperventilation, is felt to be the most characteristic feature of asthma (Boushey et al., 1980). Hyperreactivity of the lower airways was formerly thought to represent an intrinsic, probably neural, defect, which led to the asthmatic condition (Szentivanyi, 1968; Henderson et al., 1979). More recent investigations, however, have linked this phenomenon to antigen-induced, lower airway inflammation (Cockroft et al., 1977; Sotomayor et al., 1984; Laitinen et al., 1985). Although asthmatic subjects, even when asymptomatic, usually demonstrate increased nonspecific reactivity to inhaled methacholine or histamine, patients with seasonal allergic rhinitis, when out of the pollen season, do not seem to differ from normal controls with regard to their physiological response to intranasal administration of these agents (McLean et al., 1977). Part of this discrepancy may be due to the fact that even asymptomatic asthmatics demonstrate evidence of ongoing inflammation in BAL fluids (Liu et al., 1990), whereas no inflammatory abnormalities can be detected in asymptomatic rhinitis (Hastie et al., 1979).

When patients with perennial rhinitis are studied, however, their secretory nasal response to methacholine is greater than in normals (Borum, 1979). In our hands, the symptoms and the vascular permeability in response to intranasal histamine provocation are greatly enhanced in individuals with perennial allergic rhinitis compared to normal controls. In patients with seasonal allergic rhinitis who are asymptomatic and out of the pollen season, the reactivity to histamine and to methacholine is increased after antigen challenge (Andersson et al., 1989; Baroody et al., 1990; Walden et al., 1991). This can be abolished by prior treatment with topical steroids (Andersson et al., 1989; Baroody et al., 1990). The induction of nasal hyperreactivity correlates with the antigen-induced inflammation as assessed by the influx of eosinophils, neutrophils, and alcian blue–positive cells in nasal lavages, 24 hr after antigen challenge (Walden et al., 1991). However, nasal nonspecific hyperreactivity is different from nasal priming to antigen: the former assumes that the target organ in the mucosa, such as the gland or vessel, overreacts to a stimulus, such as an inflammatory mediator, whereas the latter, in addition to hyperreactivity, involves the production of more mediators in response to antigen.

It is not clear whether natural antigenic exposure during the pollen season will result in nonspecific nasal mucosal hyperreactivity. Bedard and his colleagues (1989) report that the reactivity to histamine, as assessed by nasal airway resistance, is higher in patients with nasal pollinosis, during the allergy season, compared to a group of normal subjects. In Naclerio's hands, however, the seasonal antigenic exposure to ragweed increased only the baseline nasal vascular permeability, but did not seem to shift the histamine dose-response curve to the left (Naclerio et al., 1989a).

In several studies we have demonstrated that a number of individuals develop rhinorrhea and nasal congestion when they inhale dry air through the nose and have shown that inflammatory mediators, some of which are mast cell derived, are released in nasal secretions during this reaction (Togias et al., 1985, 1986a). A discussion of the mechanism of this phenomenon is beyond the scope of this review, but our evidence points toward a role of increased osmolality of the epithelium lining fluid resulting from the drying effect of inhaled air and leading to mast cell activation and to neuronal reflex activity (Togias et al., 1988; Cruz et al., in press). Recent data demonstrate that, 24 hr after nasal antigen challenge, allergic individuals who had minimal responsiveness to dry air at baseline develop a significantly more pronounced reaction to the same stimulus (unpublished observations). We have also found that the nasal response to inhalation of cold, dry air is enhanced in patients with perennial disease compared to normal controls (unpublished observations). The nasal dry air reaction cannot be characterized as nonspecific, since it seems to involve a specific, quite complex, mechanism. It represents the only example of a physical stimulus leading to a nasal response that can be potentiated by inflammation. From that aspect, it can also be used as a tool to understand how antigen-induced inflammation may affect the clinical presentation of allergic rhinitis.

D. Known and Missing Links Between the Early and Late, Antigen-Induced, Inflammatory Phenomena

It is clear that the antigen-IgE interaction on the surface of mast cells in nasal epithelium initiates the acute allergic response and that both preformed and newly generated mast cell mediators are responsible for the induction of the acute symptoms. Histamine seems to play a major role in this inflammatory phase since it can mimic the acute symptoms of allergic rhinitis and since all H_1 receptor antagonists demonstrate impressive efficacy in inhibiting the early response (Togias et al., 1986b; Naclerio et al., 1989b, 1990). Our understanding of the pathogenesis of the late events following antigen provocation is much less developed. The significant knowledge that has been recently acquired is still rather descriptive. The mechanisms behind the infiltration of eosinophils and basophils and the phenomena of the late spontaneous mediator release, the late rhinitic symptoms, priming to antigen, and the development of nonspecific hyperreactivity are elusive.

It is possible that infiltration of cells, with a predominance of eosinophils (Bascom et al., 1988b) and the distinct increase in basophils, may be attributed to some of the acutely released inflammatory mediators. PAF is a potent eosinophil chemoattractant (Wardlaw et al., 1986), and LTB_4 has the same effect on neutrophils (Palmblad et al., 1981). Bochner et al. (1990) recently showed that interleukin (IL)-1, a known promoter of cellular recruitment and a cytokine that potentiates mediator release, is released locally, during the cutaneous allergic late-phase reaction. Il-1 activates vascular endothelium and induces the expression of adhesion molecules for leukocytes, including ELAM-1, ICAM-1, and VCAM-1 (Bochner et al., 1990). Preliminary data from the skin blister model suggest that additional cytokines such as IL-3 and GM-CSF, which have marked proinflammatory effects on basophils and eosinophils, including activation, priming, and prolongation of survival, are also present during the late-phase reaction (unpublished observations). Unfortunately, such data are not available in the nose at this time.

The spontaneous release of mediators during late inflammation, probably from basophils and eosinophils, is another unexplained phenomenon. Both basophils and eosinophils from late fluids have acquired the so-called "hypodense" phenotype, which implies a state of activation (unpublished observations). Blood basophils from patients with asthma demonstrate increased releasability to certain stimuli (Findlay and Lichtenstein, 1980). Recently, similar findings were reported for the basophils of patients with symptomatic allergic rhinitis (Casolaro et al., 1990). In studies in our laboratory designed to answer questions on the mechanism of late mediator release, nasal lavages obtained during the late inflammatory stage contained histamine-releasing factors (HRF) with characteristics similar to those from cultured human alveolar macrophages (Schulman et al., 1985). Several forms of HRF have been described, some of them IgE dependent (MacDonald and Lichtenstein, 1990). Since purification and characterization of these factors have not been yet accomplished, their source in nasal secretions and the stimulus for their release are totally unknown. However, they may play an important role in providing the missing link between early antigen challenge and the late mediator release.

The mechanisms of nasal priming can be diverse. The presence of additional target cells, such as basophils, increased releasability of resident cells, increased penetration of antigen through a disrupted epithelium, and reduction in the ability of the mucosa to catabolize mediators are some, theoretically plausible, causes. Since, however, nonspecific mucosal hyperreactivity also occurs following antigen challenge, the primed clinical response to antigen may be partly due to this phenomenon, as well. The mechanisms of antigen-induced hyperreactivity have not been examined. Two specific questions need to be addressed. First, hyperreactivity needs to be characterized with regard to each of the mucosal end-organs. Specific methods to evaluate the responses of vessels, glands, and irritant receptors should be developed. Second, each inflammatory element, especially the eosinophil leukocyte, requires closer investigation with regard to its potential effects on the end-organs. This type of investigation can be more easily performed in the nasal mucosa than in the lower airways. Therefore, the nose will serve as a model in our efforts to understand basic elements of the pathogenesis of lower airway disease.

E. A Reappraisal of the Clinical Picture of Allergic Rhinitis

Based on our recently acquired knowledge on the events that follow nasal antigen challenge in patients with allergic rhinitis, it is important to review the clinical features of the natural disease and attempt to provide a more complete hypothesis on their pathogenesis.

The bouts of sneezing, facial pruritus, lacrimation, watery rhinorrhea, and nasal congestion that constitute part of the clinical picture can be attributed to the acute inhalation of a relatively high dose of antigen that is deposited on the nasal mucosa and generates an early-phase reaction. It has been estimated that, during a typical ragweed season, approximately 63 pollen grains enter the nasal cavities every hour, the level reaching 350 at the peak of the season (Marsh, 1975). However, when patients with seasonal rhinitis are challenged with antigen in the laboratory, out of the pollen season, it is unusual to detect a significant clinical response or inflammatory mediators in lavage fluids with insufflation of less than 10,000 grains of pollen (Wachs et al., 1989). This large discrepancy may be explained by introducing the concept of priming into the pathogenetic model. In Wachs's study, in which nasal provocation was repeated daily for 3 days, several individuals released inflammatory mediators when challenge with only 100 pollen grains, even on the second day (Wachs et al., 1989). As mentioned earlier, priming probably also explains the 1–2-week lag phenomenon in symptom reduction observed while the pollen counts are decreasing (Norman et al., 1988).

The symptoms that patients with allergic rhinitis frequently attribute to environmental irritants may be explained by the development of nonspecific mucosal hyperreactivity, as a result of antigen-induced inflammation. These complaints are more common in patients with perennial allergic rhinitis, which is a more severe and resistant form of the disease. One would expect, for example, that cigarette smoke, which is known to activate irritant receptors (Barnes, 1986), will result in more potent reflex activity in the inflamed nose, compared to the normal condition. The same may be true for gases such as ammonia, sulfur dioxide, and ozone. Furthermore, if the inflammatory hyperreactivity affects not only the irritant receptors but also the targets of the reflex arc, such as the submucosal glands and the nasal vessels, one would expect that the end result of the irritant response will be even more potentiated in the presence of inflammation. The same may be true for stimuli other than environmental irritants, which patients frequently describe under the category of "weather, temperature, or humidity changes." The nasal reactivity to dry air is a well-established example.

As we previously emphasized, the chronic symptomatology of patients with allergic rhinitis differs from the acute bouts of rhinitic symptoms and resembles more the symptomatology appearing in the late stages after experimental antigen provocation. This symptomatology, as well as the elevated mediator levels during the late inflammatory stage, are almost totally inhibited by a 3-day pretreatment with 60 mg of oral prednisone, whereas the early response to antigen remains unaffected (Pipkorn et al., 1987a). These observations emphasize the clinical importance of the late-phase symptomatology and its pathogenesis. It is, therefore, conceivable that the chronic symptoms of the disease are, at least in part, manifestations of multiple, antigen-induced, late reactions, interwoven with sporadic acute reactions to inhalation of relatively higher doses of antigen. Adding the nonspecific irritant responses to this picture creates a much more complex, but probably more realistic, model. There is little doubt that the common denominator in this model is the chronic, antigen-induced, nasal mucosal inflammation.

IV. Rationalizing the Approach to the Management of Allergic Rhinitis

It was not the intention of this chapter to cover the details of managing allergic rhinitis. We would like, however, to emphasize certain concepts. Allergic rhinitis should be regarded as a chronic inflammatory condition and should be treated as such. This approach directs our emphasis to any form of treatment that can resolve or, most important, prevent the development of inflammation. In this respect, allergen avoidance and local treatment with glucocorticosteroids should play strategic roles in the management of the disease.

The emphasis with regard to allergen avoidance should be mainly directed to the indoor environment and, therefore, to the allergens from dust mites, cockroaches, pets, and fungi. Not only are indoor allergens more amenable to some control, but, at least with regard to the lower airways, their avoidance has been clearly associated with symptomatic improvement and with reduction of inflammatory correlates such as hyperreactivity to methacholine (Platts-Mills et al., 1982, 1987, 1988; Kang et al., 1989; Owen et al., 1990). Unfortunately, the increasing impact of indoor allergens is to a great extent secondary to the changing life-style of the industrialized world population: not only does this population spend progressively more time indoors, but the air quality of the indoor environment is clearly deteriorating, in closed, poorly ventilated buildings (Samet et al., 1987).

Apart from reducing the exposure to the etiological agents, preventing inflammation involves several steps. To the extent that the basic, mast cell–bound IgE-antigen interaction leads not only to acute symptomatology, but also to the late stages of inflammation, inhibition of mast cell activation may be of major importance in the management of the disease. Unfortunately, a definitive link between mast cell activation and late inflammation has not been established. In theory, some of the known properties of the mediators released during the acute response to antigen can be regarded as promoting inflammation, with vascular dilatation and increased permeability having a central role. Although this concept has not been clinically examined in detail, it is conceivable that even a simple antihistamine may play a role in inhibiting the development of inflammation. If that is the case, the attitude of administering these agents on an "as needed" basis, in order to simply antagonize some of the acute symptomatology of allergic rhinitis, may be inadequate, and continuous treatment with antihistamines may be more effective. The same concept should apply to the antagonists against other acute mediators, which are currently being developed.

The anti-inflammatory properties of steroids are well established, but their mechanism(s) of action in allergic diseases is not entirely known. Several known effects of steroids may be crucial in their antiallergic activity. For example, these agents may be able to reduce the number of mast cells in the nasal mucosa, when applied topically, for prolonged periods of time (Okuda et al., 1983). In vitro incubation of human basophils with steroids inhibits the IgE-dependent release of histamine and LTC_4 (Schleimer et al., 1981). This property becomes very important as the role of basophils in the late stages of the antigen-induced inflammatory response is appreciated. Steroids reduce the chemotactic and the adherence abilities of eosinophils (Clark et al., 1979; Altman et al., 1981), and have inhibitory effects on the production and the activity of several cytokines that seem to be central in regulating the inflammatory response (Schleimer, 1990). In our hands, topical nasal steroids have very potent and diverse actions. One week of pretreatment with flunisolide inhibits mediator release and the symptoms of the early reaction to antigen (Pipkorn et al., 1987b). Furthermore, it prevents the late elevations in lavage fluid mediator levels and inhibits the symptoms of the late reaction (Pipkorn et al., 1987b). The infiltration of eosinophils and basophils is also inhibited (Bascom et al., 1988a,b). In the same study, flunisolide inhibited the priming response to antigen 12 hr after the first challenge (Pipkorn et al., 1987b), and in another study, beclomethasone diproprionate inhibited the antigen-induced increase in nasal reactivity to histamine (Baroody et al., 1990). Most recently, we have found that the seasonal increase in both the serum ragweed-specific IgE and the nasal secretion IgE in patients with ragweed pollinosis was inhibited by treatment with topical triamcinolone throughout the pollen season (unpublished observations). These findings clearly demonstrate the multilevel effectiveness of topical steroids in allergic rhinitis. It is worth emphasizing that the prevention of all indices of antigen-induced inflammation was the dominant characteristic in these studies, so that the clinical approach should be the same: patients with seasonal rhinitis should be placed on such treatment before the pollen appears in the air.

Acknowledgments

This work was supported by Grants AI 08270, HL 37119, and AI 07290 from the National Institutes of Health, Bethesda, Maryland.

Discussion

Casale: When were the lavages done after antigen challenge of the lungs? If they were performed prior to or during the late phase reaction (LPR), is it fair to state that the cells were clinically important in causing the LPR?

Lichtenstein: The lavages were done 18–24 hr after the initial lavage. As it is impossible to do close kinetics in the lungs, we have to rely on data derived from all three in vivo systems.

Kaplan: I was surprised to see that corticosteroids (CCS) did not affect neutrophil migration in the skin model.

Schleimer: In the nasal and skin models, oral CCS inhibits the infiltration of eosinophils and basophils, but not neutrophils. Topical CCS inhibits neutrophil infiltration as well. These selective differences between the routes of CCS administration might relate to the eosinopenia and basopenia seen after oral CCS or to the inhibition of VCAM (an endothelial adhesion molecule that selectively binds eosinophils and basophils, but not neutrophils) expression.

Claman: The inhibition of neutrophil influx into the skin was demonstrated by Dale and Fauci using skin windows. The results you present in the airway are different, perhaps indicating that each target organ will have to be assessed individually.

Schwartz: The major site of PGD_2 synthetase may be antigen-processing cells in the skin and other tissues. Can you really tell if mast cells are the major source of PGD_2?
Lichtenstein: We do not know which other cells may be contributing PGD_2.
Stevens: Will the ratio of LTC_4/PGD_2 production by mast cells change with repeated allergen challenges?
Lichtenstein: We cannot repeatedly challenge mast cells or basophils in vitro because they become desensitized.
Lee: Do basophils infiltrate the mucosa after cold, dry air challenge?
Lichtenstein: We have not looked.
Casale: In the skin model you showed that increased IL-1 and the number of basophils paralleled each other. If you believe that the IL-1 is important in induction of increased basophil adherence to newly expressed adhesion molecules, wouldn't you have expected the IL-1 to increase first, as it takes hours for the adhesion molecules to be expressed?
Lichtenstein: When you begin to see an inflammatory marker in the supernatant, it may have been in the tissues much earlier.
Schleimer: The source of IL-1 in the blister model is unknown and may well be mononuclear cells that infiltrate during the LPR. It is known that ELAM expression occurs within 2–4 hr after antigen challenge. These data suggest that IL-1 or other tissue activator (such as TNF) is released rapidly after antigen challenge.
Denburg: Basophils and eosinophils found in LPR may also arise from progenitor cells among the chronic inflammatory cells. The accepted phenotypes of mast cells and basophils may be altered under the inflamed conditions found after repeated allergen challenges and might actually appear to be intermediate forms, for which no established criteria for absolute identification exist.
Dvorak: Published studies employing plastic-embedded sections have shown that mature basophils and eosinophils marginate and migrate into the skin during LPR.
Claman: In Colorado, the rhinorrhea seen after cold-air challenge is called "skier's nose." My colleague, Bill Silvers, treats this condition with topical ipratropium, suggesting that it is mediated through the parasympathetic system. Can you comment?
Lichtenstein: Atropine partially inhibits the response to cold, dry air but not antigen.

References

Ackerman, S. J., Kephart, G. M., Habermann, T. M., Greipp, P. R., and Gleich, G. J. (1983). Localization of eosinophil granule major basic protein in human basophils. *J. Exp. Med.* 158:946.

Altman, L. C., Hills, J. S., Hairfield, W. M., and Mullarkey, M. F. (1981). Effects of corticosteroids on eosinophil chemotaxis and adherence. *J. Clin. Invest.* 67:28.

Andersson, M., Andersson, P., and Pipkorn, U. (1989). Allergen-induced specific and non-specific nasal reactions. Reciprocal relationship and inhibition by topical glucocorticosteroids. *Acta Otolaryngol.* (*Stockh.*) 107:270.

Arnoux, B., David, D., and Benveniste, J. (1980). Release of platelet activating factor (Paf-acether) from alveolar macrophages by the calcium ionophore A23187 and phagocytosis. *Eur. J. Clin. Invest.* 10:437.

Bacon, J. R., McLean, J. A., Mathews, K. P., and Banas, J. M. (1981). Priming of the nasal mucosa by ragweed extract or by an irritant (ammonia). *J. Allergy Clin. Immunol.* 67:111.

Baraniuk, J. N., Lundgren, J. D., Mizoguchi, H., et al. (1990). Bradykinin and respiratory mucus membranes. Analysis of bradykinin binding site distribution and secretory responses in vitro and in vivo. *Am. Rev. Respir. Dis.* 141:706.

Barnes, P. J. (1986). Neural control of human airways in health and disease. *Am. Rev. Respir. Dis.* 134:1289.

Baroody, F., Lichtenstein, L. M., Kagey-Sobotka, A., Proud, D., and Naclerio, R. M. (1990). Topical steroids inhibit antigen-induced nasal hyperreactivity to histamine. *J. Allergy Clin. Immunol.* 85:163 (abstract).

Bascom, R., Wachs, M., Naclerio, R. M., Pipkorn, U., Galli, S. J., and Lichtenstein, L. M. (1988a). Basophil influx occurs after nasal antigen challenge: Effects of topical corticosteroid pretreatment. *J. Allergy Clin. Immunol.* 81:580.

Bascom, R., Pipkorn, U., Lichtenstein, L. M., and Naclerio, R. M. (1988b). The influx of inflammatory cells into nasal washings during the late response to antigen challenge. Effect of steroid pretreatment. *Am. Rev. Respir. Dis.* 138:406.

Bascom, R., Pipkorn, U., Proud, D., et al. (1989). Major basic protein and eosinophil-derived neurotoxin concentrations in nasal lavage fluid after antigen challenge: Effect of systemic corticosteroids and relationship to eosinophil influx. *J. Allergy Clin. Immunol.* 84:338.

Baumgarten, C. R., Togias, A. G., Naclerio, R. M., Lichtenstein, L. M., Norman, P. S., and Proud, D. (1985). Influx of kininogens into nasal secretions following antigen challenge of allergic individuals. *J. Clin. Invest.* 76:191.

Baumgarten, C. R., Nichols, R. C., Naclerio, R. M., Lichtenstein, L. M., Norman, P. S., and Proud, D. (1986). Plasma kallikrein during experimentally induced allergic rhinitis: Role of kinin formation and contribution to TAME-esterase activity in nasal secretions. *J. Immunol.* 137:977.

Bedard, P. M., Jobin, M., Clement, L., Mourad, W., and Hebert, J. (1989). Evaluation of nonspecific nasal reactivity to histamine during and after natural ragweed pollen exposure. *Am. J. Rhinol.* 3:211.

Bernstein, I. L., and Safferman, R. (1973). Clinical sensitivity to green algae demonstrated by nasal challenge and in vitro tests of immediate hypersensitivity. *J. Allergy Clin. Immunol.* 51:22.

Bienenstock, J., Befus, A. D., Pearce, F., Denburg, J., and Goodacre, R. (1982). Mast cell heterogeneity: Derivation and function with emphasis on the intestine. *J. Allergy Clin. Immunol.* 70:407.

Bisgaard, H., Olsson, P., and Bende, M. (1984). Leukotriene D_4 increases nasal blood flow in humans. *Prostaglandins* 27:599.

Blackley, C. H. (1873). Experimental researches on the cause and nature of catarrhus aestivus (hay fever or hay asthma). Bailliere, Tindell and Cox; reprinted 1959 by Dawson's of Pall Mall, London, pp. 77.

Bochner, B. S., Lamas, A. M., Benenati, S. V., and Schleimer, R. P. (1990). On the central role of vascular endothelium in allergic reactions. In *Late Phase Allergic Reactions*. Edited by R. Dorsh. Boca Raton, FL, CRC Press, pp. 221.

Bochner, B. S., Charlesworth, E. N., Lichtenstein, L. M., et al. (1990). Interleukin-1 is released at sites of human cutaneous allergic reactions. *J. Allergy Clin. Immunol.* 86:830.

Booij-Nord, H., Orie, N. G. M., and de Vries, K. (1971). Immediate and late bronchial obstructive reactions to inhalation of house dust and protective effect of disodium cromoglycate and prednisolone. *J. Allergy Clin. Immunol.* 48:344.

Borum, P. (1979). Nasal methacholine challenge. A test for the measurement of nasal reactivity. *J. Allergy Clin. Immunol.* 63:253.

Boushey, H. A., Holtzman, M. J., Sheller, J. R., and Nadel, J. A. (1980). Bronchial hyperreactivity. *Am. Rev. Respir. Dis.* 121:389.

Brown, M., Peters, S. P., Adkinson, N. F., Jr., et al. (1987). Arachidonic acid metabolites during nasal challenge. *Arch. Otol–Head Neck Surg.* 113:179.

Capron, A., Dessaint, J. P., Capron, M., and Joseph, M. (1983). IgE receptors on different cell lines and their role in triggering different immunologic mechanisms. In *Proceedings of the XII Congress of European Academy of Allergology and Clinical Immunology*. Rome, OIC Medical, pp. 17.

Capron, M., Spiegelberg, H. L., Prin, L., Bennich, H., Butterworth, A. G., and Pierce, R. J. (1984). Role of IgE receptors in effector function of human eosinophils. *J. Immunol.* 132:462.

Casolaro, V., Spadaro, G., and Marone, G. (1990). Human basophil releasability. VI. Changes in basophil releasability in patients with allergic rhinitis or bronchial asthma. *Am. Rev. Respir. Dis.* 142:1108.

Castells, M., and Schwartz, L. B. (1988). Tryptase levels in nasal-lavage fluid as an indicator of the immediate allergic response. *J. Allergy Clin. Immunol.* 82:348.

Chan-Yeung, M., Kinsella, M., Chan, H., Lam, S., Tse, K. S., and Salari, H. (1988). Release of histamine, prostaglandins, and leukotrienes after antigen challenge in hayfever subjects. *Am. J. Rhinol.* 2:183.

Charlesworth, E. N., Hood, A. F., Soter, N. A., Kagey-Sobotka, A., Norman, P. S., and Lichtenstein, L. M. (1989). Cutaneous late-phase response to allergen. Mediator release and inflammatory cell infiltration. *J. Clin. Invest.* 83:1519.

Clark, R. A. F., Gallin, J. I., and Fauci, A. S. (1979). Effects of in vivo prednisone on in vitro eosinophil and neutrophil adherence and chemotaxis. *Blood* 53:633.

Cockroft, D. W., Ruffin, R. E., Dolovich, J., and Hargreave, F. E. (1977). Allergen-induced increase in nonallergic bronchial reactivity. *Clin. Allergy* 7:503.

Cohan, V. L., Massey, W. A., Gittlen, S. D., et al. (1989). The heterogeneity of human histamine containing cells. In *Mast Cell and Basophil Differentiation and Function in Health and Disease*. Edited by S. J. Galli and K. F. Austen. New York, Raven Press, pp. 149.

Collins, J. G. (1988). Prevalence of selected chronic conditions, United States, 1983–85. Advance Data from Vital and Health Statistics, 1988; No. 155, DHHS Pub. No. (PHS) 88-1250. Hyattsville, MD, Public Health Service.

Connell, J. T. (1967). Quantitative intranasal pollen challenges. I. Apparatus design and technique. *J. Allergy* 39:358.

Connell, J. T. (1968). Quantitative intranasal pollen challenges. II. Effect of daily pollen challenge, environmental pollen exposure and placebo challenge on the nasal membrane. *J. Allergy* 41:123.

Connell, J. T. (1969). Quantitative intranasal pollen challenges: III. The priming effect in allergic rhinitis. *J. Allergy* 43:33.

Creticos, P. S., Peters, S. P., Adkinson, N. F., Jr., Naclerio, R. M., Norman, P. S., and Lichtenstein, L. M. (1984). Peptide leukotriene release after antigen challenge in patients sensitive to ragweed. *N. Engl. J. Med.* 310:1626.

Cruz, A. A., Naclerio, R. M., Lichtenstein, L. M., and Togias, A. G. (1990). Further support for the role of hypertonicity on mast cell activation during nasal dry air reactions. *Clin. Res.* 38:484A (abstract).

Cruz, A. A., Togias, A. G., Lichtenstein, L. M., Kagey-Sobotka, A., Proud, D., and Naclerio, R. M. Local application of atropine attenuates the upper airway reaction to cold, dry air. *Am. Rev. Respir. Dis.* (in press).

Dale, H. H., and Laidlaw, P. P. (1910). The physiological action of **b**-imidazolylethylamine. *J. Physiol.* 41:318.

Dale, H. H., and Laidlaw, P. P. (1919). Histamine shock. *J. Physiol.* 52:355.

Dolovich, J., Bach, N., and Arbesman, C. (1970). Kinin-like activity in nasal secretions of allergic patients. *Int. Arch. Allergy Appl. Immunol.* 38:337.

Dolovich, J., Hargreave, F. E., Chalmers, R., Shier, K. J., Gauldie, J., and Bienenstock, J. (1973). Late cutaneous allergic responses in isolated IgE-dependent reactions. *J. Allergy* 52:38.

Doyle, W. J., Skoner, D. P., and Boehm, S. (1989). Human responses to intranasal challenge with bradykinin, histamine, prostaglandin D_2 and PGF_{2a}. In *Proceedings of the VIII International Symposium on Infection and Allergy of the Nose*. Baltimore, abst. #139.

Dvoracek, J. E., Yunginger, J. W., Kerr, E. B., Hyatt, R. E., and Gleich, G. J. (1984). Induction of nasal late phase reactions by insufflation of ragweed pollen extract. *J. Allergy Clin. Immunol.* 73:363.

Eggleston, P., Hendley, J., Gwaltney, J., Eggleston, A., and Leavell, B. (1978). Histamine in nasal secretions. *Int. Arch. Allergy Appl. Immunol.* 57:193.

Enerback, L. (1981). The gut mucosal mast cell. *Monogr. Allergy* 17:222.

Findlay, S. R., and Lichtenstein, L. M. (1980). Basophil "releasability" in patients with asthma. *Am. Rev. Respir. Dis.* 122:53.

Freeland, H. S., Pipkorn, U., Schleimer, R. P., et al. (1989). Leukotriene B_4 as a mediator of early and late reactions to antigen in humans. The effect of systemic glucocorticoid treatment in vivo. *J. Allergy Clin. Immunol.* 83:634.

Friedman, M. M., and Kaliner, M. (1985). In situ degranulation of human nasal mucosal mast cells: Ultrastructural features and cell-cell associations. *J. Allergy Clin. Immunol.* 76:70.

Galli, S. J., Dvorak, A. M., and Dvorak, H. F. (1984). Basophils and mast cells:

Okazaki, T., Reisman, R., and Arbesman, C. (1977). Prostaglandin E in the secretions of allergic rhinitis. *Prostaglandins* 13:681.

Okuda, M., and Otsuka, H. (1977). Basophilic cells in allergic nasal secretions. *Arch. Oto-Rhino-Laryngol.* 214:283.

Okuda, M., and Otsuka, H. (1987). Heterogeneity of human nasal mast cell. In *Immunobiology, Histophysiology and Tumor Immunology in Otolaryngology*. Proceedings 2nd International Academic Conference. Amsterdam/Berkeley, Kugler Publications. pp. 317.

Okuda, M., Kawabori, S., and Otsuka, H. (1978). Electron microscope study of basophilic cells in allergic nasal secretions. *Arch. Otolaryngol.* 221:215.

Okuda, M., Sakaguchi, K., and Otsuka, H. (1983). Intranasal beclomethasone: mode of action in nasal allergy. *Ann. Allergy* 50:116.

Okuda, M., Otsuka, H., and Kawabori, S. (1985). Characteristics and role of the surface basophilic cells in nasal allergy. In *Immunobiology, Autoimmunity and Transplantation in Otorhinolaryngology*. Edited by B. Veldman, et al. Amsterdam/Berkeley, Kugler Publications, pp. 267.

Ophir, D., Fink, A., Eliraz, A., Tabachnik, E., and Bentwich, Z. (1988). Allergen-induced leukotriene production by nasal mucosa and peripheral blood leukocytes. *Arch. Otolaryngol. Head Neck Surg.* 114:522.

Owen, S., Morganstern, M., Hepworth, J., and Woodcock, A. (1990). Control of house dust mite antigen in bedding. *Lancet* 335:396.

Palmblad, J., Malmsten, C. L., Uden, A-M., Radmark, O., Engstedt, L., and Samuelsson, B. (1981). Leukotriene B_4 is a potent and stereospecific stimulator of neutrophil chemotaxis and adherence. *Blood* 58:658.

Pelican, Z. (1978). Late and delayed responses of the nasal mucosa to allergen challenge. *Ann. Allergy* 41:37.

Peters, S. P., MacGlashan, D. W., Schulman, E. S., et al. (1984). Arachidonic acid metabolism in purified human lung mast cells. *J. Immunol.* 132:1972.

Pipkorn, U., Karlsson, G., and Bake, B. (1984). Effect of platelet activating factor on the human nasal mucosa. *Allergy* 39:141.

Pipkorn, U., Proud, D., Lichtenstein, L. M., et al. (1987a). Effect of short-term systemic glucocorticoid treatment on human nasal mediator release after antigen challenge. *J. Clin. Invest.* 80:957.

Pipkorn, U., Proud, D., Lichtenstein, L. M., Kagey-Sobotka, A., Norman, P. S., and Naclerio, R. M. (1987b). Inhibition of mediator release in allergic rhinitis by pretreatment with topical glucocorticosteroids. *N. Engl. J. Med.* 316:1506.

Platts-Mills, T. A. E., Mitchell, E. B., Nock, P., Tovey, E. R., Moszoro, H., and Wilkins, S. R. (1982). Reduction of bronchial hyperreactivity during prolonged allergen avoidance. *Lancet* 2:675.

Platts-Mills, T. A. E., and Chapman, M. D. (1987). Dust mite: Immunology, allergic disease, and environmental control. *J. Allergy Clin. Immunol.* 80:755.

Platts-Mills, T. A. E., Mitchell, E. B., Chapman, M. D., and Heymann, P. W. (1988). Dust mite allergy: Its clinical significance. *Hosp. Practice* February 15:167.

Price, J. A., Pollock, I., Little, S. A., Longbottom, J. L., and Warner, J. O. (1990). Measurement of airborne mite antigen in homes of asthmatic children. *Lancet* 336:895.

Proud, D., Togias, A., Naclerio, R. M., Crush, S. A., Norman, P. S., and Lichtenstein, L. M. (1983). Kinins are generated in vivo following nasal airway challenge of allergic individuals with allergen. *J. Clin. Invest.* 72:1678.

Proud, D., Reynolds, C. J., Lacarpa, S., Kagey-Sobotka, A., Lichtenstein, L. M., and Naclerio, R. M. (1988). Nasal provocation with bradykinin induces symptoms of rhinitis and a sore throat. *Am. Rev. Respir. Dis.* 137:613.

Rankin, J. A., Hitchcock, M., Merrill, W., Bach, M. K., Brashler, J. R., and Askenase, P. W. (1982). IgE-dependent release of leukotriene C_4 from alveolar macrophages. *Nature* 297:329.

Ricketti, A. J. (1985). Allergic rhinitis. In *Allergic Diseases. Diagnosis and Management*. Edited by R. Patterson. Philadelphia, Lippincott, pp. 207.

Robertson, D. J., Kerigan, A. T., Hargreave, F. E., Chalmers, R., and Dolovich, J. (1974). Late asthmatic responses induced by ragweed pollen allergen. *J. Allergy Clin. Immunol.* 54:244.

Salvaggio, J. E., Cavanaugh, J. J. A., Lowell, F. C., and Leskowitz, S. (1964). A comparison of the immunologic responses of normal and atopic individuals to intranasally administered antigen. *J. Allergy* 35:62.

Samet, J. M., Marbury, M. C., and Spengler, J. D. (1987). Health effects and sources of indoor air pollution. Part I. *Am. Rev. Respir. Dis.* 136:1486.

Schleimer, R. P. (1990). Effects of glucocorticosteroids on inflammatory cells relevant to their therapeutic applications in asthma. *Am. Rev. Respir. Dis.* 141:S59.

Schleimer, R. P., Lichtenstein, L. M., and Gillespie, E. (1981). Inhibition of basophil histamine release by antiinflammatory steroids. *Nature* 292:454.

Schulman, E. S., Proud, D., Liu, M. C., MacGlashan, D. W., Lichtenstein, L. M., and Plaut, M. (1985). Human lung macrophages induce histamine release from basophils and mast cells. *Am. Rev. Respir. Dis.* 131:230.

Schumacher, M. J., and Pain, M. C. F. (1979). Nasal challenge testing in grass pollen hay fever. *J. Allergy Clin. Immunol.* 64:202.

Schwartz, L. B., and Austen, K. F. (1988). The mast cell and mediators of immediate hypersensitivity. In *Immunological Diseases*. Edited by M. Samter, T. W. Talmage, M. M. Frank, K. F. Austen, and H. N. Claman. Boston, Little, Brown, pp. 157.

Schwartz, L. B., Kawahara, M. S., Hugli, T. E., Vik, D., Fearon, D. T., and Austen, K. F. (1983). Generation of C3a anaphylatoxin from human C3 by human mast cell tryptase. *J. Immunol.* 130:1891.

Secher, C., Kirkegaard, J., Borum, P., Maansson, A., Osterhammel, P., and Mygind, N. (1982). Significance of H_1 and H_2 receptors in the human nose: rationale for topical use of combined antihistamine preparations. *J. Allergy Clin. Immunol.* 70:211.

Sekizawa, C., Caughey, G. H., Lazarus, S. C., Gold, W. M., and Nadel, J. A. (1989). Mast cell tryptase causes airway smooth muscle hyperresponsiveness in dogs. *J. Clin. Invest.* 83:175.

Shaw, R. J., Fitzharris, P., Cromwell, O., Wardlaw, A. J., and Kay, A. B. (1985). Allergen-induced release of sulphidopeptide leukotrienes (SRS-A) and LTB_4 in allergic rhinitis. *Allergy* 40:1.

Silberstein, D. S., Owen, W. F., Gasson, J. C., et al. (1986). Enhancement of human

eosinophil cytotoxicity and leukotriene synthesis by biosynthetic (recombinant) granulocyte-macrophage colony-stimulating factor. *J. Immunol.* 137:3290.
Siraganian, R. P., and Hook, W. A. (1977). Mechanism of histamine release by formyl methionine-containing peptides. *J. Immunol.* 119:2078.
Skoner, D. P., Doyle, W. J., Boehm, S., and Fireman, P. (1989). Priming of the nose and eustachian tube during natural pollen exposure. *Am. J. Rhinol.* 3:53.
Solley, G. O., Gleich, G. J., Jordan, R. E., and Schroeter, A. L. (1976). The late phase of the immediate wheal and flare skin reaction. Its dependence upon IgE antibodies. *J. Clin. Invest.* 58:408.
Sotomayor, H., Badier, M., Vervloet, D., et al. (1984). Seasonal increase of carbachol airway responsiveness in patients allergic to grass pollen. *Am. Rev. Respir. Dis.* 130:56.
Sporik, R., Holgate, S. T., Platts-Mills, T. A. E., and Cogswell, J. J. (1990). Exposure to house-dust mite allergen (*Der pI*) and the development of asthma in childhood. A prospective study. *N. Engl. J. Med.* 323:502.
Szentivanyi, A. (1968). The beta-adrenergic theory of the atopic abnormality in bronchial sthma. *J. Allergy* 42:203.
Taylor, G., and Shivalka, P. R. (1971). "Arthus-type" reactivity in the nasal airways and skin in pollen sensitive subjects. *Clin. Allergy* 1:407.
Togias, A. G., Naclerio, R. M., Proud, D., et al. (1985). Nasal challenge with cold, dry air results in the production of inflammatory mediators: Possible mast cell involvement. *J. Clin. Invest.* 76:1375.
Togias, A. G., Naclerio, R. M., Peters, S. P., et al. (1986a). Local generation of sulfidopeptide leukotrienes upon nasal provocation with cold, dry air. *Am. Rev. Respir. Dis.* 133:1133.
Togias, A. G., Naclerio, R. M., Warner, J., et al. (1986b). Demonstration of inhibition of mediator release from human mast cells by azatadine base. In vivo and in vitro evaluation. *JAMA* 255:225.
Togias, A. G., Proud, D., Kagey-Sobotka, A., Norman, P. S., Lichtenstein, L. M., and Naclerio, R. M. (1987). The effect of a topical tricyclic antihistamine on the response of the nasal mucosa to challenge with cold, dry air and histamine. *J. Allergy Clin. Immunol.* 79:599.
Togias, A., Proud, D., Lichtenstein, L. M., et al. (1988). The osmolality of nasal secretions increases when inflammatory mediators are released in response to inhalation of cold dry air. *Am. Rev. Respir. Dis.* 137:625.
Tonnesen, P., Hindberg, I., Schaffalitzky, O. B., and Mygind, N. (1988). Effect of nasal allergen challenge on serotonin, substance P and vasoactive intestinal peptide in plasma and nasal secretions. *Allergy* 43:310.
Triggiani, M., Hubbard, W. C., and Chilton, F. H. (1990). Synthesis of 1-acyl-2acetyl-sn-glycero-3-phosphocholine by an enriched preparation of the human lung mast cell. *J. Immunol.* 144:4773.
Turkeltaub, P. C., and Gergen, P. J. (1988). The prevalence of allergic and non-allergic respiratory symptoms in the U.S. population: Data from the national health and nutrition examination survey, 1976–80 (NHANES II). *J. Allergy Clin. Immunol.* 81:305 (abstract).
Volovitz, V., Osur, S. L., Bernstein, J. M., and Ogra, P. L. (1988). Leukotriene C_4

release in upper respiratory mucosa during natural exposure to ragweed in ragweed-sensitive children. *J. Allergy Clin. Immunol.* 82:414.

Wachs, M., Proud, D., Lichtenstein, L. M., Kagey-Sobotka, A., Norman, P. S., and Naclerio, R. M. (1989). Observations on the pathogenesis of nasal priming. *J. Allergy Clin. Immunol.* 84:492.

Walden, S. M., Proud, D., Lichtenstein, L. M., Kagey-Sobotka, A., and Naclerio, R. M. (1991). Antigen-provoked increase in histamine reactivity: Observations on mechanisms. *Am. Rev. Respir. Dis.* 144:642.

Wardlaw, A. J., Moqbel, R., Cromwell, O., and Kay, A. B. (1986). Platelet-activating factor. A potent chemotactic and chemokinetic factor for human eosinophils. *J. Clin. Invest.* 78:1701.

Williams, J. D., Czop, J. K., and Austen, K. F. (1984). Release of leukotrienes by human monocytes on stimulation of their phagocytic receptor for particular activations. *J. Immunol.* 132:3034.

22

Mast Cells in Asthma

THOMAS SCOTT and MICHAEL KALINER

National Institute of Allergy and Infectious Diseases
National Institutes of Health
Bethesda, Maryland

I. Introduction

Over 15 million Americans (about 7% of the U.S. population) suffer from bronchial asthma. Of those aged 30 years or younger, 90% are allergic. Asthmatics more than 40 years old are allergic in half the cases. Since most cells play a central role in allergic diseases, studies have focused on their basic and clinical function.

II. Mast Cell Development

Human mast cells can be grown in culture from bone marrow, cord blood, and fetal liver cells (Denberg, 1990; Yuen et al., 1988). Human hematopoietic cells bearing the CD34 marker develop into metachromatic cells (mast cells/basophils) in vitro when cultured on agarose or 3T3 fibroblasts, plus interleukin-3 (IL-3) (Kirshenbaum et al., 1991; Furitsu et al., 1989). Further development of these precursor cells is likely influenced by additional cytokines. For instance, it appears that CD34+ cells under the influence of IL-3, granulocyte-macrophage colony-stimulating factor (GM-CSF), IL-5, and IL-8 develop into basophils rather than mast cells (Denberg, 1990). IL-3 is required for the growth and maturation of mast cells; however it is postulated that IL-4 and other products of stromal cells influence the development of mast cell precursors. Once committed, these precursor cells might migrate via the circulation to their target tissue where local factors influence terminal differentiation.

III. Mast Cell Distribution

Mast cells are found in the connective tissue of virtually every organ system in the body. They tend to congregate around nerves, blood vessels, and lymphatic vessels. Mast cells are most abundant in the skin, conjunctiva, and gastrointestinal, genitourinary, and respiratory tracts (Metcalfe, 1981). In the lungs, they are located in the intra-alveolar septa, trachea, bronchioles, and bronchi. Human lung mast cells comprise less than 1% of total lung cells (Wasserman, 1980; van Overveld, 1989) and 0.5–3% of cells recovered at bronchoalveolar lavage (BAL) (Flint et al., 1985; Wardlaw et al., 1986). About half of lung mast cells reside in the intra-alveolar septa, with the remainder dispersed in the mucosa and submucosa of the bronchioles and bronchi.

IV. Mast Cell Morphology

Human mast cells are heterogeneous in shape. In sections of lung tissue they may appear oval, round, or trapezoidal, with a mean diameter of 10–12 μ. Some mast cells may assume an alongated shape up to 20 μ in length. The surface of the mast cell has short, filamentous folds. Mast cells are characteristically mononuclear. The cytoplasm contains filaments, Golgi apparatus ribosomes, lipid bodies, and mitochondria. Numerous granules of varying size are found in the cyoplasm. They are smaller more numerous, and more varied in shape than those of basophils. Moreover, the mast cell granule structure shows heterogeneous patterns (scrolls, lattices) when examined by electron microscopy (Fox et al., 1981; Tsao et al., 1977). Each granule is surrounded by a limiting membrane. These features undergo changes when mast cells are activated (Dvorak et al., 1983, 1985; Trotter and Orr, 1973). In early activation, the granules swell within minutes of stimulation. The membranes surrrounding the granules fuse to form channels in the cytoplasm. These channels ultimately form a communication with the cell exterior by fusing with the plasma membrane. The structure of the granule matrix alters once inside the degranulation channels. In the lung, the characteristic mast cell granule structure is that of scrolls that progressively solubilize through intermediate reticular shapes before expulsion as a soluble material.

A recovery period follows these events. The intracytoplasmic channels are sealed. Channel membranes are remodeled and reconstructed. Granule matrix then condenses within the membranes, leading to the restoration of recognizable crystalline structure. The actual mechanism which granule condensation takes place is not yet known (Dvorak, 1991; Dvorak et al., 1987; Caufield, 1980).

V. Mast Cell Heterogeneity

Human mast cells can display phenotypic variation morphologically, histochemically, and functionally (Schulman et al., 1990; Schwartz et al., 1987; Patterson et al., 1980). Strobel and colleagues (1981) noted that the method of fixation affected the numbers of mast cells visualized from specimens. Specifically, human mucosal mast cells fixed in formalin failed to stain metachromatically, a phenomenon described previously in the mouse mucosal mast cell. The use of special fixatives such as Carnoy's or Alcian blue results in better presentation of mast cells for staining (Enerback, 1981). It has been shown that human mast cells contain unique neutral proteases, tryptase, chymase, and carboxypeptidase (Goldstein et al., 1989). Two populations of human mast cells were defined immunohistochemically, one with tryptase and the other with tryptase and chymase (Irani et al., 1986). These neutral proteases are virtually absent in basophils (Castells, 1986). Variability in granule ultrastructure (lattice, scroll) was attributed to graded stages of mast cell activation. However, Craig and Associates (1988, 1989) have shown that scrolls were found in granules from tryptase-positive mast cells, and granules of chymase/tryptase-positive mast cells had a lattice or grating structure. Human lung mast cells are predominantly, but not exclusively, tryptase-positive cells with scroll-like patterns in their granules. Ninety-nine percent of mast cells in the bronchial epithelium, 93% in the alveoli, and 77% in the submucosa contain tryptase only (Irani and Schwartz, 1989).

VI. Mast Cell Secretagogues

The classic method by which mast cells are activated involves cross-linkage of membrane-bound IgE by antigen (Ishizaka et al., 1972; Segal et al., 1977). Monomeric IgE will not trigger the cell. Preparations of oligomers of cross-linked IgE causes receptor aggregation and then mast cell activation. The receptor for IgE ($Fc_\epsilon RI$) has high affinity for IgE. There are about 300,000 high-affinity receptors per mast cell. However, aggregation of only about 100 receptors is required for detectable responses, and maximal histamine release occurs when 10% of receptors are aggregated. IgE, therefore, provides a mechanism for specific antigen-mediated mast cell degranulation.

$FC_\epsilon RI$ aggregation interacts with multiple cellular components in signal transduction. Several reactions have been shown to occur in triggering mast cell degranulation. The enzyme phospholipase C is activated, starting a cascade of reactions leading to hydrolysis of phosphatidylinositol (IP_3). The products of PI hydrolysis [1,2-diacylglycerol (DAG) and inositol 1,4,5-triphosphate] then trigger production of prostaglandins/leukotrienes, activate the enzyme protein kinase C (DAG), and mobilize intracellular calcium (IP_3). Adenylate cyclase is activated by phospholipase C, leading to cAMP production. Cyclic AMP activates phospholipase A_2, an enzyme also thought to be important in histamine release. The exact timing and sequence of these complex reactions have yet to be determined.

In studies of human skin mast cells (predominantly MC_{TC}) a number of nonimmunological agents were found to activate mast cells: poly-L-lysine, compound 48/80 (Morrison and Henson, 1978), complement components C3a and C5a (Gorski et al., 1979), substance P (Hägermark et al., 1978), opiates (Casale et al., 1984), iodinated contrast media, curare, and Ca^{2+} ionophore (A23187) (Foreman et al., 1973). Certain antibiotics and muscle relaxants also act as mast cell secretagogues. Adenosine has been shown to augment IgE-dependent mediator (histamine, leukotriene) release from human lung mast cells by acting at the adenosine (A_2) receptor. This effect is antagonized by theophylline, causing a reduction in IgE-mediated LTC_4 release, but not that of histamine (Peachell et al., 1988; Foreman, 1987). Histamine-releasing factors (HRF) are a heterogeneous group of substances from various sources (macrophages, platelets, eosinophils, granulocytes, endothelial cells, and nasal washings) (White, 1988, 1989; White and Kaliner, 1987; Orchard, 1986; Schulman, 1985; Theuson, 1987). HRFs cause non-IgE-dependent degranulation of mast cells. Many HRFs have been described, with varying characteristics (Alam, 1990; Baeza et al., 1989; MacDonald et al., 1987). Cytokines Il-1, IL-3, IL-8, and GM-CSF also stimulate degranulation of human basophils, albeit weakly. Human lung mast cells (mainly MC_T) have thus far not shown responses to nonimmunological factors (Tharp et al., 1987; Lowman et al., 1988). Human lung and nasal mast cells will degranulate after exposure to hyperosmotic stimuli, the proposed mechanism by which cold dry air induces bronchospasm in asthmatics (Eggleston, 1984; Silber et al., 1988; Togias et al., 1985).

VII. Pathological Changes in Asthma

Information regarding pathological changes seen in asthma came initially from analyses of sputum and from autopsies. In those individuals who died in status asthmaticus, the lung is overdistended, despite relaxation of smooth muscle postmortem. This failure of the lung to collapse postmortem is due to fixed airway obstruction from thickened swollen bronchial walls with inspissated mucus. Cutz and Associates (1978) compared lung biopsies from chronically asthmatic children to those of children who had died from asthma. Both groups displayed thickened basement membranes and extensive mucus plugs consisting of degenerating macrophages, epithelial cells, and cell fragments. Mast cells were found in various stages of degranulation scattered between epithelial cells. The airways were edematous, and edema fluid was found in the lumen. Excessive mucus production by goblet cells and hyperplastic, hypertrophic submucosal glands contributed to the airway obstruction. This mucus is enriched not only with cellular debris, but with plasma proteins. The resultant thick mucus is difficult for the mucociliary elevator to eliminate from the airway.

In studies using bronchoscopic biopsies and bronchoalveolar lavage, epithelial fragility was also apparent in the form of denuded surface epithelium on biopsy specimens and abundant epithelial cells in BAL fluid from mild and severe asthmatics (Lozewicz et al., 1990; Jeffery et al., 1989; Beasley et al., 1989; Laitinen et al., 1985; Djukanovic et al., 1990a). Clumps of some cells recovered at BAL had intact tight junctions and ciliary function (Djukanovic et al., 1990b; Beasley et al., 1989), suggesting that inflammation at the basal cell layer or basement membrane may produce disruption of ciliated cells. Eosinophils infiltrate into the mucosal and submucosal layers of the airway. These cells release their products when activated and are associated with epithelial damage (Bousquet, 1990). The loss of normal epithelium impairs mucociliary clearance. Replacement of epithelium by hypertrophied, hyperplastic goblet cells results in the elaboration of more tenacious, thick secretions that are difficult to remove. In the remaining cells, ciliary dysfunction and damage has been demonstrated (Laitinen et al., 1985).

Another pathological feature of asthma is the appearance of thickened basement membranes on light microscopy (Hogg, 1986). The true basement membrane in asthmatics is of normal thickness. Electron microscopic and immunohistochemical analyses document the presence of interstitial collagens (types I, III, and V) and fibronectin in the abnormally thickened lamina reticularis. These subepithelial deposits are devoid of collagen type IV and laminin, normal constituents of the basement membrane. Fibroblasts may be responsible for producing additional aberrant deposits found beneath the true basement membrane in asthmatic airways (Roche et al., 1989; Brewster et al., 1990). These changes can be attributed to long-standing inflammation and probably contribute to the irreversible small airway narrowing seen late in the course of some chronic asthmatics (Sobonya, 1984). Stimuli mitogenic for fibroblasts may be released by mast cells and other inflammatory cells (macrophages, eosinophils, bronchial epithelium) and interact to influence collagen deposition in inflammed airways. Smooth muscle hypertrophy and mucosal edema, known features of asthmatic airways, further exacerbate luminal narrowing seen during bronchospasm. In airways thickened by chronic inflammation, edema, and smooth muscle hypertrophy, only marginal bronchial smooth muscle contraction may be required for bronchial obstruction (James et al., 1989; Desai et al., 1988).

Mixed cellular infiltrates are commonly seen in those who die with asthma (Kaliner et al., 1976). Eosinophils, lymphocytes, and neutrophils can be found with degranulated mast cells in the mucosa and the submucosa of asthmatics. These changes may also be found in moderate and mild asthmatics, differing only in the degree of involvement. Eosinophils and their products are associated with the development of injury to bronchial mucosal epithelium (Bousquet, 1990; Gleich et al., 1987). Eosinophils and activated T lymphocytes (CD25+)

were identified in bronchoscopic biopsies using monoclonal antibodies and immunohistochemical staining (Azzawi et al., 1990). In biopsies of asthmatics, the number of mastcells has not been shown to increase after allergen provocation. However, when compared to nonasthmatic controls, the mast cells of asthmatics were degranulated (Beasley et al., 1989; Laitinen et al., 1985). In BAL fluids obtained from asthmatics, mast cell numbers were increased compared to nonasthmatics, suggesting migration of mast cells to the luminal surface of the bronchial mucosa (Tomioka et al., 1984).

VIII. Mast Cell Mediators

Human mast cell mediators may be performed, newly generated, or granule associated. Preformed mediators are packaged in granules and released after activation of mast cells. Histamine, the best studied of mast cell products, is prepackaged in granules after its synthesis from histidine in the cytosol of mast cells (Wood-Baker and Church, 1990). It exists in close association with proteoglycans within the granule matrix. Histamine comprises 5–10% of mast cell granule content. The biological effects of histamine are mediated via histamine receptors. H_1 receptor stimulation causes phosphoinositol metabolism, with subsequent elevation of intracellular calcium, formation of inositol triphosphate, and the generation of cyclic GMP. H_1 stimulation results in smooth muscle contraction, increased vascular permeability, pruritus, prostaglandin generation, tachycardia (by reducing AV nodal conduction time), and vagal afferent nerve stimulation. H_2 receptors are coupled to adenylate cyclase. Cyclic AMP levels rise after stimulation of this receptor, producing secretion of gastric acid and airway mucus, esophageal contraction, and stimulation of suppressor T lymphocytes (Beer et al., 1982). Dual stimulation of H_1 and H_2 receptors causes headache, flushing, hypotension, and tachycardia (White, 1990; Barnes et al., 1988).

Chemotactic factors (eosinophil and neutrophil chemotactic factors) have been described that are released from mast cells as preformed mediators. ECF-a attracts eosinophils to sites of inflammation. However, ECF-a is not as potent an eosinophil chemotactic agent as PAF or LTB_4 (Wardlaw et al., 1986) or lymphocyte chemotactic factor (Rand et al., 1991). A neutrophil chemotactic factor is also released early in the course of mast cell activation. This 600-kDa protein is released after allergic and exercise challenges of asthmatics (Atkins et al., 1978). However, NCF-a is also released in response to other nonallergic, inflammatory conditions such as urticaria (Atkins and Zweiman, 1981; Lee et al., 1983; Nagy et al., 1982) and lower respiratory tract infections (Cundell et al., 1984).

Neutral proteases tryptase and chymase are enzymes associated within the granule matrix of mast cells only. Tryptase exists as a tetraner with a MW of 134 kDa. Each subunit has an active site, which functions as a serine protease.

Purified in 1981, tryptase can be found in all mast cells; however, most human lung mast cells do not contain chymase. Twenty percent (12 pg tryptase/60 pg granule protein) of the protein found in human lung mast cell granules is composed of tryptase (Schwartz et al., 1981). In 1983, chymase was isolated and purified from human cutaneous mast cells (Schechter et al., 1983). Chymase is also a serine protease found exclusively in mast cells. Skin mast cells contain up to 1 pg chymase/mast cell. Chymase has been isolated from purified human lung mast cells; however, human skin mast cells contain 10-fold more chymase (Wintroub et al., 1986). Chymase is a monomer with a MW of 28–30 kDa. Chymase and tryptase are not inhibited by classic inhibitors of serine proteases. Both are bound in an active state to heparin within the granule. The activity of these enzymes is reduced by binding to proteoglycan and by the acidic milieu of the mast cell (Lagunoff and Rickard, 1983; Metcalfe et al., 1979). When mast cell degranulation occurs, both are released into the local environment in an active state; no cleavage of a proenzyme has been described. Tryptase dissociates into monomers after it separates from heparin. Without heparin, the enzymatic activity of tryptase rapidly falls. The role of neutral proteases in asthma is not yet known. However, tryptase does cleave C3 (to C3a), kallikrein, fibrinogen, and vasoactive peptide (VIP), and it may be the kininogenase released from mast cells at degranulation. Chymase also converts angiotensinogen to angiotensin (Wintroub et al., 1984). A group of lysosomal enzymes are released early at mast cell degranulation. Arylsulfatase A degrades leukotrienes, though this is of undetermined significance. The biological role of lysosomal enzymes in asthma is not known at present. Heparin and chondroitin sulfate E are the principal proteoglycans found in mast cell granules (Hisamoto et al., 1987). These highly sulfated molecules are responsible for metachromatic staining properties of basophils and mast cells (Lagunoff, 1974). Apart from their role in binding mediators within granules of mast cells and basophils, little is known about their effects in asthmatics.

Arachidonic acid metabolites are another group of newly generated mediators that are not stored but produced de novo after mast cell degranulation (Kaliner, 1980). This category of mediators includes leukotrienes, prostaglandins, adenosine, and platelet-activating factor. Activation of mast cells results in activation of phospholipase A_2. This enzyme cleaves arachidonic acid from lipids in the plasma membrane. The eicosanoids that are subsequently synthesized depend on which of a number of enzymes are present to act on it (O'Byrne, 1990). The action of cyclooxygenase results in production of the cyclic endoperoxides PGG_2 and PGH_2 from arachidonic acid. PGD_2 is subsequently formed by the degradation of PGH_2 and the major product produced by mast cells. After it is activated by 5-lipooxygenase-activating protein (FLAP), 5-lipooxygenase catalyzes the C-5 oxygenation of arachidonic acid. The product of this enzymatic step is 5-hydroperoxyeicosatetraenoic acid (5-HPETE), the immediate precursor of the leukotriene series of mediators (Henderson, 1991).

PGD_2 and LTC_4 are the eicosanoids synthesized and released preferentially from human lung mast cells (Enerback, 1981; Lewis et al., 1982; Holgate et al., 1984; Schleimer et al., 1986; Cohan et al., 1989; van Overveld, et al., 1989). Smaller quantities of thromboxane A_2 (TXA_2), monohydroxyacids (HETEs), LTB_4, LTD_4, and LTE_4 are also released. These eicosanoids display a variety of potent effects on airways that mimic the features of asthma (Burka and Patterson, 1980; Chilton and Lichtenstein, 1990). More is mentioned about these eicosanoids below.

Platelet-activating factor (PAF) is a short-lived, but powerful, mediator with multiple biological actions. PAF is also synthesized by the action of the enzyme phospholipase A_2 on arachidonic acid. Human lung mast cells (and other inflammatory cells) produce PAF and lyso-PAF. The latter is inactive. PAF is rapidly inactivated by phosphatidyl-2-acetyl hydrolase conversion to lyso-PAF. PAF is the most potent chemotactic factor for eosinophils. It also attracts neutrophils, aggregates platelets, and stimulates increased vascular permeability by its action on endothelial cells. PAF contracts bronchial smooth muscle directly by acting at PAF receptors on muscle fibers. It causes bronchospasm indirectly by inducing production of other mediators, perhaps histamine and leukotrienes (Cuss et al., 1986; Henderson, 1987; Smith et al., 1988). It is postulated that asthmatics are chronically exposed to PAF, resulting in the development of tachyphylaxis to exogenous PAF (Rubin et al., 1987). PAF augments airway secretion by its effects on vascular permeability, stimulates bronchial mucus secretion, and slows mucociliary transport; these actions may be due to the secondary generation of LTC_4 (Lundgren et al., 1990). PAF may play a role in asthma. It is capable of producing all four pathophysiological features of asthma (bronchospasm, mucosal edema, mucous secretion, and mucosal inflammation). However, PAF synthesized in lung mast cells is released in negligible amounts. The role of intracellular PAF has yet to be determined (Lynch and Henson, 1986; Sturk et al., 1989). It is likely that other cells, such as macrophages, eosinophils, platelets, and endothelial cells, are the source of PAF.

Reactive oxygen species are generated as a result of inflammation by granulocytes and eosinophils. Mast cells also may release superoxide, hydrogen peroxide, and hydroxyl radicals when activated (Henderson and Kaliner, 1978). These substances injure cells by inhibiting enzyme systems, damaging DNA, or causing formation of lipid peroxides (Junod, 1987). In bovine airways, H_2O_2 produces bronchospasm, vasodilation, and increased vascular permeability. The effects on airway tissue can be inhibited by pretreatment with indomethacin, suggesting that H_2O_2 induces release of arachidonic acid metabolites (Barnes and Rhoden, 1987). Oxygen radicals may also alter beta-adrenergic function on smooth muscles, enhancing bronchoconstriction (Engel et al., 1985).

Adenosine is a purine released after mast cell activation by cleavage of

AMP. When released extracellularly, adenosine behaves like an autocoid on target cells, stimulating purinoceptors (A_1 or A_2) linked to adenylate cyclase. The A_1 adenosine receptor inhibits and the A_2 receptor stimulates adenylate cyclase (Wolfe et al., 1981). By interacting with purinoceptors, adenosine produces bronchospasm and increases vascular permeability in airway mucosal tissues (Polosa et al., 1990). The bronchoconstrictor effects of adenosine appear to be partially mediated via the A_2 receptor. Adenosine will potentiate IgE-dependent histamine and leukotriene release from mast cells (Marquardt et al., 1978; Peachell et al., 1988). Since the actions of adenosine as a smooth muscle agonist are relatively weak (Church et al., 1986), it is likely that adenosine acts predominantly by its autocoid effects on mast cell secretion of vasoactive, inflammatory mediators.

Recently, it has been shown that mast cells are rich sources of cytokines. Most of these studies were performed on murine mast cells, revealing production of IL-3,-4,-5,-6, GM-CSF, and tumor necrosis factor alpha (TNF_α). In humans, $TNF\alpha$ mRNA and protein has been demonstrated in mast cells (Steffen et al., 1989). It is likely that other cytokines made by murine mast cells are also produced in humans. Cytokine production by mast cells generally occurs about 6 hr after activation. However, some preformed TNF is released early with granule-associated mediators. Elaboration of cytokines by mast cells indicates that they may play a wider role in the pathogenesis of asthma. These roles may include proliferation of mast cells after IgE-dependent activation, through elaboration of IL-3 and IL-4. IL-4 also may promote production of IgE by B lymphocytes in the local mucosal milieu. IL-5 is thought to potentiate IL-4 effects on B lymphocytes and to promote the reactions and survival of eosinophils. Mast cells have been shown to express mRNA for IL-5. Release of these cytokine/growth factors suggests that mast cells may fundamentally influence the development of an allergic diathesis in susceptible, sensitized individuals. Interestingly, pretreatment with cyclosporin A inhibits IL-3-dependent mast cell proliferation in culture (Costa, 1990). Proinflammatory cytokines released from mast cells would further enhance the spectrum of mast cell responses in allergic and inflammatory disorders. Although it is not known for certain that human lung mast cells possess this repertoire of cytokine responses, murine models have been good predictors of analogous processes (Johnson and Holgate, 1990).

IX. Mast Cell Mediators and Bronchial Obstruction

Airway obstruction in asthma can be attributed to (1) muscle spasm, (2) mucosal edema, (3) mucosal inflammation, and (4) mucus secretion. Mast cells, through secretion of mediators, contributes directly (or indirectly by recruitment of inflammatory cells) to the development of airway obstruction in asthma (Wasserman, 1989). Bronchospasm following mast cell activation results from the degranulation of rapid-acting, preformed mediators. Histamine is the first mediator released from mast cells. Histamine release is one-half maximal at 2 min following activation of purified human mast cells (Schleimer et al., 1986; Flint et al., 1985). Histamine-induced bronchoconstriction is mediated by stimulation of the H_1 receptor on smooth muscle fibers. A few H_2 receptors, which mediate smooth muscle relaxation, can be found in the human airway (Vincenc et al., 1984). However, the ineffectiveness of H_2 antagonists in vivo in reversing bronchospasm suggests that if present, they are not important. In vitro, histamine causes contraction of large and small human airways (Finney et al., 1984). Inhaled histamine causes bronchospasm in asthmatic, but not normal, subjects (Curry, 1946). Studies of histamine levels in BAL fluid are frequently utilized as an index of human lung mast cell degranulation. BAL in patients with various lung conditions revealed direct correlations between the absolute BAL mast cell count and BAL fluid histamine levels (Agius et al., 1985). Asthmatics challenged with allergen respond with elevations in BAL histamine. BAL fluid histamine levels exceeding 100 pg/ml were inversely correlated with bronchial hyperresponsiveness (Casale et al., 1987a). In another study, instillation of allergen via bronchoscopy into a subsegmental airway of asthmatic subjects produced visible changes in the airway: blanching, hyperemia, edema, and narrowing. These changes were accompanied by significant increases in BAL fluid histamine levels. Such changes did not occur in normals subjected to the same procedure. Instillation of cold saline into the airway of asthmatic subjects failed to reproduce these findings (Casale et al., 1987b). These studies provide evidence of mast cell activation, histamine release, and subsequent bronchospasm in response to allergen.

Within minutes of histamine release, products of arachidonic acid metabolism are secreted from mast cells. Histamine, via H_1 receptor stimulation, is responsible for 50% of the prostaglandins generated (Platshon and Kaliner, 1978). Human lung mast cells synthesize and release prostaglandins (PGD_2) and leukotrienes (LTC_4) (Holgate et al., 1984; Gravelyn et al., 1988). Both substances contribute to bronchospasm in asthma. PGD_2, a potent bronchoconstrictor, achieves one-half maximal release within 5 min of IgE-dependent activation of purified lung mast cells (Schleimer et al., 1986). $PGF2_{\alpha}$, also a powerful bronchoconstrictor, and PGD_2 were elevated 12–22-fold in BAL fluid from mild asthmatics compared to nonatopic controls, and 10-fold when compared to atopic nonasthmatics (Liu et al., 1990). PGD_2 is the major cyclooxygenase metabolite of arachidonic acid in human lung mast cells in vitro (Peters et al., 1984) and in vivo (Murray et al., 1986). PGD_2 and its metabolite 9a,11b-PGF_2 are 30 times more potent than histamine in producing bronchospasm (Beasley et al., 1989). Not only is PGD_2 more potent than histamine, its duration of action is longer (Hardy et al., 1984). PGD_2 causes bronchospasm by acting directly via stimulation of receptors and indirectly by inducing presynaptic acetylcholine release from cholinergic nerves in the airway (Munoz et al., 1986). Even subthreshold levels of PGD_2 produce bronchial hyperreactivity to histamine and methacholine (Fuller et al., 1986).

The compounds now known as LTC_4, LTD_4, and LTE_4 were formerly called slow-reacting substance of anaphylaxis (SRS-a) (Lewis and Austen, 1984). LTC_4 is the predominant leukotriene made and released by human lung mast cells. LTC_4 can be enzymatically converted to LTD_4 by the action of glutamyltranspeptidase and to LTE_4 by a dipeptidase. All are potent bronchoconstrictors of human airways in vitro. LTE_4, while causing longer-lasting bronchoconstriction, is generally less potent that LTC_4 or LTD_4 (Davidson et al., 1987). Leukotrienes are 100–1000 times more potent than histamine or methacholine in causing muscle contraction (Dahlen et al., 1980; Griffin et al., 1983; Adelroth et al., 1986). LTC_4 is released later than histamine and PGD_2 (one-half maximum release 10–20 min) from mast cells after activation (Schleimer et al., 1986). Wardlaw and colleagues (1989) found elevated levels of LTC_4 in BAL fluid from symptomatic asthmatics. At baseline and after allergen challenge, histamine, PGD_2, and LTC_4 levels were increased in BAL fluids of allergic asthmatics (Wenzel et al., 1990). Miadonna and colleagues (1990) also found increases in all of these three mast cell mediators in BAL washings after allergen provocations of asthmatics and atopic nonasthmatics, but not nonatopic, nonasthmatic controls. Inhaled LTC_4 and LTD_4 are potent bronchoconstrictors of asthmatic and normal subjects (Griffin et al., 1983; Adelroth et al., 1986; Smith et al., 1985, 1987), with a longer duration than inhaled histamine (Barnes et al., 1984). In vivo studies comparing the effects of inhaled leukotrienes and histamine in normal and asthmatic airways are less consistent (Roberts et al., 1987). Although these agents are potent, there did not appear to be as great a difference in bronchial reactivity between histamine and leukotrienes (Griffin et al., 1983) or in comparing normals with ashmatics (Adelroth et al., 1986). In other studies, precontraction of the airways with LTD_4 increases bronchial reactivity (Kern et al., 1986; Bel et al., 1987). In asthmatics challenged with inhaled LTE_4, a unique sensitivity to its bronchospastic effects was found, which was not seen in nonasthmatics (Arm et al., 1988). Enzymatic conversion of LTC_4 to LTE_4 may in part account for the extended actions of leukotrienes at the site of airway contraction (Sautebin et al., 1985).

Adenosine is produced from AMP (Fain and Malbon, 1979) and released within minutes of mast cell activation. Both the purine and nucleoside produce bronchoconstriction in atopics and asthmatics, but not in normals, when inhaled (Cushley et al., 1983). This effect is maximal by 2–5 min, resolves within an hour, and is antagonized by theophylline (Cushley et al., 1984). By acting at the A_2 receptor on mast cells, it also enhances histamine and other mediator release (Marquardt et al., 1978; Peachell et al., 1988). Interestingly, cromolyn sodium and nedocromil blocked the bronchoconstrictor effects of inhaled adenosine in asthmatics (Altounyan et al., 1986), presumably by stabilizing mast cells. H_1 antagonists terfenadine and astemizole also inhibited AMP-induced bronchospasm (Phillips et al., 1987), as did indomethacin (Crimi et al., 1989). These studies suggest contractile agonists released from mast cells mediate adenosine-induced muscle contraction. Their direct actions on smooth muscle fibers may not be as important as their indirect effects on mast cells in asthmatics.

Mucosal edema contributes to obstruction of the airway in asthmatics. Increases in airway edema are caused by increased vascular permeability (Chung et al., 1990). Bronchial biopsies of asthmatics reveal gaps between venule endothelial cells (Laitinen et al., 1985). These cells contain actin and myosin. When the cells are stimulated, contraction of these filaments may cause gaps to form between endothelial cells (Becker and Nachman, 1973). An unfiltered flow of plasma and protein into the interstitium follows this increase in permeability (Persson, 1991). The edema fluid is rapidly transported into the lumen via a periepithelial cell elevator system. As serum proteins mix with secreted mucoglycoproteins, the character of mucous is altered, producing a stickier, gel-like consistency that contributes to airway obstruction. Several mast cell products are capable of mediating these changes in capillary permeability. Histamine, via H_1 receptors, causes leakage in bronchial vascular endothelium. Tachyphylaxis to these effects develops in vitro after continuous infusion of histamine. It is unlikely that histamine alone can sustain the increased permeability and edema seen in asthmatic inflammation. Histamine may stimulate release of neuropeptides (substance P) from sensory nerves in the lung, which acts to increase vascular permeability (Kowalski and Kaliner, 1988). Also, increased plasma flow caused by early histamine release results in an influx of proteins that may influence airway inflammation. High-molecular-weight kininogen, which can be enzymatically converted to bradykinin by a mast cell enzyme, possibly tryptase (Robinson and Holgate, 1985), is one of these proteins. Bradykinin may also be generated from low-molecular-weight kininogen, which has been recovered in BAL fluid of asthmatics (Christiansen et al., 1987). Bradykinin is a potent inducer of vascular permeability and vasodilation (Proud et al., 1985). The vascular effects of bradykinin may be due in part to prostaglandins. Bradykinin infusions have been shown to release PGI_2 in humans (Barrow et al., 1986). Leukotrienes B_4, C_4, D_4, and E_4 also cause increased vascular permeability and edema. LTC_4 and LTD_4 are 100–1000 times as potent as histamine in this regard (Woodward et al., 1983). Leukotrienes act directly on endothelial cells in postcapillary venules (Joris et al., 1987). Vascular changes induced by LTB_4 may be related to an interaction of neutrophils with vascular endothelial cells (Bray et al., 1981; Bjork et al., 1982). PAF is known to induce microvascular leakage in airway tissues at doses 1000-fold less than histamine (Evans et al.,

1987). PAF receptors on endothelial cells (Bussolino et al., 1988) may permit direct stimulation of the vasculature by PAF. Specific PAF inhibitors, but no histamine antagonists, leukotriene inhibitors, or cyclooxygenase antagonists, block changes in permeability caused by PAF (Chung et al., 1987; Hellewell and Williams, 1986). Adenosine, PGD_2, and $PGF_{2\alpha}$ also raise vascular permeability in the bronchial vasculature, but further study will be needed to define their roles in causing vascular changes in asthma.

Mucus secretion contributes to bronchial obstruction in asthmatics. This contribution can be quite significant when one considers that the airway lumen is also narrowed by bronchospasm and increased airway thickness (edema, muscular hypertrophy). Increased secretion may occur in stable as well as severe asthmatics, limiting airflow by plugging the lumen of small airways (Cutz et al., 1978; Messer et al., 1960). The primary sources of the mucus component of these secretions are goblet cells and submucosal glands. Secretion from these sources appears to be under humoral or neural control (or both) in human airways (Richardson and Peutfield, 1987). Submucosal gland hypertrophy and hyperplasia is a feature of asthma. These glands receive innervation from parasympathetic and sympathetic sources. Vagal stimulation produces a mixed (mucus and serous) secretion, while sympathetic stimulation causes some selective serous secretion from submucosal glands. Goblet cells appear not to be under direct neural control (Kaliner et al., 1982). Nonadrenergic, noncholinergic nerves may modulate mucus secretion by releasing neuropeptides with secretagogue activity (calcitonin gene–related peptide, SP, gastrin-releasing peptide) (Rogers et al., 1989, 1990; Baraniuk et al., 1990; Lundgren et al., 1988). Substance P is known to be a potent mucus secretagogue in human airways (Barnes et al., 1986). Receptors for substance P can be found on human submucosal glands (Carstairs and Barnes, 1986). Mast cell products play a role in control of mucus secretion in human airways also. Histamine, acting by H_2 receptor stimulation, produces secretion from the submucosal glands. This may be blocked with H_2 antagonists. Additionally, histamine produces reflex cholinergic stimulation, which induces glandular secretion. PGD_2 and $PGF_{2\alpha}$ are more potent stimulators of mucus secretion than histamine. PDE_2 inhibits mucus secretion (Lopez-Vidreiro et al., 1977). Of the mast cell prostanoids, $PGF_{2\alpha}$ and PGD_2 were of equivalent potency. However, leukotrienes are the most potent mucus secretagogues released from human mast cells (Shelhamer et al., 1981; Marom, 1981). 15-HETEs also function as powerful secretagogues. Made spontaneously by airway epithelium, they appear to be intermediate in potency between leukotrienes and prostaglandins (Lai et al., 1990). The role of HETEs in the control of airway secretion may be one of regulation since they are constantly released by the airway, whereas leukotrienes and prostaglandins may be responsible for mucorrhea after allergenic stimulation of the mast cell. Cells recruited or activated by mast cells also contain mediators that act as secretagogues. Eosinophils release

(Beasley, 1989). It appears that many cells play a role in producing chronic mucosal inflammation. Eosinophil products are quite toxic to epithelial cells. ECP, eosinophil-derived neurotoxin, PAF, MBP, and oxygen radical products cause mast cell degranulation and epithelial cell disruption and promote inflammation (O'Donnell et al., 1983). Eosinophils can persist for days in the bronchial mucosa after the onset of allergen-induced inflammation.

The mast cell and eosinophil are the predominant cells found to increase significantly in BAL fluid obtained after allergen challenge of asthmatic, but not normal, subjects. Diaz et al., (1989), however, found that basophils in BAL fluid from asthmatics during the late-phase allergic response were increased 200-fold. However, the numbers of basophils in the BAL fluid obtained during the late phase represented only 1% of cells. This change was associated with rises in permeability, kinin levels, PGE_2, and $PGF_{2\alpha}$. Mast cells from atopic patients with asthma appear to display various stages of degranulation, suggesting low levels of constant mediator release in the airway mucosa (Broide et al., 1991).

Biopsies and bronchial washings of asthmatics often reveal lymphocytic infiltration (Gonzales et al., 1987). The presence of activated T lymphocytes (bearing Il-2 receptors or CD-25+) suggests that these cells play an important regulatory role in the allergic inflammation. These CD-25+ cells have been associated with eosinophilic infiltration and degranulation in biopsies from airways of asthmatics (Bradley et al., 1991). Cytokines elaborated by T lymphocytes may promote mast cell degranulation, IgE production by B lymphocytes, and differentiation and recruitment of eosinophils, and support ongoing inflammation (Kay et al., 1989, 1991). However, cytokines may be produced by mast cells (Plaut et al., 1989; Steffen et al., 1989) at a time that coincides with the occurrence of the late allergic response (about 6 hr after activation). Indirect evidence of mast cell involvement in asthma is suggested by inhibition of early and late allergic reactions by disodium cromoglycate. The attenuation of the late-phase reaction with immunotherapy (Warner, 1976; Warner et al., 1978) or after passive administration of antigen-specific IgG (Behrens, 1984) implies that IgE-dependent mast cell activation remains important to its pathogenesis (Booij-Noord et al., 1972; Boulet et al., 1984; Burrows et al., 1989).

Mast cells play a pivotal role in the pathophysiology of asthma. Mast cells and their mediators are capable of generating all the cardinal features of asthma: bronchospasm, mucous secretion, mucosal edema, and mucosal inflammation. The early actions of the activated mast cell initiate the airway inflammatory response to inhaled stimuli. Later, other inflammatory cells appear to amplify this response. Mast cell mediators may not act alone in causing mucosal inflammation, but their activity is critical to the development of early and late allergic responses in asthma. Moreover, the regulation of airway inflammation in asthma may be modulated by elaboration of cytokines by mast cells in concert with T lymphocytes.

Discussion

Casale: Do you feel that the increases in vascular permeability seen in vivo in asthmatics occur independently of cells migrating through the epithelium?
Kaliner: Yes, the data indicate that acute responses are due to mast cell or inflammatory mediators directly causing postcapillary venules to become permeable. This change occurs in the absence of inflammatory cells, although inflammation may augment the reaction.
Schleimer: Are cytokines mucus secretagogues?
Kaliner: We have examined IL-1, IL-2, and IL-4 in vitro on human respiratory epithelium and failed to find any mucus secretions. We have also studied patients receiving IL-2 and/or IL-4 in vivo for cancer chemotherapy and again have failed to find mucus secretions. We have not instilled any cytokines directly onto the nasal mucosa in vivo.
Schleimer: Is there unidirectional secretory flow?
Kaliner: Increased plasma protein and fluid leak into the interstium leads to unidirectional flow of fluid from the tissue into the airway lumen. At the time of this unidirectional flow, there is no increased mucosal permeability for markers instilled on the luminal surface. Thus, the flow is unidirectional.
Schwartz: Do the plasma proteins alter mucus viscoelasticity?
Kaliner: Plasma proteins and DNA mix with mucous glycoproteins and serous secretions to produce the viscid mucus characteristically seen in asthma.
Casale: Have you examined the effects of alpha-adrenergic agents on mediator-induced vascular permeability?
Kaliner: It seems logical and predictable that vasoconstrictors would reduce vascular permeability. However, Carl Persson has studied alpha agonists and found that they did not affect vascular responses in vivo in a guinea pig model system.
Casale: Would you advocate the use of α_1 agonists or NPY for the emergency treatment of asthma, given their effects on the vasculature?
Kaliner: Although both these suggestions have hypothetical merit, neither has been studied, and I would have to await clinical experience before I could consider their position in the treatment of asthma.
Schleimer: Carl Persson has suggested that increased vascular permeability may have a role in host defense. What is your opinion?
Kaliner: We agree with Persson. The acute reaction to injury, be it allergic or inflammatory, is the outpouring of plasma proteins.
Kaplan: Has mucus been stained for fibrin or fibrinogen?
Kaliner: Secretions contain both fibrin and fibrinogen, and it is conceivable that these proteins could "clot" and lead to airway occlusion.

References

Adelroth, E., Morris, M. M., Hargreave, F. E., and O'Bryne, P. M. (1986). Airway responsiveness to leukotrienes C_4 and D_4 and to methacholine in patients with asthma and normal controls. *N. Engl. J. Med.* 315:480–484.

Adventier, C., Cerrina, J., Dukroux, P., Floch, A., Pradel, J., and Renier, A. (1983). Sodium cromoglycate, verampamil and nicardipine antagonism to leukotriene D_4 bronchoconstriction. *Br. J. Pharmacol.* 78:301–306.

Agius, R. M., Godfrey, R. C., and Holgate, S. T. (1985). Mast cell and histamine content of human bronchoalveolar lavage fluid. *Thorax* 40:760–767.

Alam, R. (1990). Cytokines and bronchial hyperreactivity. *Agents Actions* (Suppl. 31):147–162.

Altounyan, R. E. C. (1970). Changes in histamine and atropine responsiveness as a guide to diagnosis and evaluation of therapy in obstructive airways disease. In *Disodium Cromoglycate in Allergic Airways Disease*. Edited by J. Pepys and A. W. Frankland. London, Butterworth, pp. 105–120.

Altounyan, R. E. C., Lee, T. B., Rocchiccioli, K. M. S., and Shaw, C. L. (1986). A comparison of inhibitory effect of nedocromil sodium and sodium cromoglycate on adenosine monophophate induced bronchoconstriction in atopic subjects. *Eur. J. Respir. Dis.* 69(Suppl. 147):277–279.

Andersson, M., Andersson, P., and Pipkorn, U. (1988). Topical glucocorticoids and allergen-induced increase in nasal reactivity: Relationship between treatment time and inhibitory effect. *J. Allergy Clin. Immunol.* 82:1019–1026.

Arm, J. P., Spur, B. W., and Lee, T. H. (1988). The effect of inhaled leukotriene E_4 on the airway responsiveness to histamine in asthmatic and normal subjects. *J. Allergy Clin. Immunol.* 82:654.

Atkins, P. C., and Zweiman, B. (1981). Mediator release in local heat urticaria. *J. Allergy Clin. Immunol.* 68:286–289.

Atkins, P. C., Norman, M. E., and Zweiman, B. (1978). Antigen induced neutrophil chemotactic activity in man. Correlation with bronchospasm and inhibition by disodium cromoglycate. *J. Allergy Clin. Immunol.* 62:149–155.

Azzawi, M., Bradley, B., Jeffery, P. K., Frew, A. J., Wardlaw, A. J., Knowles, G., Assoufi, B., Collins, J. V., Durham, S., and Kay, A. B. (1990). Identification of activated T lymphocytes and eosinophils in bronchial biopsies in stable atopic asthma. *Am. Rev. Respir. Dis.* 142:1407–1413.

Baeza, M. L., Reddigarri, S., Haak-Frendscho, M., and Kaplan, A. P. (1989). Purification and further characterization of human mononuclear cell histamine releasing factor. *J. Clin. Invest.* 83:1204–1210.

Baraniuk, J. N., Lundgren, J. D., Goft, J., Peden, D., Merida, M., Shelhamer, J., and Kaliner, M. (1990). Gastrin releasing peptide (GRP) in human nasal mucosa. *J. Clin. Invest.* 85:998–1005.

Barnes, N. C., Piper, P. J., and Costello, J. F. (1984). Comparative effects of inhaled leukotriene C_4, leukotriene D_4, and histamine in normal human subjects. *Thorax* 39:697.

Barnes, P. J. (1991). Histamine receptors in the lung. *Agents Actions* (Suppl. 33):103–122.

Barnes, P. J., and Rhoden, K. J. (1987). The effect of oxygen-derived free radicals on smooth muscle responses. *Br. J. Pharmacol.* 90:142P

Barnes, P. J., Dewar, A., and Rogers, D. F. (1986). Human bronchial secretion: effect of substance P, muscarinic and adrenergic stimulation in vitro. *Br. J. Pharmacol.* 89:76P.

Barnes, P. J., Chung, K. F., and Page, C. P. (1988). Inflammatory mediators in asthma. *Pharmacol. Rev.* 40:49–84.

Barrow, S. E., Dollery, C. T., Heavey, D. J., Hickling, N. C., Ritter, J. M., and Vial, J. (1986). Effect of vasoactive peptides on prostacyclin synthesis in man. *Br. J. Pharmacol.* 87:243–248.

Bascom, R., Wachs, M., Naclerio, R. M., Pipkorn, U., Galli, S. J., and Lichtenstein, L. M. (1988). Basophil influx occurs after nasal antigen challenge: Effects of topical corticosteroid pretreatment. *J. Allergy Clin. Immunol.* 81:580–589.

Baur, X., Dorsch, W., and Becker, T. (1980). Levels of complement factors in human serum during immediate and late asthmatic reactions and during acute hypersensitivity pneumonitis. *Allergy* 35:383–390.

Beasley, R., Roche, W. R., Roberts, J. A., and Holgate, S. T. (1989). Cellular Events in the bronchi in mild asthma and after bronchial provocation. *Am. Rev. Respir. Dis.* 139:806–817.

Becker, C. G., and Nachman, R. L. (1973). Contractile proteis of endothelial cells, platelets and smooth muscle. *Am. J. Pathol.* 71:1–22.

Beer, D. J., Osband, M. E., McCaffrey, R. P., Soter, N. A., and Rocklin, R. E. (1982). Abnormal histamine-induced suppressor cell function in atopic subjects. *N. Engl. J. Med.* 306:454–458.

Behrens, B. L., Clark, A. F., Marsh, W., and Larsen, G. (1984). Modulation of the late asthmatic response by antigen-specific immunoglobulin G in an animal model. *Am. Rev. Respir. Dis.* 130:1134–1139.

Bel, E. H., van der Veen, H., Kramps, J. A., Dijkman, J. H., and Sterk, P. J. (1987). Maximal airway narrowing to inhaled leukotriene D_4 in normal subjects. Comparison and interactions with methacholine. *Am. Rev. Respir. Dis.* 136:979–984.

Bjork, J., Hedqvist, P., and Afors, K-E. (1982). Increase of vascular permeability induced by leukotriene B_4 and the role of polymorphonuclear leukocytes. *Inflammation* 6:189–200.

Booij-Noord, H., de Vries, K., Sluiter, H. J., and Orie, N. G. (1972). Late bronchial obstructive reaction to experimental inhalation of house dust extract. *Clin. Allergy* 2:43–61.

Boulet, L. P., Roberts, R. S., Dolovich, J., and Hargreave, F. E. (1984). Prediction of late asthmatic responses to inhaled allergen. *Clin. Allergy* 14:379–385.

Bousquet, J. (1990). Microscopic anatomy of bronchial asthma and its implications regarding pathogenesis. *Insights Allergy* Aug. 5(4).

Bousquet, J., Chanez, P., Lacoste, J. Y., Barneon, G., Ghavanian, N., Enander, I., Venge, P., Ahlstedt, S., Simony-Lafontaine, J., Godard, P., and Michel, F-B. (1990). Eosinophilic inflammation in asthma. *N. Engl. J. Med.* 323: 1033–1039.

Bradley, B. L., Azzawi, M., Jacobson, M., Assoufi, B., Collins, J. V., Irani, A-M., Schwartz, L. B., Durham, S. D., Jeffery, P. K., and Kay, A. B. (1991). Eosinophils, T-lymphocytes, mast cells, neutrophils, and macrophages in bronchial biopsy specimens from atopic subjects without asthma and normal control subjects and relationship to bronchial hyperresponsiveness. *J. Allergy Clin. Immunol.* 88:661–674.

Bray, M. A., Cunningham, F. M., Ford-Hutchinson, A. W., and Smith, M. J. H. (1981). Leukotriene B_4; a mediator of vascular permeability. *Br. J. Pharmacol.* 72:483–486.

Brewster, C. E. P., Howarth, P. H., Djukanovic, R., Wilson, J., Holgate, S. T., and Roche, W. R. (1990). Myofibroblasts and subepithelial fibrosis in bronchial asthma. *Am. J. Respir. Cell. Mol. Biol.* 3:507–511.

Broide, D. H., Gleich, G. J., Cuomo, A. J., Coburn, D. A., Federman, E. C., Schwartz, L. B., and Wasserman, S. I. (1991). Evidence of ongoing mast cell and eosinophil degranulation in symptomatic asthma airway. *J. Allergy Clin. Immunol.* 88:637–648.

Burge, P. S., Efthimioiu, J., Turner-Warwick, M., and Nelmes, P. T. J., (1982). Double blind trial of inhaled beclomethasone diproprionate and flucortin butyl ester in allergen induced immediate and late asthmatic reactions. *Clin. Allergy* 12:523–531.

Burka, J. F., and Patterson, N. A. M. (1980). Evidence for lipooxygenase pathway involvement in allergic tracheal contraction. *Prostaglandins* 19:499–515.

Burrows, B., Martinez, F. D., Halonen, M., Barbee, R. A., and Cline, M. G. (1989). Association of asthma with serum IgE levels and skin-test reactivity to allergens. *N. Engl. J. Med.* 320:271–277.

Bussolino, F., Cammussi, G., Aglieta, M., Braquet, P., Bosia, A., Pescarmona, G., Sanavio, F., D'Urso, N., and Marchisio, P. C. (1988). Human endothelial cells are targets for platelet activating factor (PAF). I. PAF induces changes in cytoskeleton structures. *J. Immunol.*

Carstairs, J. R., and Barnes, P. J. (1986). Autoradiographic mapping of substance P receptors in the lung. *Eur. J. Pharmacol.* 127:295–296.

Casale, T. B., Bowman, S., and Kaliner, M. (1984). Induction of human cutaneous mast cell degranulation by opiates and endogenous opioid peptides: Evidence for opiate and nonopiate receptor participation. *J. Allergy Clin. Immunol.* 73:775–780.

Casale, T. B., Keahey, T. M., and Kaliner, M. (1986). Exercise induced anaphylactic syndromes. *JAMA* 255:2049–2053.

Casale, T. B., Wood, D., Richerson, H. B., Trapp, S., Metzger, W. J., Zavala, D., and Hunninghake, G. (1987a). Elevated bronchoalveolar lavage fluid histamine levels in allergic asthmatics are associated with methacholine bronchial hyperresponsiveness. *J. Clin. Invest.* 79:1197–1203.

Casale, T. B., Wood, D., Richerson, H. B., Zehr, B., Zavala, D., and Hunninghake, G. W. (1987b). Direct evidence for a role for mast cells in the pathogenesis of antigen-induced bronchoconstriction. *J. Clin. Invest.* 80:1507–1511.

Castells, M. C., Irani, A-M., and Schwartz, L. B. (1986). Evaluation of human peripheral blood leukocytes for mast cell tryptase. *J. Immunol.* 138:2184–2189.

Caufield, J. P., Lewis, R. A., Hein, A., and Austen, K. F. (1980). Secretion in dissociated human pulmonary mast cells. *J. Cell. Biol.* 85:299–311.

Chilton, F. H., and Lichtenstein, L. M. (1990). Lipid mediators of the allergic reaction.

In: 1939–1989: Fifty Years Progress in Allergy. Waksman, B. H. (ed.) *Chem. Immunol.* 49:173–205.

Christiansen, S. C., Proud, D., and Cochrane, C. G. (1987). Detection of tissue kallikrein in the bronchoalveolar lavage fluid of asthmatic patients. *J. Clin. Invest.* 79:188–197.

Chung, K. F., Dent, G., McCusker, M., Guinot, P., Page, C. P., and Nadel, J. A. (1987). Effect of a ginkgolide mixture (BN 52063) in antagonising skin and platelet responses to platelet activating factor in man. *Lancet* 1:248–251.

Chung, K. F., Rogers, D. F., Barnes, P. J., and Evans, T. W. (1990). The role of increased airway microvascular permeability and plasma exudation in asthma. *Eur. Respir. J.* 3:329–337.

Church, M. K., Featherstone, R. L., Cushley, M. J., et al. (1986). Relationship between adenosine, cyclic nucleotides and xanthines in asthma. *J. Allergy Clin. Immunol.* 78:670–676.

Clee, M. D., Ingram, C. G., Reid, P. C., and Robertson, A. S. (1984). The effects of astemizole on exercise-induced asthma. *Br. J. Dis. Chest* 78:180–183.

Cochran, C. G. and Muller-Eberhard, H. J. (1968). The derivation of the two distinct anaphylatoxin activities from the third and fifth components of human complement. *J. Exp. Med.* 127:371–377.

Cockroft, D. W., Killian, D. N., Mellan, J. J. A., and Hargreave, F. E. (1977). Protective effects of drugs on histamine-induced asthma. *Thorax* 32:429–437.

Cockroft, W. D., and Murdock, K. Y. (1987). Comparative effects of inhaled salbutamol, sodium cromoglycate, and beclomethasone dipropionate on allergen-induced early asthmatic responses, late asthmatic responses, and increased bronchial responsiveness to histamine. *J. Allergy Clin. Immunol.* 79:734–740.

Cohan, V., McKenzie-Wite, J., Triggiani, M., Massey, W., Kagey-Sobotka, A., and Lichtenstein, L. (1989). Heterogeneity of human mast cells and basophils. *Biochem. Pharmacol.* 38(24):4455–4459.

Costa, J. (1990). Mast cells and cytokines: New insights into the pathogenesis of allergic diseases. *Insights Allergy* Dec. 5(6).

Craig, S. S., Schechter, N. M., and Schwartz, L. B. (1988). Ultrastructural analysis of human T and TC mast cells identified by immunoelectron microscopy. *Lab. Invest.* 58:682.

Craig, S. S., Shechter, N. M., and Schwartz, L. B. (1989). Ultrastructural analysis of maturing human T and TC mast cells in situ. *Lab. Invest.* 60:147.

Crimi, N., Palermo, F., Polosa, R., et al. (1989). Effect of indomethacin on adenosine induced bronchoconstriction. *J. Allergy Clin. Immunol.* 83:921–925.

Cundell, D. R., Morgan, D. J. R., and Davis, R. J. (1984). N.C.F.—A mast cell specific chemotactic factor? *Clin. Sci.* 66:50P.

Curry, J. J. (1946). The action of histamine on the respiratory tract in normal and asthmatic subjects. *J. Clin. Invest.* 25:785–791.

Cushley, M. J., Tattersfield, A. E., and Holgate, S. T. (1983). Inhaled adenosine and guanosine on airway resistance in normal and asthmatic subjects. *Br. J. Clin. Pharmacol.* 15:161–165.

Cushley, M. J., Tattersfield, A. E., and Holgate, S. T. (1984). Adenosine-induced bronchoconstriction in asthma. *Am. Rev. Respir. Dis.* 129:380–384.

Cuss, F. M., Dixon, C. M. S., and Barnes, P. J. (1986). Effect of inhaled platelet activating factor on pulmonary function and bronchoresponsiveness in humans. *Lancet* 2:189–192.

Cutz, E., Levison, H., and Cooper, D. M. (1978). Ultrastructure of airways in children with asthma. *Histopathology* 2:407–421.

Dahlen, S. E., Hedqvist, P., Hammarstrom, S., and Samuelsson, B. (1980). Leukotrienes are potent constrictors of human bronchi. *Nature* 288:484–486.

Davidson, A. B., Lee, T. H., Scamon, P. D., Solway, J., McFadden, E. R., Ingram, R. H., Corey, E. J., Austen, K. F., and Drazen, J. M. (1987). Bronchoconstrictor effects of leukotriene E_4 in normal and asthmatic subjects. *Am. Rev. Respir. Dis.* 135:333–337.

Dawson, W., Boot, J. R., Cockerell, A. F., Mallen, D. N. B., and Osbourne, D. J. (1976). The release of novel prostaglandins and thromboxanes after immunologic challenge of guinea pig lung. *Nature* 262:699–703.

De Monchy, J. G. R., Kauffman, H. F., Venge, P., Koeter, G. H., Jansen, H. M., Sluiter, H. J., and De Vries, K. (1985). Bronchoalveolar eosinophils during allergen-induced late asthmatic reactions. *Am. Rev. Respir. Dis.* 131:373–376.

Denberg, J. A. (1990). Cytokine-induced human basophil/mast cell growth and differentiation in vitro. *Springer Semin. Immunopathol.* 12:401–414.

Desai, S. J., and Figueroa, W. G. (1988). Clinical correlation of a thickened basement membrane in asthma. *Immunol. Allergy Practice* 10(2):11–15.

Diaz, P., Gonzales, C., Galleguillos, F. R., Ancic, P., Cromwell, O., Shepherd, D., Durham, S. R., Gleich, G. J., and Kay, A. B. (1989). Leukocytes and mediators in bronchoalveolar lavage during allergen-induced late-phase asthmatic reactions. *Am. Rev. Respir. Dis.* 139:1383–1389.

Dixon, M., Jackson, D. M., and Richards, I. M. (1980). The action of sodium cromoglycate on the "C" fiber endings in the dog lung. *Br. J. Pharmacol.* 70:11–13.

Dixon, W. A., (1979). One-year's trials of Intal compound in 24 children with severe asthma. In *Disodium Cromoglycate in Allergic Airways Disease*. Edited by J. Pepys and A. W. Frankland. London, Butterworth, pp. 105–120.

Djukanovic, R., Wilson, J. W., Britten, K. M., Wilson, S. J., Walls, A. F., Roche, W. R., Howarth, P. H., and Holgate, S. T. (1990a). Quantitation of mast cells and eosinophils in the bronchial mucosa of symptomatic atopic asthmatics and healthy control subjects using immunohistochemistry. *Am. Rev. Respir. Dis.* 142:863–871.

Djukanovic, R., Roche, W. R., Wilson, J. W., Beasley, C. R. W., Twentyman, O. P., Howarth, P. H., and Holgate, S. T. (1990b). Mucosal inflammation in asthma. *Am. Rev. Respir. Dis.* 142:434–457.

Dvorak, A. M. (1991). Human mast cells. *Adv. Anat. Embryol. Cell. Biol.* 114:1–109.

Dvorak, A. M., Galli, S. J., Schulman, E. S., Lichtenstein, L. M., and Dvorak, H. F. (1983). Basophil and mast cell degranulation: ultrastructural analysis of mechanisms of mediator release. *Fed. Proc.* 2:2510–2515.

Dvorak, A. M., Schulman, E. S., Peters, S. P., MacGlashan, D. W., Jr., Newball, H. H., Schleimer, R. P., and Lichtenstein, L. M. (1985). Immunoglobulin E-mediated degranulation of isolated human mast cells. *Lab. Invest.* 53:45–56.

Dvorak, A. M., Schleimer, R. P., and Lichtenstein, L. M. (1987). Morphologic mast cell cycles. *Cell. Immunol.* 105:199–204.

Eggleston, P. A., Kagey-Sobotka, A., Schleimer, R., and Lichtenstein, L. M. (1984). Interaction between hyperosmolar and IgE-induced histamine release from basophils and mast cells. *Am. Rev. Respir. Dis.* 130:86–91.

Eiser, N. M., Mills, J., Snashall, P. D., and Guz, A. (1981). The role ofhistamine receptor antagonists in normal and asthmatic subjects. *Thorax* 35:428–434.

Enerback, L. (1981). The gut mucosal mast cell. *Monogr. Allergy* 17:222–232.

Engel, F., Oosting, R. S., and Nijkamp, F. P. (1985). Pulmonary macrophages induce deterioration of guinea pig tracheal beta-adrenergic function through release of oxygen radicals. *Eur. J. Pharmacol.* 111:143–144.

Evans, T. W., Chung, K. F., Rodgers, D. F., and Barnes, P. J. (1987). Effect of platelet activating factor on airway vascular permeability: possible mechanisms. *J. Appl. Physiol.* 63:479–484.

Fain, J. N., and Malbon, C. C. (1979). Regulation of adenylate cyclase by adenosine. *Mol. Cell. Biochem.* 25:143–169.

Feldman, C. H., Fox, J., Kraut, E., Feldman, B. R., and Davies, W. J. (1982). Exercise induced asthma [EIA]: Treatment for early and late responses. *Am. Rev. Respir. Dis.* 125 Pt 2:191 (abstract).

Fick, R. B. Jr., Richerson, H. B., Zavala, D. C., and Hunninghake, G. W. (1987). Bronchoalveolar lavage in allergic asthmatics. *Am. Rev. Respir. Dis.* 135:1204–1209.

Finney, M. J. B., Karlsson, J-A., and Persson, C. G. A. (1984). Effects of bronchoconstrictors and bronchodilators on a novel human small airway preparation. *Br. J. Pharmacol.* 85:29–36.

Flint, K. C., Leung, K. B. P., Pearce, F. L., Hudsmith, B. N., Brostoff, J., and Johnson, McI. N. (1985). Human mast cells recovered by bronchoalveolar lavage: Their morphology, histamine release and the effects of sodium cromoglycate. *Clin. Sci.* 68:427–432.

Foreman, J. C., Mongar, J. L., and Gomperts, B. D. (1973). Calcium ionophores and movement of calcium ions following physiologic stimulus to a secretory process. *Nature (Lond.)* 245:249–251.

Fox, B., Bull, T. B., and Guz, A. (1981). Mast cells in the human alveolar wall: An electron microscopic study. *J. Clin. Pathol.* 34:1333–1342.

Fox, C. C., Wolf, E. J., Kagey-Sobotka, A., and Lichtenstein, L. M. (1988). Comparison of human lung and intestinal mast cells. *J. Allergy Clin. Immunol.* 81:89–94.

Franz, T., McMurrain, K. D., Brooks, S., and Bernstein, I. L. (1971). Clinical, immunologic and physiologic observations in factory workers exposed to *B. fragilis* enzyme dust. *J. Allergy* 47:170–180.

Freeland, H. S., Schleimer, R. P., Schulman, E. S., Lichtenstein, L. M., and Peters, S. P. (1988). Generation of leukotriene B_4 by humans lung fragments and purified lung mast cells. *Am. Rev. Respir. Dis.* 138:389–394.

Friedman, M. M., and Kaliner, M. A. (1987). Mast cells and asthma. *Am. Rev. Respir. Dis.* 135:157–164.

Fuller, R. W., and Collier, J. C. (1984). Sodium cromoglycate and atropine block the fall in FEV_1 but not the cough induced by hypotonic mist. *Thorax* 39:766–770.

Fuller, R. W., Dixon, C. M. S., Dollery, C. T., and Barnes, P. J. (1986). Prostaglandin D_2 potentiates airway responsiveness to histamine and methacholine. *Am. Rev. Respir. Dis.* 133:252–254.

Fuller, R. W., Dixon, C. M. S., Cuss, F. M. C., and Barnes, P. J. (1987). Bradykinin induced bronchoconstriction in humans. *Am. Rev. Respir. Dis.* 135:175–180.

Furitsu, T., Saito, H., Dvorak, A. M., Schwartz, L. B., Irani, A-M., Burdick, J. F., Ishizaka, K., and Ishizaka, T. (1989). *Proc. Natl. Acad. Sci. USA* 86:10039–10043.

Gleich, G. J., Motojima, S., Frigas, E., Kephart, G. M., Fujisawa, T., and Kravis, L. P. (1987). The eosinophilic leukocyte and the pathology of fatal bronchial asthma: Evidence for pathologic heterogeneity. *J. Allergy Clin. Immunol.* 80 (3 Pt 2):412–414.

Gobel, P. P. (1978). The protective effect of ketotifen in bronchial asthma. *J. Int. Med. Res.* 6:79–8

Godden, D., Jamieson, S., and Higenbottan, T. (1983). "Fog" induced bronchoconstriction is inhibited by sodium cromoglycate but not lignocaine or ipratropium. *Thorax* 38:226–227.

Goldstein, S. M., Kaempfer, C. E., Kealey, J. T., and Wintroub, B. U. (1989). Human mast cell carboxypeptidase. *J. Clin. Invest.* 83:1630–1636.

Gonzalez, M. C., Diaz, P., Galleguillos, F. R., Ancic, P., Cromwell, O., and Kay, A. B. (1987). Allergen-induced recruitment of bronchoalveolar helper (OKT4) and suppressor (OKT8) T-cells in asthma. *Am. Rev. Respir. Dis.* 136:600–604.

Gorski, J. P., Hugli, T. E., and Muller-Eberhard, H. J. (1979). The third anaphylatoxin of the human complement system. *Prosc. Natl. Acad. Sci. USA* 76:5299–5304.

Goswami, S. K., Ohashi, M., Panangiotis, S., and Marom, Z. (1987). Platelet-activating factor enhances mucous glycoprotein release from human airways in vitro. *Am. Rev. Respir. Dis.* 135:A159

Gravelyn, T. R., Pan, P. M., and Eschenbacher, W. L. (1986). Mediator release in an isolated airway segment in subjects with asthma. *Am. Rev. Respir. Dis.* 137:641–646.

Griffin, M., Weiss, J. W., Leitch, A. G., McFadden, E. R. Jr., Corey, E. J., Austen, K. F., and Drazen, J. M. (1983). Effects of leukotriene D on the airways in asthma. *N. Engl. J. Med.* 308:436–439.

Haas, F., and Bergofski, E. H. (1972). Role of the mast cell in the pulmonary pressor response to hypoxia. *J. Clin. Invest.* 51:3143–3162.

Hägermark, O. E., Hoekfelt, T., and Pernow, B. (1978). Flare and itch induced by substance P in human skin. *J. Invest. Dermatol.* 71:233–235.

Hardy, C. C., Robinson, C., Tattersfield, A. E., and Holgate, S. T. (1984). Bronchoconstrictor response to inhaled PGD_2 in normal and asthmatic man. *N. Engl. J. Med.* 311:209–213.

Harries, M. G. (1981). Bronchial irritant receptors and a possible new action for cromolyn sodium. *Ann. Allergy* 46:156–158.

Hegardt, B., Pauwels, R., and Van der Stratten, M. (1981). Inhibitory effects of KWO 2131, terbutaline and DSCG on the immediate and late allergen-induced bronchoconstriction. *Allergy* 36:115–122.

Hellewell, P. G., and Williams, T. J. (1986). A specific antagonist of platelet-activating factor suppresses oedema formation in an arthus reaction but not oedema induced by leukocyte chemoattractants in rabbit skin. *J. Immunol.* 137:302–307.

Henderson, W. R., Jr. (1987). Lipid-derived and other chemical mediators of inflammation in the lung. *J. Allergy Clin.* Immunol. 79:543–553.

Henderson, W. R. Jr. (1991). Eicosanoids and platelet-activating factor in allergi respiratory diseases. *Am. Rev. Respir. Dis.* 143:S86–S90.

Henderson, W. R., Jr., and Kaliner, M. (1978). Immunologic and nonimmunologic generation of superoxide from mast cells and basophils. *J. Clin. Invest.* 61:187–96.

Hisatomo, H., Tsuda, T., Tsurumi, N., Takai, Y., Maeda, M., Takahashi, K., and Kimura, I. (1987). Anticoagulant substance released from human lung mast cells by stimulation with anti-IgE or Ca-ionophore A23187. *Acta Med. Okayama* 41(2):85–87.

Hitchcock, M. amd Kokolis, N. A. (1981). Arachidonic acid metabolism and modulation of in vitro anaphylaxis by 5,8,11,14-eicosatetraenoic acid and 9a,12a-octadecadiynoic acid. *Br. J. Pharmacol.* 72:689–695.

Hogg, J. C. (1986). Airway structure and function in asthma. *NER Allergy Proc.* 7:228–234.

Holgate, S. T., Burns, G. B., Robinson, C., and Church, M. K. (1984). Anaphylactic and calcium-dependent generation of prostaglandin D_2 [PGD_2], thromboxane B_2, and other cyclooxygenase products of arachidonic acid by dispersed human lung cells and relationship to histamine release. *J. Immunol.* 133:375–380.

Holgate, S. T., Djukanovic, R., Wilson, J., Roche, W. R., and Holwarth, P. H. (1991). Inflammatory processes and bronchial hyperresponsiveness. *Clin. Exp. Allergy* 21 (Suppl 1):30–36.

Holland, J. A., Pritchard, K. A., Pappolla, M. A., Wolin, M. S., Rogers, N., and Stemerman, M. B. (1990). Bradykinin induces superoxide anion release from human endothelial cells. *J. Cell. Physiol.* 143:21–25.

Howarth, P. H., Durham, S. R., Kay, A. B., and Holgate, S. T. (1987). The relationship between mast cell-mediator release and bronchial reactivity in allergic asthma. *J. Allergy Clin. Immunol.* 80:703–711.

Irani, A-M., and Schwartz, L. B. (1989). Mast cell heterogeneity. *Clin. Exp. Allergy* 19:143–155.

Irani, A-M., Schechter, N. M., Craig, S. S., DeBlois, G., and Schwartz, L. B. (1986). Two types of human mast cells that have distinct neutral protease compositions. *Proc. Natl. Acad. Sci. USA* 83:4464–4468.

Ishizaka, T., Chang, T. H., Taggart, M., and Ishizaka, K. (1972). Histamine release from rat mast cells by antibodies against rat basophilic leukemia cell membrane. *J. Immunol.* 108:339–345.

James, A. L., Pare, P. D., and Hogg, J. C. (1989). The mechanics of airway narrowing in asthma. *Am. Rev. Respir. Dis.* 139:242–246.

Jeffery, P. K., Wardlaw, A. J., Nelson, F. C., Collins, J. V., and Kay, A. B. (1989). Bronchial biopsies in asthma. *Am. Rev. Respir. Dis.* 140:1745–1753.

Johnson, S. L., and Holgate, S. T. (1990). Cellular and chemical mediators—their roles in allergic diseases. *Curr. Opin. Immunol.* 2:513–524.

Joris, I., Majno, G., Corey, E. J., and Lewis, R. A. (1987). The mechanism of vascular leakage induced by leukotriene E_4: Endothelial contraction. *Am. J. Pathol.* 126:19–24.

Junod, A. P. (1987). Effects of oxygen intermediates on cellular functions. *Am. Rev. Respir. Dis.* 135:32S–34S.

Kaliner, M. A. (1980), Mast cell derived mediators and bronchial asthma. In: *Airway Reactivity*. Edited by F. E. Hargreave. Mississauga, Ontario, Canada, Astra Pharmaceuticals Canada, pp. 175–187.

Kaliner, M. (1985). Mast cell mediators and asthma. *Chest* 87S:2–5.

Kaliner, M. (1989). Asthma and mast cell activation. *J. Allergy Clin. Immunol,* 83:510–520.

Kaliner, M., Blennerhassett, J., and Austen, K. F. (1976). Bronchial asthma. In: *Textbook of Immunopathy*. Edited by P. A. Meischer and H. J. Muller-Eberhard. New York, Grune & Stratton. pp. 387–402.

Kaliner, M., Shelhamer, J. H., Davis, P. B., Smith, L. J., and Venter, J. C. (1982). Autonomic nervous system abnormalities and allergy. *Ann. Intern. Med.* 96:349–57.

Karcezewski, W., and Widdecomb, J. G. (1969). The role of the vagus nerves in the respiratory and circulatory reactions of anaphylaxis in rabbits. *J. Physiol. (Lond.)* 201:293–304.

Kay, A. B. (1991). Asthma and inflammation. *J. Allergy Clin. Immunol.* 87:893–910.

Kay, A. B. (1989). Inflammatory cells in bronchial asthma. *J. Asthma* 26:335–344.

Kay, A. B., and Barnes, P. J. (1985). Pharmacologic modulation of the asthmatic response. In: *Current Perspectives in the Immunology of Respiratory Diseases*. Edited by A. B. Kay and E. J. Goetzl. New York, Churchill Livingstone, pp. 30–38.

Keahey, T. M., Indrisano, J. M., Lavker, R. M., and Kaliner, M. A. (1987a). Delayed vibratory angioedema: Insights into pathophysiologic mechanisms. *J. Allergy Clin. Immunol.* 80:831–838.

Keahey, T. M., Yancey, K. B., and Lawley, T. J. (1987b). Immediate hypersensitivity. *J. Am. Acad. Dermatol.* 17(5 Pt. 1):826–837.

Kern, R., Smith, L. J., Patterson, R., et al (1986). Characterisation of the airway response to inhaled LTD_4 in normal subjects. *Am. Rev. Respir. Dis.* 133: 1127.

Keyzer, J. J., Kauffman, H. F., de Monchy, J. G., Keyzer-Udding, J. J., and de Vries, K. (1984). Urinary N-tau methylhistamine during early and late allergen-induced bronchial obstructive reactions. *J. Allergy Clin. Immunol.* 74:240–245.

Kirby, J. G., Hargreave, F. E., Gleich, G. J., and O'Byrne, P. M. (1987). Bronchoalveolar cell profiles of asthmatic and non-asthmatic subjects. *Am. Rev. Respir. Dis.* 136:379–383.

Kirsenbaum, A. S., Kessler, S., Goff, J., and Metcalfe, D. D. (1991). Demonstration of the origin of human mast cells from bone marrow progenitor cells. *J. Immunol.* 146:1410–1415.

Kowalski, M. L., and Kaliner, M. A. (1988). Neurogenic inflammation, vascular permeability, and mast cells. *J. Immunol.* 140:3905–3911.

Lagunoff, D. (1974). Analysis of dye binding sites in the mast cell granule. *Biochemistry* 13:3982–3986.

Lagunoff, D., and Rickard, A. (1983). Evidence for control of mast cell granule protease in situ by low pH. *Exp. Cell. Res.* 144:353–60.

Lai, C. K. W., Polosa, R., and Holgate, S. T. (1990). Effect of 15-(s)-hydroxyeicosatetraenoic acid on allergen-induced asthmatic responses. *Am. Rev. Respir. Dis.* 141:1423–1427.

Laitinen, L. A., Heino, M., Laitinen, A., Kava, T., and Haahtela, T. (1985). Damage of the airway epithelium and bronchial reactivity in patients with asthma. *Am. Rev. Respir. Dis.* 131:599–606.

Lam, S., Chan, H., LeRiche, J. C., Chan-Yeung, M., and Salari, H. (1988). Release of leukotrienes in patients with bronchial asthma. *J. Allergy Clin. Immunol.* 81:711–717.

Lamb, D., and Lumsden, A. (1982). Intra-epithelial mast cells in human airway epithelium: Evidence for smoking induced changes in their frequency. *Thorax* 37:334–42.

Lampl, K. L., Lichtenstein, L. M., and Schleimer, R. P. (1985). In vitro resistance to dexamethasone of basophils from patients receiving long term steroid therapy. *Am. Rev. Respir. Dis.* 132:1015–1018.

Lee, T. H., Nagakura, T., Papageorgiou, N., Iikuray, I., and Kay, A. B. (1983). Exercise induced late asthmatic reactions with neutrophil chemotactic activity. *N. Engl. J. Med.* 308:1502–1505.

Lemanske, R. F., and Kaliner, M. A. (1988). Late phase allergic reactions. In: *Allergy Principles and Practice,* 3rd ed. Edited by E. Middleton, C. E., Reed, E. F., Ellis, N. F. Adkinson, and J. W., Yuninger. St. Louis, Mosby.

Lewis, R. A., and Austen, K. F. (1984). The biologically active leukotrienes biosynthesis, metabolism, receptors, functions, and pharmacology. *J. Clin. Invest.* 73:889–897.

Lewis, R. A., Soter, N. A., Diamond, N., Austen, K. F., Oates, J. A., and Roberts, L. J. (1982). II. Prostaglandin D_2 generation after activation of rat and human mast cells with anti-IgE. *J. Immunol.* 129:1627–1631.

Liu, M. C., Bleeker, E. R., Lichtenstein, L. M., Kagey-Sobotka, A., Niv, Y., Mclemore, T. L., Permutt, S., Proud, D., and Hubbard, W. C. (1990). Evidence for elevated levels of histamine, prostaglandin D_2, and other bronchoconstricting prostaglandins in the airways of subjects with mild asthma. *Am. Rev. Respir. Dis.* 142:126–132.

Liu, M. C., Hubbard, W. C., Proud, D., Stealey, B. A., Galli, S. J., Kagey-Sobotka, A., Bleeker, E. R., and Lichtenstein, L. M. (1991). Immediate and late inflammatory responses to ragweed antigen challenge of the peripheral airways in allergic asthmatics. *Am. Rev. Respir. Dis.* 144:51–58.

Lopez-Vidreiro, M. I., Das, I., Smith, A. P., Picot, R., and Reid, L. (1977). Bronchial secretion from normal human airways after inhalation of prostaglandin $F_{2\alpha}$, acetylcholine, histamine, and citric acid. *Thorax* 32:734–739.

Lowhagen, O., and Rak, I. (1985). Modification of bronchial hyperreactivity after treatment with sodium cromoglycate in atopic asthmatic patients not exposed to relevant allergens. *J. Allergy Clin. Immunol.* 75:343–347.

Lowman, M. A., Rees, P. H., Benyon, R. C., and Church, M. K. (1988). Human mast cell heterogeneity: Histamine release from mast cells dispersed from skin, lung, adenoids, tonsils, and colon in response to IgE-dependent and nonimmunologic stimuli. *J. Allergy Clin. Immunol.* 81:590–597.

Lozewicz, S., Wells, C., Gomez, E., Ferguson, H., Richman, P., Devalia, J., and

Davies, R. J. (1990). Morphological integrity of the bronchial epithelium in mild asthma. *Thorax* 45:12–15.

Lundgren, J. D., Wiedermann, C. J., Logun, C., Plutchok, J., Kaliner, M., and Shelhamer, J. (1988). Substance P mediated secretion of respiratory glycoconjugate from feline airways in vitro. *Exp. Lung. Res.*

Lundgren, J. D., Kaliner, M. A., Logan, C., and Shelhamer, J. H. (1990). Platelet activating factor and tracheobronchial respiratory glycoconjugate release in feline and human explants: involvement of lipoxygenase pathways. *Agents Actions* 30:329–337.

Lundgren, J. D., Davey, R. T., Lundgren, B., Mullol, J., Marom, Z., Logun, C., Baraniuk, J., Kaliner, M. A., and Shelhamer, J. H. (1991). Eosinophil cationic protein stimulates and major basis protein inhibits airway mucus secretion. *J. Allergy Clin. Immunol.* 87:689–698.

Lynch, J. M., and Henson, P. M. (1986). The intracellular retention of newly-synthesized platelet activating factor. *J. Immunol.* 137:2653–2661.

MacDonald, S. M., Lichtenstein, L. M., Proud, D., Plaut, M., Naclerio, R. M., MacGlashan, D. W., and Kagey-Sobotka, A. (1987). Studies of IgE-dependent histamine releasing factors: Heterogeneity of IgE. *J. Immunol.* 139:506–512.

Mak, J. C. W., and Barnes, P. J. (1991). Autoradiographic visualization of bradykinin receptors in human and guinea pig lung. *Eur. J. Pharmacol.* 194:37–43.

Margo, A. M. (1974). Involvement of IgE in Con-A induced histamine release from human basophils in vitro. *Nature (Lond.)* 249:572–574.

Marom, Z., Shelhamer, J. H., and Kaliner, M. (1981). The effect of arachidonic acid, monohydroxyeicosatetraenoic acid, and prostaglandins on the release of mucous glycoprotein from human airways in vitro. *J. Clin. Invest.* 67:1695–1702.

Marone, G., Casolaro, V., Cirillo, R., Stellato, C., and Genovese, A. (1989). Pathophysiology of human basophils and mast cells in allergic disorders. *Clin. Immunol. Immunopathol.* 50:S24–S40.

Marquardt, D. L., Parker, C. W., and Sullivan, T. J. (1978). Potentiation of mast cell mediator release by adenosine. *J. Immunol.* 120:871–878.

Mattoli, S., Mattoso, V. L., Soloperto, M., Allegra, L., and Fasoli, A. (1991). Cellular and biochemical characteristics of bronchoalveolar lavage fluid in symptomatic nonallergic asthma. *J. Allergy Clin. Immunol.* 87:794–802.

Messer, J. W., Peters, G. A., and Bennett, W. A. (1960). Causes of death and pathologic findings in 304 cases of bronchial asthma. *Chest* 38:616–624.

Metcalfe, D. D., Lewis, R. A., Silbert, J. E., Rosenberg, R. D., Wasserman, S. I., and Austen, K. F. (1979). Isolation and characterization of heparin from human lung. *J. Clin. Invest.* 64:1537–1543.

Metcalfe, D. D., Kaliner, M. A., and Donlon, M. A. (1981). The mast cell. *CRC Crit. Rev. Immunol.* 3:23–74.

Metzger, W. J., Richerson, H. B., Worden, K., Monick, H., and Hunninghake, G. (1986). Bronchoalveolar lavage of allergic asthmatic patients following allergen bronchoprovocation. *Chest* 89:477–483.

Metzger, W. J., Zavala, D., Richerson, H. B., Moseley, P., Iwamota, P., Monick, M., Sjoerdsma, K., and Hunninghake, G. (1987). Local allergen challenge and bronchoalveolar lavage of allergic asthmatic lungs. *Am. Rev. Respir. Dis.* 135:433–440.

Miadonna, A., Tedeschi, A., Brasca, C., Folco, G., Sala, A., and Murphy, R. C. (1990). Mediator release after endobronchial antigen challenge in patients with respiratory allergy. *J. Allergy Clin. Immunol.* 85:906–913.

Moqbel, R., Durham, S. R., Shaw, R. J., Walsh, G. M., MacDonald, A. J., MacKay, J. A., Carroll, M., and Kay, A. B. (1986). Enhancement of leukocyte cytotoxicity after exercise-induced asthma. *Am. Rev. Respir. Dis.* 133:609–613.

Morrison, D. C., and Henson, P. M. (1978). Release of mediators from mast cells and basophils induced by different stimuli. In: *Immediate Hypersensitivity—Modern Concepts and Development*. Edited by M. K. Bach. New York, Marcel Decker, pp. 431–502.

Munoz, N. M., Shiioya, T., Murphy, T. M., Primak, S., Dame, C., Sands, M. F., and Leff, A. R. (1986). Potentiation of vagal contractile responses by thromboxane mimetic U-46619. *J. Appl. Physiol.* 61:1173–1179.

Murray, J. J., Tonnel, A. B., Brash, A. R., et al. (1986). Release of prostaglandin D_2 into human airways during acute allergen challenge. *N. Engl. J. Med.* 315:800–804.

Nagy, L., Lee, T. H., and Kay, A. B. (1982). Neutrophil chemotactic activity in antigen-induced late asthmatic reactions. *N. Engl. J. Med.* 306:497–501.

O'Byrne, P. M. (1990). Eicosanoids and inflammatory cells in asthma. *Agents Actions* (Suppl. 31):85–101.

O'Donnell, M. C., Ackerman, S. J., Gleich, G. L., and Thomas, L. L. (1983). Activation of basophil and mast cell histamine release by eosinophil granule major basic protein. *J. Exp. Med.* 157:1981–1991.

Orchard, M. A., Kagey-Sobotka, A., Proud, D., and Lichtenstein, L. M. (1986). Basophil histamine release induced by a substance from stimulated human platelets. *J. Immunol.* 136:2240–2244.

Patterson, R., Ts'ao, C-h, and Susko, I. M. (1980). Heterogeneity of bronchial lumen mast cells which are homogenous by electron microscopy. *J. Allergy Clin. Immunol.* 65:278–284.

Patterson, N. A. M., Burka, J. F., and Craig, I. D. (1981). Release of slow reacting substance of anaphylaxis from dispersed pig lung cells: effect of cyclo-oxygenase and lipoxygenase inhibitors. *J. Allergy Clin. Immunol.* 67:426–434.

Peachell, P., Columbo, M., Kagey-Sobotka, A., Lichtenstein, L. M., and Marone, G. (1988). Adenosine potentiates mediator release from human lung mast cells. *Am. Rev. Respir. Dis.* 138:1143–1151.

Persson, C. G. A. (1991). Mucosal exudation in respiratory defence:neural or non-neural control? *Int. Arch. Allergy Appl. Immunol.* 94:222–226.

Persson, C. G. A., Erjefalt, I., and Sundler, F. (1987). Airway microvascular and epithelial leakage of plasma induced by PAF-acether (PAF) and capsaicin (CAP). *Am. Rev. Respir. Dis.* 135:A401.

Peters, S. P., MacGlashan, D. W., Schulman, E. S., Schleimer, R. P., Hoyes, E. S., Rokach, J., Adkinson, N. F., Jr., and Lichtenstein, L. M. (1984). Arachidonic acid metabolism in purified human lung mast cells. *J. Immunol.* 131:1972–1979.

Phillips, G. D., Rafferty, P., Beasley, C. R. W., and Holgate, S. T. (1987). The effect of oral terfenadine on the bronchoconstrictor response to inhaled histamine and adenosine 5'-monophosphate in non-atopic asthma. *Thorax* 42:939–945.

Platshon, L., and Kaliner, M. (1978). The effect of the immunologic release of histamine upon human lung cyclic nucleotide levels and prostaglandin generation. *J. Clin. Invest.* 62:1113–1121.

Plaut, M., Pierce, J. H., Watson, C. J., Hanley-Hyde, J., Nordan, R. P., and Paul, W. E. (1989). Mast cells produce lymphokines in response to cross linkage of $Fc_{\epsilon}R$ and to calcium ionophores. *Nature* 339:64–67.

Polosa, R., Church, M. K., and Holgate, S. T. (1990). The mode of action of airway responses to adenosine in asthma. *Immunol. Allergy Clin. North Am.* 10(2):363–372.

Proud, D., Baumgarten, C. R., Naclerio, R. M., and Lichtenstein, L. M. (1986). The role of kinins in human allergic disease. *NER Allergy Proc.* 7:213–218.

Rand, T., Cruikshank, W. W., Center, D. M., and Weller, P. F. (1991). CD4 mediated stimulation of human eosinophils: lymphocyte chemoattractant factor and other CD4 binding ligands elicit eosinophil migration. *J. Exp. Med.* 173:1521–1528.

Richardson, P. S., and Peatfield, A. C. (1987). The control of airway mucus secretion. *Eur. J. Respir. Dis.* 71(Suppl. 153):43–51.

Roberts, J. A., Rodger, I. W., and Thomson, N. C. (1987). In vivo and in vitro human airway responsiveness to leukotriene D_4 in patients without asthma. *J. Allergy Clin. Immunol.* 80:688–694.

Robertson, D. G., Kerigan, A. T., Hargreave, F. E., Chalmers, R., and Dolovich, J. (1974). Late asthmatic responses induced by ragweed pollen allergen. *J. Allergy Clin. Immunol.* 54:244–254.

Robinson, C., and Holgate, S. T. (1985). Mast cell-dependent inflammatory mediators and their putative role in bronchial asthma. *Clin. Sci.* 68:103–112.

Roche, W. R., Beasley, R., Williams, J., and Holgate, S. T. (1989). Subepithelial fibrosis in the bronchi of asthmatics. *Lancet* 1:520–524.

Rogers, D. F., and Dewar, A. (1990). Neural control of airway mucus secretion. *Biochem. Pharmacother.* 44:447–453.

Rogers, D. F., Aursudkij, B., and Barnes, P. J. (1989). Effects of tachykinins on mucus secretion in human bronchi in vitro. *Eur. J. Pharmacol.* 174:283–286.

Rosenthal, R. R., Norman, P. S., Summer, W. R., and Permutt, S. (1977). Role of the parasympathetic system in antigen-induced bronchospasm. *J. Appl. Physiol.* 42:600–606.

Rubin, A-H. E., Smith, L. J., and Patterson, R. (1987). The bronchoconstrictor properties of platelet activating factor in humans. *Am. Rev. Respir. Dis.* 136:1145–1151.

Sautebin, L., Vitgano, T., Grassi, E., et al. (1985). Release of leukotrienes, induced by the Ca^{++} ionophore A23187, from human lung parenchyma in vitro. *J. Pharmacol. Exp. Ther.* 234:217

Schechter, N. M., Fraki, J. E., Geesin, J. C., and Lazarus, G. S. (1983). Human skin chymotryptic protease isolation and relation to cathepsin G and rat mast cell proteinase I. *J. Biol. Chem.* 258:2973–2978.

Schleimer, R. P., MacGlashan, D. W. Jr., Peters, S. P., Pinckard, R. N., Adkinson, N. F., Jr., and Lichtenstein, L. M. (1986). Characterization of inflammatory mediator release from purified human lung mast cells. *Am. Rev. Respir. Dis.* 133: 614–617.

Schulman, E. S., Newball, H. H., Demers, L. M., Fitzpatrick, F. A., and Adkinson, N. F., Jr. (1981). Anaphylactic release of thromboxane A_2, prostaglandin D_2, and prostacyclin from lung parenchyma. *Am. Rev. Respir. Dis.* 124:402–406.

Schulman, E. S., Liu, M. C., Proud, D., MacGlashan, D. W., Lichtenstein, L. M., and Plaut, M. (1985). Human lung macrophages induce histamine release from basophils and mast cells. *Am. Rev. Respir. Dis.* 131:230–235.

Schulman, E. S., Pollack, R. B., Post, T. J., and Peters, S. P. (1990). Histochemical heterogeneity of dispersed human mast cells. *J. Immunol.* 144:4195–4201.

Schwartz, L. B., Lewis, R. A., and Austen, K. F. (1981). Tryptase from human pulmonary mast cells: purification and characterization. *J. Biol. Chem.* 256:11939–11943.

Schwartz, L. B., Irani, A-M., Roller, K., Castells, M. C., and Schechter, N. M. (1987). Quantitation of histamine, tryptase, and chymase in dispersed human T and TC mast cells. *J. Immunol.* 138:2611–2615.

Segal, D. M., Taurog, J. D., and Metzger, H. (1977). Dimeric immunoglobulin E serves as a unit signal for mast cell degranulation. *Proc. Natl. Acad. Sci. USA* 74:2993–2998.

Shelhamer, J. H., Marom, Z., and Kaliner, M. (1980). Immunologic and neuropharmacologic stimulation of mucous glycoprotein release from human airways in vitro. *J. Clin. Invest.* 66:1400–1408.

Shelhamer, J. H., Marom, Z., Sun, F., Black, M. K., and Kaliner, M. (1981). The effects of arachinoids and leukotrienes on the release of mucus from human airways. *Chest* 81S:36–37.

Silber, G., Proud, D., Warner, J., Naclerio, R., Kagey-Sobotka, A., Lichtenstein, L. M., and Eggleston, P. (1988). In vivo release of inflammatory mediators by hyperosmolar solutions.

Smith, L. J., Kern, R., Patterson, R., Krell, R. D., and Bernstein, P. R. (1987). Mechanism of leukotriene D_4-induced bronchoconstriction in normal subjects. *J. Allergy Clin. Immunol.* 80:338–345.

Smith, L. J., Greenberger, P. A., Patterson, R., Krell, R. D., and Bernstein, P. R. (1985). The effect of leukotriene D_4 in humans. *Am. Rev. Respir. Dis.* 131:368–372.

Smith, L. J., Rubin, A. E., and Patterson, R. (1988). Mechanisms of platelet activating factor induced bronchoconstriction in humans. *Am. Rev. Respir. Dis.* 137:1015–1019.

Sobonya, R. E. (1984). Quantitative structural alterations in long-standing allergic asthma. *Am. Rev. Respir. Dis.* 130:289–292.

Spannhake, E. W., Hyman, A. L., and Kadowitz, P. J. (1981). Bronchoactive metabolites of arachidonic acid and their role in airway function. *Prostaglandins* 22:1013–1026.

Sperber, K., Goswami, S. K., Gollub,. E., Mayer, L., and Marom, Z. (1991). Mucus secretagogue production by a human macrophage hybridoma. *J. Allergy Clin. Immunol.* 87:490–498.

Stalenheim, G., and Machado, L. (1985). Late allergic bronchial reactions and the effect of allergen provocation on the complement system. *J. Allergy Clin. Immunol.* 75:508–512.

Steel, L., and Kaliner, M. (1981). Prostaglandin-generating factor of anaphylaxis—identification and isolation. *J. Biol. Chem.* 256:12592–12598.

Steel, L., Platshon, L., and Kaliner, M. (1979). Prostaglandin generation by human and guinea pig lung tissue: comparison of parenchymal and airway responses. *J. Allergy Clin. Immunol.* 64:287–293.

Steffen, M., Abboud, M., Potter, G. K., Yung, Y. P., and Moore, M. A. S. (1989). Presence of tumour necrosis factor or a related factor in human basophil/mast cells. *Immunology* 66:445–450.

Strobel, S., Miller, H. R. P., and Ferguson, A. (1981). Human intestinal mast cells: evaluation of fixation and staining techniques. *J. Clin. Pathol.* 34:841–858.

Sturk, A., Wouten ten Cate, J., Hosford, D., and Nencia-Huerta. (1989). The synthesis, catabolism, and pathophysiological role of platelet activating factor. *Adv. Lipid Res.* 23:219–276.

Tannenbaum, S., Oertel, H., Henderson, W., and Kaliner, M. (1980). The biologic activity of mast cell granules. I. Elicitation of inflammatory responses in rat skin. *J. Immunol.* 125:325–335.

Tharp, M. D., Kagey-Sobotka, A., Fox, C. C., Marone, G., Lichtenstein, L. M., and Sullivan, T. J. (1987). *J. Allergy Clin. Immunol.* 79:646–653.

Theuson, D. O., Speck, L. S., Lett-Brown, A., and Grant, J. A. (1979). Histamine releasing activity (HRA). I. Production by mitogen or antigen stimulated human mononuclear cells. *J. Immunol.* 123:626–632.

Togias, A. S., Naclerio, R. M., Proud, D., Fish, J. E., Adkinson, N. F., Jr., Kagey-Sobotka, A., Norman, P. S., and Lichtenstein, L. M. (1985). Nasal challenge with cold, dry air results in release of inflammatory mediators. Possible mast cell involvement. *J. Clin. Invest.* 76:1375–1381.

Tomioka, M., Ida, S., Shindoh, Y., Ishisara, T., and Takishima, T. (1984). Mast cells in bronchoalveolar lumen of patients with bronchial asthma. *Am. Rev. Respit. Dis.* 129:1000–1005.

Trotter, C. M., and Orr, R. S. C. (1973). A fine structure study of some cellular components in allergic reactions. *Clin. Allergy* 3:411–425.

Ts'ao, C., Patterson, R., McKenna, J. M., and Suzko, I. M. (1977). Ultrastructural identification of mast cells obtained from human bronchial lumens. *J. Allergy Clin. Immunol.* 59:320–326.

van Overveld, F. J. (1989). Mediator release from human lung mast cell subtypes in chronic bronchitis and emphysema. *Agents Actions* 27:97–100.

van Overveld, F. J., Houben, A. M. J., Schmitz du Moulin, F. E. M., Bruijnzeel, P. L. B., Raaijmakers, J. A. M., and Terpstra, G. K. (1989). Mast cell heterogeneity in human lung tissue. *Clin. Sci.* 77:297–304.

Vincenc, K., Black, J., and Shaw, J. (1984). Relaxation and contraction responses to histamine in human lung parenchymal strips. *Eur. J. Pharmacol.* 84:201–210.

Wardlaw, A. J., Cromwell, O., Celestino, D., Fitzharris, P., Geddes, D. M., Collins, J. V., and Kay, A. B. (1986). Morphologic and secretory properties of bronchoalveolar lavage mast cells in respiratory diseases. *Clin. Allergy* 16:163–173.

Wardlaw, A. J., Dunnette, S., Gleich, G. J., Collins, J. V., and Kay, A. B. (1988). Eosinophils and mast cells in bronchoalveolar lavage in subjects with mild asthma. Relationship to bronchial hyperreactivity. *Am. Rev. Respir. Dis.* 137:62–69.

Wardlaw, A. J., Hay, H., Cromwell, O., Collins, J. V., and Kay, A. B. (1989). Leukotrienes, LTC_4 and LTB_4 in bronchoalveolar lavage in bronchial asthma and other respiratory diseases. *J. Allergy Clin. Immunol.* 84:19–24.

Warner, J. O. (1976). Significance of late reactions after bronchial challenge with house dust mite. *Arch. Dis. Child.* 51:905–911.

Warner, J. O., Soothill, J. F., Price, J. F., and Hey, E. N. (1978). Controlled trial of hyposensitization to dermatophagoides pteronyssius in children with asthma. *Lancet* 2:912–915.

Wasserman, S. I. (1980). The lung mast cell: Its physiology and potential relevance to defense of the lung. *Environ. Health Perspect.* 35:153–164.

Wasserman, S. I. (1987). The regulation of inflammatory mediator production by mast cell products. *Am. Rev. Respir. Dis.* 135:S46–S48.

Wasserman, S. I. (1989). Mast cell-mediated inflammation in asthma. *Ann. Allergy.* 63:546–550.

Wenzel, S. E., Fowler, A. A., and Schwartz, L. B. (1988). Activation of pulmonary mast cells by bronchoalveolar lavage challenge: In vivo release of histamine and tryptase in atopic subjects with and without asthma. *Am. Rev. Respir. Dis.* 137:1002–1008.

Wenzel, S. E., Wescott, J. Y., Smith, H. R., and Larsen, G. L. (1989). Spectrum of prostanoid release after bronchoalveolar allergen challenge in atopic asthmatics as in control groups. *Am. Rev. Respir. Dis.* 139:450–457.

Wenzel, S. E., Larsen, G. L., Johnston, K., Voelkel, N. F., and Westcott, J. Y. (1990). Elevated levels of leukotriene C_4 in bronchoalveolar lavage fluid from atopic asthmatics after endobronchial allergen challenge. *Am. Rev. Respir. Dis.* 142:112–119.

White, M. V. (1990). The role of histamine in allergic diseases. *J. Allergy Clin. Immunol.* 86:599–605.

White, M. V., and Kaliner, M. A. (1987). Neutrophils and mast cells. I. Human neutrophil-derived histamine-releasing activity. *J. Immunol.* 139:1624–1630.

White, M. V., Kaplan, A. P., Haak-Frendscho, M., and Kaliner, M. (1988). Neutrophils and mast cells. Comparison of cells responsive to neutrophil derived histamine releasing activity (HRA-N) with other histamine releasing factors. *J. Immunol.* 141:3575–3583.

White, M. V., Kowalski, M., and Kaliner, M. A. Mast cell secretagogues. In: *Biochemistry of the Acute Allergic Reaction,* Fifth International Symposium. Edited by B. Wintroub, F. Tauber, and A. S. Simon. New York, Alan R. Liss.

Wintroub, B. U., Schechter, N. M., Lazarus, G. S., Kaempfer, C. E., and Schwartz, L. B. (1984). Angiotensin I conversion by human and rat mast cell chymotryptic proteinases. *J. Invest. Dermatol.* 83:336–339.

Wintroub, B. U., Kaempfer, C. E., Schechter, N. M., and Proud, D. (1986). A human lung mast cell chymotrypsin-like enzyme. *J. Clin. Invest.* 77:196–201.

Wolfe, J., Londos, C., and Cooper, D. M. R. (1981). Adenosine receptors and the regulation of adenylate cyclase. *Adv. Cyclic Nucleotide Res.* 14:199–214.

Wood-Baker, R., and Church, M. K. (1990). Histamine and asthma. *Immunol. Allergy Clin. North Am.* 10(2):329–336.

Woodward, D. F., Weichman, B. M., Gill, C. A., and Wasserman, M. A. (1983). The effect of synthetic leukotrienes on tracheal microvascular permeability. *Prostaglandins* 25:131.

Yuen, E., Brown, R. B., van der Lubbe, L., Rickard, K. A., and Kronenberg, H. (1988). Identification and characterization of human hemopoietic mast cell colonies. *Exp. Hematol.* 16:896–902.

23

Mast Cell Involvement in Food Allergy

HUGH A. SAMPSON

The Johns Hopkins University School of Medicine
Baltimore, Maryland

I. Introduction

A. Prevalence of Food Hypersensitivity

Although food allergic reactions were first documented over 2000 years ago, the prevalence of this disorder is still unknown. A recent survey of American households found that at least one member of the family was believed to suffer from food allergies in one-third of households (Sloan and Powers, 1986). In a prospective study of 501 newborns followed in a general pediatric practice through their third birthday, parents reported adverse food reactions in 28% of the infants (Bock, 1987). As recorded in the *Federal Register,* the U.S. Department of Agriculture estimated that "some 15% of the population may be allergic to some food ingredients or ingredient" (U.S. Dept. of Agriculture, 1983).

While the "perceived prevalence" of food allergic reactions is quite high, most medical texts suggest that the "true prevalence" of food allergy is less than 1% of the population. In fact, virtually no data exist to address this issue. In Bock's study, 480/501 children were followed until their third birthday. Of 133 reported to have experienced an adverse reaction to a food, only 38 cases (or 8% overall) could be confirmed by oral food challenge (Bock, 1987). This study demonstrated that "perceived" food allergy is much greater than true food allergy, but also suggests that true allergy (at least in this age group) may be more prevalent than previously believed. Appropriate epidemiological studies in older individuals are obviously needed.

B. Potential Mechanisms of Mast Cell Activation by Food Antigens

As shown in Table 1, there are a variety of potential mechanisms by which food antigens may activate mast cells. The type I, IgE-mediated hypersensitivity reaction to foods is the only mechanism that is clearly established. The generation of the anaphylatoxins C3a and C5a following the formation of food antigen-antibody complexes has been suggested as a likely cause of mast cell activation, but has not been demonstrated in clinical trials (Sampson, 1988). Major basic protein, which has been shown to activate mast cells in vitro (Gleich and Leiferman, 1986), is deposited in the skin of some patients with atopic dermatitis following oral food challenges (Sampson, 1988). Mononuclear cells from patients with food allergy have been shown to secrete histamine-releasing factors in vitro that activate basophils via surface-bound IgE (Sampson et al., 1989a) and perhaps mast cells. Similarly, neuropeptides such as gastrin have been shown to activate mast cells in vitro. Whether any of these cytokines play a pathogenic role in food hypersensitivity in humans remains speculative.

II. Antigen Handling by the Gastrointestinal Tract

A. Gastrointestinal Barrier

The main function of the gastrointestinal tract is to process ingested food into basic components that can be absorbed and utilized for energy and cell growth. Food represents the greatest antigenic load confronting the body and therefore must be converted into a nonimmunogenic state. As shown in Table 2, a variety of physiological and immunological mechanisms are used to prevent antigens/allergens from entering the body (Walker, 1981). A series of enzymes are present to degrade glycoproteins to amino acids, small peptides, and sugars.

Table 1 Potential Mechanisms of Food Antigen–Induced Mast Cell Activation

1. Type I, IgE-mediated hypersensitivity
2. ? Type III, antigen-antibody complex activation with generation of C3a and C5a
3. ? Major basic protein release from eosinophils
4. ? Mononuclear cell generation of HRFs
5. ? Release of neuropeptides (e.g., gastrin)
6. ? Food lectin-IgE activation of mast cells

Table 2 Barriers to Ingested Food Antigens

Physiological
Breakdown ingested antigens
Gastric acid and pepsins
Pancreatic enzymes
Intestinal enzymes
Intestinal epithelial cell lysozyme activity
Block penetration of ingested antigens
Intestinal peristalsis
Intestinal mucus coat (glycocalyx)
Intestinal microvillus membrane composition
Immunological
Block penetration of ingested antigens
Antigen-specific s-IgA in gut lumen
Clear penetrating antigens
Serum antigen-specific IgA and IgG
Reticuloendothelial system

Specialized mucosal epithelial cells selectively absorb amino acids and small peptides and possess lysozymal activity to further degrade small peptides into amino acids. The intestinal peristaltic activity, mucus layer (glycocalyx), and microvillus membrane composition all serve to block entry of foreign antigen. Antigen-specific s-IgA is produced by the gut-associated lymphoid tissue and secreted into the intestinal lumen, where it "ties up" foreign antigens, blocking their penetration of the gut wall. Antigen-specific IgG and IgA is present to bind antigens that enter the body proper, making them readily susceptible to clearing by the reticuloendothelial system.

B. Antigen Penetration of the Gastrointestinal Barrier

Despite the elaborate gastrointestinal barrier network present in humans, early studies clearly demonstrated that immunologically intact food proteins enter the circulation and are distributed throughout the body. The principle of passive sensitization, first demonstrated by Prausnitz and Kustner, was exploited by several investigators to demonstrate that immunologically intact food antigens penetrated the gut barrier. In a classic case of self-experimentation, Freeman injected the mucosa of one side of his nose with serum from an egg-allergic patient (Freeman, 1925). Later he ingested an egg and noted stuffiness and pruritus on that side of his nose for several hours.

In a series of experiments, Walzer and his colleagues utilized sera from egg-and-fish-allergic patients to passively sensitize volunteers. Adult volunteers were given an intradermal injection of 0.05 ml of patient and control sera. Approximately 24 hr later they were fed fish or eggs (Walzer, 1927). Within several minutes to 1 hr after ingestion, a wheal and erythema were noted at the sensitized site but not the control site in over 90% of subjects. Within 1–8 hr, the reaction completely subsided. Utilizing a similar protocol in 14 subjects, it was shown that peanut antigen was rapidly absorbed from different locations in the gastrointestinal tract: oral–24.3 min, duodenum—18.6 min, and rectum—18.7 min (Gray and Walzer, 1940). Overall, it was demonstrated that food antigens were most readily absorbed from the small intestine, colon, and rectum and somewhat more slowly from the esophagus and stomach. Several factors, including increased stomach acidity, the presence of other food, and kaolin, decreased antigen absorption, while increased absorption resulted from decreased stomach acidity and alcohol (Walzer, 1941). Passive sensitization of rectal, colonic, and ileal mucosa was carried out in normal volunteers and patients with ileostomies and colostomies. Oral ingestion of the specific food allergen resulted in pallor at the sensitized site initially, followed rapidly by edema, hyperemia, and marked mucus secretion (Walzer, 1941). Interestingly, allergen reaching the sensitized tissues by the systemic route provoked a greater reaction than larger quantities of antigen applied topically to the sensitized site. Overall, this series of experiments proved unequivocally that food antigens/allergens are rapidly adsorbed from the gastrointestinal tract and transported via the circulation to intestinal and extraintestinal mast cells.

III. Food-Induced Mast Cell Activation in the Gut

A. Animal Studies of IgE-Mediated Food Hypersensitivity

The IgE-mediated gastrointestinal reaction in the rat has proven to be a useful model of immediate food hypersensitivity. Gall and co-workers demonstrated several physiological changes in the gastrointestinal tract following the ingestion of a food allergen, as shown in Table 3 (Perdue et al., 1984; Scott et al., 1988). In the stomach there is a sharp increase in gastric acid secretions, delayed gastric emptying, and mast cell degranulation with increased intraluminal histamine and serum rat mast cell protein II (RMCP-II). In the intestine, Na^+, Cl^-, and water absorption decreases sharply, while markedly increased aboral contractility leads to diarrhea. Intestinal mast cells appear degranulated, and intraluminal histamine and serum RMCP-II increase significantly. The mucosal architecture appears largely unchanged following a reaction, but significant disruption of the basement membrane and underlying collagenous matrix is apparent by ultrastructural examination (Patrick et al., 1988). None of these responses are blocked by cromolyn sodium, H_1 antihistamines, or H_2 antihistamines (Perdue and Gall, 1985).

Table 3 IgE-Mediated Gastrointestinal Reaction in the Rat

Stomach
↑ Gastric acid secretion
Delayed gastric emptying
MC degranulation in gastric mucosa
↑ Intraluminal release of histamine
↑ Serum RMCP-II
Intestine
↓ Na^+, Cl^-, & H_2O absorption
↑ Aboral contractility and diarrhea
Not blocked by Na cromolyn, H_1 or H_2 antagonists

Source: Gall et al. IgE-mediated GI reaction in the rat.

Using a similar model in rats sensitized with ovalbumin, Turner and co-workers demonstrated the effects of repeated daily ingestion of ovalbumin (Turner et al., 1990). Serum RMCP-II levels were approximately 16 times normal following the ovalbumin challenge on the first day and ranged between 2 and 5 times normal on the subsequent 4 days. Interestingly, after the rats were rested 9 days before rechallenge with ovalbumin, serum RMCP-II levels again rose to only 5 times normal concentrations. In the sensitized rats, the initial allergen exposure led to a marked mast cell activation (release of RMCP-II and probably other mast cell mediators), followed by a period of partial desensitization. Subsequent allergen exposures after brief periods of avoidance result in smaller (but significant) amounts of mediator release. These studies lend support to the observation in humans that an extended period of food avoidance is desirable to elicit a distinctive response to oral food challenge. In addition, they provide an explanation for why it is often difficult to observe obvious symptoms in a food-allergic individuals ingesting a food allergen on a regular basis.

B. Human Studies of IgE-Mediated Food Hypersensitivity

Early studies focused on the roentgenological changes associated with the ingestion of a food allergen. Eyermann studied a wheat-sensitive patient following a deliberate feeding of wheat. He noted hypertonicity in the transverse and pelvic colon and hypotonicity in the cecum and ascending colon (Eyermann, 1927). Rowe studied four patients after administering barium mixtures containing specific allergens. He observed gastric retention, hypermotility of the intestine, and colonic spasm (Rowe, 1933). Utilizing a single-blind protocol, a comparative fluoroscopic study of barium sulfate meals with and without food allergen was conducted in 12 food-allergic children (Fries, 1937). The most prominent findings included gastric hypotonia and retention of the allergen test meal, prominent pylorospasm, and increased or decreased peristaltic activity of the intestines.

In the late 1930s, several investigators utilized the rigid gastroscope to observe allergic reactions in the stomach. Pollard and Stuart studied six patients with gastrointestinal food allergy, four patients who had asthma symptoms exacerbated by food ingestion, and three controls (Pollard and Stuart, 1942). Food allergen was applied to the gastric mucosa of patients and revisualized 30 min later. As seen at passively sensitized intestinal mucosal sites in the studies of Walzer, the gastric mucosa was markedly hyperemic and edematous, with patches of thick, gray mucous and scattered petechiae. In patients with wheezing provoked by food ingestion, mild hyperemia of the gastric mucosa was noted. More recent studies of intragastric provocation under endoscopic control (IPEC) by Reimann and Lewin have verified the observations of Pollard. In addition, they demonstrated that food-allergic patients have increased tissue mast cell counts prior to challenge compared to normal controls and have significant decreases in tissue histamine content and stainable mast cells following food challenge (Reimann and Lewin, 1988). The specificity of IPEC for symptomatic food allergy remains unclear, however, because no investigators have evaluated patients with positive skin tests to foods and no evidence of clinical reactivity. As shown in Table 4, Selbekk compared IPEC to the results of prick skin tests, RAST, and in vitro mast cell degranulation from mucosal biopsies in 15 patients (Selbekk, 1985). This study demonstrated that prick skin tests and RASTs showed poor correlation with the results of IPECs in patients with predominantly gastrointestinal symptoms.

C. Signs and Symptoms of Mast Cell-Mediated Hypersensitivity in Humans

A variety of syndromes are associated with food-induced, IgE-mediated mast cell activation in humans. This mechanism is well established in oral anaphylaxis, gastrointestinal anaphylaxis, and a subgroup of allergic eosino-

Table 4 Comparison of IPEC, MMCD, PST, and RAST in Patients with Gastrointestinal Allergy

	MMCD		PST		RAST	
IPEC	+	–	+	–	+	–
+	13	1	5	9	1	11
–	4	18	3	16	1	19

Source: Selbekk (1985).

philic gastroenteropathy, but its role in food-induced enterocolitis syndrome and a subgroup of infantile colic remains to be confirmed.

Oral Allergy Syndrome

The oral allergy syndrome is similar to contact urticaria except that symptoms are confined almost exclusively to the oropharynx and rarely involve other target organs. Symptoms are most commonly associated with the ingestion of various fresh fruits and vegetables and consist of pruritus and edema of the lips, tongue, palate, and throat (Ortaloni et al., 1989). Respiratory allergy secondary to certain airborne pollens is frequently associated with this syndrome. For example, patients sensitive to birch pollen may develop oral symptoms following the ingestion of raw potatoes, carrots, celery, apples, and hazelnuts; patients allergic to ragweed may experience symptoms following contact with melons (watermelon, cantalope, honeydew, etc.) and bananas.

Gastrointestinal Anaphylaxis

A variety of food-induced IgE-mediated gastrointestinal symptoms have been confirmed by oral food challenge (Sampson, 1989a). These symptoms generally develop within minutes to 2 h of consuming a food allergen and consist of nausea, abdominal pain, cramps, vomiting, and/or diarrhea. There is some evidence that frequent ingestion of a responsible food allergen leads to partial desensitization of gastrointestinal mast cells and less prominent symptoms, such as poor appetite and periodic abdominal pain.

Allergic Eosinophilic Gastroenteropathy

In a subset of patients with allergic eosinophilic gastroenteropathy syndrome, food-induced, IgE-mediated mast cell activation is responsible for symptoms. Patients with this syndrome commonly present with postprandial nausea and vomiting, abdominal pain, diarrhea, occasionally steatorrhea, and weight loss in adults or failure to thrive in young infants (Kettlehut and Metcalfe, 1988). Patients with food-induced symptoms generally have the mucosal form of this syndrome, other atopic disorders, elevated serum IgE levels, positive prick skin tests to a variety of foods and inhalants, peripheral blood eosinophilia, iron deficiency anemia, and hypoalbuminemia. Generalized edema secondary to hypoalbuminemia may occur in some infants with marked protein-losing enteropathy, often in the presence of minimal gastrointestinal symptoms, such as occasional vomiting and diarrhea (Waldman et al., 1967). Rarely allergic eosinophilic gastroenteropathy may present in infants as pyloric stenosis with outlet obstruction (Snyder et al., 1987). Elimination of the responsible food allergen from the diet for up to 12 weeks may be necessary to bring about resolution of symptoms and normalization of intestinal histology.

Food-Induced Enterocolitis Syndrome

Food-induced enterocolitis syndrome is most commonly seen in young infants sensitive to cow milk or soy protein, but also has been reported in older individuals with egg sensitivity. Infants generally present between 1 week and 3 months with protracted vomiting and diarrhea, which not infrequently results in dehydration (Powell, 1978). Stools generally contain occult blood, polymorphonuclear neutrophils, and eosinophils and are frequently positive for reducing substances (malabsorbed sugars). Prick skin tests to the responsible food allergen are characteristically negative. Food challenges generally result in vomiting and diarrhea within minutes to 4 hr and occasionally can lead to shock (Goldman et al., 1963). Although the immunopathogenic mechanism responsible for this syndrome is unknown, there is some recent evidence that localized IgE-mediated gastrointestinal mast cell activation may be involved. In several patients with symptoms compatible with this syndrome described by Selbekk (1985) and Nolte and co-workers (1989), food antigen–induced degranulation of intestinal mast cells obtained by endoscopy correlated well with the outcome of oral challenge, whereas the results of prick skin tests and RASTs correlated poorly. Further controlled studies are necessary to establish the etiology of the food-induced entercolitis syndrome.

Infantile Colic

Infantile colic is an ill-defined syndrome of paroxysmal fussiness characterized by inconsonable crying, drawing up of the legs, abdominal distention, and excessive gas. It generally develops in the first 2–4 weeks of life and persists through the third to fourth months of life. A recent double-blind crossover trial implicated IgE-mediated hypersensitivity as a pathogenic factor in some infants (Lothe, 1989). As reviewed elsewhere, this mechanism probably accounts for about 15% of colicky infants (Sampson, 1989b).

IV. Extraintestinal Food-Induced Mast Cell Activation

A. Respiratory Reactions

Both upper and lower respiratory reactions have been provoked during double-blind, placebo-controlled oral food challenges (DBPCFC). Within minutes to 2 hr of ingestion, food allergens may induce typical signs and symptoms of rhinoconjunctivitis, although isolated upper airway symptoms are uncommon (Bock and Atkins, 1990). These include periocular erythema and pruritus, and tearing, as well as nasal congestion, pruritus, sneezing, and rhinorrhea. Utilizing a protocol of nasal lavage during DBPCFCs, lavage fluid histamine was found to rise significantly with the onset of nasal symptoms, as shown in Figure 1 (Silber and Sampson, 1988), strongly implicating a pathogenic role for nasal mast cell activation. Similarly, spirometric measurements during DBPCFCs have demon-

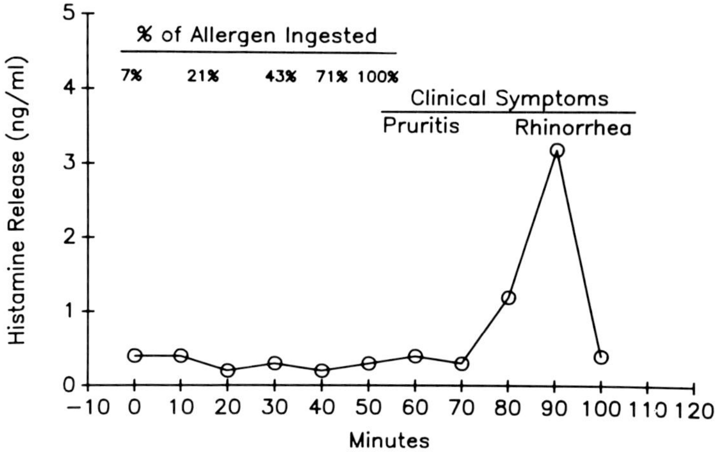

Figure 1 Histamine content of nasal lavage fluid obtained from a patient experiencing a positive DBPCFC. Symptoms began shortly after the patient had ingested 10 g of the lyophilized test antigen.

strated significant drops in FVC, FEV_1, and MMEF during a positive food challenge, as shown in Figure 2 (Sampson et al., 1989b).

Ingestion of food allergens rarely may be the main aggravating factor in chronic rhinoconjunctivitis and asthma. There is some evidence that ingestion of food antigens can lead to bronchial hyperreactivity (Silverman and Wilson, 1986). Two studies have evaluated large series of asthmatic patients followed in pulmonary clinics. In one survey, 300 patients between the ages of 8 months and 80 years were evaluated for food allergy by history, prick skin tests, and/or RASTs. Findings suggestive of food-induced symptoms were evaluated by blinded food challenges (Onarato et al., 1986). Overall, six patients (2%) had wheezing provoked by the food challenge. In the second series, 140 children with asthma were screened and eight (6%) were found to have wheezing induced by oral food challenge (November et al., 1988). Interestingly, all asthmatic children with food-induced wheezing had either atopic dermatitis or a history of eczema.

B. Cutaneous Reactions

The skin is a common target organ in IgE-mediated food hypersensitivity reactions. Ingestion of food allergens may lead to the rapid onset of cutaneous symptoms or aggravate more chronic conditions.

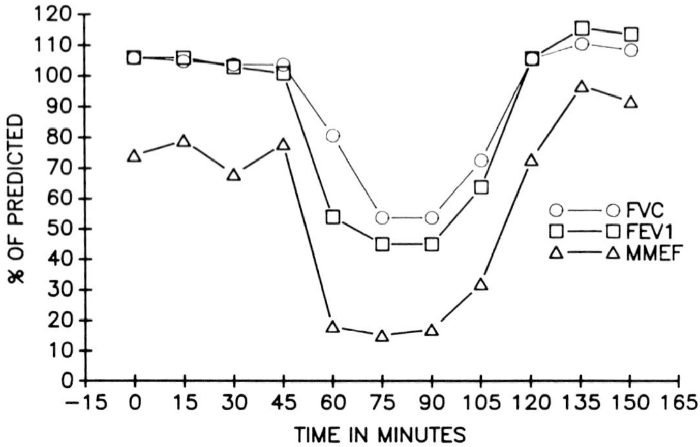

Figure 2 Spirometric evaluation of a patient experiencing a positive DBPCFC. Dyspnea and audible wheezing developed shortly after the patient had ingested about 50% of the lyophilized test material. The patient received nebulized metaproterenol prior to the "60 min" pulmonary function tests.

Urticaria/Angioedema

It is believed that acute urticaria and angioedema are among the most common symptoms of food allergic reactions. However, the prevalence of these reactions is unknown. In most cases, the onset of symptoms follows within minutes of ingesting the responsible allergen, and the cause-and-effect nature of the reaction is apparent to the patient. Consequently, most individuals with these reactions do not seek medical assistance nor do they necessarily report them to their physicians. The foods most commonly incriminated in children include eggs, milk, peanuts, and nuts, and in adults fish, shellfish, nuts, and peanuts. Although the prevalence of acute contact urticaria to foods is unknown, it is probably relatively common and most often the result of contact with raw meats, fish, vegetables, and fruits (Winton and Lewis, 1982).

The significance of food hypersensitivity in chronic urticaria and angioedema (symptoms lasting greater than 6 weeks) is subject to debate. However, most evidence suggests that food allergy is rarely responsible for chronic symptoms. In one series of 554 adult patients with chronic urticaria, food allergy was implicated in 1.4% (Champion et al., 1969).

Atopic Dermatitis

The pathogenic role of food hypersensitivity in atopic dermatitis has been debated for more than 75 years (Schloss, 1915). Utilizing DBPCFCs in children referred for evaluation of chronic, severe atopic dermatitis, we have established that IgE-mediated mast cell activation is responsible at least in part for cutaneous symptoms in approximately 60% of children studied. The prevalence of food hypersensitivity in this select group is twice that seen in a more general population of patients seen by dermatologists and allergists (Burks et al., 1988). As discussed below, a single ingestion of food allergen does not provoke an eczematous lesion, but repeated positive challenges do result in typical changes of atopic dermatitis.

To date, we have evaluated 271 patients with atopic dermatitis, ranging in age from 6 months to 25 years (median—4.7 years) for evidence to food hypersensitivity. These patients are highly atopic: 85% have elevated total serum IgE concentrations (median—3,400 IU/ml), 93% have positive family histories for atopic disease, and 45% have both asthma and allergic rhinitis at the time of evaluation (only 23% had atopic dermatitis alone at the initiation of study). DBPCFCs provoked a variety of symptoms within minutes to 2 hrs. Cutaneous reactions developed in 75% of positive challenges, but symptoms were confined to the skin alone in only 30% of positive responses. In the initial evaluation, cutaneous symptoms generally consisted of a markedly pruritic, erythematous, morbilliform rash in predilection sites for atopic dermatitis, and urticarial lesions were rarely seen. In follow-up challenges after 1–2 years on an appropriate allergen elimination diet, patients who had experienced clearing of their eczema but who remained food sensitive frequently developed urticaria in response to food challenge. Gastrointestinal complaints other than poor appetite were rarely evident in patient histories, yet 41% of patients experienced gastrointestinal symptoms; nausea, abdominal cramping, vomiting, and/or diarrhea. Nearly one-third of challenges provoked upper respiratory symptoms, especially laryngeal edema (sensation of itching and tightness in the throat, persistent throat clearing with dry hacking cough, and hoarseness), and about 10% resulted in wheezing.

In a series of studies utilizing the DBPCFC, we have been able to document both immediate and late-phase effects of ingested food allergens (Sampson and Jolie, 1984; Sampson and McCaskill, 1985; Sampson et al., 1989a; Leiferman et al. 1986). As noted above, a markedly pruritic, erythematous morbilliform rash develops within minutes to 2 hr of the oral challenge. The rash is generally abrupt in onset and persists for 30–120 min. Several laboratory findings implicate IgE-mediated cutaneous mast cell activation as the cause of symptoms: (1) sharp rise in plasma histamine concentration only in conjunction with positive DBPCFCs, (2) slight rise in plasma tryptase in patients with positive food challenges (unpublished), (3) no significant change in plasma C3a or C5a associated with a positive challenge, and (4) no evidence of immediate activation of circulating basophils as evidenced by no change in circulating basophil number, total histamine content, or spontaneous basophil histamine release in vitro in concert with a positive food challenge. Several lines of evidence implicate an IgE-mediated, late-phase component in conjunction with positive DBPCFCs. Approximately 4–8 hr following initial skin symptoms, many patients develop diffuse pruritus and, less frequently, an erythematous macular rash. In 14/15 patients experiencing a positive challenge, a significant rise in circulating polymorphonuclear neutrophils was seen (median—5904 versus 3196 cells/mm^3; $p < 0.01$) as well as a marked drop in circulating eosinophils (unpublished). In three patients studied to date, circulating eosinophils changed from a prechallenge normodense to postchallenge hypodense profile, as determined by percoll density gradients (unpublished). Biophies obtained at the site of a challenge-induced morbilliform lesion 8–14 hr following a positive challenge revealed eosinophil infiltration and deposition of major basic protein.

In patients with atopic dermatitis and food hypersensitivity, the continued ingestion of food allergens provokes the spontaneous production of histamine-releasing factor (HRF) from mononuclear cells in vitro, and most likely *in vivo* (Sampson et al., 1989a). The generation of HRF is associated with increased spontaneous basophil histamine release in vitro, increased basophil releasibility in vitro, and increased cutaneous hyperirritability (state of increased reactivity to a variety of minor, nonspecific stimuli, e.g., heat, cold, detergents, etc.). When the food allergens are identified and removed from the diet, spontaneous generation of HRF falls to background levels over a 6–9-month period, spontaneous basophil histamine release returns to background levels, basophil releasibility normalizes, and cutaneous hyperirritability diminishes. Changes associated with allergen elimination are not confined to the skin in these patients. Children ingesting food allergens were found to have increased lactulose absorption, which resolved when the responsible food allergens were eliminated from the diet (Flick et al., 1988). This study indicated that food-allergic patients with atopic dermatitis have subclinical malabsorption, which is reversed when food allergens are removed from the diet.

In follow-up studies of 75 children, it was noted that patients developed tolerance to nearly one-third of symptomatic food hypersensitivities after 1–2 years of a strict elimination of the responsible food allergen. The probability of developing tolerance was dependent on the antigen in question; i.e., development of tolerance to soy was common whereas development of tolerance to peanut was rare. Interestingly, results of prick skin tests remained virtually unchanged. The response of cutaneous mast cells to contact with various allergens was assessed by introducing food allergens into skin blister chambers. The chamber blister fluid was then monitored for changes in mediator and cell content (Charlesworth et al., 1991). No differences in immediate and late-phase histamine or PGD_2 concentrations were seen between "relevant" (food antigen to which the patient was skin test and challenge positive) and "irrelevant" (food antigen to which the patient was skin test positive and challenge negative) food allergens. Based on this study and the studies of Walzer noted above, the difference between sensitized patients with or without clinical reactivity appears to be the result of factors intervening between the gut and target organ, e.g., antibody clearing.

C. Generalized Anaphylaxis

The prevalence of food-induced anaphylaxis is unknown. Recently Yunginger and co-workers brought attention to this problem by reporting seven food-induced anaphylactic deaths reviewed over a period of 14 months (Yunginger, 1988). In all but possibly one case, the victim unknowingly ingested a food that had provoked a previous allergic reaction. In the past 9 months, the author has reviewed five fatal and six near-fatal food-induced anaphylactic reactions in children (aged 2–17 years) (Sampson et al., 1991). Common factors in these cases included the following: (1) all patients had asthma, (2) all patients had experienced previous allergic reactions to the incriminated food, (3) all patients had unknowingly ingested the food allergen, and (4) all patients experienced immediate symptoms and then most had a quiescent period prior to a major respiratory collapse. None of the patients in either series who died received epinephrine immediately. However, three patients with near-fatal reactions did receive epinephrine within 15 min of developing symptoms but still went on to develop respiratory collapse and hypotension requiring mechanical ventilation and pressor support (12 hr to 2 weeks).

V. Conclusions

Despite a number of physiological and immunological barriers, up to 2% of ingested food may penetrate the gastrointestinal tract and circulate throughout the body proper (Mowat, 1987). In a small minority of individuals, normal immunological tolerance fails to develop, resulting in various hypersensitivity disorders. Many of these disorders involve activation of cutaneous, gastrointestinal, and/or respiratory tract mast cells, primarily through surface-bound, allergen-specific IgE molecules. Our current understanding of these food-allergic disorders is far from complete, our diagnostic methods are frequently inaccurate (skin tests and RASTs) or time consuming and cumbersome (DBPCFC), and our therapy (allergen elimination) is at best inconvenient, and in reality, often impossible. On the other hand, food allergy provides an extremely useful model to study mast cell–related hypersensitivity disorders since it presents an opportunity where exposure to allergen can be largely controlled.

Acknowledgments

This work is supported by Grants AI24439 from the National Institute of Allergy and Infectious Diseases and RR00052 from the Division of Research Resources, National Institutes of Health.

Discussion

Hanifin: Do cold foods cause urticaria?
Sampson: Lip swelling, e.g., to ice cream, is common, and tongue and pharyngeal swelling can occur, but are rare. The reaction does not go beyond that and the remainder of the gastrointestinal tract is unaffected.
Hanifin: Do levels of tryptase correlate with food-allergic reactions?
Sampson: We are looking at serum tryptase levels in patients undergoing blinded challenges. Tryptase levels are elevated in some patients with positive reactions, but not to the degree that we had expected. Even in some of the patients with food-induced anaphylaxis, serum tryptase levels appear lower than in patients experiencing anaphylaxis from bee stings or parenteral drugs.
Sullivan: The kinetics of the delayed-onset (1–2-hr delay) reactions to foods are consistent with the generation of HRF from lymphocytes. Could these be cytokine-mediated reactions?
Sampson: That is certainly a possibility.
Lichtenstein: Do you see basophils on the lesions of atopic dermatitis in children eating foods they are sensitive to?
Sampson: In the few biopsies we did in lesions provoked by challenge, we did not look for basophils in a systematic way.
Kaplan: When patients have upper respiratory symptoms to foods, are they due to inhalation or systemic absorption?
Sampson: Probably to systemic absorption. In the early studies of Walzer and colleagues, they found that some passively sensitized control subjects developed wheal and flare at the sensitized site in 2 min. In our patients, many children developed distal skin symptoms prior to developing respiratory symptoms, suggesting that the food allergen is in the circulation prior to wheezing. There is no evidence of aspiration in these children.
Hanifin: Regarding the comment on delayed food reactions, many others have observed lesions appearing after 24–96 hr. Such reactions would be more consistent with the chronic lesions that characterize atopic dermatitis. Have you seen delayed responses?
Sampson: In reactions where IgE-mediated mast cell activation is implicated, we have never seen reactions occurring later than 4 hr following challenge. This

delay may be secondary to retention of food in the stomach, where absorption of antigen is much poorer than in intestine.
Metcalfe: It has been suggested that plasma histamine levels after food challenge could be used to diagnose food allergy. Do you agree?
Sampson: Because histamine is rapidly catabolized, it is unlikely that measurements of histamine in minimal or subclinical reactions will be useful.
Stevens: When you activate mouse mast cells, there is a 1–2-hr lag in the expression of most cytokine transcripts. Is there any known cytokine that might be released from an activated mast cell in sufficient quantities that could result in death of the patient?
Sampson: To my knowledge, no one has looked for cytokines in patients experiencing severe systemic anaphylaxis. Many of our patients experiencing positive food challenges develop marked lethargy and slight rise in temperature approximately 1 hr following the reaction, suggesting the possibility of some cytokine effect.

References

Bock, S. A. (1987). Prospective appraisal of complaints of adverse reaction to foods in children during the first 3 years of life. *Pediatrics* 79:683–688.

Bock, S. A., and Atkins, F. M. (1990). Patterns of food hypersensitivity during sixteen years of double-blind placebo-controlled food challenges. *J. Pediatr.* 117:561–567.

Burks, A. W., Mallory, S. B., Williams, L. W., and Shirrell, M. A. (1988). Atopic dermatitis: Clinical relevance of food hypersensitivity reactions *J. Pediatr.* 113:447–451.

Champion, R. H., Roberts, S. O., Carpenter, R. G., and Roger, J. H. (1969). Urticaria and angioedema: a review of 554 patients. *Br. J. Dermatol.* 81:588–597.

Charlesworth, E. N., Kagey-Sobotka, A., Norman, P. S., Lichtenstein, L. M., and Sampson, H. A. (1991). Cutaneous late-phase response in food allergic children with atopic dermatitis. J. Invest. Dermatol. (submitted).

Eyermann, C. H., (1927). X-ray demonstration of colonic reaction in food allergy. *J. Missouri Med. Assoc.* 24:129–132.

Flick, J. A., Sampson, H. A., and Perman, J. A. (1988). Intestinal permeability to carbohydrates in children with atopic dermatitis and food hypersensitivity. *Pediatr. Res.* 23:303A.

Freeman, J. (1925). Discussion on paroxysmal rhinorrhea. *Proc. Royal Soc. Med.* 18:29–32.

Fries, J. H., Zizmor, J. (1937). Roentgen studies of children with alimentary disturbances due to food allergy. *Am. J. Dis. Child.* 54:1239–1251.

Gleich, G. J., and Leiferman, K. M. (1986). Eosinophils and hypersensitivity disease. In *Proceedings of the XIIth International Congress of Allergology and Clinical Immunology*. Edited by C. E. Reed. St. Louis, Mosby, pp. 124–130.

Goldman, A. S., Anderson, D. W., Sellars, W. A., Saperstein, S., Kniker, W. T., Holpern, S. R., and collaborators. (1963). Milk allergy. Il Oral challenge with milk and isolated milk proteins in allergic children. 32:425–443.

Gray, I., Walzer, M. (1940). Studies in absorption of undigested proteins in human beings. VIII. Absorption from the rectum and a comparative study of absorption following oral, duodenal, and rectal administrations. *J. Allergy*. 11:245–250.

Kettlehut, B. V., and Metcalfe, D. D. (1988). Adverse reactions to foods. In *Allergy: Principles and Practice,* 3rd ed. Edited by E. Middleton, C. E. Reed, E. F., Ellis, N. F. Adkinson, J. W. Yunglinger. St. Louis, Mosby, pp. 1481–1502.

Leiferman, K. M., Ackerman, S. J., Sampson, H. A., Haugen, H. S., Venencie, P. Y., and Gleich, G. J. (1986). Dermal deposition of eosinophil granule major basic protein in atopic dermatitis. Comparison with onchocerciasis. *N. Engl. J. Med.* 313:282–285.

Lothe, I., Lindberg, T. (1989). Cow's milk whey protein elicits symptoms of infantile colic in colicky formula-fed infants: a double-blind crossover study. *Pediatr.* 83:262–266.

Mowat, A. M. (1987). The regulation of immune responses to dietary protein antigens. *Immunol. Today* 8:93–98.

Nolte, H, Schiotz, P. O., Kruse, A., and Skov, P. S. (1989). Comparison of intestinal mast cell and basophil histamine release in children with food allergic reactions. *Allergy* 44:554–463.

Novembre, E., de Martino, M., and Vierucci, A. (1988). Roods and respiratory allergy. *J. Allergy Clin. Immunol.* 81:1059–1065.

Onarato, J., Merland, N., Terral, C., Michel, F. B., and Bousquet, J. (1986). Placebo-controlled double-blind food challenge in asthma. *J. Allergy Clin. Immunol.* 78:1139–1146.

Ortaloni, C., Ispano, M., Pastorello, E. A., Ansaloni, R., and Magri, G. C. (1989). Comparison of results of skin prick tests (with fresh foods and commercial food extracts) and RAST in 100 patients with oral allergy syndrome. *J. Allergy Clin. Immunol.* 83:683–690.

Patrick, M. K., Dunn, I. J., Buret, A., Miller, H. R. P., Huntley, J. F., Gibson, S., and Gall, D. G. (1988). Mast cell protease release and mucosal ultrastructure during intestinal anaphylaxis in the rat. *Gastroenterology* 94:1–9.

Perdue, M. H., and Gall, G. (1985). Transport abnormalities during intestinal anaphylaxis in the rat: Effect of antiallergic agents. *J. Allergy Clin. Immunol.* 76:498–503.

Perdue, M. H., Chung, M., and Gall, D. G. (1984). Effect of intestinal anaphylaxis on gut function in the rat. *Gastroenterology* 86:391–397.

Pollard, H. M., and Stuart, G. J. (1942). Experimental reproduction of gastric allergy in human beings with controlled observations on the mucosa. *J. Allergy* 13:467–473.

Powell, G. K., (1978). Milk and soy induced enterocolitis of infancy: clinical features and standardization of challenge. J. Pediatr. 93:553–560.

Reimann, H. J., and Lewin, J. (1988). Gastric mucosal reactions in patients with food allergy. *Am. J. Gastroenterol.* 83:1212–1219.

Rowe, A. H. (1933). Roentgen studies of patients with gastrointestinal food allergy. *JAMA* 100:394–400.

Sampson, H. A. (1988). The role of food allergy and mediator release in atopic dermatitis. *J. Allergy Clin. Immunol.* 81:635–645.
Sampson, H. A. (1989a). Food allergy. *J. Allergy Clin. Immunol.* 84:1062–1067.
Sampson, H. A. (1989b). Infantile colic and food allergy: Fact or fiction? *J. Pediatr.* 115:583–584.
Sampson, H. A., and Jolie, P. L. (1984). Increased plasma histamine concentrations after food challenges in children with atopic dermatitis. *N. Engl. J. Med.* 321:228–232.
Sampson, H. A., and McCaskill, C. M. (1985). Food hypersensitivity and atopic dermatitis: Evaluation of 113 patients. *J. Pediatr.* 107:669–675.
Sampson, H. A., Broadbent, K. R., and Bernhisel-Broadbent, J. (1989a). Spontaneous release of histamine from basophils and histamine-releasing factor in patients with atopic dermatitis and food hypersensitivity. *N. Engl. J. Med.* 321:228–232.
Sampson, H. A., Broadbent, J. B., and Scanlon, S. M. (1989b). Food-induced respiratory reactions in children with atopic dermatitis. *J. Allergy Clin. Immunol.* 83:241 (abstract).
Sampson, H. A., Mendelson, L., and Rosen, J. P. (1991). Fatal and near-fatal food anaphylaxis reactions in children. *J. Allergy Clin. Immunol.* 87 (abstract) (in press).
Schloss, O. M. (1915). Allergy to common foods. *Trans. Am. Pediatr. Soc.* 27:62–68.
Scott, R. B., Diamant, S. C., and Gall, D. G. (1988). Motility effects of intestinal anaphylaxis in the rat. *Am. J. Physiol.* 255 (*Gastrointest. Liver Physiol.* 18):G505–G511.
Selbekk, B. H. (1985). A comparison between in vitro jejunal mast cell degranulation and intragastric challenge in patients with suspected food intolerance. *Scand. J. Gastroenterol.* 20:299–303.
Silber, G. M., and Sampson, H. A. (1988). Nasal mediator release following double-blind placebo-controlled oral food challenges. *J. Allergy Clin. Immunol.* 81:185 (abstract).
Silverman, M., and Wilson, N. (1986). Clinical physiology of food intolerance in asthma. In *Proceedings of the XIIth International Congress of Allergology and Clinical Immunology*. Edited by C. E. Reed, St. Louis, Mosby, pp. 457–462.
Sloan, A. E., and Powers, M. E. (1986). A perspective on popular perceptions of adverse reactions to foods. *J. Allergy Clin. Immunol.* 78:127–133.
Snyder, J. D., Rosenblum, N., Wershil, B., Goldman, H., and Winter, H. S. (1977). Pyloric stenosis and eosinophilic gastroenteritis in infants. *J. Pediatr. Gastroenterol. Nutr.* 6:543–547.
Turner, M. W., Barnett, G. E., and Strobel, S. (1990). Mucosal mast cell activation patterns in the rat following repeated feeding of antigen. *Clin. Exp. Allergy* 20:421–427.
U.S. Department of Agriculture. (1983). *Federal Register:* Rules and regulations. 48:32749.
Waldman, T. A., Wochner, R. D., Laster, R. D., and Gordon, R. S. (1967). Allergic gastroenteropathy. A cause of excessive gastrointestinal protein loss. *N. Engl. J. Med.* 276:761–769.
Walker, W. A. (1981). Intestinal transport of macromolecules. In *Physiology of the Gastrointestinal Tract*. Edited by L. R. Johnson. New York, Raven Press, pp.

1271–1289.

Walzer, M. (1927). Studies in absorption of undigested proteins in human beings. I. A simple direct method of studying the absorption of undigested protein. *J. Immunol.* 14:143–174.

Walzer, M. (1941). Allergy of the abdominal organs. *J. Lab. Clin. Med.* 26:1867–1877.

Winton, G. B., and Lewis, C. W. (1982). Contact urticaria. *Int. J. Dermatol.* 21:573–578.

Yunginger, J. W., Sweeney, K. G., Sturner, W. O., et al. (1988). Fatal food-induced anaphylaxis. *J. Am. Med. Assoc.* 260:1450–1452.

24

Urticaria

Characterization of Two Different Pathogenic Mechanisms

ALLEN P. KAPLAN

State University of New York
Stony Brook, New York

I. Introduction

It appears that when hives are fleeting, as is seen in physically induced hives, they are caused by a rapid burst of local mast cell degranulation. There is no tissue infiltration with cells, no late-phase component to the reaction, and therapy is dependent on antihistaminics or mast cell–stabilizing agents. The nonsustained mediator release may be a result of the absence of a defined antigen, a very brief encounter with the initiating physical stimulus, and rapid removal of vasoactive substances and chemotactic factors, so that the hive disappears quickly and a chemotactic factor gradient is not sustained so as to attract cells. Chronic urticaria differs in that the hive forms slowly, disappears over many hours, and is associated with a perivascular accumulation of mononuclear cells and mast cells. These mononuclear cells appear to be critical for development of the lesion and may secondarily induce mast cell proliferation and activation. Indirect evidence in support of this is the efficacy of corticosteroids in abrogating this type of hive.

The pathogenic mechanisms that can lead to hive formation are many; thus, any discussion of the mechanism of hive formation must consider each type of hive separately. Many recent reviews approach the subject in this fashion

(Kaplan, 1985, 1988). If one attempts to develop some more general hypotheses about hives, I believe many of the urticarial disorders can be divided into those in which individual lesions form quickly and disappear within 2 hr and those that last many hours. The former group includes most physically induced hives (cold urticaria, cholinergic urticaria, dermatographism, solar urticaria, etc.) while the latter includes chronic idiopathic urticaria and delayed pressure urticaria. Common to all of these is the absence of any defined antigenic stimulus. Uriticarial reactions in which an antigen can be defined (food allergies, drug reactions, some immune complex–mediated diseases) may utilize similar (but not identical) mechanisms, and the lesions can vary greatly in duration from a few hours to 1–2 days. In this review, I will discuss disorders in which a defined antigen is absent and contrast what is known about the pathogenesis of cold urticaria with chronic idiopathic urticaria.

II. Cold Urticaria

Cold urticaria most commonly presents as a local reaction to a cold stimulus in which a flare reaction develops quickly and the lesion disappears within a few hours. This reaction is not different from that seen when a skin test is performed in an allergic subject, except for the size and shape of the lesion and the presence of a defined antigen with skin testing. When studied in patients, a two-phase reaction is seen in which a decrease in temperature initiates the reaction, but the lesion develops while the area warms back to body temperature. This is true of the ice cube test as usually performed and experimental protocols in which one hand is submerged in ice water for 5 min followed by rewarming (Kaplan et al., 1975; Wasserman et al., 1977). It has been demonstrated that mediator release from mast cells occurs concomitant with hive formation, and the time course of release occurs during the rewarming period. The mediators demonstrated include histamine, eosinophilotactic peptides, neutrophil chemotactic factor, prostaglandin D_2, and platelet-activating factor (Heavey et al., 1986; Grandel et al., 1985). This suggests that degranulation has occurred and that lipid-derived mediators are also synthesized. One would anticipate that leukotrienes C4/D4 would also be synthesized, but these have not been measured. Bradykinin formation has also been observed; this could result from release of a mast cell protease (kallikrein-like enzyme such as tryptase) that directly cleaves high-molecular-weight kininogen present in interstitial fluid or could be generated by contact activation of plasma as the wheal evolves.

When considering classic allergic reactions, the presence of specific IgE antibody is required for development of a positive skin test, and this may be followed by a late-phase reaction 2–8 hr later (Dolovich et al., 1973; Solley et al., 1976). Cold urticaria is thought to closely resemble the mechanism of hive formation induced by antigen because it too may be IgE-dependent (Houser et al., 1970). This has been shown by passive transfer studies in which the responsible factor could be destroyed by heating plasma to 56°C for 30–60 min or removed by passage of plasma over an anti-IgE immunoabsorbent substance (Kaplan et al., 1981). A role for IgE was demonstrable in only a fraction of patients tested (published reports vary from 10 to 50%); results of our own studies are approximately 10%. This may be due to insensitivity of the passive transfer test (i.e., underestimation), or other mechanisms may be operative in most patients. IgM-dependent cold urticaria has been described (Wanderer et al., 1971) and the possibility that IgM or IgG anti-IgE might be present and responsible for histamine release must also be considered (Gruber et al., 1988).

Nevertheless, a direct IgE-dependent mechanism is present in some patients. The IgE seems active as a monomer (Kaplan et al., 1981); i.e., an IgE aggregate or cryoprotein does not appear to be required. Such studies also indicate that normal mast cells can be rendered cold sensitive by exposure to the pathogenic IgE. Yet the mechanism for signal transduction by this IgE is unknown. One thesis is that the cell-bound IgE becomes perturbed in some fashion by a drop in temperature. Secretion, however, being inhibited at low temperatures, occurs when the challenged area rewarms. We have considered the possibility that this IgE is an antibody to a cold-induced antigen present in skin (presumably in proximity to cutaneous mast cells to account for the temperature dependence of the reaction), but we have been unable to demonstrate it. Since any stimulus to skin will affect sensory nerve endings (in this case, receptors for temperature), one can postulate initiation by an abnormal neural secretory product that acts directly on cutaneous mast cells or interacts with the bound IgE. However, the ability of washed skin biopsy speciments to degranulate upon a cold challenge, followed by rewarming in vitro, argues against this thesis (Kaplan et al., 1981).

It is also of interest that a late-phase reaction is *not* seen in patients with cold urticaria regardless of lesion size or intensity of stimulus. Thus, mast cell degranulation may be necessary but not sufficient for a late-phase reaction to occur. We suspect that persistence of antigen (or stimulus) may also be needed. Thus, biopsy of cold urticarial lesions reveals vasodilation, increased vascular permeability, and local mast cell degranulation, but no cellular infiltrate. Biopsy of the lesion 4–6 hr after the hive has formed might be revealing; however, there is no persistence of swelling past the 2-hr point after an ice cube test. This is true also of the lesion seen with cholinergic urticaria or dermatographism. It is possible to have associated angioedema in patients with a "physical urticaria," as seen in cold urticaria when an extremity is submerged in cold water, or when cholinergic lesions become confluent with continued exercise or occur in the deep dermis. Then the lesion can persist for many hours or even an entire day, but this is a reflection of the much larger amount of fluid that must be reabsorbed and is not indicative of a late phase.

III. Chronic Idiopathic Urticaria

Chronic urticaria is a disease of unknown origin in which there is no identifiable antigenic stimulus yet recurrent hives are seen, often on a daily basis. The lesions typically last from 4 to 72 hr and can occur on any part of the body. There may be associated angioedema, mild dermatographism, and an increased sensitivity at pressure points, although delayed pressure urticaria is clearly a distinct entity (Estes and Yang, 1981; Kaplan et al., 1978). The pathogenesis of this lesion is clearly more complex than that described for cold urticaria because mast cells are not the only cells with a critical role. Skin biopsy specimens taken from urticarial lesions of patients reveal a nonnecrotizing, perivascular infiltration of mononuclear cells (predominantly) (Natbony et al., 1983), such that the integrity of the vessel wall is preserved. When the mononuclear cell infiltrate is examined more carefully using monoclonal antibodies, there is a T-cell lymphocytosis, a monocytosis (Fig. 1), and an increased number of mast cells (Table 1) (Elias et al., 1986). The 11% mast cells shown represent about a ninefold increase compared to skin biopsies of normal subjects (Natbony et al., 1983). Early studies of induced skin blisters placed over urticarial lesions demonstrated an increased histamine content; however, this was also true of normal-appearing skin in patients with chronic urticaria. These data suggest that mast cells in chronic urticaria are hyperresponsive to a variety of stimuli, in this case the trauma of the procedure (Kaplan et al., 1978). Studies of total histamine content of skin biopsy specimens also demonstrated an increased amount of histamine in both lesional and nonlesional skin of hive patients (Phanuphak et al., 1980). Since basophil infiltration is not seen upon skin biopsy, these results all suggest an increased number of mast cells and increased responsiveness of these cells. The latter point has also been emphasized recently using codeine as a cutaneous mast cell–degranulating agent. Responsiveness of patients with chronic urticaria seems far greater than is seen in normal subjects (Cohen and Rosenstreich, 1986).

One must, therefore, consider that increased numbers of mast cells are due to a proliferative stimulus. The effect of interleukin-4, acting in conjunction with interleukin-3, is one possibility (Hamaguchi et al., 1987). Although these are primarily products of T lymphocytes, they may also be synthesized by mast cells. An alternative is that mast cells are responsive to chemotactic factors and accumulate around blood vessels. The hyperresponsiveness seen may be due to "priming" of cells. It has been shown that many cytokines can cause basophils to be more responsive to other secretagogues at concentations that do not them-

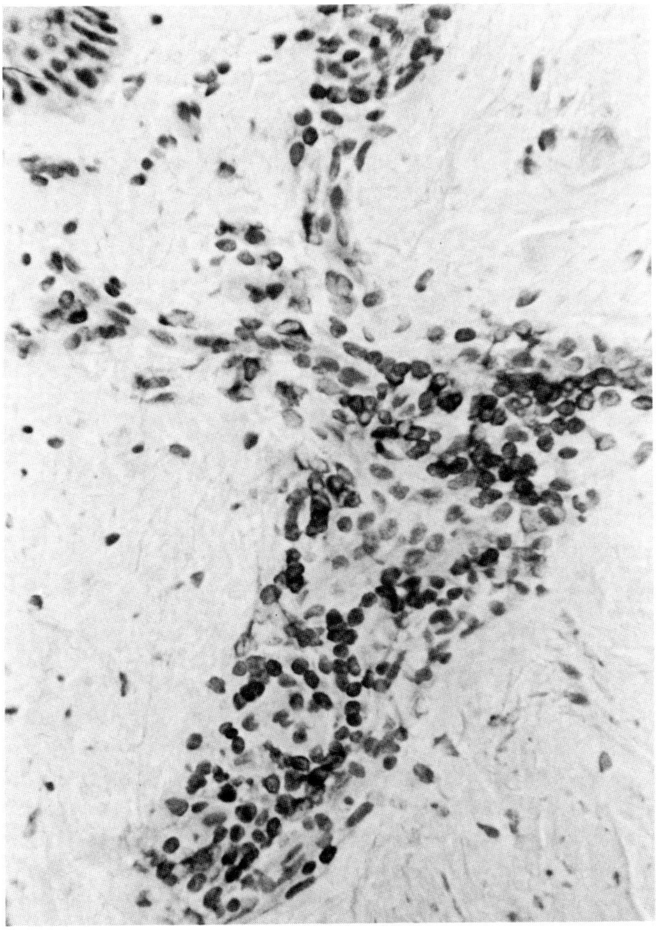

Figure 1 Immunoperioxidase staining of monocytes within the perivascular lesion of a patient with chronic idiopathic urticaria using Leu M3 monoclonal antibody. The darker positive cells can be distinguished from other mononuclear cells and account for 20% of the cellular infiltrate.

selves cause significant release. These included interferon-γ (Ida et al., 1977) and interleukin-3 (MacDonald et al., 1988). These or other cytokines may have an analogous effect on cutaneous mast cells, but this has not yet been examined. Since mast cell degranulation is seen in chronic urticaria, there must also be a stimulus for mast cell secretion. Among the cytokines capable of doing this are interleukin-3 (Haak-Frendscho et al., 1988a), granulocyte-macrophage colony-

Table 1 Percentage of Cells Counted in Skin Biopsy Specimens

Patient no.	T cells	Monocytes[a]	Mast cells[b]	Unidentified[c]
1	45	29	20	6
2	60	25	7	8
3	30	33	10	27
4	37	27	9	27
5	30	19	10	40
6	70	18	8	4
7	41	23	10	26
8	57	11	7	25
9	72	7	11	10
10	40	29	20	11
11	51	15	10	24
12	30	33	5	32
Mean	47	22	11	19

[a]Reported as Ma3-positive cells.
[b]By chloroacetate esterase.
[c]Calculated by subtracting the sum of T cells, monocytes, and mast cells from 100.
Source: Elias et al. (1986).

stimulating factor (Haak-Frendscho et al., 1988a), and, to a much lesser degree, interleukin-1 (Haak-Frendscho et al., 1988b). Nevertheless, there are histamine-releasing substances in a mononuclear cell supernatant (HRF) that are more potent and/or more plentiful than these cytokines, which are probably responsible for basophil (Thueson et al., 1979) and perhaps mast cell degranulation.

Our studies of mononuclear cell–derived HRF have led to the purification of three proteins, each of which can cause basophil histamine release. These have molecular weights of 10,000–12,000, 15,000–17,000, and 35,000–41,000 (Kaplan et al., 1986; Baeza et al., 1989). We have prepared a monoclonal antibody to the 10,000–12,000 moiety that does not react with the other two forms of HRF. Thus, we are dealing with at least two, and perhaps three, separate gene products. This monoclonal antibody could be used to isolate the 10–12-kDa form of HRF in a single step. The product was first subjected to SDS gel electrophoresis using a 15% gel to obtain improved resolution. Stained gels revealed a broad band rather than the more narrow band seen using a 23% gel. The material was next electroblotted onto nitrocellulose paper, the band was divided into an upper and lower half, and each half subjected to amino acid sequence analysis. Close homology was seen between the upper half (HRF-1) and the sequence of connective tissue activating peptide III (CTAP-III) (Baeza et al., 1990), a derivative of platelet α granules that causes activation and proliferation of fibroblasts (Castor et al., 1983). When the amino acid sequence of the lower half of the band was determined (HRF-2), it also was homologous to CTAP-III if the alignment began with residue 16. Thus, the observed broad band appeared to represent heterogeneity due to cleavage of the N-terminal 15 amino acids from the native protein (Baeza et al., 1990).

Such a cleavage has been described for CTAP-III, in which it is converted to a molecule that is a potent activator of neutrophils and designated "neutrophil activating peptide-2" (NAP-2). CTAP-III possesses little or no activity on neutrophils, and conversion of CTAP-III to NAP-2 can be accomplished using neutrophil elastase or supernatants derived from mononuclear cells (Walz and Baggiolini, 1989). We compared the ability of CTAP-III and NAP-2 to activate basophils, and preliminary data suggest they are equipotent. Since our starting material contains platelets, CTAP-III/NAP-2 may represent one form of patelet-derived HRF. It is also possible that mononuclear cells are capable of producing a similar or identical molecule. We are now characterizing the other molecular forms of HRF, and we will then determine whether any of these moieties are secreted by mononuclear cells present in the lesions of patients with chronic uritcaria.

The characteristic lesion of chronic urticaria forms more slowly than the lesions seen in physically induced hives and lasts much longer. These lesions are infiltrative, presumably due to the cells present and perhaps to fibrin disposition. But the lesion of chronic urticaria cannot be considered to be a manifestation of a late-phase reaction because there is no antecedent immediate reaction, and no antigen or other initiating stimulus has been defined.

If the mononuclear cells (T cells, monocytes) have been activated, the stimulus is not known, but I have assumed, in this discussion, that the mast cell abnormalities/secretion is mononuclear cell-dependent. It is also possible that some primary abnormality of mast cells causes an accumulation of T cells and monocytes.

IV. Therapy

Cold urticaria can be treated with antihistamines. The drug of choice appears to be cyproheptadine; however, the reason for its particular efficacy is uncertain (Wanderer and Ellis, 1971) (Fig. 2). It does not inhibit mast cell secretion and acts by receptor blockade at the end-organ (small venules). It appears that histamine is the major mediator of most physically induced hives, but it is not the only one, since a variety of vasoactive substances are released from mast cells. This may account, in part, for the variability in response in different subjects.

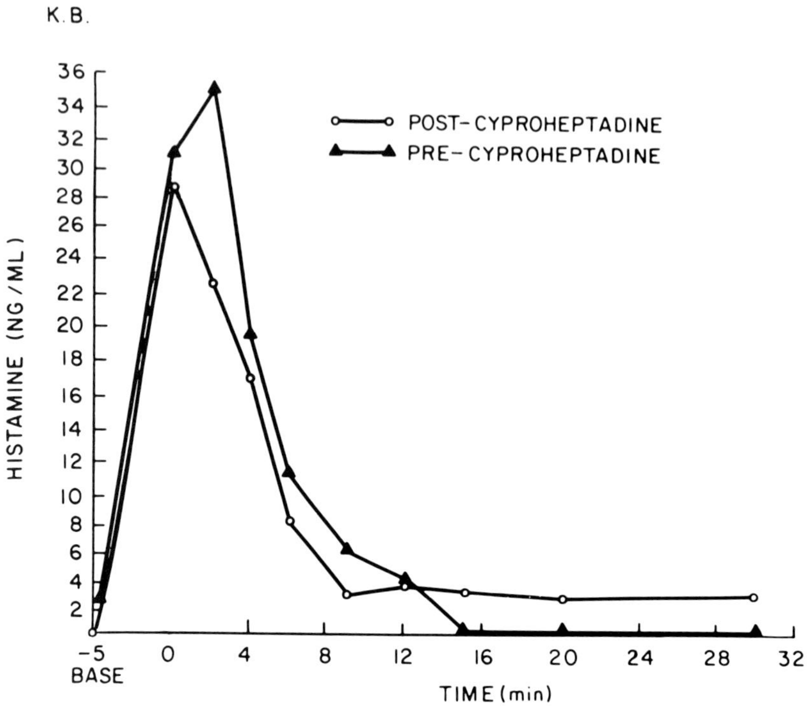

Figure 2 Histamine release into the brachial vein of a subject with cold urticaria challenged by submersion of the hand in cold water for 4 min. The response before and after therapy with periactin is shown. Although a markedly diminished clinical response is seen with this agent, it has no effect on mast cell histamine release.

Thus, any antihistamine given in sufficient quantity should be effective. This is true for dermatographism, but is less clear for cold urticaria and cholinergic urticaria, in which cyproheptadine and hydroxyzine, respectively, have particular efficacy. These disorders do not respond to corticosteroids, and this may be due to absence of a steroid effect on cutaneous mast cell degranulation. Agents that inhibit mast cell degranulation, such as ketotifen, inhibit mediator release and may have particular efficacy for the therapy of physically induced hives (Huston et al., 1986).

By contrast, antihistamines have limited effectiveness in the therapy of patients with chronic idiopathic urticaria. They relieve pruritus, may inhibit hive formation in mild cases, but are often ineffective even in very high doses. Additionally, H_2 receptor blockers are of some value in some patients, and the use of mast cell stabilizers such as ketotifen can be a promising adjunct. Corticosteroids are the only agents that inhibit formation of the lesions of chronic urticaria, however. This suggests an effect on the infiltrating mononuclear cells. Monocytes and T lymphocytes may not only be the initiators of mast cell secretion, but also may contribute to hive formation by release of vasoactive substances independent of mast cells. A protocol for the use of corticosteroids for therapy of severe cases of chronic urticaria has been described such that side effects are minimized and a gradually decreasing alternate-day dosage is utilized (Kaplan, 1985).

Discussion

Goldstein: Why no late-phase reaction?
Kaplan: I believe you need persistence of the stimulus (e.g., allergen) to see a late phase, and a single burst of mast cell secretion is inadequate regardless of magnitude.
Sullivan: Does normal skin have more mast cells and less mononuclear cells?
Kaplan: Normal-appearing skin of chronic urticaria patients has increased mast cells and higher-than-normal mononuclear cells. It is in between lesional skin and that seen in normal subjects.
Casale: Does capsaicin prevent the wheal-and-flair reaction?
Kaplan: Capsaicin will diminish the flare by depletion of substance P but has little effect on the wheal.
Dvorak: Have you used plastic embedded tissue to look for basophils?
Kaplan: Yes, we have. Basophils were not seen. Thin sections were used and were carefully scanned.
Schwartz: What is the role of IgG and IgE?
Kaplan: We have demonstrated IgM and IgG anti-IgE in some cold urticaria patients and a subpopulation of chronic urticaria patients. Its role is unknown but it is enticing that selected spontaneously occurring anti-IgE can cause histamine release. One prominent case in a cold urticaria patient was studied extensively but we were unable to demonstrate cold dependence for the histamine release reaction.
Hohman: Have you purified IgE from these patients?
Kaplan: We have taken serum from cold urticaria patients (200 ml), passed it over an anti-IgE immunoadsorbant, eluted the column, dialyzed and concentrated the eluate, and tested it for function. We could transfer cold urticaria and quantitate IgE, but when examined on gels no protein was seen.

References

Baeza, M. L., Reddigari, S., Haak-Frendscho, M., and Kaplan, A. P. (1989). Purification and further characterization of human mononuclear cell histamine releasing factor. *J. Clin. Invest.* 83:1204.

Baeza, M. L., Reddigari, S. R., Kornfeld, D., Ramani, N., Smith, E. M., Hossler, P. A., Fischer, T., Castor, C. W., Gorevic, P. G., and Kaplan, A. P. (1990). Relationship of one form of human histamine releasing factor to connective tissue activating peptide III. *J. Clin. Invest.* 85:1516.

Castor, C. W., Miller, J. W., and Walz, D. A. (1983). Structural and biological characteristics of connective tissue activating peptides (CTAP III), a major human platelet derived growth factor. *Proc. Natl. Acad. Sci. USA* 70:765.

Cohen, R. W., and Rosenstreich, D. L. (1986). Discrimination between urticaria-prone and other allergic patients by intradermal skin testing with codeine. *J. Allergy Clin. Immunol.* 77:802.

Dolovich, J., Hargreave, F. G., Chalmers, R., Shier, K. J., Gauldie, J., and Bienenstock, J. (1973). Late cutaneous allergic responses in isolated IgE-dependent reactions. *J. Allergy Clin. Immunol.* 52:38.

Elias, J., Boss, E., and Kaplan, A. P. (1986). Studies of the cellular infiltrate of chronic idiopathic urticaria: Prominence of T lymphocytes, monocytes, and mast cells. *J. Allergy Clin. Immunol.* 78:914.

Estes, S. A., and Yang, C. W. (1981). Delayed pressure urticaria: an investigation of some parameters of lesion induction. *J. Am. Acad. Dermatol.* 5:25.

Grandel, K. E., Farr, R. S., Wanderer, P. A., Eisenstadt, T. C., and Wasserman, S. I. (1985). Association of platelet-activating factor with primary acquired cold urticaria. *N. Engl. J. Med.* 313:405.

Gruber, B. L., Baeza, M. L., Marchese, M. J., Agnello, V., and Kaplan, A. P. (1988). Prevalence and functional role of anti-lgE autoantibodies in urticarial syndromes. *J. Invest. Dermatol.* 90:213.

Haak-Frendscho, M., Arai, N., Arai, K-I., Baeza, M. L., Finn, A., and Kaplan, A. P. (1988a). Human recombinant granulocyte-macrophage colony stimulating factor and interleukin 3 cause basophil histamine release. *J. Clin. Invest.* 82:17.

Haak-Frendscho, M., Dinarello, C., and Kaplan, A. P. (1988b). Recombinant human interleukin 1 beta causes histamine release from human basophils. *J. Allergy Clin. Immunol.* 82:218.

Hamaguchi, Y., Kanakura, Y., Fujita, J., Takeda, S. I., Nakano, T., Tarui, S., Honjo, T., and Kitamura, Y. (1987). Interleukin 4 as an essential factor for in vitro clonal growth of murine connective tissue-type mast cells. *J. Exp. Med.* 165:268.

Heavey, D. J., Kobza-Black, A., Barrow, S. E., Chappell, C. G., Greaves, M. W., and Dollery, C. T. (1986). Prostaglandin D_2 and histamine release in cold urticaria. *J. Allergy Clin. Immunol.* 78:458.

Houser, D. D., Arbesman, C. E., Ito, K., and Wicher, K. (1970). Cold urticaria: Immunologic studies. *Am. J. Med.* 49:23.

Huston, D. P., Bressler, R. B., Kaliner, M., Sowell, L. K., and Baylor, M. W. (1986). Prevention of mast-cell degranulation by ketotifen in patients with physical urticaria. *Ann. Intern. Med.* 204:507.

Ida, S., Hooks, J. J., Siraganian, R. P., and Notkins, A. L. (1977). Enhancement of IgE-mediated histamine release from human basophils by viruses. Role of interferon. *J. Exp. Med.* 145:892.

Kaplan, A. P. (1985). Urticaria and angioedema. In *Allergy*. New York, Churchill Livingstone, pp. 439–471.

Kaplan, A. P. (1988). Urticaria and angioedema. In Inflammation: Basic Principles and Clinical Correlates. Edited by J. I. Gallin, IN, Goldstein and R. Snyderman. New York, Raven Press, pp. 667–678.

Kaplan, A. P., Gray, L., Shaff, F. E., Horakova, Z., and Beaven, M. A. (1975). In vivo studies of mediator release in cold urticaria and cholinergic urticaria. *J. Allergy Clin. Immunol.* 55:394.

Kaplan, A. P., Horakora, Z., and Katz, S. I. (1978). Assessment of tissue fluid histamine levels in patients with urticaria. *J. Allergy Clin. Immunol.* 6:350.

Kaplan, A. P., Garofalo, J., Sigler, R., and Hauber, T. (1981). Idiopathic cold urticaria: In vivo demonstration of histamine release upon challenge of skin biopsies. *N. Engl. J. Med.* 305:1074.

Kaplan, A. P., Haak-Frendscho, M., Fauci, A., Dinarello C., and Halbert E. (1986). A histamine releasing factor from activated human mononuclear cells. *J. Immunol.* 135:2027.

MacDonald, S. M., Kagey-Sobotka, A., and Gillis, S. (1988). Human recombinant interleukin 3 induces histamine release from basophils. *J. Allergy Clin. Immunol.* 81:31 (abstract).

Natbony, S. F., Phillips, M., Elias, J. M., Godfrey, H. P., and Kaplan, A. P. (1983). Histologic studies of chronic idiopathic urticaria. *J. Allergy Clin. Immunol.* 71:177.

Phanuphak, P., Schocket, A. L., Arroyave, C. M., and Kohler, P. F. (1980). Skin histamine in chronic urticaria. *J. Allergy Clin. Immunol.* 65:371.

Solley, G. O., Gleich, G. J., Jordan, R. E., and Schroeter, A. L. (1976). The late phase of the immediate wheal and flare reaction. *J. Clin. Invest.* 58:408.

Thueson, D. O., Speck, L. S., Lett-Brown, M. A., and Grant, J. A. (1979). Histamine releasing activity (HRA). I. Production by mitogen or antigen-stimulated human mononuclear cells. *J. Immunol.* 123:626.

Walz, A., and Baggiolini, M. (1989). A novel cleavage product of b thromboglobulin formed in cultures of stimulated mononuclear cells activates human neutrophils. *Biochem. Biophys. Res. Commun.* 159:969.

Wanderer, A. P., and Ellis, E. F. (1971). Treatment of cold urticaria with cyproheptadine. *J. Allergy Clin. Immunol.* 48:366.

Wanderer, A. A., Maselli, R., Ellis, E. F., and Ishizaka, K. (1971). Immunologic characterization of serum factors responsible for cold urticaria. *J. Allergy Clin. Immunol.* 48:13.

Wasserman, S. I., Soter, N. A., Center, D. M., and Austen, K. F. (1977). Cold urticaria: Recognition and characterization of a neutrophil chemotactic factor of anaphylaxis during cold challenge. *J. Clin. Invest.* 60:189.

25

Do Mast Cells Play a Role in Atopic Dermatitis?

JON M. HANIFIN

Oregon Health Sciences University
Portland, Oregon

I. Introduction

Atopic dermatitis is a chronic cutaneous inflammatory disease characterized by recurrent flares of bright erythema, severe pruritus, and papulated edema. Rubbing and scratching lead to secondary weeping, excoriation, and lichenification. The face, neck, and flexors of elbows and knees are most commonly involved, but the condition may be generalized or may affect only a local area such as the hands. Affected individuals usually have accompanying allergic respiratory disease, but the 20% who have no apparent atopy show no differences in cutaneous disease.

Histologically, the acute lesion shows the characteristic intercellular epidermal edema, known as spongiosis, which typifies all the eczematous diseases (Mihm et al., 1976). An inflammatory infiltrate of lymphocytes and histiocytes is evident around superficial vessels and in some areas of the epidermis. Eosinophils are seldom prominent, but Leiferman et al. (1985) have used monoclonal antibodies and immunofluorescence to demonstrate specific cationic protein residuals from infiltrating eosinophils. Mast cell numbers are not increased in early lesions, but, as discussed below, increased numbers are evident in chronic lesions, which are characterized by epidermal hyperplasia and increased lymphohistiocytic dermal infiltrate.

The case for a mast cell role in the pathogenesis of atopic dermatitis rests on a number of seemingly reasonable assumptions combined with several experimental investigations that partially support the assumptions. Perhaps the most reasonable of these assumptions is that histamine is the only known mediator of itch, and mast cells are the most likely source. Another prominent assumption is that, since atopic dermatitis travels with allergic rhinitis (AR) and AR is initiated by mast cells, then atopic dermatitis must also be initiated by mast cells. This thought train also assumes that protein antigens and IgE have pathological relevance to atopic dermatitis. For many years this concept has provided a plausible mechanism to explain the lability and pruritus that are so prominent in atopic dermatitis.

All of the assumptions await proof, however, and new, evolving information raises an equally plausible case for T-lymphocyte initiation of the atopic dermatitis lesion (Plaut, 1990). T-cell cytokines from a putative Th-2 subset, e.g., interleukins-3 and -4 (IL-3, Il-4), may, if a murine analogy holds, also serve as autocrine growth regulators for mast cells. These and other cytokines could be fundamental control factors. If there are increased mast cell proliferation and mediator releasibility in atopic dermatitis, then they may be secondary to expansion of a Th-2 lymphocyte population that secretes relevant growth factors and histamine-releasing factors. These newly developing concepts should be considered in a balanced review of the mast cell in atopic dermatitis.

II. Increased Mast Cell Numbers

Several studies agree that mast cell numbers are increased in skin from chronic, hyperplastic lesions but not from acute lesions of atopic dermatitis (Mihm et al., 1976; Mikhail and Miller-Milinska, 1964; Irani et al., 1989). Mikhail and Miller-Milinska (1964) quantitated mast cells in ethanol-fixed, toluidine blue–stained skin biopsy specimens from a large number of sites and in a variety of dermatoses. Numbers varied greatly in different locations but appeared to be significantly increased in the one case of chronic atopic dermatitis studied. Mihm et al. (1976) studied plastic-embedded, Giemsa-stained sections and likewise noted significantly increased mast cell numbers in lichenified atopic dermatitis. They also observed evidence of mast cell degranulation in acute lesions, though atopic dermatitis was not specifically compared with other conditions. Studies have also shown increased mast cell numbers in chronic psoriasis and lichen planus (Braun-Falco and Burg, 1970; Walton and DeSouza, 1983), and Brody (1984) has clearly demonstrated mast cell degranulation during acute eruptions of psoriasis. Such studies provide a context for the consideration that acute phase mast cell degranulation and chronic phase proliferation may be nonspecific concomitants of cutaneous inflammation.

Irani and colleagues (1989) have reported immunocytochemical studies that agree very well with the numbers of mast cells in normal and atopic dermatitis skin observed by Mikhail and Miller-Milinska (1964). In accord with other studies, mast cells were increased in hyperplastic lesions while normal numbers were present in acute erythematous antecubital skin. An interesting additional finding in Irani's studies was the observation that, in three of four atopic dermatitis biopsies, a variable number of the mast cells (2–17%) stained for tryptase but not chymase. This indicates the presence of mucosal-type mast cells (MC_T) in atopic dermatitis lesions. The MC_T were not seen in site-matched normal skin. These preliminary findings need to be expanded and confirmed to determine whether the finding of cutaneous MC_T in atopic dermatitis is distinctive and frequent and whether it has relevance to the development of inflammation in this disease. Conceivably, this type of mast cell, which may differ in its responses to substance P and opiates, might account for differences between urticaria and atopic dermatitis in their responses to antihistamines. Alternatively, this cell may simply represent an alternative phenotypic expression induced by the intense surrounding immunological reaction.

III. Induced Increase in Mast Cells

Mitchell et al. (1986) reported increased numbers of mast cells in biopsies from four patients with atopic dermatitis taken 6 and 10 days after repeated application of mite antigen to abraded skin. The quantitations were highly variable and not blinded, but they indicated that prolonged antigen-induced inflammation may stimulate mast cell proliferation or recruitment. The authors found increased basophil numbers in earlier biopsies at 24–48 hr and suggested that these findings are analogous to past descriptions of basophils infiltrating renal allograft and allergic contact dermatitis sites. They hypothesized that the lesions of atopic dermatitis may be cutaneous basophil hypersensitivity.

Other histological studies of aeroallergen patch test sites have provided little support for the idea of cutaneous basophil hypersensitivity. Reitamo et al. (1986) noted no increased mast cell or basophil numbers in 48-hr sites, though techniques were not optimized for such detection. Their study did have the advantage of using Finn Chamber applications to undistrubed skin. The possibility remains that the abraded patch sites used by Mitchell et al. (1986) alter conditions in favor of basophil and mast cell accumulation. Bruynzeel-Koomen et al. (1988) did note evidence of mast cell degranulation in biopsies taken 2–6 hr after patch testing to mite antigen. Gondo et al. (1986) applied mite antigen to scratched skin and noted early signs of urticaria and mast cell degranulation but did not specifically quantitate increased mast cells.

Norris et al. (1988), in a comprehensive, well-controlled study, described worsening of dermatitis after five daily applications of mite antigen in patients with atopic dermatitis. The control patients with atopy and no dermatitis developed only short-lived urticarial papulation and pruritus, with no eczematous response. The pruritus was significantly greater on antecubital test sites than on the back. The finding might be considered evidence against a mast cell role in atopic dermatitis, while the urticaria in patients with respiratory atopy alone seems likely due to mast cell mediator release.

IV. Increased Levels of Histamine and Other Mediators

In line with above-mentioned studies showing increased mast cell numbers along with mast cell degranulation in atopic dermatitis skin are studies that show elevated skin histamine concentrations (Johnson et al., 1960; Juhlin, 1967). The latter study, utilizing a histofluorescent assay, also demonstrated elevated histamine in other dermatitides. In contrast, however, Ruzicka and Gluch (1983), using the more sensitive and specific radioenzyme assay, found elevated skin histamine content in only 3 of 22 patients with atopic dermatitis. In a later study, this group noted normal histamine levels in suction blister fluid from lesional and nonlesional skin of patients with atopic dermatitis and in psoriasis controls (Ruzicka et al., 1986).

Even with high skin histamine levels, a cause/effect assumption for a specific disease is not necessarily justified, because, as pointed out by Eady et al. (1979), there is a well-established association between mast cells, histamine, and blood vessels. All may be increased in a variety of inflammatory diseases. Some investigators (Eady et al., 1979; El-Ackad and Brody, 1975) have suggested that histamine is synthesized and stored within vascular walls, hypothesizing a relationship between vessels and histamine that is independent of mast cells. Elevations of endothelial histamine might help explain the increased histamine sensitivity of face, neck, and antecubital skin—those areas so prominently affected in patients with atopic dermatitis (Williams, 1938). Likewise, this might account for the frequently observed wide variations in histamine content in different skin areas. Further studies are needed to clarify whether there is non–mast cell histamine in human skin and whether this might be the source of increased concentrations in some cases of atopic dermatitis.

As with skin, plasma histamine levels have been recorded only in some patients with atopic dermatitis (Hanifin, 1977; Ring and O'Connor, 1979). Occasionally, very high levels are seen (Hanifin, 1977), but in another study (Ring and O'Connor, 1979), only three of six patients showed increases, and these were low level. In an extension of this study, mild elevations of plasma histamine were noted in 17 of 54 patients (Ring, 1983). Longitudinal assays in seven of these patients reveled normalization during remissions.

In contrast to atopic dermatitis, both skin (Ruzicka and Gluch, 1983) and urinary histamine (Dreskin et al., 1987) levels appear to be more consistently elevated in the hyperimmunoglobulin-E syndrome. In the latter study (Dreskin et al., 1987), increased urine histamine correlated with the presence of eczematous dermatitis. Three control patients with severe atopic dermatitis were also studied, and one had modestly increased histamine levels. A larger study of 11 patients with severe atopic dermatitis revealed only one outside the range of normal values (Petersen et al., 1979).

Interpreting these diverse studies is difficult, but it does appear that intermittent histamine release occurs in some patients with atopic dermatitis. The study of Sampson and Jolie (1984), discussed below, documents relatively rapid release of histamine after positive food challenge, though the source of histamine, whether basophils, mast cells, or both, is uncertain.

V. Functional Abnormalities of Mast Cells

The inaccessibility of pure mast cell populations has precluded direct assessment of functional abnormalities in atopic dermatitis. In vivo perturbations of mast cell mediator release have been inconclusive. Voorhorst and van der Hooft–van Asbeck (1979), found no difference between atopics and normals who were skin-tested with 48/80. A study of histamine releasibility from biopsy skin fragments (Ruzicka and Gluch, 1983) likewise showed no difference between atopic dermatitis and normal skin in response to 48/80, but anti-IgE stimulated twofold greater histamine release in the atopic dermatitis specimens.

This finding is consistent with studies (Lebel et al., 1980; Butler et al., 1983; Marone et al., 1986) showing increased basophil histamine releasibility in atopic dermatitis. The basophil hyperreleasibility has been demonstrated by stimulation with concanavalin A (Butler et al., 1983), D_2O, and calcium ionophore (Marone et al., 1986), as well as anti-IgE (Lebel et al., 1980; Butler et al., 1983; Marone et al., 1986). Atopic basophils also have increased spontaneous histamine release (Marone et al., 1986; Sampson et al., 1989). Sampson et al. (1989) suggested that this defect was more pronounced in atopic dermatitis patients with food allergy and that this was associated with a unique "IgE+" in the serum as well as a mononuclear cell–derived histamine-releasing factor (HRF). It is possible that these patients' mast cells also have altered function, but this analogy cannot be proven with currently available techniques. A primary role for T cells and monocytes in the production of atypical IgE+ and HRF is an interesting focus for speculation.

The best delineated mechanism controlling mediator release from basophils and mast cells is the cyclic nucleotide system, with cyclic AMP serving a prominent inhibitory influence. Increased cyclic AMP-phosphodiesterase (PDE) activity in atopic dermatitis leukocytes correlates with histamine hyperreleasibility, which, in turn, is normalized by phosphodiesterase inhibitors in vitro (Butler et al., 1983). By analogy, mast cell mediator releasibility may also be increased in atopic dermatitis, and this could explain the inappropriate hyperreactivity that characterizes atopic dermatitis.

VI. Clinical Observations

Certain responses in patients with atopic dermatitis support a mast cell role in the evolution of skin lesions. Among the many factors that exacerbate atopic dermatitis, emotional stress and oral food challenge have given consistent responses in the experimental setting. Graham and Wolf (1953) used an emotional stress interview technique and were able to trigger erythema and itching in 14 of 15 selected patients with atopic dermatitis. These reactions were very rapid and occurred in sites of prior atopic dermatitis, consistent with a mast cell–initiated mechanism. This type of response is typical of what many patients recognize as a stress-related flare. Neuropeptides such as substance P may trigger mast cell release of mediators that act on predisposed skin to cause erythema and itch. This could well be the initiating event. Alternatively, a direct neurovascular mechanism might account for the response, especially when considering that, usually, a mast cell reaction that is brief and pruritic generates an urticarial wheal.

Food-induced reactions appear to cause responses similar to those that are stress-induced. Sampson and Jolie (1984) utilized the double-blind food challenge technique in selected atopic dermatitis patients who have skin test reactions. Positive food challenges elicit pruritic, erythematous papules, usually within an hour, and these have been correlated with increased plasma histamine levels drawn 30 min postchallenge. Antigen-IgE-triggered mast cells and/or basophils are the presumed source of histamine and other mediators that generate inflammation in the skin and, not infrequently, in gastrointestinal and respiratory mucosae as well.

These important clinical observations are perhaps the most direct evidence for a mast cell role in atopic dermatitis. Both methods elicit the erythema and itching that are hallmarks of the atopic dermatitis lesion. Again, however, a presumption is necessary to complete the model. Presumably the dermatitis is then prolonged either by repeated antigen exposure or by self-inflicted trauma such as scratching. In reality, at least in the experimental setting, the induced lesions are usually not propagated and simply fade within an hour or two. Even when lesions are prolonged, e.g., by intradermal injection of antigen to cause a late-phase reaction (LPR), the reactions are not typical of atopic dermatitis. The itch is not prolonged and the LPR histology is neutrophilic (Leiferman et al., 1989) and lacks spongiosis. The presence of eosinophil infiltration in atopic dermatitis and LPR lesions is inadequate to make the analogy if itch does not endure. Evidence cited above indicates that a truly eczematous lesion may be induced by prolonged antigen contact under patch tests kept in place for 24–48 hr. These lesions may actually be T-cell–mediated and they could develop independent of mast cells.

VII. T-Cell Modulation of Mast Cells

For many years, major support for a mast cell role in atopic dermatitis has been based on the mechanistic concept that relates elevated serum IgE and the triggering effect of food and airborne antigens. Recent information linking T cells and mast cells to IL-4 (Plaut, 1990; Brown and Hanifin, 1990) is providing an alternative conceptual framework, or at least a shift in emphasis. IL-4 plays a major role in IgE synthesis and may contribute to excessive IgE production (Pene et al., 1988; Romagnani et al., 1989). IL-4 also acts as a growth factor for murine mast cell lines, and this and other cytokines are up-regulated by crosslinking of the high-affinity IgE receptor (Plaut et al., 1989; Wodnar-Filipowicz et al., 1989). If the same holds for humans, an interactive network between T cells, IL-4, IgE, and mast cells may be of central importance to the pathogenesis of atopic disease. Recent studies have provided evidence for increased numbers of IL-4-producing T cells in the blood and skin of patients with atopic dermatitis (Romagnani et al., 1989; Brown et al., 1989). Moreover, a recent study (Wierenga et al., 1990) has demonstrated that T-cell clones raised from mite-sensitive atopics produce IL-4 but not interferon-γ in response to mite antigen. This Th-2 cytokine profile is favorable to excessive IgE production and consistent with the atopic diathesis. If this model is correct, it is conceivable that T cells may be perturbed by antigens and staphylococcal toxins/superantigens, possibly acting through epidermal antigen-presenting cells that are hyperfunctional in atopic dermatitis skin (Bruynzeel-Koomen et al., 1988; Cooper et al., 1990).

With the present, rather primitive state of knowledge, it is probably prudent to remain open to multiple mechanisms. In some instances, mast cells may initiate a flare of atopic dermatitis, while in other situations, a mast cell–independent mechanism may lead to the T-cell activation and enduring eczematous response that is so typical of atopic dermatitis.

VIII. Failure of Therapeutic Agents

The failure of mast cell–directed therapy presents a major realm of evidence against a mast cell role in atopic dermatitis. Antihistamines that work dramatically to relieve itch and wheal size in urticaria give only negligible benefit in atopic dermatitis. This inadequacy is perhaps due to the fact that numerous other, nonhistaminic inflammatory factors are released from mast cells. However, unless there is selective release in the two diseases or hyperreleasibility in atopic dermatitis versus impaired release in urticaria, the difference is difficult to understand. Inhibitors of mast cell degranulation, such as cromolyn, have likewise failed to show benefit in most well-controlled studies, though a recent study raises the possibility that topical therapy with certain vehicles may provide benefit (Kimata and Igarashi, 1990; Sampson, 1990).

Chronically applied topical corticosteroids are known to significantly deplete mast cells from normal human skin (Lavker and Schechter, 1985). Although this has not been studied in atopics, it might be anticipated that these patients would likewise be depleted by mast cells, considering the chronicity of treatment. However, they typically flare severely, even on their chronically treated, severely atrophied skin, within a few days of discontinuing corticosteroid applications.

Among the newer therapies, thymentin (TP-5) (Leung et al., 1990) and interferon-gamma (IFN-γ) (Boguniewicz et al., 1990; Schneider et al., 1991) have both recently shown effectiveness in treating patients with severe atopic dermatitis. Thymentin apparently acts to increase IFN-γ production and IFN-γ is known to block IL-4-induced IgE production. However, in the human studies to date (Boguniewicz et al., 1990; Schneider et al., 1991), no change in IgE synthesis or serum levels is evident. New information indicates that IFN-γ may reduce IL-4 effects (Gajewski and Fitch, 1990) and that it may act as a PDE inhibitor on atopic monocytes (Li et al., 1990). The possibility that these mechanisms also impinge on mast cells should be considered. Certainly PDE inhibition would be an effective control on basophil and mast cell hyperreleasibility, and newer, more potent inhibitors, administered topically or systemically, may have considerable potential for future therapeutic approaches. Cyclosporin A (CsA) was noted to provide relatively rapid reduction in pruritus when used for therapy of atopic dermatitis (Wahlgren et al., 1990). The authors considered this as evidence for a T-cell role in the pruritus of atopic dermatitis, though there is some evidence that CsA also reduces mast cell activity (Hohman and Hultsch, 1990).

IX. Conclusions

The role of mast cells in atopic dermatitis is uncertain. The numbers are increased in chronic lesions of atopic dermatitis, but also in other inflammatory skin diseases. Histamine levels in skin, plasma, and urine are increased inconsistently, suggesting that there are at least occasional episodes of mast cell or basophil degranulation. The strongest support for clinical relevancy for mast cell or basophil involvement comes from food challenge correlations with increased plasma histamine. Whether the associated skin changes regularly progress to the typical atopic dermatitis lesion remains to be determined. Perhaps multiple cells, including basophils, eosinophils, monocytes, and T cells, must be activated in order for the mast cell response to generate atopic dermatitis.

New information suggests that atopic dermatitis can develop independently of mast cells and that such aspects as mast cell proliferation, basophil and eosinophil infiltration, and increased histamine releasibility may all result from monocyte and T-cell activation, with release of cytokines such as IL-4, IL-5, IL-3, and histamine-releasing factors. The continuing lesion of atopic dermatitis has many more similarities to delayed hypersensitivity than to immediate hypersensitivity and late-phase reactions. Delayed hypersensitivity responses are rare on mucosal surfaces, and this may reflect a fundamental difference between allergic respiratory disease and atopic dermatitis. Further support for a primary T-cell role in atopic dermatitis comes from the failure of mast cell–directed therapy and the recently documented efficacy of T-cell–directed immunopharmacological modalities such as thymentin and IFN-γ. Evolving information relating to several facets of the T-cell/IL-4/IFN-γ axis encourage a more balanced reappraisal of pathogenic events in atopic dermatitis.

Discussion

Schleimer: I was interested in your focus on the lymphocyte. In collaboration with Bill Massey, we have recently shown the release of GM-CSF in our skin blister model. In one patient with atopic dermatitis, we found increased lymphokine release, and the data suggested that IL-3 was prominently released. One possible source of IL-3 might be the lymphocyte.

Hanifin: Your observation might relate to a recent observation by Dutch workers who cloned Th-2-type lymphocytes from the skin of atopic dermatitis patients. TH-2 cells might be expected to produce IL-3, IL-4, and IL-5, accounting for your finding of IL-3.

Denburg: Viennese workers have shown that melanocytes make message for and produce a variety of cytokines.

Hanifin: I agree. A variety of cytokines are produced by keratinocytes and now melanocytes. These observations suggest that the source of cytokines found in blister fluid will have to be interpreted carefully.

Bienenstock: Do you know whether the work reported by Askanase on a T-cell–derived, antigen-specific, mast cell–sensitizing factor has been repeated in humans?

Hanifin: I am not aware of any human extension of this work.

Lichtenstein: Are increased mast cells or basophils seen in atopic dermatitis?
Hanifin: This area has not been systematically investigated. However, the few data that exist suggest that basophils are increased after 24–48 hr and that mast cell increases require up to 10 days. Whether these increases apply to only atopic dermatitis or also apply to other immunological skin reactions requires much more careful study.
Schwartz: There are similarities between atopic dermatitis and asthma. Have any epidemiological studies been performed in atopic dermatitis to identify risk factors?
Hanifin: Studies such as those reported by Platts-Mills have suggested the importance of dust mites, but systematic studies have not been reported.

References

Boguniewicz, M., Sullivan, M. J., and Leung, D. Y. M. (1990). Recombinant gamma interferon in treatment of patients with atopic dermatitis and elevated IgE levels. *Am. J. Med.* 88:365–370.

Braun-Falco, O., and Burg, G. (1970). Das entzundliche infiltrat bei psoriasis vulgaris. Eine cytochemische Untersuchung. *Arch. Klin. Exp. Dermatol.* 236:297–314.

Brody, I. (1984). Mast cell degranulation in the evolution of acute eruptive guttate psoriasis vulgaris. *J. Invest. Dermatol.* 82:460–464.

Brown, M. A., and Hanifin, J. M. (1990). Atopic dermatitis. *Curr. Opin. Immunol.* 2:531–534.

Brown, M. A., Li, S. H., Chan, S. C., and Hanifin, J. M. (1989). Interleukin 4 mRNA expression by normal and atopic T lymphocytes. *Clin. Res.* 37:406A.

Bruynzeel-Koomen, C.A.F.M., VanWichen, D. F., Spry, C. J. F., Venge, P., and Bruynzeel, P. L. B. (1988). Active participation of eosinophils in patch test reactions to inhalant allergens in patients with atopic dermatitis. *Br. J. Dermatol.* 118:229–238.

Butler, J. M., Chan, S. C., Stevens, S., and Hanifin, J. M. (1983). Increased leukocyte histamine release with elevated cyclic AMP-phosphodiesterase activity in atopic dermatitis. *J. Allergy Clin. Immunol.* 71:490–497.

Cooper, K. D., Taylor, R. S., Hammerberg, C., and Chang, L. (1990). Abnormal Langerhans cell differentiation in atopic dermatitis: Increased CD36, CD1b, CD1c expression in association with increased autostimulatory capacity. *Clin. Res.* 38:835A.

Dreskin, S. C., Kaliner, M. A., and Gallin, J. I. (1987). Elevated urinary histamine in the hyperimmunoglobulin E and recurrent infection (Job's) syndrome: Association with eczematoid dermatitis and not with infection. *J. Allergy Clin. Immunol.* 79:515–522.

Eady, R. A. J., Cowen, T., Marshall, T. F., Plummer, V., and Greaves, M. W. (1979). Mast cell population density, blood vessel density and histamine content in normal human skin. *Br. J. Dermatol.* 100:623–633.

El-Ackad, T. M., and Brody, M. J. (1975). Evidence for non-mast cell histamine in the vascular wall. *Blood Vessels* 12:181.

Gajewski, T. F., and Fitch, F. W. (1990). Regulation of helper T lymphocyte activation by IFN-gamma. *J. Interferon. Res.* 10(Suppl. 1):S82.

Gondo, A., Saeki, N., and Tokuda, Y. (1986). Challenge reactions in atopic dermatitis after percutaneous entry of mite allergen. *Br. J. Dermatol.* 115:485–493.

Graham, D. T., and Wolf, S. (1953). The relation of eczema to attitude and to vascular reactions of the human skin. *J. Lab. Clin. Med.* 42:238–254.

Hanifin, J. M. (1977). Type I hypersensitivity diseases of the skin: divergent aspects of urticaria and atopic dermatitis. *Ann. Allergy* 39:153–160.

Hohman, R. J., and Hultsch, T. (1990). Cyclosporin A: New insights for cell biologists and biochemists. *New Biol.* 2:663–672.

Irani, A-M. A., Sampson, H. A., and Schwartz, L. B. (1989). Mast cells in atopic dermatitis. *Allergy* 44(Suppl. 9):31–34.

Johnson, H. H., DeOreo, G. A., Lascheid, W. P., and Mitchell, F. (1960). Skin histamine levels in chronic atopic dermatitis. *J. Invest. Dermatol.* 34:237–238.

Juhlin, L. (1967). Localization and content of histamine in normal and diseased skin. *Acta Derm. Venereol. (Stockh.)* 47:383–391.

Kimata, H., and Igarashi, M. (1990). Topical cromolyn (disodium cromoglycate) solution in the treatment of young children with atopic dermatitis. *Clin. Exp. Allergy* 20:281–283.

Lavker, R. M., and Schechter, N. M. (1985) Cutaneous mast cell depletion results from topical corticosteroid usage. *J. Immunol.* 135:2368–2373.

Lebel, B., Venecie, P. Y., Saurat, J. H., Soubrane, C., and Paupe, J. (1980). Anti-IgE-induced histamine release from basophils in children with atopic dermatitis. *Acta Derm. Venereol.* 92(Suppl.):57–59.

Leiferman, K. M., Ackerman, S. J., Sampson, H. A., Haugen, H., Venenci, P. Y., and Gleich, G. J. (1985). Dermal deposition of eosinophil-granule major basic protein in atopic dermatitis. *N. Engl. J. Med.* 313:282–285.

Leiferman, K. M., Peterson, E. A., Fujisawa, T., Gray, B. H., and Gleich, G. J. (1989). Differences between atopic dermatitis (AD) and the IgE-mediated cutaneous late phase reaction (LPR): Failure to detect neutrophil degranulation in AD. *Clin. Res.* 37:737A.

Leung, D. Y. M., Hirsch, R. L., Schneider, L., Moody, C., Takaoka, R., Li, S. H., Meyerson, L. A., Mariam, S. G., Goldstein, G., and Hanifin, J. M. (1990). Thymopentin therapy reduces the clinical severity of atopic dermatitis. *J. Allergy Clin. Immunol.* 85:927–933.

Li, S. H., Chan, S. C., and Hanifin, J. M. (1990). IFN-gamma modulates monocyte cyclic AMP-phosphodiesterase activity: Differential effect on normal and atopic cells. *J. Interferon Res.* 10(Suppl. 1):S169.

Marone, G., Giugliano, R., Lembo, G., and Ayala, F. (1986). Human basophil releasability. II. Changes in basophil releasability in patients with atopic dermatitis. *J. Invest. Dermatol.* 87:19–23.

Mihm, M., Jr., Soter, N., Dvorak, H., and Austen, K. F. (1976). The structure of normal skin and the morphology of atopic eczema. *J. Invest. Dermatol.* 67:305–312.

Mikhail, G. R., and Miller-Milinska, A. (1964). Mast cell population in human skin. *J. Invest. Dermatol.* 43:249–254.

Mitchell, E. B., Crow, J., Williams, G., and Platts-Mills, T. A. E. (1986). Increase in skin mast cells following chronic house dust mite exposure. *Br. J. Dermatol.* 114:65–73.

Norris, P. G., Schofield, O., and Camp, R. D. R. (1988). A study of the role of house dust mite in atopic dermatitis. *Br. J. Dermatol.* 118:435–440.

Pene, J., Rousset, F., Briere, F., Chretien, I., Bonnefoy, J-Y., Spits, H., Yokota, T., Arai, N., Arai, K-I., Banchereau, J., and DeVries, J. (1988). IgE production by normal human lymphocytes is induced by interleukin 4 and suppressed by interferons γ and α and prostaglandin E_2. *Proc. Natl. Acad. Sci. USA* 85:6880–6884.

Petersen, H. O., Thormann, J., and Zachariae, H. (1979). Urinary histamine in severe atopic dermatitis. *Arch. Dermatol. Res.* 264:193–195.

Plaut, M. (1990). Antigen-specific lymphokine secretory patterns in atopic disease. *J. Immunol.* 144:4497–4500.

Plaut, M., Pierce, J. H., Watson, C. J., Hanley-Hyde, J., Nordan, R. P., and Paul, W. E. (1989). Mast cell lines produce lymphokines in response to cross-linkage of $Fc_{\epsilon}RI$ or to calcium ionophores. *Nature* 339:64–67.

Reitamo, S., Visa, K., Kahonen, K., Kayhko, K., Stubb, S., and Salo, O. P. (1986). Eczematous reactions in atopic patients caused by epicutaneous testing with inhalant allergens. *Br. J. Dermatol.* 114:303–309.

Ring, J. (1983). Plasma histamine concentrations in atopic eczema. *Clin. Allergy* 13:545–552.

Ring, J., and O'Connor, R. (1979). In vitro histamine and serotonin release studies in atopic dermatitis. *Int. Arch. Allergy Appl. Immunol.* 58:322–330.

Romagnani, S., DelPrete, G. F., Maggi, E., Parronchi, P., Tiri, A., Macchia, D., Giudizi, M. G., Almerigogna, F., and Ricci, M. (1989). Role of interleukins in induction and regulation of human IgE synthesis. *Clin. Immunol. Immunopathol.* 50:S13–23.

Ruzicka, T., and Gluch, S. (1983). Cutaneous histamine levels and histamine releasability in the skin in atopic dermatitis and hyper-IgE syndrome. *Arch. Dermatol. Res.* 275:41–44.

Ruzicka, T., Simmet, T., Peskar, B. A., and Ring, J. (1986). Skin levels of arachidonic acid–derived inflammatory mediators and histamine in atopic dermatitis and psoriasis. *J. Invest. Dermatol.* 86:105–108.

Sampson, H. A. (1990). Atopic dermatitis and cromolyn. *Clin. Exp. Allergy* 20:243–244.

Sampson, H. A., and Jolie, P. L. (1984). Increased plasma histamine concentrations after food challenges in children with atopic dermatitis. *N. Engl. J. Med.* 311:372.

Sampson, H. A., Broadbent, K. R., and Bernhisel-Broadbent, J. (1989). Spontaneous release of histamine from basophils and histamine-releasing factor in patients with atopic dermatitis and food hypersensitivity. *N. Engl. J. Med.* 321:228–232.

Schneider, L. C., Hanifin, J. M., Cooper, K., Boguniewicz, M., Milgrom, H., Jaffe, H. S., Izu, A. E., Bucalo, L. R., and Leung, D. Y. M. (1991). Recombinant interferon-gamma (rIFN-γ) therapy reduces the clinical severity of atopic dermatitis (AD). *J. Allergy Clin. Immunol.* (abstract) *J. Allergy Clin. Immunol.* 87:235.

Voorhorst, R., and van der Hooft–van Asbeck, M. C. (1979). Atopic skin test re-evaluated. VI. Skin reactions to compound 48/80 and histamine in patients with atopic and non-atopic chronic respiratory complaints and in normal volunteers. *Ann. Allergy* 42:185–186.

Wahlgren, C-F., Scheynius, A., and Hagermark, O. (1990). Antipruritic effect of oral cyclosporin A in atopic dermatitis. *Acta Derm. Venereol. (Stockh.)* 70:323–329.

Walton, S., and DeSouza, E. J. (1983). Variation in mast cell numbers in psoriasis and lichen planus: Comparisons with normal skin. *Dermatologica* 166:236–239.

Wierenga, E. A., Snoek, M., deGroot, C., Chretien, L., Bos, J. D., Jansen, H. M., and Kapsenberg, M. I. (1990). Evidence for compartmentalization of functional subsets of $CD4^+$T lymphocytes in atopic patients. *J. Immunol.* 144:4651–4653.

Williams, D. H. (1938). Skin temperature reaction to histamine in atopic dermatitis (disseminated neurodermatitis). *J. Invest. Dermatol.* 1:119–129.

Wodnar-Filipowicz, A., and Heusser, C. H., and Moroni, C. (1989). Production of the haemopoietic growth factors GM-CSF and interleukin-3 by mast cells in response to IgE receptor-mediated activation. *Nature* 339:150–152.

26

Mast Cells and Fibrosis

Hints from Graft-Versus-Host Disease and Scleroderma

HENRY N. CLAMAN

University of Colorado
Denver, Colorado

I. Introduction

The mast cell is considered to be at the center of IgE-triggered allergic reactions, including both the immediate and the late-phase constituents (Holgate et al., 1988). Indeed, exploration of this central position in allergy has uncovered a surprising plethora of mast cell activities, far exceeding in complexity the classic and simple pathway of histamine release (Gordon et al., 1990).

Recently, however, the mast cell seems to be appearing in other biological reactions in which IgE is not essential. This review will focus on the role of the mast cell in fibrosis. I will discuss the evidence that mast cells contribute to fibroblast activation and collagen production in vitro and also in vivo. The latter phase will gather together some observations on chronic graft-versus-host disease (GVHD) in the laboratory and on scleroderma at the bedside. I will include a hypothesis implicating the mast cell in the pathogenesis of scleroderma and will point out other experimental and clinical links between mast cells and fibrosis.

II. Mast Cell–Fibroblast Relationships In Vitro

A. Mast Cell Growth Facilitation by Fibroblasts and Cytokines

Ehrlich, who discovered the mast cell, commented on its prominence in chronic inflammation (quoted by Riley, 1959). Although fibrosis is a characteristic of chronic inflammation, possible mast cell–fibroblast interactions were neither appreciated nor explored for many years. A major obstacle was the inability to develop or maintain mast cells in tissue culture. A big step forward was the observation that mast cells could be cultured from mouse thymus, but only in the presence of embryonic fibroblasts (Ginsburg and Sachs, 1963).

Experiments showing the differentiation of mast cells from antigen-stimulated lymphoid tissue in cultures containing fibroblast monolayers (Ginsburg and Lagunoff, 1967) were followed by studies showing that mast cell growth and differentiation can be promoted by the presence of conditioned medium (Razin et al., 1981; Schrader et al., 1981). A critical growth factor was later identified as IL-3 (Ihle et al., 1983). In general, the mast cells that grow out in such mouse cell cultures have the characteristics of mucosal mast cells (MMC), i.e., failure to stain with safranin, low content of histamine and carboxypeptidase A, and preferential synthesis of chondroitin sulfate-E. Fibroblast layers are particularly useful in growing rodent mast cells (Levi-Schaffer et al., 1985, 1986). Further studies (Dayton et al., 1988) showed that cloned IL-3-dependent mouse MC, when cultured with 3T3 fibroblasts, change their phenotype to that of connective tissue mast cells (CTMC), i.e., show increased staining with safranin and increased histamine and heparin content.

Thus, careful manipulation of cells, cytokines, and culture conditions allows mast cell precursors to change their pathways of differentiation (Kobayashi et al., 1986).

B. Mast Cell Influences on Fibroblasts

From the standpoint of this chapter, I am even more interested in what influence the mast cell may have on the fibroblast, perhaps leading to fibrosis. Mast cells can transfer their granules to fibroblasts (Greenberg and Burnstock, 1983; Subba Rao et al., 1983). Histamine is known to stimulate fibroblast growth in vitro (Norrby, 1973; Russell et al., 1977), an effect mediated by H_2 receptors (Jordana et al., 1988). Whether these observations are clinically relevant is moot, as conditions in which histamine release is repetitive, such as IgE-mediated asthma or urticaria pigmentosa, are not ones where fibrosis is prominent. Recent studies have shown that IL-3 activated mouse BMMC stimulate the growth of mouse fibroblasts (Dayton et al., 1989). However, as BMMC lysates were ineffective, histamine may not be the fibroblast regulator. It is possible that tryptase, a prominent constituent of many mast cell granules, is also a fibroblast growth factor (G. H. Caughey, personal communication).

In summary, tissue culture studies show that mast cells thrive on fibroblast layers and that fibroblasts may be stimulated by mast cells and their products. The exact mechanisms for this two-way interaction will undoubtedly come to light soon.

III. Mast Cell Activation In Vivo—Murine GVHD

Our attention was drawn to the possible role of mast cells in fibrosis by our studies on chronic murine GVHD across minor histocompatibility barriers (Jaffee and Claman, 1983). We had developed this model because of clinical and laboratory reports indicating that chronic GVHD resembled scleroderma. We had been looking for a mouse model of scleroderma.

A. Mast Cell Counts—Disappearance and Recovery

By accident, we noticed that mast cells were very hard to find in the skin of mice with chronic GVHD (Claman et al., 1985). Merely counting toluidine blue CTMCs showed that there was a slow "disappearance" of these cells from the skin as GVHD progressed over a period of several weeks (Claman, 1985). We believed it was significant that the skin was also the major site of inflammation and fibrosis in these mice. [It is of interest that a "dropout" of stainable mast cells had previously been seen in similar models of murine chronic GVHD (Charley et al., 1983) but no connection had been made with fibrosis.] The "disappearance" of mast cells from GVHD skin was dramatic (Fig. 1) (Claman et al., 1986). Furthermore, mast cell counts slowly returned to normal, then became supranormal, and finally returned to the normal range (Lee Choi et al., 1987). From the standpoint of fibrosis, this was an interesting kinetic development, as it was similar to what happens to mast cell counts in experimental would healing in rat skin (used as a model of fibrosis). In that situation, there is also an early disappearance of mast cells close to the wound edge, followed by mast cell recovery, mast cell hyperplasia, and finally normalization of mast cell counts (Wichmann, 1955; Persinger et al., 1983). Of course, the whole sequence is much more rapid in the rat skin wound model than it is in chronic murine GVHD with fibrosis.

B. Mast Cell Ultrastructure in Chronic Murine GVHD

What was the basis of the "mast cell disappearance reaction" in the mouse GVHD model? Did the mast cells die, or leave the skin, or were there other

(itchy) skin of the forearm showed numerous mast cells, many of which had a bizarre appearance (Fig. 2B). These cells were themselves edematous, their cell membranes were indistinct, and their granules looked "motheaten." The appearance of the granules is reminiscent of "piecemeal degranulation," described by Dvorak and colleagues as characteristic of a slow activation process (Chapter 1, this volume). Another biopsy was taken 1 year later, after the disease had been greatly improved by high-dose corticosteroid treatment. This specimen was from shoulder skin that was thickened but neither itchy nor edematous, and it showed normal-appearing mast cells (Fig. 2A).

Both the above cases show that significant (albeit different) changes in mast cell ultrastructure occur in aggressive scleroderma. Similar changes are not seen in late or quiescent disease.

C. Degranulated, Activated ("Phantom") Mast Cells in Scleroderma

Using the double-fluorescent method to detect granulated and degranulated "phantom" mast cells, we again explored paired biopsies from progressing and regressing scleroderma patients, each patient yielding a sample of "involved" and "uninvolved" skin (Seibold et al., 1990). In this study, mast cell membranes were stained with a monoclonal antibody and mast cell granules were stained with avidin. The results (Fig. 3) show the following:

1. All scleroderma biopsies showed far more mast cells than control biopsies.
2. There were greater numbers of phantom mast cells in early disease, in both involved and uninvolved skin. In general, these patients with early disease were getting worse, clinically.
3. In late disease, there were more mast cells than normal in involved and uninvolved skin, but more phantoms only in uninvolved skin. As these patients were, in general, improving clinically, the uninvolved skin might better be called "previously involved" skin.
4. Most important, in the 2 years following the biopsies from the early cases, the uninvolved skin became fibrotic and tethered in 10/11 cases. Thus, the increased numbers of both granulated and activated (phantom) mast cells in uninvolved skin in early disease *preceded* the clinical fibrosis and tethering.

These findings are important and surprising for several reasons: (1) They represent the first systematic study of clinically uninvolved skin in progressive systemic sclerosis (scleroderma). (2) They show that biopsies of normal-appearing skin in these patients have changes (with regard to mast cell numbers and activation) that are indistinguishable from those in "involved" skin. (3) They

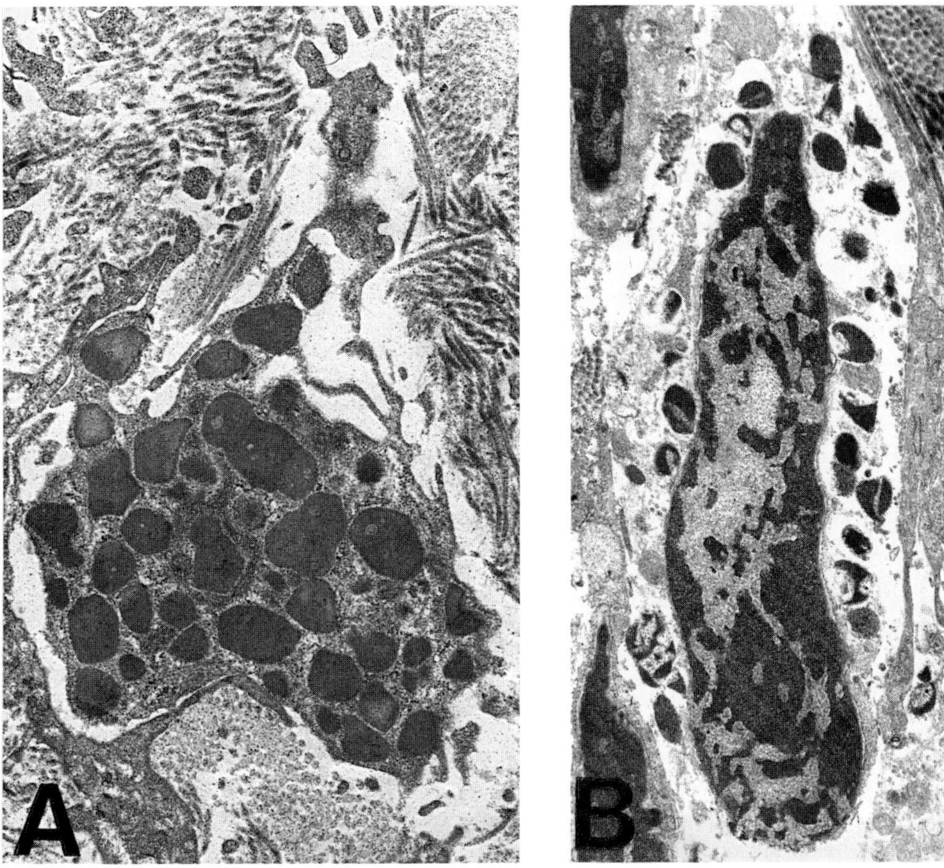

Figure 2 Electron photomicrographs of the skin of a woman with aggressive scleroderma. A. A mature, relatively quiescent mast cell in skin after treatment. The cell membrane is intact and granules are uniform. B. A mast cell from an earlier biopsy when the disease was very active. The mast cell looks edematous, and its cell membrane is not visible. Granules show a "motheaten" appearance with fragmentation. (17,356x)

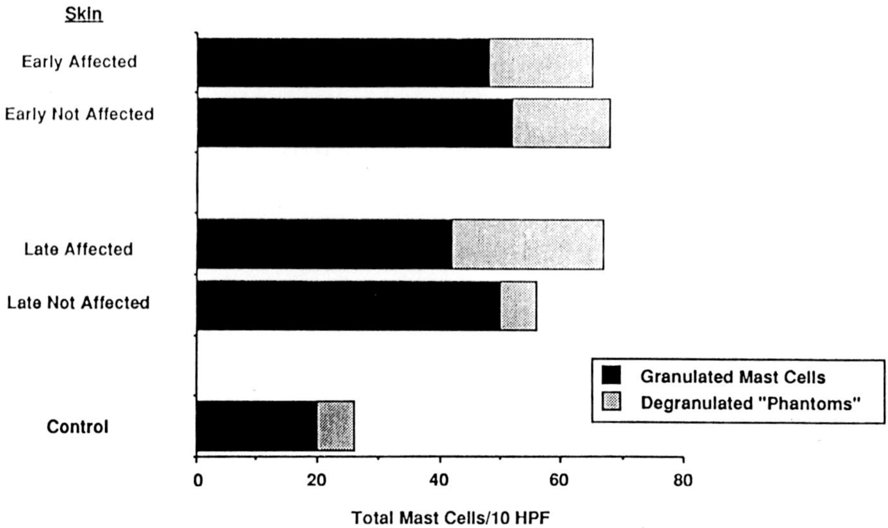

Figure 3 Mast cell counts from skin biopsies from scleroderma patients and normal controls. Early disease (11 patients with scleroderma for <3 years). Late disease (8 patients with scleroderma for >3 years). Seven normal controls. Mast cells were detected by staining with a monoclonal antibody to mast cell membranes. Granulated mast cells also stained with avidin-rhodamine. Degranulated "phantom" mast cells stained with the monoclonal antibody but not with avidin-rhodamine.

indicate that mast cell activation and hyperplasia *precede* clinical fibrosis. Newer data from the same biopsies show that endothelial activation and the formation of new, unprocessed procollagen are also more pronounced in scleroderma than in control normal skin. Again, there is no difference between involved and uninvolved skin; both show the same abnormalities (Claman et al, 1991).

These findings raise several interesting questions. First, if uninvolved dermis is just as abnormal as involved dermis, then the disease may be far more widespread in the skin—perhaps universal—then has been suspected by the clinician. These results call into question such concepts as "limited scleroderma." Second, if uninvolved and involved dermis look similar, why is the involved skin bound down and sclerotic, while the uninvolved skin is soft and mobile? It is likely that the differences are due to changes in the subcutaneous tissue, which is well out of the grasp of the 4-mm punch biopsy, the usual tool for skin biopsies in these patients. Subcutaneous changes have been described in scleroderma skin (Fleischmajer et al., 1972), but these changes have not been compared in involved and uninvolved specimens.

D. A Schema for the Pathogenesis of Scleroderma

We have tried to develop a comprehensive schema for the development of scleroderma. As the disease shows changes in the blood vessels as well as in the mast cells and fibroblasts, we developed a hypothesis linking these three cells (Fig. 4). The schema suggests that fibroblast activation leading to excess collagen production and endothelial activation leading to vascular instability (Raynaud's?), occlusion, and tissue hypoxia might both be promoted by mast cells via their production of heparin. Heparin, in turn, stabilizes and potentiates a number of heparin-binding growth factors, including acidic and basic fibroblast growth factors (FGFs), endothelial cell–derived growth factor (ECGF), and

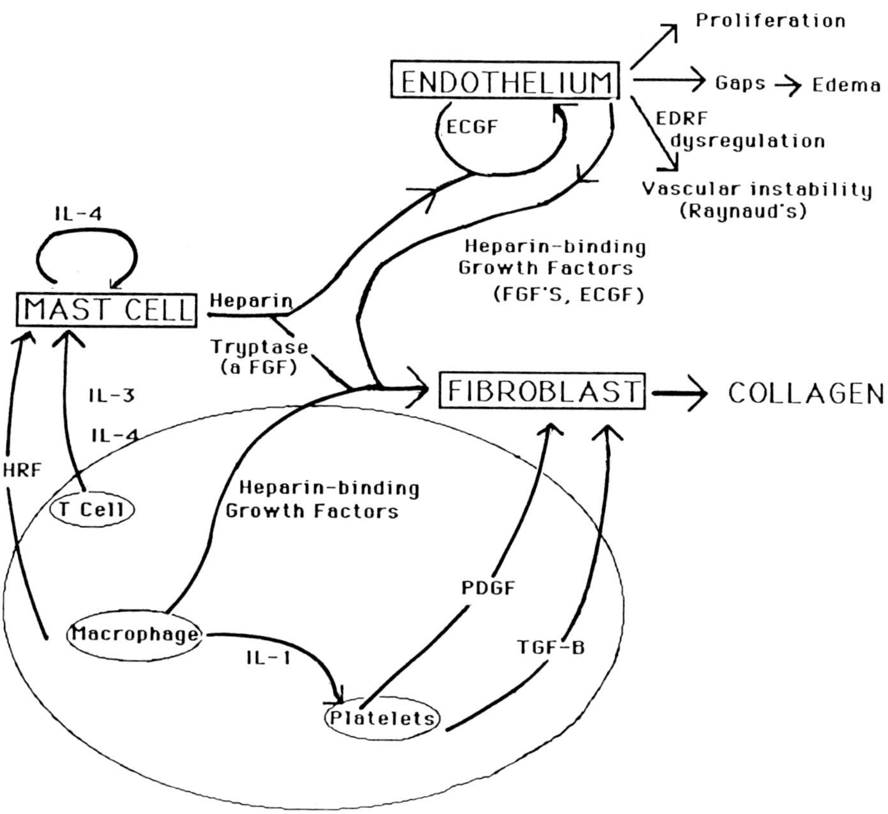

Figure 4 A schema for the development of scleroderma, showing the interactions of mast cells, fibroblasts and endothelial cells. Also shown are contributions from T cells, macrophages and platelets (adapted from J.A.M.A., *262*, Sept. 1, 1989, p. 1206. Copyright 1989, American Medical Association).

perhaps mast cell tryptase. As scleroderma also shows many properties common to autoimmune diseases, T-cell activation and other cells and cell products are brought into the picture for the sake of comprehensiveness. It should be recognized, however, that there is little evidence as yet for the direct participation of the various cytokines in scleroderma.

V. Mast Cell Involvement in Other Fibrotic States

There are many situations where mast cells have been noted to be prominent in fibrotic processes. It is unlikely that searching the literature for this kind of coincidence will provide a crisp analysis of mast cell–fibroblast interactions. Nevertheless, it is instructive to point out the variety of fibrotic situations in which mast cell hyperplasia has been seen. We should note that most of the studies merely notice or count metachromatically stained mature mast cells. A few studies show mast cell activation by electron microscopy. No papers, other than the ones on murine GVHD and scleroderma from our laboratory (noted above), provide data on degranulated "phantom" mast cells.

A. Experimental Fibrosis

Many experimental models of fibrosis have excess numbers of mast cells. In the rat lung, both bleomycin (Goto et al., 1984) and ionizing radiation (Watanabe et al., 1974) produce fibrosis with mast cell hyperplasia. This is also true in radiation-induced myocardial fibrosis (Fajardo and Stewart, 1973). Mast cells are prominent in corneal allograft reactions, and they appear before the fibrosis is marked (Smith and Basu, 1970). Experimental allergic neuritis, a peripheral nervous system analog of experimental allergic encephalomyelitis) is a chronic inflammatory and fibrotic condition in which mast cell hyperplasia occurs (Powell et al., 1983; Brosman et al., 1985).

An interesting genetic model of fibrosis occurs in the "tight skin" (Tsk) mouse. This animal has multiple skeletal changes but also shows diffuse fibrosis. The fibrotic areas have excess numbers of mast cells, many of which can be seen to be degranulating by metachromatic staining (Walker et al., 1985).

B. Clinical Fibrosis

In his comprehensive monograph, Fernex (1968) pointed out that mast cell hyperplasia occurs, together with fibrotic lesions, in parasitic infections such as onchocerciasis, filariasis, and schistosomiasis. The cardiac fibrosis seen in the carcinoid syndrome contains numerous mast cells (McDonald and Robbins, 1957). Mast cell hyperplasia is seen in keloids (Sylven, 1945; Smith et al., 1987) as well as in hypertrophic scars (Kirscher and Bailey, 1972). Rheumatoid synovitis and pannus formation are associated with mast cell hyperplasia (Hanes and McDonald, 1948; Crisp et al., 1984), as in chronic heliodermatitis (Lavker and Kligman, 1988). Mast cells are prominent in interstitial pulmonary fibrosis (etiology unspecified), and it is interesting that the ultrastructure of the lesions suggested that there was *slow* mast cell activation (Kawanami et al., 1979). This feature should be noted, because our hypothesis about mast cells and fibrosis is based mainly on experimental murine GVHD and on scleroderma. Both these situations reflect *chronic* processes in which one would expect that mast cell activation would be slow and prolonged (perhaps "piecemeal") and not of the rapid IgE-triggered variety.

Neurofibromas contain many more mast cells than expected (Pineda, 1965; Riccardi, Eichner, 1986), and the tumors often itch. In the Spanish toxic oil syndrome, which includes pulmonary inflammation in the acute phase and a scleroderma-like picture in the chronic phase, mast cells are excessive in the skin in the latter situation (Fonseca and Solis, 1985). In eosinophilic fasciitis, which resembles both scleroderma and the toxic oil syndrome, mast cell hyperplasia is considerable (Gabrielli et al., 1983).

Systemic mastocytosis should be an important situation in which to explore mast cell-fibroblast relationships, and when this is done, there appears to be a discrepancy. In the skin, fibrosis is not a feature of urticaria pigmentosa. However, autopsy reports indicate that fibrosis of the liver, spleen, and bone marrow may be severe (Lennert et al., 1956; Brunning et al., 1983; Horny et al., 1985). How is this discordance to be resolved? Possible reasons include the heterogeneity of mast cells and of their products (reviewed elsewhere in this volume). The skin mast cells in urticaria pigmentosa represent connective tissue mast cells in which histamine is a prominent mediator. Although histamine has been shown to stimulate fibroblasts in vitro, it is not a powerful profibrotic agent; in bronchial asthma, a condition where histamine release is repetitive, fibrosis is not prominent. The mast cells in the viscera of mastocytosis may be different (? musocal type) and may secrete other cytokines, e.g., heparin and IL-4, which are more profibrotic. This discrepancy, i.e, visceral fibrosis without skin fibrosis seen in mastocytosis, requires further study.

VI. Summary

Mast cell hyperplasia and mast cell activation are both seen in a variety of clinical and experimental situations where fibrosis is prominent. This chapter has stressed the mast cell involvement in two situations. Murine chronic graft-versus-host disease is a T-cell–mediated process where mast cell activation is intense in the skin where inflammation and fibrosis occur. Scleroderma is thought to be autoimmune, and mast cell activation is prominent in involved skin and normal-appearing (but soon-to-be-involved) skin. A hypothesis is put forth for the pathogenesis of scleroderma. This schema links mast cells, endothelial cells, and fibroblasts via heparin and heparin-binding growth factors.

Acknowledgments

This work was supported in part by the Scleroderma Research Foundation, Santa Barbara, California, NIH Grant CA-47657, and the RGK Foundation. I am grateful for the support of Dr. Ralph Giorno, Dr. James R. Seibold, Mrs. Janet Lieber, and Ms. Kathryn Utschinski.

References

Brosman, C. F., Lyman, W. D., Tansey, F. A., and Carter, T. H. (1985). Quantitation of mast cells in experimental allergic neuritis. *J. Neuropathol. Exp. Neurol.* 44:196–203.

Brunning, R. D., McKenna, R. W., Rosai, J., Parkin, J. L., and Risdall, R. (1983). Systemic mastocytosis. *Am. J. Surg. Pathol.* 7:425–438.

Charley, M. R., Bangert, J. L., Hamilton, B. L., Gilliam, J. N., and Sontheimer, R. D. (1983). Murine graft-versus-host skin disease: A chronologic and quantitative analysis of two histologic patterns. *J. Invest. Dermatol.* 81:412–417.

Claman, H. N. (1985). Mast cell depletion in murine chronic graft-versus-host disease. *J. Invest. Dermatol.* 84:246–248.

Claman, H. N. (1989). Mast cell changes in a case of rapidly progressive scleroderma—Ultrastructural analysis. *J. Invest. Dermatol.* 92:290.

Claman, H. N. (1990). Mast cells and fibrosis: The relevance to scleroderma. *Rheum. Clin. North Am.* 16:141–151.

Claman H. N., Giorno, R. C., and Seibold, J. R. (1991). Endothelial and fibroblastic activation in scleroderma. The myth of the "uninvolved skin." *Arth. Rheum.* 34:1495–1501.

Claman, H. N., Jaffee, B. D., Huff, J. C., and Clark, R. A. F. (1985). Chronic graft-versus-host disease (GVHD) as a model for scleroderma. II. Mast cell depletion with deposition of immunoglobulins in the skin and fibrosis. *Cell Immunol.* 94:73–84.

Claman, H. N., Lee Choi, I., Sujansky, W., and Vatter, A. E. (1986). Mast cell "disappearance" in chronic murine graft-vs.-host disease (GVHD)—Ultrastructural demonstration of "phantom mast cells." *J. Immunol.* 137:2009–2013.

Crisp, A. J., Chapman, C. M., Kirkham, S. E., Schiller, A. L., and Krane, S. M. (1984). Articular mastocytosis in rheumatoid arthritis. *Arthritis Rheum.* 27:845–851.

Dayton, E. T., Pharr, P., Ogawa, M., Serafin, W. E., Austen, K. F., Levi-Schaffer, F., and Stevens, R. L. (1988). 3T3 fibroblasts induce cloned interleukin 3-dependent mouse mast cells to resemble connective tissue mast cells in granular constituency. *Proc. Natl. Acad. Sci. USA* 85:569–572.

Dayton, E. T., Caulfield, J. P., Hein, A., Austen, K. F., and Stevens, R. L. (1989).

Regulation of the growth rate of mouse fibroblasts by IL-3-activated mouse bone marrow-derived mast cells. *J. Immunol.* 142:4307–4313.

Fajardo, L. F., and Stewart, J. R. (1973). Pathogenesis of radiation-induced myocardial fibrosis. *Lab. Invest.* 29:244–254.

Fernex, M. (1968). *The Mast-Cell System: Its Relationship to Atherosclerosis. Fibrosis and Eosinophils.* Baltimore, Williams & Wilkins, pp. 1–212.

Fleischmajer, R., Damiano, V., and Nedwich, A. (1972). Alteration of subcutaneous tissue in systemic scleroderma. *Arch. Dermatol.* 105:59–66.

Fonseca, E., and Solis, J. (1985). Mast cells in the Skin: Progressive systemic sclerosis and the toxic oil syndrome. *Ann. Intern. Med.* 102:864–865.

Gabrielli, A., DeNictolis, M., Campanati, G., and Cinti, S. (1983). Eosinophilic fasciitis: A mast cell disorder? *Clin. Exp. Rheumatol.* 1:75–80.

Ginsburg, H., and Lagunoff, D. (1967). The in vitro differentiation of mast cells. Culture of cells from immunized mouse lymph nodes and thoracic duct lymph on fibroblast monolayers. *J. Cell. Biol.* 35:685.

Ginsburg, H., and Sachs, L. (1963). Formation of pure suspensions of mast cells in tissue culture by differentiation of lymphoid cells from the mouse thymus. *J. Natl. Cancer Inst.* 31:1–39.

Giorno, R., Lee Choi, K., and Claman, H. N. (1987). Simultaneous in situ detectors of IgE receptors and cytoplasmic granules in murine cutaneous mast cells. *J. Immunol. Meth.* 99:163–166.

Gordon, J. R., Burd, P. R., and Galli, S. J. (1990). Mast cells as a source of multifunctional cytokines. *Immunol. Today* 11:458–464.

Goto, T., Befus, D., Low, R., and Bienenstock, J. (1984). Mast cell heterogeneity and hyperplasia in bleomycin-induced pulmonary fibrosis in rats *Am. Rev. Respir. Dis.* 130:797–802.

Greenberg, I., and Burnstock, G. (1983). A novel cell-to-cell interaction between mast cells and other cell types. *Exp. Cell. Res.* 147:1–13.

Hawkins, R. A., Claman, H. N., Clark, R. A. F., and Steigerwald, J. C. (1985). Increased dermal mast cell populations in progressive systemic sclerosis: A link in chronic fibrosis. *Ann. Intern. Med.* 102:182–186.

Holgate, S. T., Robinson, C., and Church, M. K. (1988). The contribution of mast cell mediators to acure allergic reactions in human skin and airways. *Allergy* 43(Suppl. 5):22–31.

Horny, H-P., Parwaresch, M. R., and Lennert, K. (1985). Bone marrow findings in systemic mastocytosis. *Hum. Pathol.* 16:808–814.

Ihle, J. N., Keller, J., Oroszlan, S., Henderson, L. E., Copeland, T. D., Fitch, F., Prystowsky, M. B., Goldwasser, E., Schrader, J. W., Palasyzynski, E., Dy, M., and Lebel, B. (1983). Biologic properties of homogeneous interleukin-3. I. Demonstration of Wehi-3 growth factor activity, mast cell growth factor activity, P cell–stimulating factor activity, colony-stimulating factor activity and histamine-producing cell-stimulating factor activity. *J. Immunol.* 131:282–287.

Jaffee, B. D., and Claman, H. N. (1983). Chronic graft-versus-host disease (GVHD) as a model for scleroderma. I. Description of model systems. *Cell. Immunol.* 77:1–12.

Janes, J., and McDonald, J. R. (1948). Mast cells: Their distribution in various human tissues. *Arch. Pathol.* 45:622–634.

Jordana, M., Befus, A. D., Newhouse, M. T., Bienenstock, J., and Gauldie, J. (1988).

Effect of histamine on proliferation of normal human adult lung fibroblasts. *Thorax* 43:552–558.

Kawanami, O., Ferrans, V. J., Fulmer, J. D., and Crystal, R. G. (1979). Ultrastructure of pulmonary mast cells in patients with fibrotic lung disorders. *Lab. Invest.* 40:717–734.

Kirscher, C. W., and Bailey, J. F. (1972). The mast cell in hypertrophic scars. *Tex. Rep. Biol. Med.* 30:327–338.

Kobayashi, T., Nakano, T., Nakahata, T., Asai, H., Tagi, Y., Tsiji, K., Komiyama, A., Ababane, T., Kajima, S., and Kitamura, Y. (1986). Formation of mast cell colonies in methylcellulose by mouse peritoneal cells and differentiation of these cloned cells in both the skin and gastric mucosa of W/W^v mice: Evidence that a common precursor can give use to "connective-tissue type" and "mucosal" mast cells. *J. Immunol.* 136:1378–1384.

Lavker, R. M., and Kligman, A. M. (1988). Chronic heliodermatitis: A morphologic evaluation of chronic actinic dermal damage with emphasis on the role of mast cells. *J. Invest. Dermatol.* 90:325–330.

Lee Choi, K., Giorno, R., and Claman, H. N. (1987). Cutaneous mast cell depletion and recovery in murine graft-vs.-host disease. *J. Immunol.* 138:4093–4101.

Lennert, K., Koster, E., and Martin, H. (1956). Uber die mastzellenleukamie. *Acta Haematol. (Basel)* 16:255–272.

Levi-Schaffer, F., Austen, K. F., Caulfield, J. P., Hein, A., Bloes, W. F., and Stevens, R. L. (1985). Fibroblasts maintain the phenotype and viability of the rat heparin-containing mast cell in vitro. *J. Immunol.* 135:3454–3462.

Levi-Schaffer, F., Austen, K. F., Gravallese, P. M., and Stevens, R. L. (1986). Coculture of interleukin 3-dependent mouse mast cells with fibroblasts results in a phenotypic change in the mast cells. *Proc. Natl. Acad. Sci. USA* 83:6485–6488.

McDonald, R. A., and Robbins, S. L. (1957). Pathology of the heart in the carcinoid syndrome—A comparative study. *Arch. Pathol.* 63:103–112.

Nishioka, K., Kobayashi, Y., Katayama, I., and Takijiri, C. (1987). Mast cell numbers in diffuse scleroderma. *Arch. Dermatol.* 123:205–208.

Norrby, K. (1973). Effect of heparin, histamine and serotonin on the density-dependent inhibiton of replication in two fibroblastic cell lines. *Virchows Arch. B Cell. Pathol.* 15:75–93.

Persinger, M. A., Lepage, P., Simard, J-P., and Parker, G. H. (1983). Mast cell numbers in incisional wounds in rat skin as a function of distance, time and treatment. *Br. J. Dermatol.* 108:179–187.

Pineda, A. (1965). Their presence and ultrastructural characteristics in peripheral nerve tumors. *Arth. Neurol.* 13:372–283.

Powell, H. C., Braheny, S. L., Myers, R. R., Rodriguez, M., and Lampert, P. W. (1983). Early changes in experimental allergic neuritis. *Lab. Invest.* 48:332–338.

Razin, E., Cordon-Cardo, C., and Good, R. A. (1981). Growth of pure population of mouse mast cells in vitro with conditioned medium derived from Concanavalin A stimulated splenocytes. *Proc. Natl. Acad. Sci. USA* 78:2559–2562.

Riccardi, V. M., and Eichner, J. E. (1986). *Neurofibromatosis: Phenotype, Natural History, and Pathogenesis.* Baltimore, Johns Hopkins University Press, pp. 209–213.

Riley, J. F. (1959). *The Mast Cells*. Edinburgh, E. & S. Livingston, pp. 1–182.

Russell, J. D., Russell, S. B., and Trupin, K. M. (1977). The effect of histamine on the growth of cultured fibroblasts isolated from formal and keloid tissue. *J. Cell. Physiol,* 93:389–394.

Schrader, J. W., Lewis, S. J., Clark-Lewis, I., and Culvenor, J. G. (1981). The persisting (P) cell: Histamine content, regulation by a T-cell derived factor, origin from a bone-marrow precursor and relationship to mast cells. *Proc. Natl. Acad. Sci. USA* 78:323.

Seibold, J. R., Giorno, R. C., and Claman, H. N. (1990). Dermal mast cell degranulation in systemic sclerosis. *Arth. Rheum.* 33:1702–1709.

Smith, C. J., Smith, J. C., and Finn, M. C. (1987). The possible role of mast cells (allergy) in the production of keloid and hypertrophic scarring. *J. Burn Care Rehab.* 8:126–131.

Smith, S. S., and Basu, P. K. (1970). Mast cells in corneal immune reactions. *Can. J. Ophthalmol.* 5:175–183.

Subba-Rao, P. V., Friedman, M. M., Atkins, F. M., and Metcalfe, D. D. (1983). Phagocytosis of mast cell granules by cultured fibroblasts. *J. Immunol.* 130:341–349.

Sylven, B. (1945). Ester sulphuric acids of high molecular weight and mast cells in mesenchymal tumors. *Acta Radiolog. (Scand.)* (Suppl. 59): 1–99.

Walker, M., Harley, R., Maize, J., DeLustro, F., and LeRoy, E. C. (1985). Mast cells and their degranulation with TSK mouse model of scleroderma. *Proc. Soc. Exp. Biol. Med.* 180:323.

Watanabe, S., Watanabe, K., Ohishi, T., Aiba, M., and Kageyama, K. (1974). Mast cells in the rat alveolar septa undergoing fibrosis after ionizing irradiation. *Lab. Invest.* 31:555–567.

Wichmann, B-E. (1955). The mast cell count during the process of wound healing. *Acta Pathol. Microbiol. Scand.* (Suppl. 108):1–35.

27

Mast Cells and Their Role in Parasitic Helminth Infection

THOMAS B. NUTMAN

National Institute of Allergy and Infectious Diseases
National Institutes of Health
Bethesda, Maryland

I. Introduction

Although major strides have been made in controlling certain helminth parasitic infections, through either transmission control schemes or new chemotherapeutic agents, these parasitic diseases continue to cause morbidity and mortality throughout the developing world. Gastrointestinal parasites such as *Ascaris lumbricoides,* hookworm, and *Strongyloides stercoralis* are estimated to affect >1.2 billion individuals worldwide; another ~300 million individuals are infected with schistosome or filarial parasites. The reason for the high prevalence and continued transmission of these parasitic infections is, in part, due to the inability to find methods to induce protective immunity to these parasites. As the impact of these parasite infections is significant in terms of their effects on individual health as well as on the socioeconomic status of communities at large, emphasis has been placed on investigating the unique relationship between the parasite and the host immune system.

Helminth parasites, like the atopic state, induce immune effector mechanisms that are associated with immediate hypersensitivity. These are charac-

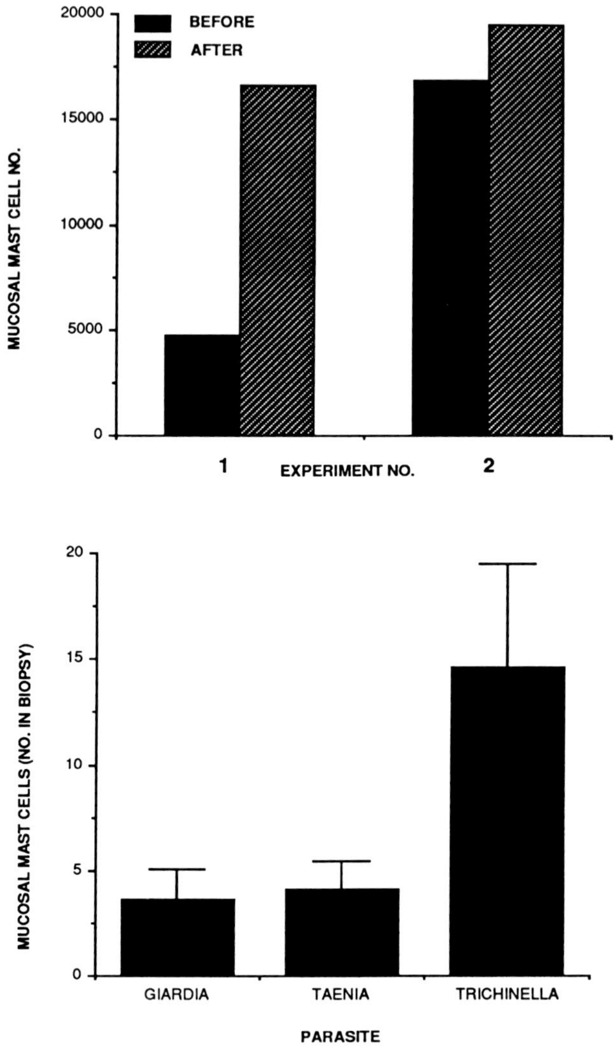

Figure 1 Mast cell hyperplasia in nonhuman and human primates. (Top) Mucosal mast cell number in intestinal biopsy specimens of monkeys before (dark bars) and after (hatched bars) infection with *S. stercoralis*. (Bottom) Mean mucosal mast cell number in biopsy specimens of humans infected with *Giardia, Taenia,* and *Trichinella*. [Data adapted from Barrett et al. (1988) and Gustowska et al. (1983).]

ate, clonally expand, and produce locally acting growth factors for mucosal mast cells.

IV. Mast Cells and the Nonpermissive State

For a large number of helminth parasites, a phenomenon of nonpermissiveness exists; this state is characterized by the inability of the parasite to establish a chronic infection. In rodents, certain nematodes are rapidly expelled from the host; thus this relatively "rapid expulsion" of helminth larvae or adult parasites has led to an examination of the factors responsible for the failure of a parasite to establish a patent infection (self-cure). It has been postulated that the proliferation and activation of mast cells is one of the major effector mechanisms whereby parasites are rejected (Bienenstock, 1986; Miller, 1984; Woodbury et al., 1984). Released mast cell mediators have clearly been shown to damage parasites (Henderson et al., 1986) and augment the expulsion of helminths either directly or by recruitment of other effector cells, such as eosinophils (Anwar et al., 1980; Moqbel, 1986; Moqbel et al., 1983) or cells found in the intestinal epithelium (Befus, 1986).

A. Mast Cells and Rapid Expulsion Phenomenon

That the mast cell plays a major role in the phenomenon of rapid expulsion of pathogenic helminth parasites was suggested by the observation that the survival of *T. spiralis* in the intestine of infected rodents was prolonged by the administration of drugs that diminish degranulation of mast cells. However, the role of the mast cell in rapid expulsion has been shown most definitively in studies utilizing immunodeficient strains of mice (Table 1), particularly those that are mast cell deficient (W/W^v and Sl/Sl^d).

Initially, these mast cell–deficient mice were infected with either *T. spiralis* (Alizadeh and Wakelin, 1982a; Ha et al., 1983; Kamiya et al., 1985) or *S. ratti* (Itayama et al., 1987), and the time to expulsion of these parasites was compared to that in normal congenic littermates. In all cases there was a delay in the parasite expulsion. This delayed expulsion could be reconstituted by normal bone marrow (Abe and Nawa, 1987; Nawa et al., 1985; Oku et al., 1984), normal bone marrow–derived cultured mast cells (Abe and Nawa, 1987), and spleen cells from normal mice (Oku et al., 1984). In the nude mouse infected with *S. ratti*, there was also a delay in the expulsion of the parasites (Vos et al., 1983), here felt to reflect the T-lymphocyte–dependent absence of mucosal mast cells. In this situation, repetitive IL-3 administration was able to restore the rapid expulsion phenomenon, presumably by increasing the number of mucosal mast cells found in the small intestine (Abe and Nawa, 1988b).

Table 1 Studies on Expulsion of Intestinal Parasites in Immunodeficient Mice

Genetic background	Parasite	Expulsion	Reconstitution leading to rapid expulsion	Reference
W/W^v	*Trichinella spiralis*	Delayed		Alizadeh and Wakelin, 1982a
W/W^v	*Trichinella spiralis*	Delayed		Ha et al., 1983
W/W^v	*Trichinella spiralis*	Delayed	Bone marrow	Nawa et al., 1985
W/W^v	*Trichinella spiralis*	Delayed		Kamiya et al., 1985
W/W^v	*Trichinella spiralis*	Delayed	Bone marrow	Abe and Nawa, 1987
W/W^v	*Strongyloides ratti*	Delayed	Bone marrow Spleen	Itayama et al., 1987
Sl/Sl^d	*Trichinella spiralis*	Delayed		Oku et al., 1984
W/W^v	*Strongyloides ratti*	Delayed	Bone marrow Cultured mast cells	Vos et al., 1983
Nu/Nu	*Strongyloides ratti*	Delayed	IL-3	Abe and Nawa, 1988a

The mechanism underlying the establishment of the nonpermissive state is not well understood. It is clear, however, that mast cell activation occurs during the rapid expulsion of helminth parasites, as determined by the measurement of mucosal mast cell–derived mediators such as RMCP-II (Huntley, 1987, 1990; Miller et al., 1983; Woodbury et al., 1984) and serotonin (Parmentier et al., 1987). In addition, use of the serotonin antagonists methylsergide and ketanserin in *T. spiralis*–infected mice was associated with both inhibition of the mucosal mast cell response to antigen and diminution of the recruitment of eosinophils, goblet cell hyperplasia, and villous atrophy (Parmentier et al., 1987).

The physiological basis for the rapid expulsion phenomenon has been addressed in animals infected with either *T. spiralis* (Castro et al., 1987; Harari and Castro 1989; Harari et al., 1987; Parmentier et al., 1987; Russell, 1986) or *Nippostrongylus brasiliensis* (Perdue et al., 1990). In the *T. spiralis* model, IgE-mediated mast cell activation (and the mediators released by such activation) has been shown to alter ion transport (particularly Cl^-) across the intestinal epithelium that may mediate parasite rejection (Harari et al., 1987). In a more recent study, however, neural interactions with mast cells (as opposed to mast cell activation per se) have been implicated as the stimulus for ion transport alterations (Perdue et al., 1990).

B. Genetic Control of the Nonpermissive State

Within a given species, there is evidence for genetic control of the nonpermissive state (Wakelin, 1978a, 1984, 1986, 1989). When the rapid expulsion phenomenon of *T. spiralis* was followed after primary infection in different inbred mouse strains, there were clear-cut differences in the duration of infection among the various strains (Wakelin, 1978a, 1984). This differential responsiveness to primary infection appears to come under the control of major histocompatibility complex (MHC) linked genes as well as other non-MHC-linked genes, and the relative contribution of each set of genes to the expulsion phenomenon varies among strains (reviewed in (Wakelin, 1984)).

The role of the non-MHC linked genes in controlling the intestinal response to *T. spiralis*, at least, has been addressed using reciprocal adoptive transfer of mesenteric lymph node cells and bone marrow cells between histocompatible mice with differing abilities to clear infection (Wakelin and Donachie, 1981). The results of these and similar studies (Alizadeh and Wakelin, 1982b) suggested that the non-MHC-linked genes control the nature of myeloid cells and thereby influence the generation of the intestinal inflammation.

The role of the MHC-linked genes on the expulsion of adult *T. spiralis* has been studied extensively, as well (Wassom et al., 1983, 1984), using sets of H-2 congenic and recombinant mice. Using such mice, the two sets of genes controlling the expulsion were able to be mapped to specific loci within the MHC locus. Alleles of these loci have been associated with relative susceptibility and resistance (so-called Ts-1 locus), as well as the ability to influence T cells whose function is to provide T-cell help for the generation of an intestinal inflammatory response (Ts-2 locus).

The fact that the nonpermissive state is, in part, under genetic control augurs poorly for finding methods for inducing such a state in a permissive host. Little progress has been made, to date, in significantly altering the expression of genetically controlled immune responses, and thus an additional layer of complexity is added to the attempts to control infections whose consequences are pathological.

V. Role of the Mast Cell in Pathogenesis

A. Proinflammatory Responses

Antigen Nonspecific Effects

Parasites by themselves or as a consequence of their interaction with immune effector cells can clearly cause pathological responses associated with mast cell degranulation. One mechanism by which helminth infection could have an effect on the manifestation of infection involves the nonspecific degranulation of mast cell by parasite-derived antigens, and several pieces of experimental evidence point to this as a plausible theory. Factors have been identified in worm extracts that cause histamine release from the mast cells of unsensitized animals (Thompson, 1972; Tolone et al., 1972, 1974; Unvas et al., 1960; Unvas and Wold, 1967). From *Ascaris* spp., low-molecular-weight [2–3 kDa (Unvas and Wold, 1967) and 8–9 kDa (Thompson, 1972)] factors and a higher-molecular-weight molecule [25–40 kDa (Tolone et al., 1974)] have been isolated that induce mast cell degranulation nonspecifically. In schistosome parasites, studies have shown that the infective cercariae contain a component in their preacetabular glands capable of degranulating mast cells from nonsensitized hosts (Catto et al., 1980) and that extracts from these same parasites have the ability to generate an "anaphylatoxin" from serum complement that also nonspecifically causes mast cell degranulation (Gazzinelli et al., 1969; Mazinque et al., 1980). In addition, a proteolytic enzyme from adult schistosome worms has been shown to induce a histamine skin reaction (Senft and Maddison, 1975).

Another mechanism hypothesized to explain immediate allergic reactivity to helminth infection involves sensitization of the parasite-infected individual to the effects of histamine (reviewed by Jarrett and Miller, 1982). This theory has been extrapolated from work performed in animals given *Bordatella pertussis*, which causes experimental animals to become much more responsive than normal animals to the pathophysiological consequences of histamine, such that small doses of histamine in the presence of *B. pertussis* lead to anaphylaxis and death (Munoz and Bergman, 1968). This type of finding engendered similar studies in mice infected with *T. spiralis* showing that these infected mice had a markedly increased sensitivity to both serotonin and histamine (Briggs and DeGiusti, 1970). In another study, this sensitization by *T. spiralis* was shown to render the animals approximately 100 times more sensitive to the effect of histamine than uninfected animals (Munoz et al., 1974).

Antigen-Specific, Mast Cell–Based Pathological Reactions

Despite the possible beneficial effects of mast cell proliferation and activation with respect to the rapid expulsion of primary infections (see above) and perhaps resistance to reinfection (see below), there is also evidence that the accumulation and triggering of mast cells leads to inflammation whose consequences are injurious to the host. Intestinal inflammation occurs in response to parasitic infection both in humans and in animal models. Infection with gastrointestinal-dwelling helminth parasites characteristically alters the integrity of the mucosal surface and leads to a cellular infiltrative lesion in which a number of inflammatory cells participate (Moqbel, 1986), including mast cells, eosinophils, neutrophils, platelets, and macrophages (Capron et al., 1977; Joseph et al., 1983). In that the mast cells that accumulate in the intestine in response to helminth infection are sensitized with parasite-specific IgE, it stands to reason that mast cell activation occurs, resulting in the generation and/or release of a wide variety of mediators—including leukotrienes B_4, C_4, D_4, HETEs, PAF-acether, histamine, proteolytic enzymes, prostaglandins, and serotonin. Several of these mediators, by themselves, can cause epithelial damage, intestinal mucosal edema, changes in peristalisis and mucus production, and recruitment of other inflammatory cells (Moqbel, 1986; Moqbel et al., 1986, 1987).

Mast Cells and Associated Pathological Reactions in Disease States

There have been few histopathological studies, particularly in higher primates, examining the role of mast cells in parasitic helminth infections. Nevertheless, mast cells, together with eosinophils, have been seen surrounding schistosomula in the epidermis of primates (Hsu et al., 1979) and some egg-induced granulomas of schistosome-infected livers (Epstein et al., 1979). Further, depletion of mast cells has been shown to abrogate inflammatory responses against schistosomula (Capron et al., 1978). Perhaps more important, in a study of biopsy specimens from lymphedematous skin of 25 patients with filarial elephantiasis, 15 (60%) had increased numbers of mast cells; (at least twice those of controls—either normal individuals or individuals with nonfilarial lymphedema); of these 15, eight showed marked increases in degranulated mast cells and histological evidence of extracellular mast cell products (Dumont et al., 1983). This finding suggests that mast cell degranulation by altering local capillary permeability would result in the local accumulation of protein-rich interstitial fluid (lymphedema) and ultimately fibrosis (Dumont et al., 1983), a finding supported in another filarial infection, onchocerciasis (Wolfe et al., 1974).

B. Modulation of These Responses

Characteristically, patients with tissue-invasive helminth infections have all the components that contribute to immediate hypersensitivity (i.e., high levels of parasite-specific and polyclonal IgE, eosinophilia, and tissue-dwelling mast cells sensitized to parasite antigens) though they rarely show any clinically evident immediate-type hypersensitivity reactions to the parasite antigens (Ottesen, 1985). Work done by several investigators has suggested that this immediate hypersensitivity responsiveness is tightly modulated in helminth infections. Several mechanisms have been proposed, including: (1) competition for the high-affinity $Fc_{\epsilon}RI$ by 'irrelevant' (non-parasite-specific) IgE; (2) inhibition of mast cell mediator release by shed parasite antigens (Mazinque et al., 1980); and (3) the presence of so-called "blocking" antibodies, that is, IgG antibodies directed against the same antigens that are being recognized by antibodies of the IgE isotype (Ottesen et al., 1981).

Although IgE antibody responses, in most individuals, are regulated both quantitatively and qualitatively (Marsh et al., 1974), the presence of helminth infection appears to overcome these regulatory mechanisms so that high levels of IgE are consistently produced in vivo. Furthermore, most of the IgE produced is not parasite-specific and is therefore felt to represent nonspecific potentiation of a normally well-controlled immune response (Jarrett and Bazin, 1974; Jarrett and Stewart, 1972; Turner et al., 1979). This potentiating effect seem to be selective for the IgE isotype (Jarrett, 1978). This was demonstrated most definitively in studies in which animals previously sensitized to a nonparasite antigen (e.g., ovalbumin) were subsequently infected with a helminth parasite; they produced IgE antibodies directed not only against the parasite, but also against the non-parasite antigen (Jarrett and Bazin, 1974; Orr and Cox, 1969; Orr et al., 1971).

Elevated total serum IgE levels in parasitized patients have been documented in many studies (Hussain et al., 1981; Kojima et al., 1972). Characteristically, patients with invasive helminth infections have serum IgE levels approaching 100 times those of normal individuals (Ottesen, 1985). The factors responsible for this degree of elevation are not well defined; however, there seems to be not only quantitative differences in these parasitized individuals, but also qualitative ones. Although atopic individuals have moderate elevations of IgE, characteristically their IgE responses are restricted to a small number of antigens. In marked contrast, patients with invasive helminth infection produce IgE antibodies with specificity against an incredibly broad range of parasite antigens (Hussain and Ottesen, 1985). Thus, it has been proposed that this potentiated, antigen-nonspecific response leads to the production of irrelevant IgE that saturates the mast cells' $Fc_{\epsilon}RIs$ and renders them unable to be triggered by parasite antigen.

Parasite-derived inhibitors of mast cell degranulation have also been proposed as a mechanism for the modulation of the hypersensitivity response to helminth parasites. Although there is little evidence for such a mechanism, in one study a "factor" derived from *Schistosoma mansoni* was shown to inhibit mast cell degranulation both in vitro and in vivo (Mazinque et al., 1980).

A final mechanism for the modulation of the mast cell response is the production of IgG blocking antibodies that occur in great abundance during chronic helminth infection and function, similar to those blocking antibodies that develop during immunotherapy. Further, in a qualitative study of the immune response (both IgG and IgE) to filarial parasite antigen using Western blotting techniques (Hussain and Ottesen, 1985), dual recognition of antigens by IgG and IgE antibodies has been shown. The relative magnitude of IgG to IgE then can be used to give a plausible explanation for why patients with invasive helminth infections have so little allergic reactivity in the face of IgE elevations. While the nature of these blocking antibodies and their relationship to the regulation of IgE response to parasite antigens are still being delineated, recent evidence showing that this blocking antibody is of the IgG4 subclass and is the subclass responsible for the antigen recognition that parallels IgE may provide the link necessary to explain the blocking phenomenon (Hussain and Ottesen, 1991).

VI. Role of the Mast Cell in Protective Immunity to Parasitic Infection

Almost all the helminth parasites pathogenic for humans establish a patent and often chronic infection. These infections, however, engender an immune response that provides, to some degree, a protective response to reinfection. Most illustrative of this situation is the concept of *concomitant immunity*, which occurs in schistosome-infected individuals (Smithers and Terry, 1969). This is a state in which adult worms are and remain very well established in the host, but in which these same schistosomes induce an immune response that limits further infection by the infective stages of the life cycle.

Although the accumulation of mast cells in parasitized tissues has been used as an argument in favor of the mast cells' role in protective immunity, it is not certain that these cells serve a protective function in parasite infection. Nevertheless, animal models of immunity to challenge infection have provided some experimental evidence for a salutary role of the mast cell. These types of secondary challenge studies have provided evidence that mast cells are responsible for the prevention of reinfection (Rothwell and Dineen, 1972) in gastrointestinal parasites and for the cytotoxicity against early schistosomula in the epidermis of previously vaccinated primates (Hsu et al., 1979). Further, depletion of mast cells has been shown to abrogate the cytotoxic responses against schistosomula (Capron et al., 1978). In vitro, mast cells, in concert with peroxidase and iodide, have also been shown capable of mediating cytotoxicity to schistosomula (Henderson et al., 1986).

Particularly striking has been the use of these models to study the mechanisms underlying the protective response to reinfection with gastrointestinal parasites (Befus, 1986). Because such a secondary response has been felt to reflect immediate-type hypersensitivity reactions, attention has been focused on evidence of mast cell activation and the local consequences of activation (Miller, 1984; Wakelin 1978b)—edema, mucus hypersecretion, and increased peristalsis. Release of leukotrienes and high levels of RMCP-II have been found in tissues and serum of rats immune to *T. spiralis* infection (Moqbel et al., 1987). These and other mediators are felt to contribute to the expulsion of the parasites, often within 6–20 hr after a challenge infection. These vasoactive mediators have been implicated in gut and vascular permeability, enhanced peristalsis and mucus secretion. It is the latter that likely plays a major effector function in resistance to reinfection.

Mucus secretion has been shown to physically entrap larvae (Miller et al., 1981); further, molecules (with some of the properties of the leukotrienes) functioning to inhibit migration of *Trichostrongylus colubriformis* larvae have been found in the mucus of *T. colubriformis*–immune sheep (Douch et al., 1983). The microenvironment (intestinal inflammation) clearly causes worm damage, a finding that is a feature of resistance to reinfection (reviewed by Miller, 1984, 1987; Miller and Huntley, 1982). This damage, however, is reversible if the worms are transferred from the immune animal to the gut of a naïve animal (Moqbel, 1986; Moqbel et al., 1980) and suggests that helminth-induced gastrointestinal inflammation as a consequence of antigen-specific release of mast cell mediators induces nonspecific mechanisms, such as mucus hypersecretion and enhanced peristalsis, that cause damage to the parasite or at least prevent the parasite from establishing an infection.

VII. Conclusion

For reasons of survival, helminth parasites have evolved mechanisms to avoid the consequences of host immune response. How to overcome this evolutionary adaptation remains the ultimate objective in studying the immune response parasitic infection. Unfortunately, the nature of the effector mechanisms as they act in vivo (especially with reference to human infection) is still not elucidated entirely. However, it is clear that the immune interactions that are called into play to eradicate invasive helminth parasites are extremely complex and require antibodies of particular isotypes and specificities and the recruitment of multiple types of effector cells activated appropriately.

Discussion

Lichtenstein: For the many years during which I have examined allergic mechanisms, it has always been claimed, but never proven, that allergic mechanisms exist in order to fight parasitic diseases. Can you comment?
Nutman: There is still no direct proof of the importance of mast cells or the other cells involved in allergic reactions in mediating resistance to parasitic infections.
Sullivan: Studies by Hsu et al. in the early 1980s presented evidence that mast cells regulated protective immunity by attracting eosinophils and allowing both immunoglobulins and complement to reach the site of an allergic reaction. Can you comment on this set of experiments?
Nutman: Despite the attractiveness of the hypothesis, most individuals who become parasitized develop a chronic infection. There is no evidence that the IgE–mast cell–eosinophil interaction limits infection.
Galli: I agree that the usual parasitic infection and host response are so complex

that it is impossible to examine any single component. However, in animal systems, it has been possible to show that the absence of effector mechanisms results in diminished responses. Examples include *Trichinella spiralis* and *Haemaphysalis longicornis* in mast-cell–deficient mice and the response to ticks in guinea pigs.
Nutman: I agree.

References

Abe, T., and Nawa, Y. (1987). Reconstitution of mucosal mast cells in *W/WV* mice by adoptive transfer of bone marrow-derived cultured mast cells and its effects on the protective capacity to *Strongyloides ratti*-infection. *Parasite Immunol.* 9:31–38.

Abe, T., and Nawa, Y. (1988a). Kinetic study of mast-cell growth factor production by lymphocytes during the course of *Strongyloides ratti* infection in mice. *Parasitol Res.* 74:484–488.

Abe, T., and Nawa, Y. (1988b). Worm expulsion and mucosal mast cell response induced by repetitive IL-3 administration in *Strongyloides ratti*–infected nude mice. *Immunology* 63:181–185.

Alizadeh, H., and Wakelin, D. (1982a). Comparison of rapid expulsion of *Trichinella spiralis* in mice and rats. *Int. J. Parasitol.* 12:65–73.

Alizadeh, H., and Wakelin, D. (1982b). Genetic factors controlling the intestinal mast cell response in mice infected with *Trichinella spiralis*. *Clin. Exp. Immunol.* 49:331–337.

Anwar, A. R., McKean, J. R., Smithers, S. R., and Kay, A. B. (1980). Human eosinophil- and neutrophil-mediated killing of schistosomula of *Schistosoma mansoni* in vitro. I. Enhancement of complement-dependent damage by mast cell–derived mediators and formyl methionyl peptides. *J. Immunol.* 124:1122–1129.

Askenase, P. W. (1977). Immune inflammatory responses to parasites: The role of basophils, mast cells and vasoactive amines. *Am. J. Trop. Med. Hyg.*

Askenase, P. W. (1980). Immunopathology of parasitic diseases: Involvement of mast cells and basophils. *Springer Semin. Immunopathol.* 2:417–442.

Barrett, K. E., Neva, F. A., Gam, A. A., Cicmanec, J., London, W. T., Phillips, J. M., and Metcalfe, D. D. (1988). The immune response to nematode parasites: Modulation of mast cell numbers and function during *Strongyloides stercoralis* infections in nonhuman primates. *Am. J. Trop. Med. Hyg.* 38:574–581.

Beaven, M. A. (1978). Histamine: Its role in physiological and pathological processes. *Monogr. Allergy* 13:1–113.

Befus, D. (1986). Immunity in intestinal helminth infections: Present concepts, future directions. *Trans. R. Soc. Trop. Med. Hyg.* 80:735–741.

Bienenstock, J. (1986). Mucosal immunological protection mechanisms in the airways. *Eur. J. Respir. Dis.* (Suppl.) 147:62–71.

Briggs, N. T., and DeGiusti, D. L. (1970). Increased sensitivity of *Trichinella*-infected mice to serotonin and histamine. *Life Sci.* 9:797–802.

Capron, A., Dessaint, J. P., Joseph, M., Rousseaux, R., Capron, M., and Bazin, H.

(1977). Interaction between IgE complexes and macrophages in the rat: A new mechanism of macrophage activation. *Eur. J. Immunol.* 1:315–325.

Capron, M., Rousseaux, J., Mazingue, C., Bazin, H., and Capron, A. (1978). Rat mast cell–eosinophil interactions in antibody-dependent eosinophil cytotoxicity to *Schistosoma mansoni* schistosomula. *J. Immunol.* 126:468.

Castro, G. A. (1982). Immunological regulation of epithelial function. *Am. J. Physiol.* 243:G321–329.

Castro, G. A., Harari, Y., and Russell, D. (1987). Mediators of anaphylaxis-induced ion transport changes in small intestine. *Am. J. Physiol.* 253 (Pt.1): G540–548.

Catto, B. A., Lewis, F. A., and Ottesen, E. A. (1980). Cercaria-induced histamine release: A factor in the pathogenesis of schistosome dermatitis? *Am. J. Trop. Med. Hyg.* 29:886–889.

Damonneville, M., Auriault, C., Verwaerde, C., Delanoye, A., Pierce, R., and Capron, A. (1986). Protection against experimental *Schistosoma mansoni* schistosomiasis achieved by immunization with schistosomula released products antigens (SRP-A): Role of IgE antibodies. *Clin. Exp. Immunol.* 65:244–252.

Dessein, A. J., Parker, W. L., James, S. L., and David, J. R. (1981). IgE antibody and resistance to infection. I. Selective suppression of the IgE antibody response in rats diminishes the resistance and the eosinophil response to *Trichinella spiralis* infection. *J. Exp. Med.* 153:423–436.

Dillon, S. B., and MacDonald, T. T. (1986). Limit dilution of mast cell precursor frequency in the gut epithelium of normal and *Trichinella spiralis* infected mice. *Parasite Immunol.* 8:503–511.

Douch, P. G., Harrison, G. B., Buchanan, L. L., and Greer, K. S. (1983). In vitro bioassay of sheep gastrointestinal mucus for nematode paralysing activity mediated by substances with some properties characteristic of SRS-A. *Int. J. Parasitol.* 13:207–212.

Dumont, A. E., Fazzini, E., and Jamal, S. (1983). Metachromatic cells in filarial lymphoedema. *Lancet* 2:543 (letter).

Epstein, W. K., Fukyama, K. F., Danno, K., and Kwan-Wong, E. (1979). Granulomatous inflammation in normal and athymic mice infected with *Schistosoma mansoni* schistosomula: an ultrastructural study. *J. Pathol.* 127:207.

Gazzinelli, G., Ramalho, P. F., and Silva, W. d. (1969). *Schistosoma mansoni*: Generation of anaphylatoxin by cercarial extracts. *Exp. Parasitol.* 26:86–91.

Gleich, G. J., Olson, G. M., and Loegering, D. A. (1979). The effect of ablation of eosinophils on immediate-type hypersensitivity reactions. *Immunology* 38:343–353.

Gustowska, L., Ruitenberg, E. J., Elgersma, A., and Koci:ecka, W. (1983). Increase of mucosal mast cells in the jejunum of patients infected with *Trichinella spiralis*. *Int. Arch. Allergy Appl. Immunol.* 71:304–308.

Guy-Grand, D., Dy, M., Luffau, G., and Vassalli, P. (1984). Gut mucosal mast cells. Origin, traffic, and differentiation. *J. Exp. Med.* 160:12–28.

Guy-Grand, D., Dy, M., Luffau, G., and Vassalli, P. (1986). Gut mucosal mast cells: Origin, traffic and differentiation in mice and rats. *Ann. Inst. Pasteur Immunol.* 137:215–222.

Ha, T. Y., Reed, N. D., and Crowle, P. K. (1983). Delayed expulsion of adult Trichinella spiralis by mast cell–deficient *W/Wv* mice. *Infect. Immun.* 41:445–447.

Haig, D. M., Jarrett, E. E., and Tas, J. (1984). In vitro studies on mast cell proliferation in *N. brasiliensis* infection. *Immunology* 51:643–651.

Harari, Y., and Castro, G. A. (1989). Simulation of parasite-induced gut hypersensitivity: Implications for vaccination. *Immunology* 66:302–307.

Harari, Y., Russell, D. A., and Castro, G. A. (1987). Anaphylaxis-mediated epithelial Cl-secretion and parasite rejection in rat intestine. *J. Immunol.* 138:1250–1255.

Henderson, W. R., Chi, E. Y., Jong, E. C., and Klebanoff, S. J. (1986). Mast cell mediated toxicity to schistosomula of *Schistosoma mansoni*: Potentiation by exogenase peroxidase. *J. Immunol.* 137:2695.

Horowitz, S., Smolarsky, M., and Arnon, R. (1982). Protection against *Schistosoma mansoni* achieved by immunization with sonicated parasite. *Eur. J. Immunol.* 12:327–332.

Hsu, Y. L., Hsu, H. F., Pennick, G. D., Hanson, H. O., Schiller, H. J., and Cheng, H. F. (1979). Immunoglobulin E, mast cells and eosinophils in the skin of rhesus monkeys immunized with X-irraciated cercariae of *Schistosoma japonicum*. *Int. Arch. Allergy Appl. Immunol.* 59:383–390.

Huntley, J. F., Gibson, S., Brown, D., Smith, W. D., Jackson, F., and Miller, H. R. (1987). Systemic release of a mast cell proteinase following nematode infections in sheep. *Parasite Immunol.* 9:603–614.

Huntley, J. F., Gooden, C., Newlands, G. F., Mackellar, A., Lammas, D. A., Wakelin, D., Tuohy, M., Woodbury, R. G., and Miller, H. R. (1990). Distribution of intestinal mast cell proteinase in blood and tissues of normal and *Trichinella*-infected mice. *Parasite Immunol.* 12:85–95.

Hussain, R., and Ottesen, E. A. (1985). IgE responses in human filariasis. III. Specificities of IgE and IgG antibodies compared by immunoblot analysis. *J. Immunol.* 135:1415–1420.

Hussain, R., and Ottesen, E. (1992). The IgG4 isotype acts as the blocking antibody in human lymphatic filariasis. *J. Immunol.* (in press).

Hussain, R., Hamilton, R. G., Kumaraswami, V., Adkinson, N. J., and Ottesen, E. A. (1981). IgE responses in human filariasis. I. Quantitation of filaria-specific IgE. *J. Immunol.* 127:1623–1629.

Itayama, H., Oku, Y., and Kamiya, M. (1987). Longevity and fecundity of *Trichinella spiralis* in mast cell–deficient *Sl/Sld* mice. *Jpn. J. Vet. Res.* 35:195–207.

Jarrett, E. (1978). Stimuli for the production and control of IgE in rats. *Immunol. Rev.* 41:52.

Jarrett, E. E. E., and Bazin, H. (1974). Elevation of total serum IgE in rats following helminth parasite infection. *Nature* 251:541.

Jarrett, E. E., and Miller, H. R. (1982). Production and activities of IgE in helminth infection. *Prog. Allergy* 31:178–233.

Jarrett, E. E. E., and Stewart, D. C. (1972). Potentiation of rat reaginic (IgE) antibody by helminth infection. Simultaneous potentiation of separate reagins. *Immunology* 23:749.

Joseph, M., Auriault, C., Capron, A., Vorng, H., and Viens, P. A. (1983). New function for platelets: IgE-dependent killing of schistosomes. *Nature* 303: 810–813.

Kamiya, M., Oku, Y., Itayama, H., and Ohbayashi, M. (1985). Prolonged expulsion of adult *Trichinella spiralis* and eosinophil infiltration in mast cell–deficient *W/Wv* mice. *J. Helminthol.* 59:233–239.

Kay, A. B. (1979). The role of the eosinophil. *J. Allergy Clin. Immunol.* 64:90–104.

Kay, A. B. (1985). Eosinophils: Role in asthma, allergy and parasite immunity. *N. Engl. Reg. Allergy Proc.* 6:341–345.

Kojima, S., Yokagawa, M., and Tada, T. (1972). Raised levels of serum IgE levels in human helminthiasis. *Am. J. Trop. Med. Hyg.* 21:913.

Mahmoud, A. A., Warren, K. S., and Peters, P. A. (1975). A role for the eosinophil in acquired resistance to *Schistosoma mansoni* infection as determined by anti-eosinophil serum. *J. Exp. Med.* 142:805–813.

Marsh, D. G., Bico, W. B., and Ishizaka, K. (1974). Genetic control of basal serum IgE level and its effect on specific reagin sensitivity. *Proc. Natl. Acad. Sci. USA* 71:3588.

Mazinque, C., Camus, D., Dessaint, J. P., Capron, M., and Capron, A. (1980). In vitro and in vivo inhibition of mast cell degranulation by a factor from *Schistosoma mansoni. Int. Arch. Allergy Appl. Immunol.* 63:178.

Miller, H. R. (1980). Expulsion of *Nippostrongylus brasiliensis* from rats protected with serum. I. The efficacy of sera from singly and multiply infected donors related to time of administration and volume of serum injected. *Immunology* 40:325–334.

Miller, H. R. (1984). The protective mucosal response against gastrointestinal nematodes in ruminants and laboratory animals. *Vet. Immunol. Immunopathol.* 6:167–259.

Miller, H. R. (1987). Gastrointestinal mucus, a medium for survival and for elimination of parasitic nematodes and protozoa. *Parasitology.* 94(Suppl.):577–100.

Miller, H. R., and Huntley, J. F. (1982). Protection against nematodes by intestinal mucus. *Adv. Exp. Med. Biol.* 144:243–245.

Miller, H. R., Huntley, J. F., and Wallace, G. R. (1981). Immune exclusion and mucus trapping during the rapid expulsion of *Nippostrongylus brasiliensis* from primed rats. *Immunology* 44:419–429.

Miller, H. R., Woodbury, R. G., Huntley, J. F., and Newlands, G. (1983). Systemic release of mucosal mast-cell protease in primed rats challenged with *Nippostrongylus brasiliensis. Immunology* 49:471–479.

Moqbel, R. (1986). Helminth-induced intestinal inflammation. *Trans. R. Soc. Trop. Med. Hyg.* 80:719–727.

Moqbel, R., McLaren, D. J., and Wakelin, D. (1980). *Strongyloides ratti*: Reversibility of immune damage to adult worms. *Exp. Parasitol.* 49:153–166.

Moqbel, R., Sass, K. S., Goetzl, E. J., and Kay, A. B. (1983). Enhancement of neutrophil- and eosinophil-mediated complement-dependent killing of schistosomula of *Schistosoma mansoni* in vitro by leukotriene B4. *Clin. Exp. Immunol.* 52:519–527.

Moqbel, R., King, S. J., MacDonald, A. J., Miller, H. R., Cromwell, O., Shaw, R. J., and Kay, A. B. (1986). Enteral and systemic release of leukotrienes during anaphylaxis of *Nippostrongylus brasiliensis*–primed rats. *J. Immunol.* 137:296–301.

Moqbel, R., Wakelin, D., MacDonald, A. J., King, S. J., Grencis, R. K., and Kay, A. B. (1987). Release of leukotrienes during rapid expulsion of *Trichinella spiralis* from immune rats. *Immunology* 60:425–430.

Munoz, J., and Bergman, R. K. (1968). Histamine-sensitizing factors from microbial agents, with special reference to *Bordetella pertussis*. *Bacteriol. Rev.* 32:103–126.

Munoz, J. J., Sogandares, B. F., and Bergman, R. K. (1974). Histamine sensitization of mice by *Trichinella spiralis* infection. *Proc. Soc. Exp. Biol. Med.* 147:524–526.

Nawa, Y., Kiyota, M., Korenaga, M., and Kotani, M. (1985). Defective protective capacity of *W/Wv* mice against *Strongyloides ratti* infection and its reconstitution with bone marrow cells. *Parasite Immunol.* 7:429–438.

Oku, Y., Itayama, H., and Kamiya, M. (1984). Expulsion of *Trichinella spiralis* from the intestine of *W/Wv* mice reconstituted with haematopoietic and lymphopoietic cells and origin of mucosal mast cells. *Immunology* 53:337–344.

Orr, T. S., and Cox, J. S. (1969). Disodium cromoglycate, an inhibitor of mas cell degranulation and histamine release induced by phospholipase A. *Nature* 223:197–198.

Orr, T. S., Hall, D. E., Gwilliam, J. M., and Cox, O. S. (1971). The effect of disodium cromoglycate on the release of histamine and degranulation of rat mast cells induced by compound 48–80. *Life Sci.* (*i*) 10:805–812.

Ottesen, E. (1985). Parasite infections and allergic reaction—How each affects the other. In *Bronchial Asthma: Mechanisms and Therapeutics*, 2nd ed. New York, Little Brown.

Ottesen, E. A., Kumaraswami, V., Paranjape, R., Poindexter, R. W., and Tripathy, S. P. (1981). Naturally occurring blocking antibodies modulate immediate hypersensitivity responses in human filariasis. *J. Immunol.* 127:2014–2020.

Parmentier, H. K., V. C., de Ruitenberg, E. J., and Van Loveren, H. (1987). Involvement of serotonin in intestinal mastocytopoiesis and inflammation during a *Trichinella spiralis* infection in mice. *Int. Arch. Allergy Appl. Immunol.* 83:31–38.

Perdue, M. H., Marshall, J., and Masson, S. (1990). Ion transport abnormalities in inflamed rat jejunum. Involvement of mast cells and nerves. *Gastroenterology* 98:561–567.

Ridel, P. R., Auriault, C., Darcy, F., Pierce, R. J., Leite, P., Santoro, F., Neyrinck, J. L., Kusnierz, J. P., and Capron, A. (1988). Protective role of IgE in immunocompromised rat toxoplasmosis. *J. Immunol.* 141:978–983.

Rothwell, T. L. W., and Dineen, J. K. (1972). Cellular reactins in guinea pigs following primary and secondary challenge with *Trichostrongylus colubriformis*, with special reference to the roles played by eosinophils and basophils in the rejection of the parasite. *Immunology* 22:733.

Ruitenberg, E. J., and Elgersma, A. (1976). Absence of intestinal mast cell response in congenitally athymic mice during *Trichinella spiralis* infection. *Nature* 264:258–260.

Russell, D. A. (1986). Mast cells in the regulation of intestinal electrolyte transport. *Am. J. Physiol.* 251 (Pt.1): G253–262.

Senft, A. W., and Maddison, S. E. (1975). Hypersensitivity to parasite proteolytic enzyme in schistosomiasis. *Am. J. Trop. Med. Hyg.* 24:83–89.

Smithers, S. R., and Terry, R. J. (1969). Immunity in schistosomiasis. *Ann. NY Acad. Sci.* 160:826.

Teppema, J., Blomjous, F., Elgersma, A., and Ruitenberg, E. (1981). *Trichenella pseudospiralis* and *T. spiralis* infections in monkeys. III. Pathological aspects.

Proc. 5th Int. Conf. on Trichinellosis, Noordwijk aan Zee 1981. Chertsey, Reedbooks, pp. 209–214.

Thompson, A. (1972). Isolation and characterization of a mast cell degranulating substance from *Ascaris suis*. *Biochem. Biophys. Acta*. 261:245–257.

Tolone, G., Brai, M., Bonasera, L., Bellavia, A., and Pontieri, G. M. (1972). Role of mast cells and eosinophils in tissue injury caused by injection of *Ascaris* fluid in the rat. *Pathol. Microbiol. (Basel)* 38:192–199.

Tolone, G., Bonasera, L., Brai, M., Ferina, F., and Pontieri, G. M. (1974). Isolation of mast cell degranulators from the celomatic fluid of *Parascaris equorum*. *Pathol. Microbiol. (Basel)* 41:41–50.

Turner, K. J., Feddema, L., and Quinn, E. H. (1979). Non-specific potentiation of IgE by parasitic infections in man. *Int. Arch. Allergy Appl. Immunol*. 58:232–236.

Unvas, B., and Wold, J. K. (1967). Isolation of mast cell-degranulating polypeptide from *Ascaris suis*. *Acta Physiol. Scand*. 70:269–276.

Unvas, B., Diamant, B., Hogberg, B., and Thon, I. (1960). Mechanism of mast cell disruption induced by a principle extracted from *Ascaris suis*. *Am. J. Physiol*. 199:575–578.

Vos, J. G., Ruitenberg, E. J., Van, B. N., Buys, J., Elgersma, A., and Kruizinga, W. (1983). The athymic nude rat. IV. Immunocytochemical study to detect T-cells, and immunological and histopathological reactions against *Trichinella spiralis*. *Parasite Immunol*. 5:195–215.

Wakelin, D. (1978a). Genetic control of susceptibility and resistance to parasitic infection. *Adv. Parasitol*. 16:219–308.

Wakelin, D. (1978b). Immunity to intestinal parasites. *Nature* 273:617–620.

Wakelin, D. (1984). Evasion of the immune response: survival within low responder individuals of the host population. *Parasitology*. 88 (Pt.4): 639–657.

Wakelin, D. (1986). Genetic and other constraints on resistance to infection with gastrointestinal nematodes. *Trans. R. Soc. Trop. Med. Hyg*. 80:742–747.

Wakelin, D. (1989). Nature and nurture: overcoming constraints on immunity. *Parasitology*. 99(Suppl.):521–35.

Wakelin, D., and Donachie, A. M. (1981). Genetic control of immunity to *Trichinella spiralis*. Donor bone marrow cells determine responses to infection in mouse radiation chimaeras. *Immunology* 43:787–792.

Wassom, D., Brooks, B., Bavisch, J., and Dacid, C. (1983). A gene mapping between the S and D regions of the H-2 complex influences resistance to *Trichinella spiralis* infections. *J. Immunogenet*. 101:625–631.

Wassom, D. L., Wakelin, D., Brooks, B. O., Krco, C. J., and David, C. S. (1984). Genetic control of immunity to *Trichinella spiralis* infections of mice. Hypothesis to explain the role of H-2 genes in primary and challenge infections. *Immunology* 51:625–631.

Wolfe, M. S., Petersen, J. L., Neafie, R. C., Connor, D. H., and Purtilo, D. T. (1974). Onchocerciasis presenting with swelling of limb. *Am. J. Trop. Med. Hyg*. 23:361–368.

Woodbury, R. G., Miller, H. R., Huntley, J. F., Newlands, G. F., Palliser, A. C., and Wakelin, D. (1984). Mucosal mast cells are functionally active during spontaneous expulsion of intestinal nematode infections in rat. *Nature* 312:450–452.

28

Mast Cells and the Nervous System

J. BIENENSTOCK, R. H. STEAD, AND JEAN S. MARSHALL

McMaster University,
Hamilton, Ontario, Canada

I. Introduction

A sizable body of information has documented (to a variable degree of the readers' satisfaction) that the nervous and immune systems communicate. This information ranges from morphological and morphometric observations at the light and electron microscopic level to functional evidence. Anyone interested in single-source references covering these areas is referred to recent reviews (Ader et al., 1990; Blalock, 1989). We ourselves have been engaged for a few years in a study of these interactions. Our studies (Stead et al., 1987a; Stanisz et al., 1986) began with an examination of the effects of various neuropeptides on several different immune parameters, including lymphocyte function and activity, both in vivo and in vitro. These studies were also extended to an examination of the effects of neuropeptides on mast cells (Shanahan et al., 1985). Since at that time we were describing the functional and other characteristics of mucosal mast cells that rendered them distinct from their connective tissue counterparts, it was interesting to us that only substance P, of all the neuropeptides tested, had any effect on degranulation of mucosal mast cells. Since that time we have published extensively on the subject of interactions between the nervous system and mast cells (Stead and Bienenstock, 1990). We review some of these observations in this contribution. We believe that these studies and examples reflect a broader biological reality whereby a variety of cell types, particularly those of the immune and inflammatory series, can interact with, influence, and be influenced by the nervous system, both peripheral and central.

II. Morphological and Functional Relationships

Enerback and associates showed a bouton-like association between an enteric nerve and a rat mucosal mast cell in the intestine of a rat infected with the nematode parasite *Nippostrongylus brasiliensis* (Newson et al., 1983). We have rarely seen such an event ourselves although we have reported and documented such a finding in a similar set of circumstances in the rat (Stead and Bienenstock, 1990). Much more common, however, is the association of a membrane/membrane character that occurs between enteric nerves and mast cells in the intestine in the *Nippostrongylus*-infected rat. This also occurs in noninfected animals, and analysis of these associations suggests that they occurred five times more frequently than would be expected by chance alone (Stead et al., 1987a). It was evident on examination by immunohistochemistry that the nerves in association with mast cells most frequently contained substance P (SP) and calcitonin gene–related peptide (CGRP).

We have more recently extended these studies to the human, using resection specimens of the small and large bowel, as well as the appendix, and have found a similar degree of mucosal mast cell/nerve association (Stead et al., 1989). Most recently, Arizono et al. (1990) have confirmed these associations for the rat intestinal mucosa and have extended them to include association with eosinophils and plasma cells.

We have reviewed the literature around this area elsewhere (Stead et al., 1990), and a number of other tissue sites in the body have revealed similar associations. It is not our purpose in this chapter to review the functional studies that support these morphological and morphometric observations. Suffice it to say that work by Ganguly and associates (Ganguly and Gopinath, 1979; Ganguly et al., 1978) showed that mast cells in rats' stomachs increased in granularity after vagotomy, and that pylorus ligation decreased the amount of tissue histamine present, which in turn was preventable by vagal section. Field stimulation in rat ileum caused local histamine release and decreased mast cell staining, and this was blocked by atropine and tetrodotoxin, again suggesting that stimulation of nerves could cause mast cell functional effects (Bani-Sacchi et al., 1986). The work of Kowalski and Kaliner (1988) showed that mast cell degranulation occurred only after stimulation of the saphenous nerve in the rat after prolonged stimulation. Other studies by this group have extended these observations. There is at the same time considerable literature (Foreman, 1987; Kiernan, 1986;

Lembeck and Holzer, 1979) which suggests that neurogenic inflammation can occur as a result of stimulation of nerves. This literature applies to both skin and lungs, and these data, taken together, appear at first sight to be at odds.

Most recently, electrical stimulation at various current intensities of the trigeminal ganglion in the rat and subsequent light and electron microscopic examination of mast cells in the dura mater and tongue supplied by this nerve have shown a number of interesting observations. First, the effects were current dependent. Second, at the light microscopic level changes were apparent in mast cell staining characteristics (Dimitriadou et al., 1991). Mast cells originally showing characteristic red staining with safranin (classic connective tissue mast cells) slowly, over the time course examined, changed their staining characteristics to a blue staining, with alcian blue, even though safranin was still present in the staining procedure. These changes were accompanied by alterations clearly apparent in the electron microscope, both scanning and transmission. Initially, the observations suggested loss of granularity without obvious channel formation, classically seen with degranulation. Exocytosis eventually occurred after prolonged stimulation, compatible with the observations of Kowalski and Kaliner (1988). These results are important because they provide the missing piece of information that may explain the apparently discrepant results referred to earlier.

Thus prolonged or intense nerve stimulation may cause degranulation of mast cells, but degranulation as such is not the only effect potentially observed as a consequence of nerve stimulation. This may also explain the relatively high concentrations of tachykinins that appear to be required to cause degranulation of mast cells and is compatible also with the data of Levi-Schaffer and Shalit (1989). They examined rat peritoneal mast cells and showed that there could be discriminatory release of mediators as a result of the action of different mast cell secretagogues, including SP. Further, Church et al. commented on similar discriminatory effects of different stimuli, including neuropeptides, on activation and secretion by human skin mast cells (Church et al., 1989). In the experiments of Levi-Schaffer, SP, as well as other neurotransmitters, were effective as histamine releasers but induced little synthesis of prostaglandin D_2. These types of results will be particularly interesting to apply to the whole question of cytokine generation and secretion by mast cells.

All in all, these experiments clearly indicate some effects of nerve stimulation on mast cells that depend on the mode of examination of the tissues as well as the exact mechanism whereby the nerve is stimulated.

Well-documented physiological evidence exists for a homeostatic unit between mast cells, nerves, and epithelium (Crowe et al., 1990; Perdue et al., 1991). Antigen introduced on the luminal side of both intestine and trachea causes antigen-specific, mast cell– and nerve-dependent chloride ion secretion by the epithelium, as judged bt Ussing chamber and perfusion experiments (Crowe et al., 1990; Sestini et al., 1990). The mediators involved are not completely characterized but, depending on the species (i.e., rat and guinea pig), include products of the arachidonic acid metabolism pathway, histamine, serotonin, and unknown neurotransmitters, since the whole system was inhibited by tetrodotoxin. The conclusion that mast cells were involved in this system was obtained by indirect means using different pharmacological agents. However, recent experiments have very adequately supported the mast cell as playing a central role in these systems. Perdue and co-workers (1991) have shown in the mast cell–deficient mouse strains (*Sl*^{d}/*Sl*^{d} and *W*/*W*^{v} strains) that the deficient animals are also deficient in their ability to respond in such systems relative to their +/+ littermates. Furthermore, in the *W*/*W*^{v} strain, where bone marrow can be injected to reconstitute the animals' mast cell numbers, the Ussing chamber response to antigen is restored to the control levels.

III. Mast Cell Cytokine Production and Nerve Mast Cell Interaction

Recent evidence from a number of groups has indicated that mast cells may produce a wide variety of cytokines following ionophore- or IgE-mediated activation (Plaut et al., 1989; Wodnar-Filipowicz et al., 1989). Mast cell lines in the mouse have been shown to produce IL-3, IL-4, IL-5, IL-6, GM-CSF, TNF-α, TGF-β, and a number of other cytokines (Gordon et al., 1991). In vivo evidence of cytokine production is more limited, with clear data available only for TNF-α and IL-3. However, in the mouse model the difficulty in obtaining highly purified mast cells may be limiting to the rate of progress in defining in vivo cytokine production.

We recently examined cultured mucosal mast cell–like cells in the rat for the production of cytokines that may play a role in neuronal development. Leukemia inhibitory factor (LIF) has been shown to have an important role in the differentiation, but not growth, of neurons in the rat heart and was cloned in the rat by a group investigating this cholinergic neuronal differentiation factor activity (Yamamori et al., 1989). This molecule also has a number of other important biological activities, which has led to its being described by a number of other names, including human interleukin for DA cells, differentiation inhibitory activity, and hepatocyte-stimulating factor III owing to its ability to activate the acute-phase response. Another cytokine thought to play a role in neuronal development is IL-6. As one of its many bioactivities, this factor has been shown to induce neurite outgrowth from PC12 cells (Satoh et al., 1988). IL-6 is also known to be a potent activator of the acute-phase response in the liver (Gauldie et al., 1987).

In our experiments we examined the rat basophilic leukemia cell RBL.2H3 Ca 10.7 and the peritoneal cell–derived, mucosal mast cell–like cell line RCMC9 (a generous gift from Dr. Arnold Froese, Winnipeg). Both these cell lines produce a hepatocyte-stimulating activity constitutively, which can be detected using a rat hepatocyte assay system (Gauldie et al., 1987; Baumann and Wong, in press). The production of alpha-2-macroglobulin by freshly isolated hepatocytes is used as a measure of induction of an acute-phase response. When RBL cells are activated with the calcium ionophore A23187, the amount of HSF activity produced by these cells is increased. Examination of supernatants of RBL and RCMC9 cells for IL-6 activity using the highly sensitive B9 hybridoma growth factor activity assay (Koj et al., 1984) failed to demonstrate the presence of this cytokine. Northern blot analysis of the RNA extracted from both ionophore-activated and control cells also did not reveal any IL-6 mRNA, while rat fibroblasts demonstrated a strong IL-6 signal. In view of these results, total RNA from activated and control cells was examined for the production of LIF mRNA, and this was detected in both cell lines. These results support the conclusion that rat IMMC-like cells produce LIF and do not produce significant quantities of IL-6 following ionophore stimulation. These results are in contrast to results obtained by others using mouse mast cell lines in which IL-6 mRNA was detected but LIF production has not been reported.

There are several possible implications for these findings and those of others examining mast cell cytokine production in the context of interactions between the mast cell and the nervous system. It remains to be clarified whether activation of mast cells by neuropeptides or nerve growth factor can stimulate mast cell cytokine production, but this is now a very reasonable possibility. Through such a mechanism, the nervous system could potentially affect many aspects of immunoregulation via the mast cell. Our observation of LIF production by mast cells may suggest a regulatory role for the mast cell in neuronal differentiation and development, which could be of particular importance in circumstances where tissue damage occurs involving mast cell activation, such as in allergic or other inflammatory diseases.

IV. Nerve Growth Factor

Because of our interest in mast cell association with nerves, especially in the intestinal mucosa, we have investigated the action of nerve growth factor (NGF) on a variety of cell types. Work by Aloe and Levi-Montalcini (1977) showed that injection of NGF into neonatal animals caused mast cell hyperplasia. We have extended these observations and shown that the phenotype of the mast cells that increased is appropriate to the tissues studied; i.e., mucosal mast cells were found in the intestine and connective tissue–type mast cells in the tongue. Since NGF is such a potent mast cell–degranulating agent (Bruni et al., 1982; Pearce and Thompson, 1986; Tomioka et al., 1988) Marshall et al., (1990) postulated that the degranulation itself might directly or indirectly be causing the mast cell hyperplasia found upon NGF administration. Accordingly, neonatal rats were given NGF alone or in the presence of disodium cromoglycate, which stabilizes connective tissue mast cells in rat skin. The animals so treated had very little connective tissue mast cell hyperplasia; however, the RMCP-II levels were significantly increased in rats after NGF treatment, with or without this pharmacological agent. The data clearly suggested that there was an autocrine-like effect of connective tissue mast cell hyperplasia as a result of NGF degranulation, but that the NGF effect on mucosal mast cells might be indirect. This fits the observations we have made on NGF injections into thymus-less (nude) rats in which both connective tissue and mucosal mast cell numbers increased although the increase of IMC was of questionable statistical significance ($p = 0.06$). Thus it is likely that the NGF is, through degranulation of mast cells, causing cytokine release, which promotes connective tissue mast cell hyperplasia. The dependency of mucosal mast cells on T-cell-derived IL-3 for proliferation may account for the findings. In other experiments we have shown that NGF causes the growth of hemopoietic stem cell colonies from human peripheral blood in methylcellulose cultures (Matsuda et al., 1988) and that this effect is T-cell dependent. That this system is complex and depends on interactions of multiple factors is further suggested by our recent studies that suggest that NGF can synergize with GM-CSF and Il-5, but not IL-3, in the human system (Tsuda et al., 1991).

Thus we believe that NGF may play a role in promoting mast cell growth in any area where repair and inflammation is occurring, especially in areas where nerve remodeling is taking place. It is known from the work of Heumann and Thoenen that IL-1 appears to be very important in the up-regulation of messenger RNA for NGF and NGF receptors in nerve tissue (Lindholm et al., 1987). In this respect, the synthesis and secretion of NGF and the expression of NGF receptors are known to change in the course of inflammation. Indeed, substance-P receptors increase dramatically in intestinal tissues involved in inflammatory events (Mantyh et al., 1988).

V. Neuronal Remodeling

As a consequence of these types of studies, we wondered whether nerve remodeling could be occurring in tissues involved in inflammation. These would alter nerve-target relationships (Purves et al., 1988; Brown et al., 1981), and were there to be an involvement of mast cells, this would clearly alter those functional relationships as well. We accordingly examined the intestine of rats in the course of *Nippostrongylus* infection, and after a period of time, when the tissue inflammation has disappeared but there is still a massive mast cell infiltration, we subjected the tissue to examination for nerve-related antigens such as neuron-specific enolase and growth-associated protein 43 (GAP-43), which has been described as being associated with the growth cones of remodeling axons (Benowitz and Routtenberg, 1987; Skene, 1989). These extensive studies, which are reported elsewhere (Stead, et al., 1991), have clearly shown an increase in the proportion of small GAP-43 immunoreactive nerve fibers 2–3 weeks after *Nippostrongylus* infection, consistent with nerve regeneration. The number of nerves per villus and the nerve density were also found to subsequently increase, being still 30% greater than those of control animals 7 weeks after infection. Thus it is apparent that nerves, at least in this situation, can and do change and remodel in the course of inflammation.

VI. Conclusions

Since we have shown elsewhere that psychological conditioning experiments can be used to demonstrate that mast cells will secrete RMCP-II in response to the conditioning stimulus alone in sensitized animals, the role of the central nervous system in these types of models cannot be excluded (MacQueen et al., 1989). Furthermore, we have elsewhere described in detail interactions between mast cells and nerves in tissue culture, with consequent physiological effects on both mast cells and nerves (Blennerhassett and Bienenstock, 1991; Janiszewski et al., 1990). We believe it is extremely likely that there is a bidirectional communication between mast cells and nerves, much as has been suggested by Blalock (1989) in regard to lymphocytes. The evidence for this has been reviewed in this chapter, and the consequences of these interactions are yet to be fully understood. We have concentrated primarily on what appear to be positive events in which the nervous system may be promoting the functional activities that are being read out as indicators.

There is also evidence for some negative effects of nerves, which involve mast cells. In the experiments reported by Miura et al (1990), these have been perhaps best described. Here bilateral vagal stimulation in cats sensitive to *Ascaris* antigen, and which had received atropine and propranolol, prevented the rise seen in control animals of pulmonary resistance and plasma histamine. The fact that nervous stimulation of the vagal nerves caused inhibition of histamine increase and bronchial constriction induced by antigen inhalation in sensitized animals must be interpreted as a clear demonstration of nonadrenergic, noncholinergic nerves. This may also help explain some of the negative results previously seen by peripheral nerve stimulation using a particular current level for stimulation in the rat (Kowalski and Kaliner, 1988).

The functional significance of all these observations is not completely understood at present, but they certainly suggest strongly that mast cells, which, after all, can be sensitized passively to acquire different antigen specificity, may, through release of mediators, not only change the local environment, through stimulation of nerves, but also communicate these interactions with the spinal cord and central nervous system. How these signals are then processed and the consequences of this processing still are not completely understood, but it is interesting that psychological conditioning can itself influence mast cells at the periphery. It can reasonably be expected that with the growth of new knowledge in these areas over the next few years, the importance of these observations will become increasingly obvious.

Acknowledgments

We thank the Medical Research Council of Canada for its continuing support of the research described in this chapter.

Discussion

Kaliner: It appears that the culture system you employed to show neural interactions with mast cells involved norepinephrine-containing sympathetic nerves. Moreover, in the cat, you demonstrated nerves stopping histamine release. These data appear to be consistent with observations by Kowalski that antidromic nerve stimulation failed to activate skin or airway mast cells in vivo. Any comments?
Bienenstock: The studies you describe are based on examination of vascular permeability, while ours employ changes in epithelial chloride fluxes. It may be that we are seeing different aspects of nerve–mast cell interactions and that both inhibition and activation of mast cells may be seen, depending on the model system employed.
Hohman: You demonstrated that when a nerve attaches to an RBL cell in culture, the granules change in appearance. What do you think is happening?
Bienenstock: RBL mitosis is inhibited, but their phenotype does not change. In other words, if they have PMCR protease II, they continue to express this specific protease and not PMCR protease I.
Rivera: Do you also get any change in the RBL IgE receptors in culture?
Bienenstock: We have not looked.

References

Ader, R., Felten, D. L., and Cohen, N. (1990). Interactions between the brain and the immune system. *Annu. Rev. Pharmacol. Toxicol.* 30:561–602.

Aloe, L., and Levi-Montalcini, R. (1977). Mast cells increase in tissues of neonatal rats injected with the nerve growth factor. *Brain Res.* 133:358–366.

Arizono, N., Matsuda, S., Hattori, T., Kojima, Y., Maeda, T., and Galli, S. J. (1990). Anatomical variation in mast cell nerve associations in the rat small intestine, heart, lung, and skin: Similarities of distances between neural processes and mast cells, eosinophils, or plasma cells in the jejunal lamina propria. *Lab. Invest.* 62:626–634.

Bani-Sacchi, T., Barattini, M., Bianchi, S., Blandina, P., Brunelleschi, S., Fantozzi, R., Mannaioni, P. F., and Masini, E. (1986). The release of histamine by parasympathetic stimulation in guinea-pig auricle and rat ileum. *J. Physiol.* 371:29–43.

Baumann, H., and Wong, G. G. Hepatocyte stimulating factor III shows structural and functional identity with leukaemia inhibitory factors. *J. Immunol.* (in press).

Benowitz, L. I., and Routtenberg, A. (1987). A membrane phosphoprotein associated with neural development, axonal regeneration, phospholipid metabolism, and synaptic plasticity. *TINS* 10:527–532.

Blalock, J. E. (1989). A molecular basis for bidirectional communication between the immune and neuroendocrine systems. *Physiol. Rev.* 69:1–32.

Blennerhassett, M. G., and Bienenstock, J. (1991) Apparent innervation of rat basophilic leukaemia (RBL-2H3) cells by sympathetic nerves in vitro. *Neurosci. Lett.* (in press).

Brown, M. C., Holland, R. L., and Hopkins, W. G. (1981). Motor nerve sprouting. *Annu. Rev. Neurosci.* 4:17–42.

Bruni, A., Bigon, E., Boarato, E., Mietto, L., Leon, A., and Toffano, G. (1982). Interaction between nerve growth factor and lysophosphatidylserine on rat peritoneal mast cells. *FEBS Lett.* 138:1990–192.

Church, M. K., Lowman, M. A., Robinson, C., Holgate, S. T., and Benyon, R. C. (1989). Interaction of neuropeptides with human mast cells. *Int. Arch. Allergy Appl. Immunol.* 88:70–78.

Crowe, S. E., Sestini, P., and Perdue, M. H. (1990). Allergic reactions of rat jejunal mucosa. Ion transport responses to luminal antigen and inflammatory mediators. *Gastroenterology* 99:74–82.

Dimitriadou, V., Buzzi, M. G., Moskowitz, M. A., and Theoharides, T. C. (1991). Trigeminal sensory fibre stimulation induces morphological changes reflecting secretion in rat dura mater mast cells. *J. Neurosci.* (in press).

Foreman, J. C. (1987). Peptides and neurogenic inflammation. *Br. Med. Bull.* 43:386–400.

Ganguly, A. K., and Gopinath, P. (1979). Vagus nerves and the gastric tissue histamine concentration in pylorus ligated albino rats. *Q. J. Exp. Physiol.* 64:1–6.

Ganguly, A. K., Sathiamoorthy, S. S., and Bhatnagar, O. P. (1978). Effect of subdiaphragmatic vagotomy on gastric mucosal mast cell population in pylorus ligated rats. *Q. J. Exp. Physiol.* 63:89–92.

Gauldie, J., Richards, C., Harnish, D., Lansdorp, P., and Baumann, H. (1987). Interferon β_2/B-cell stimulatory factor type 2 shares identity with monocyte-derived hepatocyte-stimulating factor and regulates the major acute phase protein response in liver cells. *Proc. Natl. Acad. Sci. USA* 84:7251–7255.

Gordon, J. R., Burd, P. R., and Galli, S. J. (1991). Mast cells as a source of multifunctional cytokines. *Immunol. Today* 11:458–465.

Janiszewski, J., Bienenstock, J., and Blennerhassett, M. G. (1990). Activation of rat peritoneal mast cells in coculture with sympathetic neurons alters neuronal physiology. *Brain Behav. Immun.* 4:139–150.

Kiernan, J. A. (1986). Stimulation of the vagus nerve causes degranulation of mast cells in the rat's trachea and bronchi. *J. Anat. (Gr. Britain & Ireland)*, pp. 247.

Koj, A., Gauldie, J., Regoeczi, E., Sauder, D. N., and Sweeney, G. G. (1984). The acute phase response of cultured rat hepatocytes. *Biochem. J.* 224:505.

Kowalski, M. L., and Kaliner, M. A. (1988). Neurogenic inflammation, vascular permeability, and mast cells. *J. Immunol.* 140:3905–3911.

Lembeck, F., and Holzer, P. (1979). Substance P as neurogenic mediator of antidromic vasodilatation and neurogenic plasma extravasation. *Naunyn-Schmiedebergs Arch. Pharmacol.* 310:175–183.

Levi-Schaffer, F., and Shalit, M. (1989). Differential release of histamine and prostaglandin D_2 in rat peritoneal mast cells activated with peptides. *Int. Arch. Allergy Appl. Immunol.* 90:352–357.

Lindholm, D., Heumann. R., Meyer, M., and Thoenen, H. (1987). Interleukin-I regulates synthesis of nerve growth factor in nonneuronal cells of rat sciatic nerve. *Nature* 330:658–659.

MacQueen, G., Marshall, J., Perdue, M. H., Siegel, S., and Bienenstock, J. (1989). Pavlovian conditioning of rat mucosal mast cells to secrete rat mast cell protease II. *Science* 243:83–85.

Mantyh, C. R., Gates, T. S., Zimmerman, R. P., Wilton, M. L., Passaro, E. P., Jr., Vigna, S. R., Maggio, J. E., Kruger, L., and Mantyh, P. W. (1988). Receptor binding sites for substance P, but not substance K or neuromedin K, are expressed in high concentrations by arterioles, venules, and lymph nodules in surgical specimens obtained from patients with ulcerative colitis and Crohn disease. *Proc. Natl. Acad. Sci. USA* 85:3235–3239.

Marshall, J. S., Stead, R. H., McSharry, C., Nielsen, L., and Bienenstock, J. (1990). The role of mast cell degranulation products in mast cell hyperplasia. I. Mechanism of action of nerve growth factor. *J. Immunol.* 144:1886–1892.

Matsuda, H., Coughlin, M. D., Bienenstock, J., and Denburg, J. A. (1988). Nerve growth factor promotes human hemopoietic colony growth and differentiation. *Proc. Natl. Acad. Sci. USA* 850:6508–6512.

Miura, M., Inoue, H., Ichinose, M., Kimura, K., Katsumata, U., and Takishima, T. (1990). Effect of nonadrenergic noncholinergic inhibitory nerve stimulation on the allergic reaction in cat airways. *Am. Rev. Respir. Dis.* 141:29–32.

Newson, B., Dahlstrom, A., Enerback, L., and Ahlman, H. (1983). Suggestive evidence for a direct innervation of mucosal mast cells. An electron microscopic study. *Neuroscience* 10:565–570.

Pearce, R. L., and Thompson, H. L. (1986). Some characteristics of histamine secretion from rat peritoneal mast cells stimulated with nerve growth factor. *J. Physiol.* 372:379–393.

Perdue, M. H., Masson, S., Wershil, B., and Galli, S. (1991). Role of mast cells in ion transport abnormalities associated with intestinal anaphylaxis. Correction of the diminished secretory response in genetically mast cell–deficient W/W^v mice by bone marrow transplantation. *J. Clin. Invest.* 87:687–693.

Plaut, M., Pierce, J. H., Watson, C. J., Hanley-Hyde, J., Nordon, R. P., and Paul, W. E. (1989). Mast cell lines produce lymphokines in response to cross linkage of FcErI or to calcium ionophores. *Nature* 339:64.

Purves, D., Snider, W., and Voyvodic, J. T. (1988). Trophic regulation of nerve cell morphology and innervation in the autonomic nervous system. *Nature* 336:123–128.

Satoh, T., Nakamura, S., Taga, T., Matsuda, T., Hirano, T., Kishimoto, T., and Kaziro, Y. (1988). Induction of neuronal differentiation in PC12 cells by B cell stimulatory factor to IL-6. *Mol. Cell. Biol.* 8:3546–3549.

Sestini, P., Bienenstock, J., Crowe, S., Marshall, J., Stead, R. H., Kakuta, Y., and Perdue, M. (1990). Ion transport in rat tracheal epithelium in vitro: Role of capsaicin-sensitive nerves in allergic reactions. *Am. Rev. Respir. Dis.* 141:393–397.

Shanahan, F., Denburg, J. A., Fox, J., Bienenstock, J., and Befus, D. (1985). Mast cell heterogeneity: Effects of neuroenteric peptides on histamine release. *J. Immunol.* 135:1331–1337.

Skene, J. H. P. (1989). Axonal growth-associated proteins. *Annu. Rev. Neurosci.* 12:127–156.

Stanisz, A. M., Befus, D., and Bienenstock, J. (1986). Differential effects of vasoactive intestinal peptide, substance P, and somatostatin on immunoglobulin synthesis and proliferations by lymphocytes from Peyer's patches, mesenteric lymph nodes, and spleen. *J. Immunol.* 136:152–156.

Stead, R. H., and Bienenstock, J. (1990). Cellular interactions between the immune and peripheral nervous systems: A normal role for mast cells? In *Cell to Cell Interaction*. Edited by M. M. Burger, B. Sordat, and R. M. Zinkernagel. Basel, Karger, pp. 170–187.

Stead, R. H., Bienenstock, J., and Stanisz, A. M. (1987a). Neuropeptide regulation of mucosal immunity. *Immunol. Rev.* 100:333–359.

Stead, R. H., Tomioka, M., Quinonez, G., Simon G. T., Felten, S. Y., and Bienenstock, J. (1987b). Intestinal mucosal mast cells in normal and nematode-infected rat intestines are in intimate contact with peptidergic nerves. *Proc. Natl. Acad. Sci. USA* 84:2975–2979.

Stead, R. H., Dixon, M. F., Bramwell, N. H., Riddell, R. H., and Bienenstock, J. (1989). Mast cells are closely apposed to nerves in the human gastrointestinal mucosa. *Gastroenterology* 97:575–585.

Stead, R. H., Perdue, M. H., Blennerhassett, M. G., Kakuta, Y., Sestini, P., and Bienenstock, J. (1990). The innervation of mast cells. In *The Neuroendocrine-Immune Network*. Edited by S. Freier. Boca Raton, FL, CRC Press, pp. 19–37.

Stead, R. H., Kosecka-Janiszenska, U., Oestreicher, A. Beate., Dixon, Michael, F., and Bienenstock, J. Remodeling of B-So (Gap-43) and NSE-immunoreactive mucosal nerves in the intestines of rats infected with nippostrongylus brasilienes, *J. Neurosci.* 11(12):3809–3821.

Tomioka, M., Stead, R. H., Nielsen, L., Coughlin, M. D., and Bienenstock, J. (1988). Nerve growth factor enhances antigen and other secretagogue-induced histamine release from rat peritoneal mast cells in the absence of phosphatidyl-serine. *J. Allergy Clin. Immunol.* 82:599–607.

Tsuda, T., Wong, D., Dolovich, J., Bienenstock, J., and Denburg, J. A. (1991). Synergistic effects of nerve growth factor and granulocyte-macrophage colony-stimulating factor on human basophilic cell differentiation. *Blood* 77:971–979.

Wodnar-Filipowicz, A., Heusser, C. H., and Moroni, C. (1989). Production of the haematopoietic growth factors GM-CSF and interleukin 3 by mast cells in response to IgE receptor mediated activation. *Nature* 339:150.

Yamamori, T., Fukada, K., Aebersold, R., Korsching, S., Fann, M-J., and Patterson, P. H. (1989). The cholinergic neuronal differentiation factor from heart cells is identical to leukemia inhibitory factor. *Science* 246:1412–1416.

29

Mast Cells in Arthritis

DANIEL G. MALONE

University of Wisconsin
Madison, Wisconsin

I. Background

A. Evidence of Synovial Mast Cell Participation in Arthritis

The pathogenesis of joint destruction in chronic arthritis is multifactorial and involves actions of many types of cells, including neutrophils, macrophages, lymphocytes, endothelial cells, synovial adherent cells, and, as recent data suggest, mast cells. It is clear that no single cell type is responsible for all the immunological and destructive changes. Knowledge of how mast cells contribute to inflammation and tissue injury in allergic diseases has led to the hypothesis that synovial mast cells contribute to the initiation and perpetuation of arthritis, and that their participation involves IgE-dependent and -independent mechanisms. Furthermore, given the close anatomical approximation of mast cells to small blood vessels and nerves in the subsynovial lining layer, it is likely that synovial mast cell interactions with synovial adherent cells, microvascular endothelial cells, and neurons are important pathways by which synovial mast cells affect synovitis. Although synovium is a mast cell–rich tissue, and there is much evidence for synovial mast cell involvement in joint injury, the data are, at best, suggestive and indirect, and much work remains to establish the nature, extent, and mechanisms of synovial mast cell participation in arthritis.

The mast cell contributes to tissue injury and inflammation in allergic diseases, and recent indirect evidence implicates mast cells in synovial inflammation as well (Malone and Metcalfe, 1988; Gruber et al., 1986; Crisp et al., 1984a; Zuraw et al., 1981). Mast cell proximity to synovial lesions and striking increases in synovial mast cell numbers in various arthritides are examples (Godfrey et al., 1984; Malone et al., 1987; Bromley et al., 1984). Mast cells are found in rheumatoid joints near damaged cartilage at the advancing edge of invading pannus (Bromley et al., 1984), suggesting their involvement in the erosive phases of the disease. A substantial percentage of lupus patients have anti-IgE autoantibodies, which correlates with arthritis in those patients (Gruber et al., 1988a), supporting previous suggestions (Crisp et al., 1984a; Malone et al., 1986) that lupus arthritis is, in part, mast cell–mediated. In addition, serum IgE rheumatoid factors from arthritis patients can sensitize human synovial mast cells to degranulate to aggregated IgG in vitro (Gruber et al., 1988b). Furthermore, concentrations of histamine that exceed normal plasma levels and intact, functioning mast cells have been detected in synovial fluid in several forms of arthritis (Malone et al., 1986). Finally, other studies have shown that in rheumatoid synovium, the number of mast cells correlates with the intensity of inflammation and infiltration by T lymphocytes bearing helper/inducer surface markers, and that mast cells may be involved in the early stages of "flareups" of arthritis (van den Broek et al., 1988; Malone et al., 1986, 1987; Malone and Metcalfe, 1988). In many ways, these findings are analogous to the mast cell–mediated, late-phase reactions of asthma and the mast cell–mediated, cutaneous, late-phase reaction in rats (Tannenbaum et al., 1980), in which inflammation with influx of eosinophils, neutrophils, lymphocytes, and monocytes is prominent. Whether the recruitment of inflammatory cells in synovitis is causally related to synovial mast cell activation is currently unknown.

The lack of clinical association between atopy and arthritis is not evidence against mast cell participation in synovitis. Mast cells in different tissues are diverse in structure and function, and, as will be shown later, rodent synovial mast cells appear to differ from other mast cells in several respects. Thus, clinical activity or inactivity of one mast cell subpopulation does not preclude or guarantee activity of another. Numerous clinical observations confirm intensive mast cell activity in one organ with little or no mast cell activity elsewhere. Not all asthmatics are atopic, nor are all persons who have anaphylactic reactions to drugs. True food allergy does not invariably occur in atopic individuals, and conversely, most persons who are prone to contact dermatitis do not have asthma, allergic rhinitis, or food allergy. It is conceivable, therefore, that there are persons with exuberant synovial mast cell activity and no other atopic signs or symptoms.

B. Mechanisms by Which Synovial Mast Cells Could Contribute to Synovitis and Tissue Degradation in Arthritis

Mast cells are well equipped to cause and amplify synovitis, since they produce and release a bewildering diversity of vasoactive and proinflammatory substances, such as histamine, serotonin, heparin, plasminogen activators (PA), and PA inhibitors (PAI) (Bartholomew and Woolley, 1988). The important cytokines interleukins-1–6, interferon-γ, and GM-CSF are also made and released by mast cells (Brown et al., 1987; Bartholomew, and Woolley, 1988; Wodnar-Filipowicz et al., 1989; Plaut et al., 1989; Burd et al., 1989). Recent evidence also suggests that stimulated mast cells increase expression of mRNA for JE, MIP-α, MIP-β, and TCA-3, the proteins of the MIP-1 (macrophage inflammatory protein-1) family of chemotactic, proinflammatory cytokines (Mican and Metcalfe, 1990; Costa et al., 1990; Burd et al., 1990). Still other substances that contribute to synovitis, prostaglandins, leukotrienes, enzymes, activators of the complement system, and chemotactic substances for a variety of inflammatory cells are also produced and released by mast cells (Wasserman, 1984; Metcalfe, 1984; Center, 1983).

Histamine, a major component of mast cell granules, is a potent vasoactive amine that affects several arms of the immune response. A subset of large CD8+ lymphocytes have histamine receptors, as do human, canine, and bovine articular chondrocytes (Taylor et al., 1985a) and canine synovial microvascular endothelial cells (Grennan, 1975). In addition to markedly enhancing vascular permeability, histamine increases neutrophil migration and stimulates cultured human synovial cells and articular chondrocytes to produce prostaglandin E2 (Taylor et al., 1986). Due to histamine's vasoactive properties, synovial mast cell degranulation probably increases synovial deposition of circulating immune complexes and/or arthritogenic antigen, as has been shown in other tissues (Cochrane and Hawkins, 1968).

Heparin, another major mast cell granule constituent, stimulates human monocyte/macrophage Il-1 production, and contributes to angiogenesis (Taylor et al., 1985b). There is also evidence that heparin affects lymphocyte responses (Frieri and Metcalfe, 1983) and enhances periarticular bone mineral loss (Crisp et al., 1984b).

Mast cells also contain and release tumor necrosis factor α (Steffen et al., 1989; Gorden and Galli 1990), which stimulates collagenase and prostaglandin production by synovial cells (Dayer et al., 1985) and stimulates procoagulant and immunological activity in endothelial cells and monocytes/macrophages, (Taylor et al., 1985b; Nawroth and Stern, 1986).

Tissue damage in arthritis is due, in large part, to the actions of several proteolytic enzymes produced by activated synoviocytes. The most noteworthy are the neutral proteases (e.g., collagenases) and metalloproteases, and it has been shown that human mass cell tryptase activates synovial fluid latent collagenase in the presence of these metalloproteases (Gruber et al., 1988c, 1989). Human mast cell tryptase also is capable of degrading a rat mesenchymal cell connective tissue matrix in an in vitro assay (Gruber and Schwartz, 1990), and human mast cell chymase may directly dissolve components of basement membrane (Gruber, 1989). Furthermore, activated mast cells release plasminogen activator (Bartholomew and Woolley, 1988), potentially giving rise to plasmin formation, and linking mast cells with the coagulation and fibrinolytic systems, both of which are closely tied to inflammation. Plasmin, an enzyme with multiple substrates, also activates latent collagenase. Thus, the pharmacopeia of the mast cell is well suited to induction and perpetuation of synovitis.

Mast cells and T lymphocytes participate in delayed-type hypersensitivity (DTH) reactions (Van Loverern et al., 1983). Rheumatoid arthritis is considered a DTH reaction in synovium, thought to be the result of antigen deposition through the relatively "leaky" synovial fenestrated capillary bed (Fassbender, 1975). As discussed above, mast cells could contribute to the process by their release of a broad variety of proinflammatory substances or by maximization of circulating immune complex (IC) (Cochrane and Hawkins, 1968) and/or arthritogenic antigen (such as bacterial cell wall peptidoglycan) deposition in synovium. It is also conceivable that mast cell–induced vasopermeability increases delivery to the circulation of constituents of damaged cells and/or joint structures, such as type II collagen, that elicit systemic antibody responses. Thus, a credible hypothesis is that degranulation of synovial mast cells augments deposition of antigen and amplifies the DTH, resulting in increased susceptibility to destructive arthritis and increased severity of the chronic disease.

C. Mast Cell–Synovial Cell and Mast Cell–Microvascular Endothelial Cell Interactions

Hypervascularity and evidence of immunological activation of several types of joint cells are important characteristic histological features of arthritis. The first detectable microscopic lesion of inflammatory synovitis in humans is perivascular collection of inflammatory cells (Schumacher and Kitridou, 1972). To initiate such a lesion, circulating immunocompetent cells must traverse capillary walls after attaching to specialized activated endothelial structures known as high endothelial venules (HEV), by interactions with a series of adhesion molecules. Synovium is one of a few nonlymphoid tissues in which HEV have been found (Jalkanen et al., 1986). Recently it has been shown, in human skin explant cultures, that mast cell activation causes a notable increase in expression of one of these adhesion molecules (Klein et al., 1989). Thus, it is reasonable to hypothesize that synovial mast cell activation up-regulates synovial adhesion molecule expression and may stimulate HEV formation by enhancing endothelial cell and/or mononuclear cell production of cytokines such as IL-1.

In situ, most synovial mast cells are situated adjacent to small neurovascular bundles, and activated capillary endothelium and mast cells both appear important in the early phases of synovitis. There is evidence in rodents that peritoneal mast cells contribute to new vessel growth (Norrby et al., 1986). Furthermore, mast cells contain heparin, which stimulates migration of endothelial cells in vitro (Folkman et al., 1979), prolongs their life in tissue culture, and avidly binds to, and protects, several endothelial cell growth factors (Schreiber et al., 1985). Mast cells also contain tumor necrosis factor α, a cytokine that stimulates procoagulant and immunological activity in endothelial cells and monocytes and macrophages and plays an important role in mast cell–induced endothelial cell adhesion molecule expression (Steffen et al., 1989; Nawroth and Stern, 1986; Klein et al., 1989). Moreover, interactions between mast cells and endothelial cells may be reciprocal, as rat microvascular endothelial cells make large quantities of GM-CSF, a factor capable of stimulating the proliferation of a murine mast cell line (Malone et al., 1988). Similarly, and because of the effects certain mast cell mediators have on synoviocytes (outlined above), synovial mast cell–synovial fibroblastoid cell interactions may be another important interaction. There is also evidence of mast cell–nervous system interaction, and innervation of joints may affect the location, pattern, and/or severity of arthritis (Levine et al., 1986, 1990; Coderre et al., 1989). The interplay of joint innervation, synovial mast cell activity, and destructive activity of articular immunocompetent cells has received relatively little research effort to date.

D. Mast Cells in Arthritis In Vivo: Animal Models

In addition to the in vitro effects and potential mechanisms of action just discussed, mast cells appear to be important participants in most in vivo rat models of chronic, erosive arthritis. Synovial mast cell degranulation occurs early in collagen-induced arthritis (Helfgott et al., 1987) and is an important factor in the acute synovitis of streptococcal cell wall–induced arthritis (Dalldorf et al., 1988) and probably in antigen-induced arthritis as well (van den Broek et al., 1988). The acute and chronic phases of rat adjuvant arthritis can be nearly eliminated by histamine receptor blockade (Al Haboubi and Zeitlin, 1982; Vickers, and Sykes, 1982), implying an important role for the mast cell granule-associated vasoactive amine in that model, and our preliminary data indicate that synovial mast cell activation exacerbates acute and chronic *Lactobacillus casei* cell wall (LCW)-induced arthritis (see below).

These findings emphasize the need for further studies in animal models on the mechanisms by which synovial mast cells contribute to chronic erosive arthritis.

II. Current Studies

A. Models

Mast Cell–Induced Arthritis in Rats

To study synovial mast cells in vivo, we developed a rat model of synovial mast cell–mediated, antigen-specific, IgE-dependent arthritis (Malone and Metcalfe, 1988). This model is ideal for examining the role of mast cells in arthritis and for defining synovial mast cell mediator release profiles and responses to pharmacological manipulation. In the following sections, I will describe briefly, first, our model of synovial mast cell–mediated arthritis, and second, LCW-induced rat arthritis, a well-established model of erosive rheumatoid arthritis that we have used in our studies of synovial mast cell effects on arthritis. Third, I will summarize work in which we have demonstrated that although a major population of synovial mast cells are connective tissue–type mast cells, they exhibit several differences from the connective tissue mast cells of rat skin and thus have their own unique biological behavior profile; fourth, that there appears to be a hyperactivity of synovial mast cells in states of hyperimmune IgE responses; and, finally, that synovial mast cell activation can exacerbate acute and chronic LCW-induced arthritis.

Ether-anesthetized rats are passively sensitized by intra-articular and intracutaneous injection of 1 μg of a mouse monoclonal IgE directed against dinitrophenol (DNP) in phosphate-buffered saline (PBS) or with hyperimmune rat serum containing high-titer, antigen-specific IgE (test-sensitized tissues). The contralateral joint (knee or ankle) and a symmetrically located contralateral skin site (sham-sensitized controls) are injected with an irrelevant monoclonal IgE, nonimmune serum or PBS. About 24 hr later, the rat is administered an intravenous (i.v.) or intra-articular injection of DNP coupled to bovine serum albumin (BSA) or other specific antigen to which the animal has been immunized. Also injected i.v. is 300 μl of 1% Evans blue dye in PBS with or without 1.11×10^5 Bq (3 μCi) of ^{125}I-labeled albumin. Within 5 min of antigen challenge, there is synovial mast cell degranulation with synovial vascular leakage in test tissues (test skin and joints swell and turn blue, and tissue water content increases), which is more accurately quantified by γ counting and calculating the ratio of [test tissue]:[control tissue] CPM/mg dry tissue weight, referred to as the "leakage ratio." The leakage ratio increases in direct proportion to vascular exudation. Full details of the original method and data referred to above have been previously published (Malone and Metcalfe, 1988).

Joint Lavage Method

To study synovial mast cell histamine, eicosanoid, and plasminogen activator/plasminogen activator inhibitor (PA/PAI) release, we developed a rapid, simple, inexpensive joint lavage method that allows collection of synovial mast cell mediators that are released into the joint cavity. Joint lavage is accomplished by insertion of two ¼-in.-long, 27-g stainless steel needles (BD Yale, #1000) into joints through adjacent sites in the infrapatellar tendon. One needle is connected by plastic tubing to a 3-ml syringe containing lavage fluid. Gentle pressure on the plunger of the syringe fills the joint with fluid, and the intra-articular pressure so created forces fluid through the joint cavity into the hub of the other needle (capacity ≈ 100–150 μl), which serves as the collection port. *A baseline lavage collection with PBS is always made before synovial mast cells are degranulated.* At several time points after antigen challenge, lavages are done on both knees. Cells are removed by centrifugation, and the supernatants are frozen at –80°C for assay. We have successfully used this technique to quantify exudation of labeled substances into the joint, to define the synovial mast cell release kinetics of histamine, to measure PA/PAI and eicosanoids from activated synovial mast cells, and to administer antigen and other stimuli of synovial mast cell degranulation (Malone, Verbsky, and Dolan, 1991). The method has many potential uses in our model and other models of animal arthritis.

Lactobacillus casei *Cell Wall (LCW)-Induced Arthritis*

(LCW)-induced arthritis, a well-established model of human RA in rats, is ideal for our experiments. A single intraperitoneal injection of sonicated cell wall fragments of *L. casei* bacteria causes an acute (1–10 days), followed by a chronic (up to 9 weeks), erosive, symmetrical polyarthritis in susceptible rat strains. The erosive phase is T-cell dependent and exhibits a pattern of joint involvement very similar to human RA (attacks small joints of the distal extremities, spares axial skeleton, hips, usually knees), from which it is histologically indistinguishable. Inbred Lewis strain (LEW/N) rats, are highly susceptible, while inbred Fischer strain (F344/N) develop acute polyarthritis, but do not develop the chronic, erosive disease. In addition, male Lewis rats get less severe erosive disease than their female counterparts. The strain susceptibilities, kinetics of arthritogenic material deposition, time course of clinical changes, histological pattern, and radiographic findings have all been reported (Lehman et al., 1983, 1984; Lehman, 1988).

B. Uniqueness of Synovial Mast Cells

In the course of early experiments with our synovial mast cell–mediated arthritis model, we noted that synovial mast cell–induced vasopermeability was decreased in rats anesthetized with Innovar Vet, a commercially available, widely used droperidol/fentanyl combination, compared to either-anesthetized rats (Fig. 1). Using the joint lavage method, we showed that this difference was due, at least in part, to a decrease in synovial mast cell histamine release into the joint

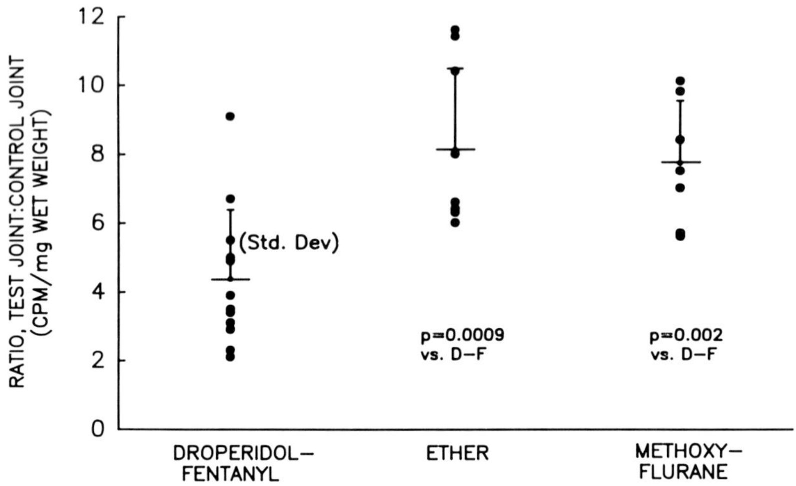

Figure 1 Effect of three anesthetic agents on rat synovial mast cell–induced vasopermeability, quantified by calculating the ratio of [test joint]:[control joint] CPM/mg wet tissue, hereafter referred to as the *LEAKAGE RATIO*. Synovium was harvested 15 min after the previously passively sensitized synovial mast cells were degranulated by i.v. injection of specific antigen and 1.11×10^5 Bq (3 μCi) of ^{125}I-albumin. Tissue samples were weighed, and the radioactivity then was determined by counting samples in a γ counter. In each group, animals were anesthetized with the indicated drug prior to the mast cell activation procedure. Each point represents one animal. Error bars show group means and standard deviations. Droperidol-fentanyl–anesthetized rats have a lower synovial leakage ratio. Differences are significant by the two-tailed Student's *t* test. (Courtesy of C. V. Mosby Co.; reprinted from Malone and Dolan, 1990.)

space (Fig. 2). Interestingly, this inhibitory effect (probably due to the droperidol) was absent in skin mast cells (Fig. 3 and 4), implying a basic difference in response between these two mast cell populations in the rat (Malone and Dolan, 1990).

C. Differential Drug Responses of Synovial Mast Cells and Involvement of Nonhistamine Mediators

These findings were confirmed and extended in another set of experiments in which we tested the effects of three nonsteroidal anti-inflammatory agents in our model (Malone et al., 1991). In these studies, ketoprofen given to rats in doses sufficient to block both cyclooxygenase and lipoxygenase arachidonic acid metabolic pathways caused a decrease in skin, but not synovial, mast cell–

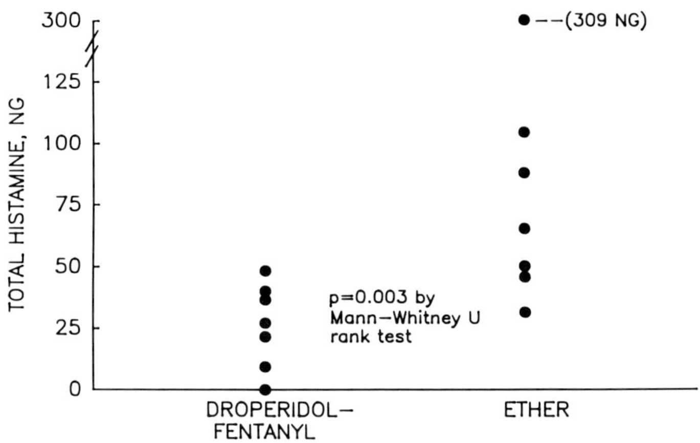

Figure 2 Intra-articular histamine release in joints of ether-anesthetized rats ($n = 7$) versus droperidol-fentanyl ($n = 7$), calculated from the total histamine content of 500 μl of rat joint lavage samples collected at 5 and 15 min after joint mast cell activation. Sensitization, activation, and rat knee lavage methods were as shown in Figure 1 and in the text describing the animal model of synovial mast cell–mediated, antigen-specific, IgE-dependent arthritis. Each point represents one animal, and error bars show group means and standard deviations. Droperidol-fentanyl–anesthetized rats released less intra-articular histamine. Differences are significant by the nonparametric Mann-Whitney U rank-sum test. (Courtesy of C. V. Mosby Co.; reprinted from Malone and Dolan, 1990.)

induced vasopermeability (Fig. 5). Furthermore, aspirin and indomethacin, which inhibit cyclooxygenase but not lipoxygenase, *increased* synovial and skin mast cell–induced vasopermeability (Figs. 6 and 7), an effect that was not reversible by concomitant H_1 and H_2 histamine receptor blockader drugs (Figs. 8 and 9). These data confirmed differences in synovial mast cell and skin mast cell behavior, suggested that mediator release profiles of these two mast cell populations differ, and suggested that the vasopermeability-enhancing effects of aspirin and indomethacin involved mechanisms other than those associated with actions of histamine. The most likely mediators responsible for the latter findings are serotonin and/or eicosanoids.

D. Synovial Mast Cell Mediator Release

It was clear that we needed more data on the biological responses, mediator and cytokine release, and subtype (connective tissue versus mucosal) of rat synovial

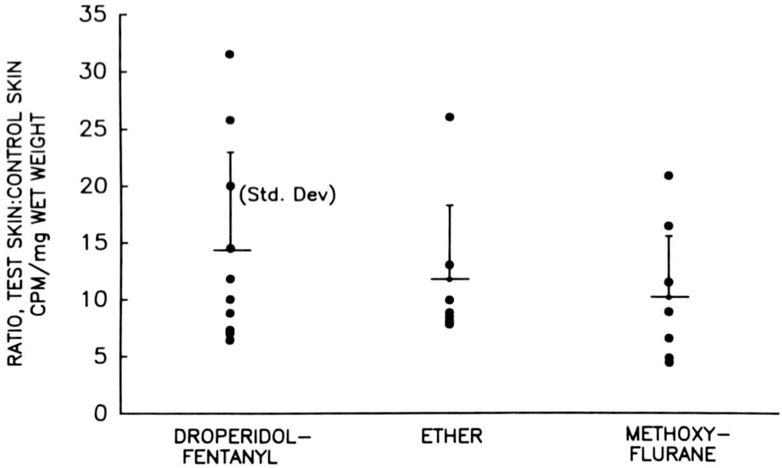

Figure 3 Effect of three anesthetic agents on rat cutaneous mast cell–induced vasopermeability, quantified by calculating the skin leakage ratio (see legend to Fig, 1). Skin samples were harvested 15 min after the previously passively sensitized mast cells were degranulated by i.v. injection of specific antigen and 1.11×10^5 Bq (3 μCi) of ^{125}I-albumin. Tissue samples were weighed, and the radioactivity then was determined by counting samples in a γ counter. In each group, animals were anesthetized with the indicated drug prior to the mast cell degranulation procedure. Each point represents one animal. Error bars show group means and standard deviations. Unlike synovium, skin leakage ratios are not significantly different (two-tailed Student's *t* test). (Courtesy of C. V. Mosby Co.; reprinted from Malone and Dolan, 1990.)

mast cells. Therefore, we used our lavage technique to establish the kinetics of synovial mast cell histamine release with five synovial mast cell challenge protocols (Malone et al., 1991). Histamine was the mediator selected for study because it is a major mast cell granule constituent, assays for its detection are operational, and it can be detected in small concentrations reliably. In experiments using the passive sensitization technique, maximum histamine appears in the joint 5 min after antigen challenge, with lower amounts present at 15 min, and much smaller differences at ≥25 min (Fig. 10). The minimal amounts in some control joints likely are due to the small increase in plasma histamine (not shown).

E. Synovial Mast Cell Classification

In experiments using other secretagogues to stimulate synovial mast cell degranulation, intra-articular instillation of a solution of compound 48/80, anti-rat

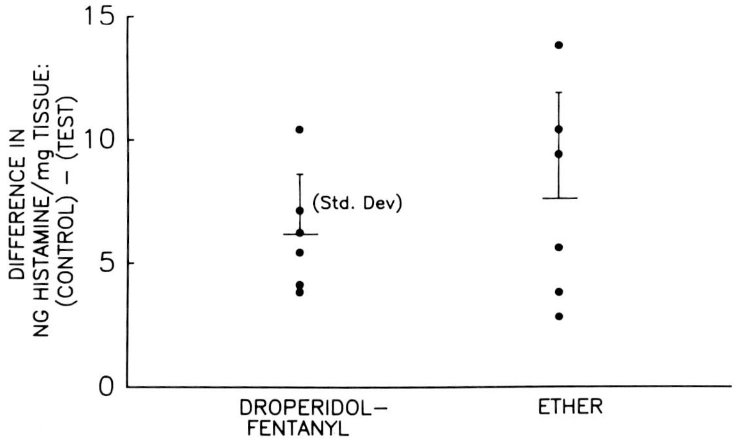

Figure 4 Total histamine release in skin in the 15 min after activation of passively sensitized rat cutaneous mast cells in droperidol-fentanyl versus ether-anesthetized animals. Values shown are the calculated difference between control and test skin total histamine content, which was determined on weighed samples by boiling them in distilled water for 20 min and assaying the histamine concentration of the supernatant on a fluorometric histamine autoanalyzer. Each point represents one animal. Error bars show group means and standard deviations. Differences are not significant (nonparametric Mann-Whitney U rank-sum test). (Courtesy of C. V. Mosby Co.; reprinted from Malone and Dolan, 1990.)

IgE, or phorbol 2-myristate 13-acetate, resulted in edema and blueing of joint tissues and evidence (by γ-counting of tissues from rats that had been injected with ^{125}I-labeled albumin) of increased vascular permeability. Since compound 48/80 activates only connective tissue–type mast cells in the rat, and since the magnitude of histamine release after intra-articular injection of this substance was equal to that in the passive sensitization experiments, the data show that connective tissue mast cells are present in rat synovium and probably account for a majority of the activity we measured (Malone et al., 1991). We also stained undecalcified methylmethacrylate-embedded rat joints with alcian blue–safranin O to distinguish connective tissue mast cells from mucosal mast cells and found an overwhelming majority of connective tissue mast cells in synovium. These findings support our theory that although synovial mast cells are probably mainly of the connective tissue type in rats, they differ in several important responses from other connective tissue–type mast cells, most notably, skin mast cells.

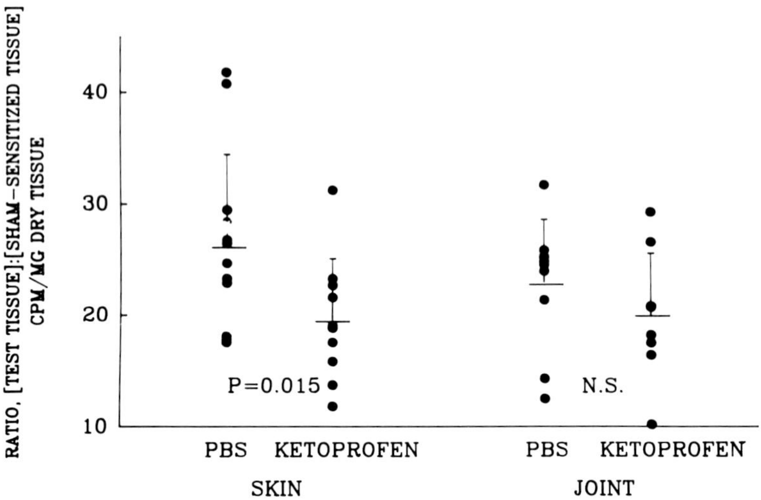

Figure 5 Effect of ketoprofen on rat synovial and skin mast cell–induced vasopermeability. Test rats got ketoprofen, 10 mg/kg orally twice a day in PBS for eight doses, and control rats got PBS orally alone. Sensitization and mast cell activation methods were as described in the legend to Figure 1 and in the text describing the animal model of synovial mast cell–mediated, antigen-specific, IgE-dependent arthritis. Tissues were harvested 15 min after the previously passively sensitized mast cells were degranulated by i.v. injection of specific antigen and 1.11×10^5 Bq (3 μCi) of ^{125}I-albumin. Tissue samples were weighed, and the radioactivity then was determined by counting samples in a γ counter. Each point is the leakage ratio of one rat, and the group means and standard deviations are shown. Ketoprofen decreased skin, but not synovium, leakage ratios. Differences are significant by the one-tailed Student's *t* test. (Courtesy of J. B. Lippincott Co.; reprinted from Malone et al., 1991.)

F. Synovial Mast Cell Hyperactivity

Our experiments with actively sensitized animals yielded an interesting and provocative observation. We found that at the peak of the serum IgE response to specific immunizing antigen (about 10–14 days after immunization), in some actively sensitized animals only, the baseline PBS lavage (before synovial mast cell activation by antigen) joint histamine levels were unusually high. In previous and subsequent experiments with passively sensitized and with normal, unsensitized rats, baseline histamine levels were never as high as those in the actively sensitized animals. Figure 11 shows a comparison of baseline joint histamine levels in actively sensitized versus unsensitized, normal rats and reveals a highly significant increase in the joints of the actively sensitized rats.

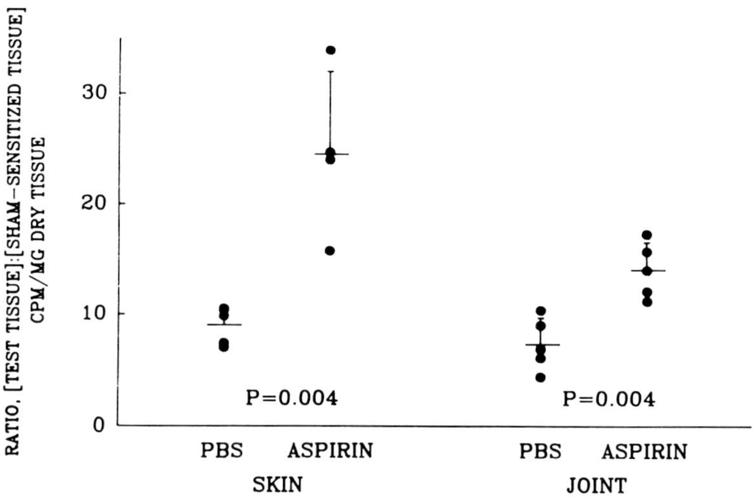

Figure 6 Effect of oral aspirin on cutaneous and synovial mast cell–mediated vasopermeability in rats. Test rats received oral aspirin, 50 mg/kg orally twice a day for eight doses, suspended in PBS, and control rats received PBS alone. Tissues were sensitized and mast cells activated as described in the legend to Figure 1 and in the text describing the animal model of synovial mast cell–mediated, antigen-specific, IgE-dependent arthritis. Tissues were harvested 15 min after the previously passively sensitized mast cells were degranulated by i.v. injection of specific antigen and 1.11×10^5 Bq (3 μCi) of ^{125}I-albumin. Tissue samples were weighed, and the radioactivity then was determined by counting samples in a γ counter. Each point represents the leakage ratio of one animal. Error bars show group means and standard deviations. Aspirin caused an increase in cutaneous and synovial leakage ratios. Differences between test and control rats are significant by the nonparametric Mann-Whitney U rank-sum test. (Courtesy of J. B. Lippincott Co.; reprinted from Malone et al., 1991).

To learn whether these high joint baseline histamine levels could be explained by high plasma histamine levels, we measured plasma histamine before active sensitization, 10–14 days after sensitization but before antigen, and again 15 min after antigen challenge. The results indicated that rats with high baseline joint histamine levels showed no increase in plasma histamine after immunization and before antigen challenge. Thus, local production apparently accounted for the high joint histamine concentration, and *not* passive diffusion of high plasma histamine levels into the joint. Furthermore, we detected plasminogen activator activity in baseline samples of actively sensitized animals (and had never detected PA in any other baseline samples), consistent with our histamine observa-

Table 1 LTB4 Levels in pg/ml Lavage Fluid in Actively and Passively Sensitized Rats

	Active	Passive
	44	<7.8
	28	11.2
	46	11.2
	34	11.2
	36	
	14	
Mean	34.7	8.4
# Joints	n = 6	n = 4

In actively sensitized rats, 10–14 days after immunization at the peak of the IgE response, 0.5 ml of PBS was washed through the knee joints before intra-articular antigen challenge. LTB4 levels in 6 joints of 3 rats are given in the left column. In passively sensitized rats, 0.5 ml PBS was washed through the knee joints before intravenous antigen challenge. LTB4 levels in lavage fluid of 4 joints in 2 rats are given in the right column.

tions. Finally, Table 1 also shows evidence of higher baseline joint LTB4 levels in actively sensitized rats than in passively sensitized rats. These findings deserve further study and present interesting possibilities regarding the role of synovial mast cells in synovitis.

G. Effects of Synovial Mast Cell Activation of Rat Arthritis

We have begun experiments combining synovial mast cell degranulation and administration of LCW to Lewis and Fischer rats, and preliminary findings clearly support a role of synovial mast cell in acute LCW arthritis. We used groups of two rats to determine the effects on acute LCW arthritis of the timing of synovial mast cell activation with respect to LCW administration. Female rats ($\approx$150 g) underwent synovial mast cell degranulation after passive sensitization in one ankle (test joints). The contralateral side underwent no mast cell activation and served as negative control. In one group of Fischer and Lewis rats, the synovial mast cells were activated simultaneously with LCW administration (5 mg total cell wall carbohydrate), and, in other groups, at 2, 6, 12, or 24 hr after LCW administration. Rats were examined daily for 7 days and twice per week

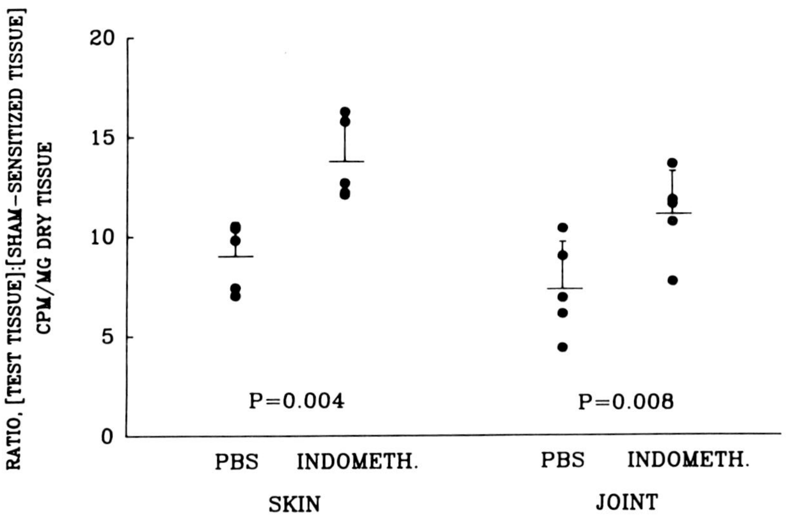

Figure 7 Effect of oral indomethacin on cutaneous and synovial mast cell–mediated vasopermeability in rats. Test rats received oral indomethacin, 2.5 mg/kg orally twice a day for eight doses, suspended in PBS, and control rats received PBS alone. Tissues were sensitized and mast cells activated as described in the legend to Figure 1 and in the text describing the animal model of synovial mast cell–mediated, antigen-specific, IgE-dependent arthritis. Tissues were harvested 15 min after the previously passively sensitized mast cells were degranulated by i.v. injection of specific antigen and 1.11×10^5 Bq (3 μCi) of ^{125}I-albumin. Tissue samples were weighed, and the radioactivity then was determined by counting samples in a γ counter. Each point represents the leakage ratio of one animal. Error bars show group means and standard deviations. Indomethacin increased cutaneous and synovial leakage ratios. Differences between test and control rats are significant by the nonparametric Mann-Whitney U rank-sum test. (Courtesy of J. B. Lippincott Co.; reprinted from Malone et al., 1991.)

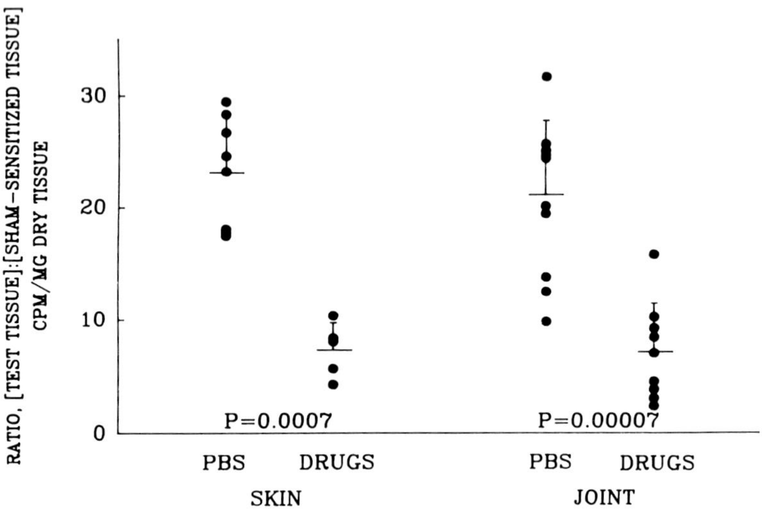

Figure 8 Effect of combined oral diphenhydramine and i.p. cimetidine on cutaneous and synovial mast cell–mediated vasopermeability in rats. Test rats received oral diphenhydramine, 50 mg/kg twice a day for three doses, and cimetidine, 200 mg/kg twice a day for three doses, and control rats received equal volumes of oral and i.p. PBS. Tissues were sensitized and mast cells activated as described in the legend to Figure 1 and in the text describing the animal model of synovial mast cell–mediated, antigen-specific, IgE-dependent arthritis. Tissues were harvested 15 min after the previously passively sensitized synovial mast cells were degranulated by i.v. injection of specific antigen and 1.11×10^5 Bq (3 μCi) of ^{125}I-albumin. Tissue samples were weighed, and the radioactivity then was determined by counting samples in a γ counter. Each point represents the leakage ratio of one animal. Error bars show group means and standard deviations. Complete H_1 and H_2 receptor blockade decreased the leakage ratios in skin and synovium. Differences between test and control rats are significant by the nonparametric Mann-Whitney U rank-sum test. (Courtesy of J. B. Lippincott Co.; reprinted from Malone et al., 1991.)

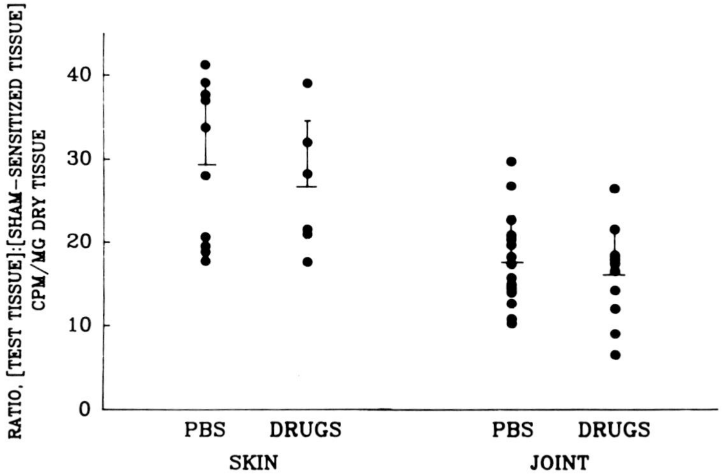

Figure 9 Effect of combined oral indomethacin, oral diphenhydramine, and i.p. cimetidine on cutaneous and synovial mast cell–mediated vasopermeability in rats. Drug doses and methods were as in legends to Figures 7 and 8. The indomethacin-induced increase in vasopermeability is unaffected by complete histamine H_1 and H_2 receptor blockade. (Courtesy of J. B. Lippincott Co.; reprinted from Malone et al., 1991.)

thereafter. Ankle swelling was graded on a scale of 0–4, where 0 = no swelling/erythema and 4 = severe swelling/erythema. In Lewis rats, there was more swelling of test ankles in the 6-hr group. In Fischer rats, however, there was more swelling of test ankles in all groups. In addition, there was evidence of ongoing swelling in some of the Fischer rats 6 weeks after LCW administration, well into the chronic phase of the disease. Fischer rats are usually resistant to chronic LCW arthritis. Control Fischer and Lewis rats (no synovial mast cell activation on either side) got symmetrical ankle swelling of lower magnitude. Figure 12, shows data on the two 6-hr Fischer rats. These findings indicate that, consistent with our hypothesis, synovial mast cell activation can exacerbate acute LCW arthritis, and that rat strain and timing of synovial mast cell activation with respect to LCW administration may be important factors governing the interaction.

It appears from our early data that, first, although connective tissue–type mast cells probably comprise a majority of synovial mast cells in the rat, they differ in several respects from the connective tissue–type mast cells of the skin. Second, mediators other than histamine appear important in synovial mast cell–induced vasopermeability in our model. Third, synovial mast cells of actively sensitized rats at the height of the serum IgE response appear hyperac-

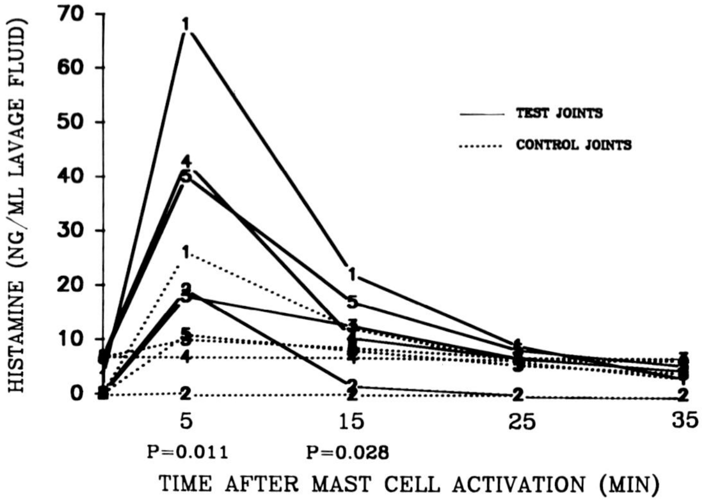

Figure 10. Release kinetics of histamine after passive sensitization with monoclonal mouse IgE anti DNP (test joints), or irrelevant IgE (control joints), and activation by i.v. antigen injection. Joint lavages were performed at the times indicated on the horizontal axis, where $t = 0$ refers to the baseline lavage, i.e., before i.v. antigen injection. Lavage fluid was collected, cells pelleted, and the supernatant was assayed for histamine content as described. Each rat, represented by a number, has two data curves: a solid line representing the test joint, and a dotted line representing the contralateral control (sham-sensitized) joint. p values refer to comparison of the test versus control joint histamine levels by the paired t test at the indicated time point. (Courtesy of C. V. Mosby Co.; reprinted from Malone et al., 1991.)

tive, and fourth, and perhaps most important, synovial mast cell activation clearly can exacerbate acute and chronic LCW arthritis.

It is likely that mast cell–associated cytokines such as interleukins 1–6, tumor necrosis factor α, and other mast cell–derived substances will be shown to mediate important mast cell effects on inflammation. Through further work on our in vivo animal models, we hope to define better the mechanisms by which synovial mast cells affect chronic, erosive arthritis.

Discussion

Dvorak: This comment relates to your observation of high baseline synovial lavage histamine levels in activley sensitized rats at the height of the serum IgE

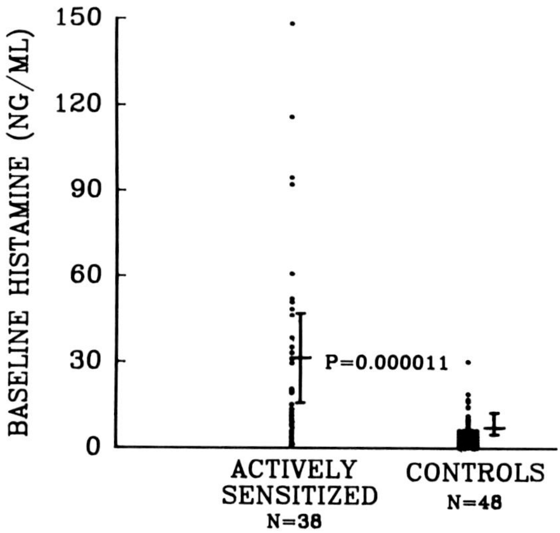

Figure 11 Comparison of baseline joint lavage fluid histamine levels in actively sensitized rats versus normal, unsensitized rats. No animal had any injection or instrumentation of joints prior to baseline lavage with PBS. The experiments were performed 10–14 days after immunization of the actively sensitized animals. The nonparametric Wilcoxon rank-sum test was used to compare the group means, which are shown with 99% confidence intervals. The highest value in the control group (≈30 ng/ml) was caused by needle insertion trauma. (Courtesy of C. V. Mosby Co.; reprinted from Malone et al., in press.)

response. I agree that your data are consistent with EM findings on isolated human synovial mast cells, in which morphological evidence of so-called "piecemeal degranulation" was seen. I think both the above-mentioned observations are suggestive of potential synovial mast cell involvement in arthritis by increased activity in states of immunological stimulation. In isolated human synovial mast cells examined by electron microscopy we have seen piecemeal degranulation. This may be of relevance to the high spontaneous histamine release you find in your rat model of cell wall–induced arthritis.

Schwartz: Do you see any differences between atopic and nonatopic subjects with rheumatoid arthritis?

Malone: I am not aware of any data that directly address this issue, but in my reading over the years I have never been impressed by any such differences. It is known that there is no increase in the prevalence of atopy in rheumatoid arthritis patients compared to the general population.

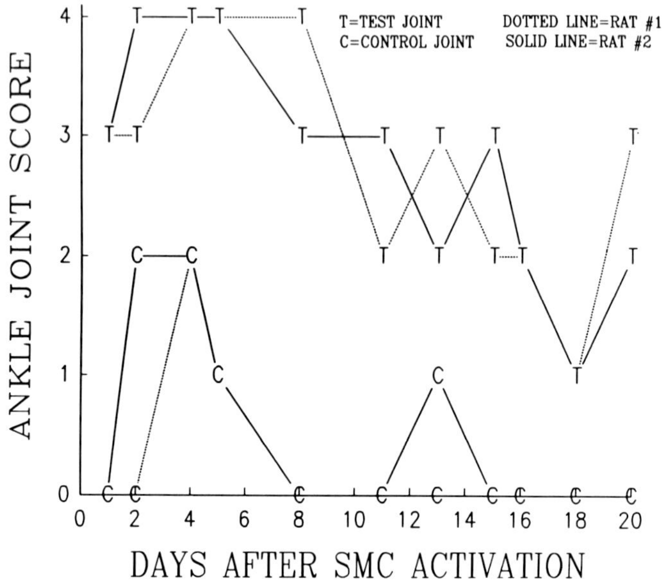

Figure 12 Exacerbation of acute *Lactobacillus casei* cell wall–induced ankle arthritis in rats by activation of ankle synovial mast cells. Bacterial cell walls (5 mg cell wall carbohydrate) were injected i.p. into 120-g female Fischer rats. Six hours later previously passively sensitized synovial mast cells were degranulated in test ankles, but not in the contralateral (control) ankles, by the methods previously cited. Rats were examined daily for a week, and joints scored on a scale of 0 (no swelling) to 4 (maximum swelling, erythema). Shown are data from two rats.

References

Al Haboubi, H. A. and Zeitlin, I. J. (1982). The actions of cimetidine hydrochloride and mepyramine maleate in rat adjuvant arthritis. *Eur. J. Pharmacol.* 78:175–185.

Bartholomew, J. S., and Woolley, D. E. (1988). Plasminogen activator release from cultured murine mast cells. *Biochem. Biophys. Res. Commun.* 153:540–544.

Bromley, M., Fisher, W. D., and Woolley, D. E. (1984). Mast cells at sites of cartilage erosion in the rheumatoid joint. *Ann. Rheum. Dis.* 43:76–79.

Brown, M. A., Pierce, J. H., Watson, C. J., Falco, J., Ihle, J. N., and Paul, W. E. (1987). B cell stimulatory factor-1/interleukin-4 MRNA is expressed by normal and transformed mast cells. *Cell* 50:809–818.

Burd, P. R., Rogers, H. W., Gordon, J. R., Martin, C. A., Jayaraman, S., Wilson, S. D., Dvorak, A. M., Galli, S. J., and Dorf, M. E. (1989). Interleukin 3-dependent and -independent mast cells stimulated with IgE and antigen express multiple cytokines. *J. Exp. Med.* 170:245–257.

Burd, P. R., Costa, J. J., Metcalfe, D. D., and Siebenlist, U. (1990). Cytokine gene expression occurs via multiple pathways in primary murine bone marrow mast cells. *FASEB J.* 4:A1705.

Center, D. M. (1983). Identification of rat mast cell–derived chemoattractant factors for lymphocytes. *J. Allergy Clin. Immunol.* 71:29–35.

Cochrane, C. G., and Hawkins, D. (1968). Studies on circulating immune complexes. 3. Factors governing the ability of circulating complexes to localize in blood vessels. *J. Exp. Med.* 127:137–157.

Coderre, T. J., Basbaum, A. I., and Levine, J. D. (1989). Neural control of vascular permeability: Interactions between primary afferents, mast cells, and sympathetic efferents. *J. Neurophysiol.* 62:48–58.

Costa, J. J., Burd, P. R., Siebenlist, U., and Metcalfe, D. D. (1990). Primary mouse bone marrow mast cell cultures transcribe multiple cytokines in response to $FC_{\epsilon}RI$ crosslinking. *FASEB J.* 4:A1943.

Crisp, A. J., Chapman, C. M., Kirkham, S. E., Schiller, A. L., and Krane, S. M. (1984a). Articular mastocytosis in rheumatoid arthritis. *Arthritis Rheum.* 27:845–851.

Crisp, A. J., Roelke, M. S., Goldring, S. R., and Krane, S. R. (1984b). Heparin modifies intracellular cAMP in human trabecular bone cells and adherent rheumatoid synovial cells. *Ann. Rheum. Dis.* 43:628–634.

Dalldorf, F. G., Anderle, S. K., Brown, R. R., and Schwab, J. H. (1988). Mast cell activation by group A streptococcal polysaccharide in the rat and its role in experimental arthritis. *Am. J. Pathol.* 132:258–264.

Dayer, J. M., Beutler, B., and Cerami, A. (1985). Cachectin/tumor necrosis factor stimulates collagenase and prostaglandin E2 production by human synovial cells and dermal fibroblasts. *J. Exp. Med.* 162:2163–2168.

Fassbender, H. G. (1975). *The Pathology of Rheumatic Diseases.* New York, Springer Verlag.

Folkman, J., Haudenshild, C. C., and Zetter, B. R. (1979). Long-term culture of capillary endothelial cells. *Proc. Natl. Acad. Sci. USA* 76:5217–5221.

Frieri, M., and Metcalfe, D. D. (1983). Analysis of the effect of mast cell granules on lymphocyte blastogenesis in the absence and presence of mitogens: Identification of heparin as a granule-associated suppressor factor. *J. Immunol.* 131:1942–1948.

Godfrey, H. P., Ilardi, C., Engber, W., and Graziano, F. M. (1984). Quantitation of human synovial mast cells in rheumatoid arthritis and other rheumatic diseases. *Arthritis Rheum.* 27:852–856.

Gorden, J. R., and Galli, S. J. (1990). Mast cells as a source of both preformed and immunologically inducible TNF-alpha/cachectin. *Nature* 346:274–276.

Grennan, D. M. (1975). Histamine receptors in the synovial microcirculation. *Eur. J. Clin. Invest.* 5:75–82.

Gruber, B. (1989). Activation of rheumatoid synovial mast cells: Role of IgE-associated globulins. *Monogr. Allergy* 26:120–134.

Gruber, B. L., and Schwartz, L. B. (1990). The mast cell as an effector of connective tissue degradation: A study of matrix susceptibility to human mast cells. *Biochem. Biophys. Res. Commun.*, 171:1272–1278.

Gruber, B., Poznansky, M., Boss, E., Partin, J., Gorevic, P., and Kaplan, A. P. (1986). Characterization and functional studies of rheumatoid synovial mast cells. Activation by secretagogues, anti-IgE, and a histamine-releasing lymphokine. *Arthritis Rheum.* 29:944–955.

Gruber, B. L., Kaufman, L. D., Marchese, M. L., Roth, W., and Kaplan, A. P. (1988a). Anti-IgE autoantibodies in systemic lupus erythematosus. Prevalence and biologic activity. *Arthritis Rheum.* 31:1000–1006.

Gruber, B., Ballan, D., and Gorevic, P. D. (1988b). IgE rheumatoid factors: quantification in synovial fluid and ability to induce synovial mast cell histamine release. *Clin. Exp. Immunol.* 71:289–294.

Gruber, B. L., Schwartz, L. B., Ramamurthy, N. S., Irani, A. M., and Marchese, M. J. (1988c). Activation of latent rheumatoid synovial collagenase by human mast cell tryptase. *J. Immunol.* 140:3936–3942.

Gruber, B. L., Marchese, M. J., Suzuki, K., Schwartz, L. B., Okada, Y., Nagase, H., and Ramamurthy, N. S. (1989). Synovial procollagenase activation by human mast cell tryptase dependence upon matrix metalloproteinase 3 activation. *J. Clin. Invest.* 84:1657–1662.

Helfgott, S., Caulfield, J.P., Hein, A., Brahn, E., Dynesius-Trentham, R. A., and Trentham, D. E. (1987). Arthritogenic factor stimulates mast cell degranulation and sequential immigration of neutrophils and monocytes into the knees of rats. *Arthritis Rheum.* 30 (Suppl.):S108 (abstract).

Jalkanen, S., Steere, A., Fox, R. I., and Butcher, E. C. (1986). A distinct endothelial cell recognition system that controls lymphocyte traffic into inflamed synovium. *Science* 233:556–558.

Klein, L. M., Lavker, R. M., Matis, W. L., and Murphy, G. F. (1989). Degranulation of human mast cells induces an endothelial antigen central to leukocyte adhesion. *Proc. Natl. Acad. Sci. USA* 86:8972–8976.

Lehman, T. J. A. (1988). *Lactobacillus casei* cell wall arthritis. In *CRC Handbook of Animal Models for the Rheumatic Diseases*. Vol. 1. Edited by H. S. Diamond and R. A. Greenwald. Boca Raton, FL., CRC Press, pp. 41–48.

Lehman, T. J. A., Allen, J. B., Plotz, P. H., and Wilder, R. L. (1983). Polyarthritis in rats following the systemic injection of *Lactobacillus casei* cell walls in aqueous suspension *Arthritis Rheum.* 26:1259–1265.

Lehman, T. J. A., Allen, J. B., Plotz, P. H., and Wilder, R. L. (1984). *Lactobacillus casei* cell wall–induced arthritis in rats: Cell wall fragment distribution and persistence in chronic arthritis-susceptible LEW/N and -resistant F344/N rats. *Arthritis Rheum.* 27:939–942.

Levine, J. D., Dardick, S. J., Roizen, M. F., Helms C., and Basbaum, A. I. (1986). Contribution of sensory afferents and sympathetic efferents to joint injury in experimental arthritis. *J. Neurosci.* 6:3423–3429.

Levine, J. D., Coderre, T. J., Covinsky, K., and Basbaum, A. I. (1990). Neural influences on synovial mast cell density in rat. *J. Neurosci. Res.* 26:301–307.

Malone, D. G., and Metcalfe, D. D. (1988). Demonstration and characterization of a transient arthritis following sensitization of synovial mast cells with antigen-specific IgE and parenteral challenge with specific antigen. *Arthritis Rheum.* 31:1063–1067.

Malone, D. G., and Dolan, P. W. (1990). Droperidol-fentanyl inhibits mast cell histamine release in rat synovium, but not skin, after immunologic activation. Evidence for mast cell heterogeneity. *J. Allergy Clin. Immunol.* 85:821–827.

Malone, D. G., Irani, A. M., Schwartz, L. B., Barrett, K. E., and Metcalfe, D. D. (1986). Mast cell numbers and histamine levels in synovial fluids from patients with diverse arthritides. *Arthritis Rheum.* 29:956–963.

Malone, D. G., Wilder, R. L., Saavedra-Delgado, A. M., and Metcalfe, D. D. (1987). Mast cell numbers in rheumatoid synovial tissues. Correlations with quantitative measures of lymphocytic infiltration and modulation by antiinflammatory therapy. *Arthritis Rheum.* 30:130–137.

Malone, D. G., Pierce, J. H., Falco, J. P., and Metcalfe, D. D. (1988). Production of granulocyte-macrophage colony-stimulating factor by primary cultures of unstimulated rat microvascular endothelial cells. *Blood* 71:684–689.

Malone, D. G., Vikingsson, A., Servi Seebruch, J., Verbsky, J. W., and Dolan, P. W. (1991). Effect of nonsteroidal anti-inflammatory drugs in vivo on rat skin and synovial mast cell-induced vasopermeability. *Arthritis Rheum.* 34:1116–1124.

Malone, D. G., Verbsky, J. W., and Dolan, P. W. (1991). A lavage method for dynamic intraarticular monitoring of animal joints in situ. Quantification and release kinetics of histamine following selective synovial mast cell activation by diverse secretagogues. *J. Lab. Clin. Med.* 118:269–279.

Metcalfe, D. D. (1984). Mast cell mediators with emphasis on intestinal mast cells. *Ann. Allergy* 53:563–575.

Mican, J. M., and Metcalfe, D. D. (1990). Arthritis and mast cell activation. *J. Allergy Clin. Immunol.* 86(pt 2):677–683.

Nawroth, P. P., and Stern, D. M. (1986). Modulation of endothelial cell hemostatic properties by tumor necrosis factor. *J. Exp. Med.* 163:740–745.

Norrby, K., Jakobsson, A., and Sörbo, J. (1986). Mast-cell-mediated angiogenesis: A novel experimental model using the rat mesentery. *Virchows Arch.* 52:195–206.

Plaut, M., Pierce, J. H., Watson, C. J., Hanley-Hyde, J., Nordan, R. P., and Paul, W. E. (1989). Mast cell lines produce lymphokines in response to cross-linkage of $Fc_{\epsilon}RI$ or to calcium ionophores. *Nature* 339:64–67.

Schreiber, A. B., Kenney. J., Kowalski, J., Thomas, K. A., Gimenez-Gallego, G., Rios-Candelore, M., Di Salvo, J., Barritault, D., Courty, J., and Courtois, Y. (1985). A unique family of endothelial cell polypeptide mitogens: the antigenic and receptor cross-reactivity of bovine endothelial cell growth factor, brain-derived acidic fibroblast growth factor, and eye-derived growth factor-II. *J. Cell Biol.* 101:1623–1626.

Schumacher, H. R., and Kitridou, R. C. (1972). Synovitis of recent onset. A clinicopathologic study during the first month of disease. *Arthritis Rheum.* 15:465–485.

Steffen, M., Abboud, M., Potter, G. K., Yung, Y. P., and Moore, M. A. S. (1989). Presence of tumour necrosis factor or a related factor in human basophil/mast cells. *Immunology* 66:445–450.

Tannenbaum, S., Oertel, H., Henderson, W. R., and Kaliner, M. (1980). The biologic activity of mast cell granules. I. Elicitation of inflammatory responses in rat skin. *J. Immunol.* 125:325–335.

Taylor, D. J., Yoffe, J. R., Brown, D. M., and Woolley, D. E. (1985a). Histamine H_2 receptors on chondrocytes derived from human, canine and bovine articular cartilage. *Biochem. J.* 225:315–319.

Taylor, D. J., Yoffe, J. R., and Woolley, D. E. (1985b). Mast-cell products and heparin stimulate the production of mononuclear-cell factor by cultured human monocyte/macrophages. *Biochem. J.* 230:83–88.

Taylor, D. J., Yoffe, J. R., Brown, D. M., and Woolley, D. E. (1986). Histamine stimulates prostaglandin E production by rheumatoid synovial cells and human articular chondrocytes in culture. *Arthritis Rheum.* 29:160–165.

van den Broek, M. F., van den Berg, W. B., and van de Putte, L. B. A. (1988). The role of mast cells in antigen induced arthritis in mice. *J. Rheumatol.* 15:544–551.

Van Loverern, H., Meade, R., and Askenase, P. W. (1983). An early component of delayed-type hypersensitivity mediated by T cells and mast cells. *J. Exp. Med.* 157:1604–1617.

Vickers, M. R., and Sykes, K. J. (1982). The effect of histamine on the development of adjuvant arthritis in the rat. *Agents Actions* 12:691–698.

Wasserman, S. I. (1984). The mast cell and synovial inflammation. Or, what's a nice cell like you doing in a joint like this? *Arthritis Rheum.* 27:841–844.

Wodnar-Filipowicz, A., Heusser, C. H., and Moroni, C. (1989). Production of the haemopoietic growth factors GM-CSF and interleukin-3 by mast cells in response to IgE receptor-mediated activation. *Nature* 33(6220):150–152.

Zuraw, B. L., O'Hair, C. H., Vaughn, J. H., Mathison, D. A., Curd, J. G., and Katz, D. H. (1981). Immunoglobulin E-rheumatoid factor in the serum of patients with rheumatoid arthritis, asthma, and other diseases. *J. Clin. Invest.* 68:1610–1613.

30

Mast Cell Disease

WILLIAM D. TRAVIS

National Cancer Institute
National Institutes of Health
Bethesda, Maryland

CHIN-YANG LI

Mayo Clinic
Rochester, Minnesota

I. Introduction

Systemic mast cell disease (SMCD) is a rare disease of unknown etiology characterized by the abnormal proliferation of mast cells with accumulation in organs such as the skin, liver, lymph node, spleen, and bone marrow (Brunning et al., 1983; Lennert and Parwaresch, 1979; Metcalfe et al. 1981; Mutter et al., 1963; Parwaresch et al., 1985; Yam et al., 1986; Webb et al., 1982). Although mast cell disease may primarily involve the skin in the form of urticaria pigmentosa (UP), this chapter will focus on SMCD.

For many years it has been known that survival in SMCD is not uniform. Most patients with SMCD have an excellent prognosis; however, a subset of patients do poorly with a survival of about 2–3 years (Lennert and Parwaresch, 1979; Webb et al., 1982). Until recently, little was known about how to predict the clinical course of SMCD. In addition, the classification of SMCD has been in a state of flux (Parwaresch et al., 1985; Lennert and Parwaresch, 1979; Sagher and Even-Paz, 1967). Recent studies performed on a group of patients from Mayo Clinic provide the basis for this review, which summarizes factors useful in predicting prognosis and addresses the issue of classification (Travis et al., 1985, 1986, 1988a, b, 1989b; Travis and Li, 1988).

II. Clinical Features

A. Urticaria Pigmentosa

UP can be divided into pediatric and adult forms (Travis et al., 1985; Myers, 1960; Mihm et al., 1973). The skin lesions of most patients with adult-onset UP diffusely involve the trunk and extremities, with a macular and/or papular appearance. Other unusual variants of UP include bullous, nodular, diffuse, pseudoxanthomatous, xanthomatous, and tumefactive UP (Travis et al., 1988b). Virtually all cases of adult UP are persistent, with only rare cases where the skin lesions appear to regress.

Pediatric UP presents most commonly as a solitary mastocytoma (Johnson and Helwig, 1961; Mihm et al., 1973; Myers, 1960). Disseminated or diffuse cutaneous forms of pediatric UP also occur (Mihm et al., 1973; Myers, 1960; Travis et al., 1988b). In approximately 80% of pediatric patients with UP, the skin lesions undergo spontaneous resolution (Travis et al., 1985). A small number of pediatric patients have diffuse cutaneous lesions, and rarely these patients may develop associated SMCD (Travis et al., 1985).

B. Systemic Mast Cell Disease

SMCD occurs in approximately 10% of patients with adult-onset UP (Sagher and Even-Paz, 1967). SMCD is very rare in children, even in those with UP (Kettelhut et al., 1985). In general, patients with SMCD are elderly, with a mean age of 56.5 years (range 17–80 years), and there is a slight male predominance. The majority of patients are between the ages of 50 and 80 years of age and virtually all patients are above 30 years of age (Fig. 1). Depending on the pattern of referral, UP can be found in 50–100% of patients with SMCD (Granerus and Roupe, 1982; Mutter et al., 1963; Travis et al., 1988b). If the referrals are collected from a dermatology clinic, UP may be found in 100% of SMCD patients (Olafsson, 1985). We found cutaneous lesions in 53% of patients, many of whom had hematological disorders (Travis et al., 1988a). Peptic ulcer disease can be found in 36% of cases, hepatomegaly in 41%, splenomegaly in 48%, and peripheral and central lymphadenopathy in 25% and 19% of cases, respectively (Fig. 2) (Travis et al., 1988b).

Patients with SMCD manifest a myriad of signs and symptoms, which can be divided into five major categories (Fig. 3) (Travis et al., 1988b). Constitutional signs and symptoms occurred in 55% of patients. Mast cell mediator–related signs and symptoms occurred in 60% of patients. Skin and bone symptoms occurred in 53% and 27.6% of patients, respectively. Anaphylactic episodes occurred in 14% of patients. The frequencies of the various types of skin and bone, mast cell mediator–related, and constitutional signs and symptoms are summarized in Figures 4–6 (Travis et al., 1988b).

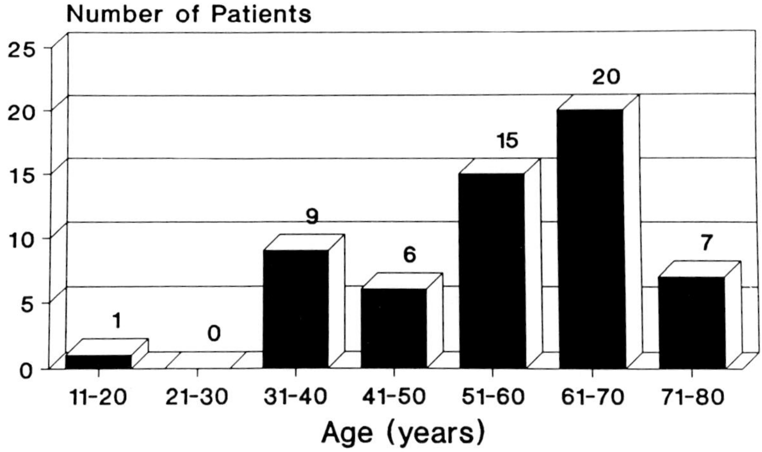

Figure 1 Age of 58 Mayo Clinic patients with SMCD by decade. [Modified from Travis et al. (1988b).]

Patients with well-differentiated forms of SMCD tend to present with more classical mast cell mediator–related signs and symptoms, while patients with more poorly differentiated forms of SMCD tend to present with more nonspecific constitutional signs and symptoms, such as fatigue, weight loss, fever, and ascites (Travis et al., 1988b).

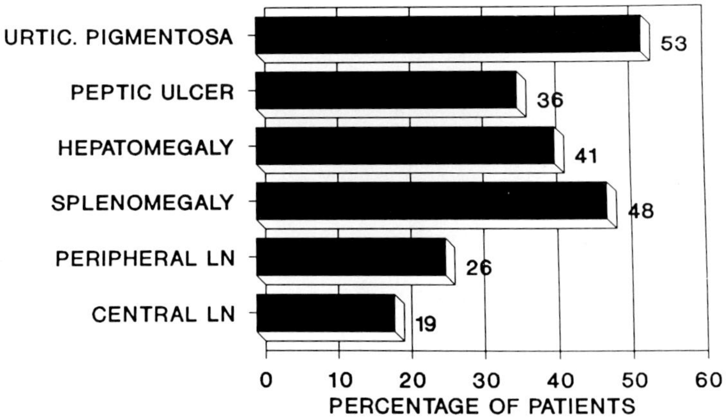

Figure 2 Percentage of SMCD patients affected by urticaria pigmentosa, peptic ulcer, hepatosplenomegaly, and lymphadenopathy. [Modified from Travis et al. (1988b).]

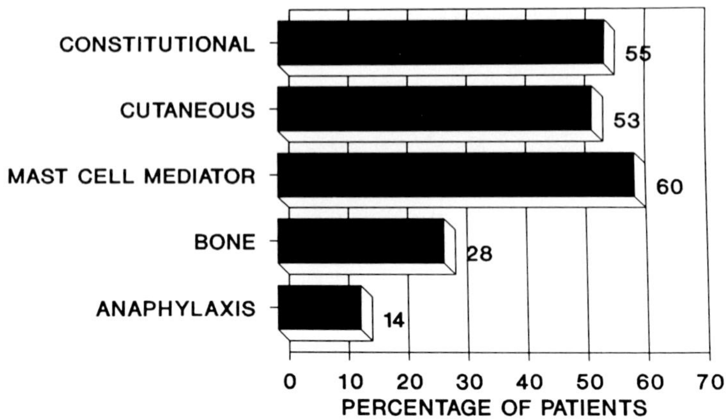

Figure 3 Percentage of SMCD patients affected by the five major categories of signs and symptoms of SMCD. [Modified from Travis et al. (1988b).]

Because of the wide variety of presenting manifestations, SMCD is often mistaken for a variety of disorders affecting the skin, bone, blood, and gastrointestinal tract. It may be confused with osteoporosis, metastatic carcinoma, chronic myelogenous leukemia, myelofibrosis, hypereosinophilic syndrome, irritable bowel, hepatitis, carcinoid syndrome, idiopathic anaphylaxis, or parasit-

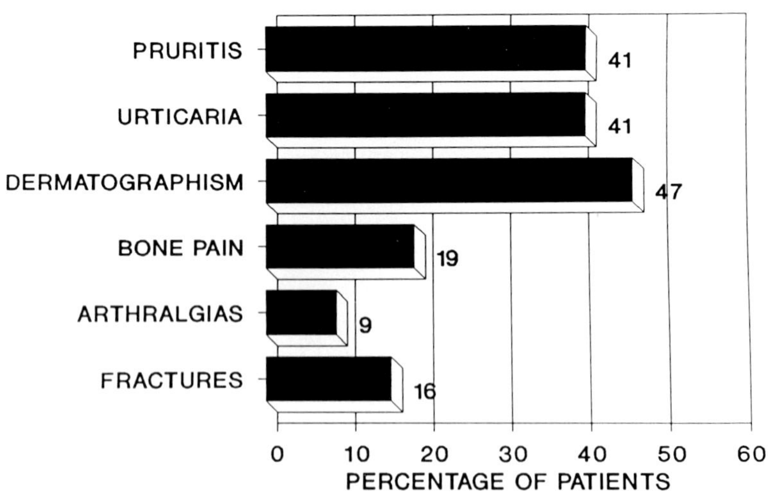

Figure 4 Percentage of SMCD patients affected by skin and bone signs and symptoms. [Modified from Travis et al. (1988b).]

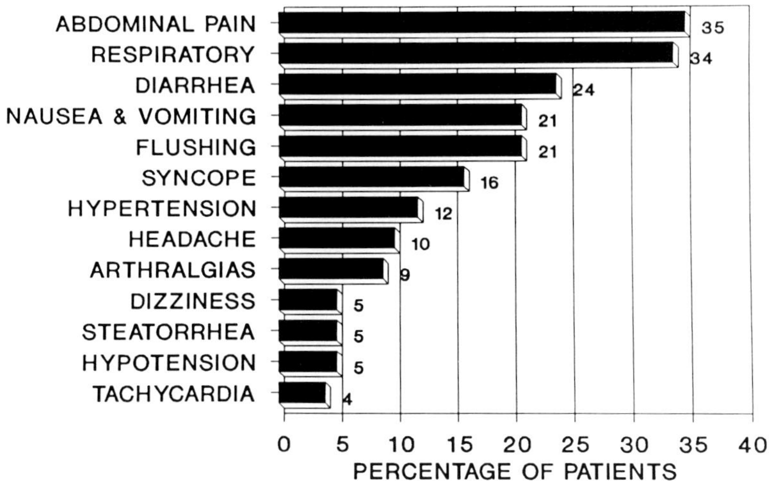

Figure 5 Percentage of patients affected by mast cell mediator–related symptoms. [Modified from Travis et al. (1988b).]

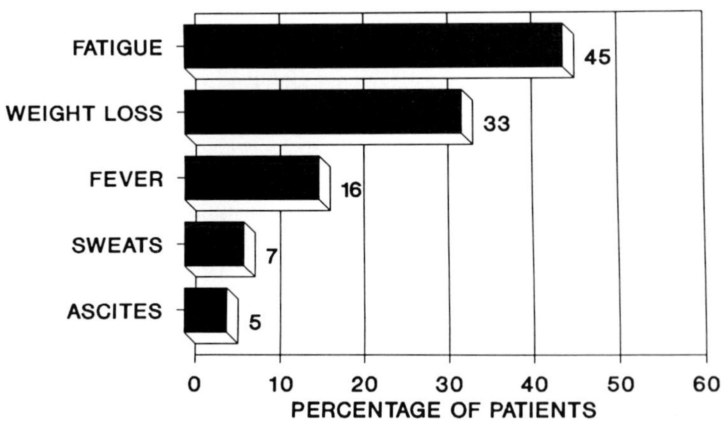

Figure 6 Percentage of SMCD patients affected by constitutional signs and symptoms. [Modified from Travis et al. (1988b).]

ic infection (Boxer, 1987; Yam et al. 1980; Travis et al., 1988b). As a result, these patients often undergo extensive medical evaluations, before the diagnosis is finally recognized.

III. Methods of Diagnosis

A. Urticaria Pigmentosa

The diagnosis of UP should be made in the appropriate clinical setting with confirmation by a skin biopsy (Travis et al., 1985; Mihm et al., 1973). Establishing the diagnosis may be relatively simple in patients with florid UP; however, the diagnosis is often overlooked in subtle cases, and other skin disorders can be confused with UP. For this reason, it is important to carefully correlate both clinical and pathological findings in a patient suspected to have UP. Interpretation of skin biopsies can be difficult since the skin of some patients demonstrates mild perivascular mast cell infiltrates. In such cases, care should be taken. It should also be considered that there is a wide variation in number of mast cells in normal skin, and increased mast cells can be found in biopsies from patients with a variety of skin conditions, including lichen planus, psoriasis, and histiocytosis X (Garriga et al., 1988; Mikhail and Miller-Milinska, 1964; Olafsson et al., 1986; Travis et al., 1988b).

B. Systemic Mast Cell Disease

Several approaches have been advocated for the diagnosis of SMCD, including clinical (Sagher and Even-Paz, 1967), pathological (Horny et al., 1985), biochemical (Friedman et al., 1989; Granerus and Roupe, 1982; Granerus et al., 1983; Granerus and Wass, 1984; Keyzer et al., 1983; Schwartz et al., 1987), radiological (Sagher et al., 1952; Huang et al., 1987), and scintigraphic (Rosenbaum et al., 1984) methods. However, since these methods do not detect abnormalities that are specific for SMCD, pathological confirmation should always be obtained. The optimal pathological specimen for demonstration of diagnostic lesions of SMCD is a bone marrow core biopsy of the iliac crest. Bone marrow aspirates seldom contain diagnostic lesions of SMCD since the aggregates of mast cells frequently remain attached to the trabeculae of bone; occasionally, SMCD lesions may be seen in bone marrow clot sections (Travis et al., 1988b; Lawrence, J., personal communication). In addition, mast cell hyperplasia frequently occurs in patients with myelodysplastic syndromes, leukemias, and lymphoproliferative disorders (Prokocimer and Polliack, 1981; Yoo and Lessin, 1982).

SMCD bone marrow infiltrates characteristically appear as focal aggregates of spindle-shaped mast cells frequently associated with eosinophils and lymphocytes (Fig. 7). The pattern of bone marrow mast cell infiltration is most commonly paratrabecular, followed by perivascular, parafollicular, and, more

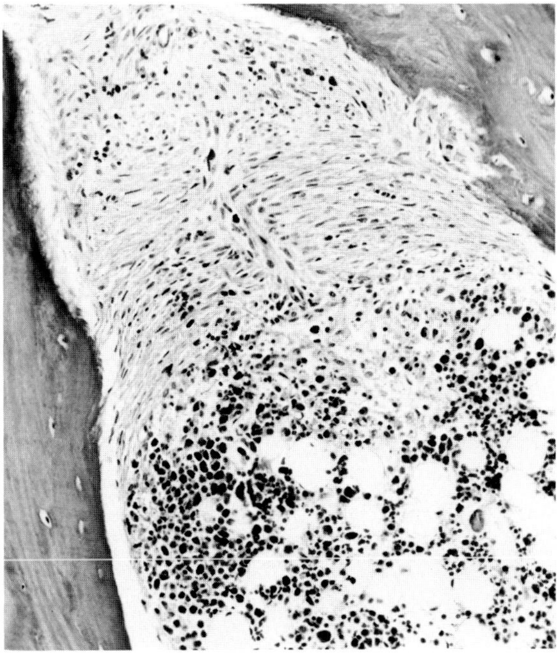

Figure 7 Photomicrograph of bone marrow from patient with indolent SMCD, demonstrating a paratrabecular aggregate of spindle-shaped mast cells. The adjacent hematopoietic marrow is normocellular. (Hematoxylin and eosin ×200).

rarely, diffuse involvement. These lesions are diagnostic of SMCD. However, they are often mistaken for other entities, such as granulomas, myelofibrosis, angioimmunoblastic lymphadenopathy, Hodgkin's disease, eosinophilic granuloma, and metastatic carcinoma. Diagnostic confusion often occurs since the metachromatic substances and enzyme activities are lost in the routine decalcification procedure used for processing bone marrow core biopsy specimens. This can be avoided if the bone marrow core biopsy is fixed in cold formalin and embedded in plastic (Travis et al., 1988b).

Not only does pathological evaluation of the bone marrow enable recognition of diagnostic SMCD infiltrates, it also provides an opportunity to identify important prognostic factors, such as decreased marrow fat, lobulated mast cell nuclei, and associated hematological disorders (Fig. 8, Table 1). While the SMCD infiltrates and the amount of marrow fat are best seen in sections of a core biopsy, the aspirate specimen is optimal for determining the presence of lobulated mast cell nuclei and for specific subclassification of hematological disorders.

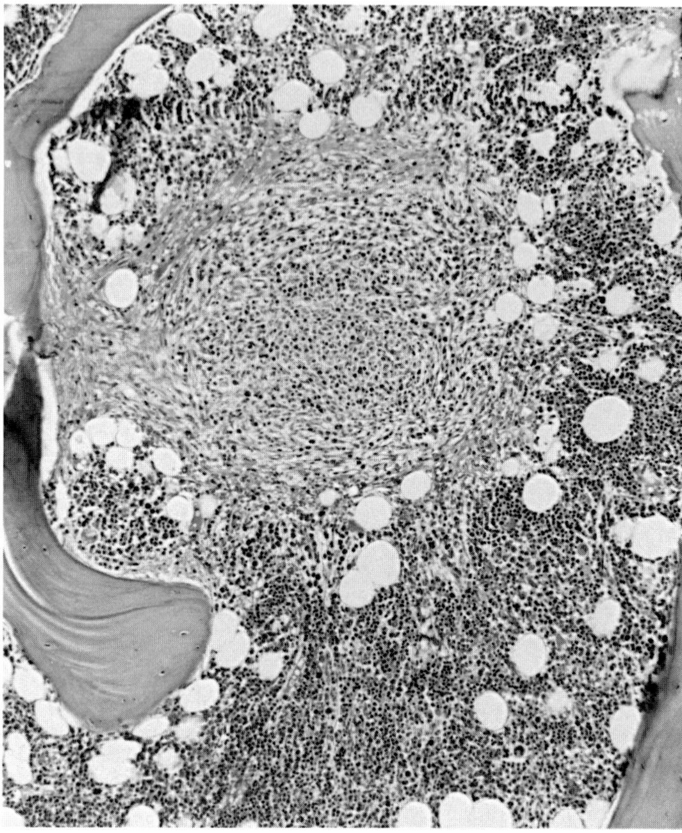

Figure 8 Photomicrograph of bone marrow from patient with SMCD and associated myelodysplastic disorder, demonstrating a nodular aggregate of oval to spindle-shaped mast cells. The adjacent hematopoietic marrow is hypercellular with a reduced number of fat cells. (Hematoxylin and eosin ×100).

The pathological diagnosis of SMCD can also be established based on specimens obtained from the lymph node, spleen, liver, and gastrointestinal tract (Travis and Li, 1988; Travis et al., 1988b). However, if biopsies of the liver or gastrointestinal tract do not reveal substantial mast cell infiltrates, a bone marrow biopsy should be performed to confirm the diagnosis, since in these organs it can be difficult to distinguish subtle infiltrates of SMCD from mast cell hyperplasia. It is not uncommon for the diagnosis of SMCD to be first recognized in specimens from the liver, lymph node, or spleen that are biopsied or removed for evaluation of unexplained hepatomegaly, lymphadenopathy, or

Table 1 Poor Prognostic Factors in SMCD Determined by Univariate Analysis

Factor	*p* (log-rank test)
Old age	0.036
Male sex	0.0029
Symptoms and signs	
Constitutional symptoms	0.0008
Absence of skin symptoms	0.018
Absence of urticaria pigmentosa	0.037
Absence of bone symptoms	0.023
Normal bone radiographically	0.022
Hepatomegaly	0.031
Splenomegaly	0.011
Laboratory findings	
Anemia	<0.0001
Thrombocytopenia	0.0005
Abnormal results on liver function tests	0.0078
Bone marrow findings	
Decreased bone marrow fat cells (<20%)	<0.0001
Lobulated mast cell nuclei (bone marrow aspirate)	0.0015
Associated hematological disorder at or before SMCD diagnosis	0.040

Source: Modified from Travis et al. (1988b).

splenectomy (Travis and Li, 1988; Horny et al., 1989; Yam et al., 1986; Norris et al., 1963).

IV. Survival and Prognostic Factors

The overall survival for SMCD patients is reduced compared to that for age- and sex-matched controls, and the majority of patients who die do so within the first 3 years, with a 3-year survival of approximately 50% (Travis et al., 1988b). Our primary goal in studying the Mayo Clinic patients with SMCD was to learn how to identify patients in this poor prognostic category at the time of initial diagnosis.

Univariate analysis revealed a group of factors that correlated with a poor survival (Table 1). Multivariate survival analysis revealed a model that identified old age, male sex, low hemoglobin, current or previous cancer, and lobulated mast cell nuclei as poor prognostic factors (Fig. 9) (Travis et al., 1989a). Using the Cox model, a score was generated for each patient based on the weighted sum of these variables. The scores for these patients were divided into three equal-sized groups, and survival curves were generated for each group (Travis

$$
\begin{aligned}
\text{SCORE} = {} & 4 + [0.02 \times \text{Age (yrs)}] \\
& - [0.3 \times \text{Hemoglobin (g/dl)}] \\
& + 1.6, \text{ if male} \\
& + 1.8, \text{ if has or has had cancer} \\
& + 0.9, \text{ if lobulated MC nuclei}
\end{aligned}
$$

Figure 9 Model derived by multivariate survival analysis allows calculation of a score for each SMCD patient based on the weighted sum of the variables. [Modified from Travis et al. (1988b).]

et al., 1988b). The differences in survival for these groups attested to the significance of the variables identified in the multivariate model (Travis et al., 1988b).

V. Classification

A. Urticaria Pigmentosa

UP can be divided into a variety of morphological forms, including macular, papular, maculopapular, bullous, nodular, diffuse, tumefactive, xanthoatous, and pseudoxanthomatous (Mihm et al., 1973; Travis et al., 1985; Travis et al., 1988b). UP can also be classified into solitary or diffuse variants and adult or pediatric subtypes (Sagher and Even-Paz, 1967; Travis et al., 1985).

B. SMCD

We recently proposed that SMCD be classified into four major categories (Travis et al., 1988b) (Table 2, Fig. 10). SMCD has previously been classified into benign and malignant forms (Horny et al., 1983, 1986; Friedman et al., 1989; Webb et al., 1982; Travis et al., 1988b). We prefer to use the term indolent rather than benign for patients with favorable prognostic features since benign implies that a patient invariably will have a good prognosis. We have seen patients in this category suffer severe symptomatic manifestations, including life-threatening anaphylaxis, and rarely these patients may subsequently develop a fatal hematological disorder. We prefer not to use the terms benign and malignant since they imply a sharp distinction; we believe that SMCD is more complex than these terms imply and that the distinction is not always clear-cut.

Table 2 Classification of SMCD

I.	Indolent SMCD
II.	SMCD with associated hematological disorders
III.	Mast cell leukemia
IV.	Aggressive SMCD

This is supported by our finding that multiple clinical, laboratory, radiographic, and pathological factors may be necessary to predict prognosis in SMCD.

Patients with indolent SMCD must be separated from those who fall into poor prognostic categories (Fig. 10). This is possible in most cases at the time of initial diagnosis using the poor prognostic factors identified in our study (Table 1, Fig. 9). The patients with poor prognostic factors in our study fell into three major categories: (1) those with hematological disorders as defined by standard clinical and histopathological criteria; (2) those with mast cell leukemia; (3) those with aggressive SMCD, who had poor prognostic factors but did not have either a recognizable hematological disorder or mast cell leukemia. Some of these patients had a lymphoma-like course with extensive lymph node infiltration while others had more nonspecific constitutional signs and symptoms, such as fatigue, weight loss, and portal hypertension with ascites. Similar patients have been recognized at the National Institutes of Health (NIH) and reported under the term "lymphadenopathic mastocytosis with eosinophilia" (Meggs et al., 1985).

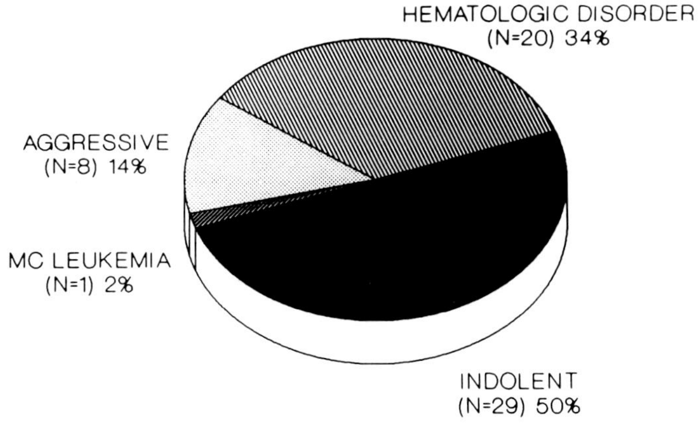

Figure 10 Percentage of patients in each category of SMCD. [Modified from Travis et al. (1988b).]

Indolent SMCD

The majority of patients with indolent SMCD will have urticaria pigmentosa and other manifestations typical of SMCD, such as bone, gastrointestinal, and mast cell mediator–related signs and symptoms. Although the absence of UP is a poor prognostic factor, a small subset of patients with indolent SMCD will not have skin involvement (Travis et al., 1988b). Patients with indolent SMCD will have a low score (less than 3.50) using the model generated by multivariate survival analysis (Fig. 9) (Travis et al., 1988b, 1989a). Most of these patients will have an excellent prognosis.

SMCD with Associated Hematological Disorders

We found distinct hematological disorders in one-third of patients with SMCD (Travis et al., 1988a). A spectrum of hematological disorders occurred, most commonly myelodysplastic disorders, followed by myeloproliferative disorders, acute nonlymphocytic leukemia, malignant lymphoma, and chronic neutropenia (Fig. 11). Thus, the myeloid hematopoietic cell line was affected in 86% of cases, and the lymphoid cell line in 14% of cases.

The hematopoietic bone marrow in these patients was typically hypercellular, with decreased marrow fat and increased hematopoietic elements (Fig. 8). In these cases the SMCD lesions were often overlooked owing to the prominent abnormalities in the adjacent marrow.

Hematological disorders were defined by previously described clinical and hematopathological criteria for classification of myelodysplastic disorders (Bennett et al., 1982; Travis and Pierre, 1985), myeloproliferative disorders

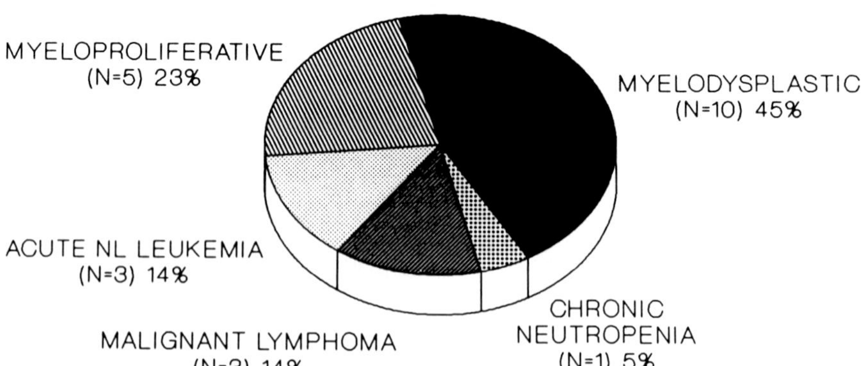

Figure 11 Different types of hematological disorders and percentage of SMCD patients with each type of disorder. [Modified from Travis et al. (1988a).]

(Laszlo, 1975), acute nonlymphocytic leukemia (Bennett et al., 1985a, b), malignant lymphoma (Non-Hodgkin's Lymphoma Pathologic Classification Project, 1982), and chronic neutropenia (Dale et al., 1979).

The 5-year survival of SMCD patients with hematological disorders as a group was 30%, compared with 60% for patients without them (Travis et al., 1988a). The significantly reduced survival for this group of patients emphasizes the importance of recognizing these hematological syndromes.

The close relationship between SMCD and hematological disorders observed in our experience supports the concept that SMCD represents a hematopoietic, stem cell–derived, myeloproliferative disorder with potential for multilineage neoplastic transformation, which appears to predominantly affect the myeloid cell line. It is also consistent with recent evidence in mice and in humans that mast cells are derived from a pluripotent hematopoietic stem cell (Denburg et al., 1983, 1986; Galli, 1987; Ishizaka et al., 1976; Horton and O'Brien, 1983; Nakano et al., 1987).

We observed not only hematological malignancies, but also solid tumors in patients with SMCD (Travis et al., 1989b). The majority of these malignancies presented before or within 12 months of the diagnosis of SMCD. Statistical analysis did not indicate that SMCD patients had an increased incidence of malignancy subsequent to the diagnosis of SMCD (Travis et al., 1989b). There are several reasons why it is important to recognize this potential association with SMCD. First, both solid and hematological malignancies can adversely affect prognosis of SMCD patients. Although the signs and symptoms of malignancy may overshadow the SMCD, recognition of SMCD is important since these patients may have skin or mast cell mediator–related symptoms that can be controlled with appropriate therapy. In a cancer patient, these symptoms might easily be overlooked and considered a complication related to their neoplasm or antineoplastic therapy. Second, while the distribution of solid malignancies appears to be random, the predominance of hematological disorders suggests that SMCD is a myeloproliferative disorder (Travis et al., 1989b).

Mast Cell Leukemia

Mast cell leukemia is the most poorly differentiated of all forms of SMCD. Based on our observations in a single case and a review of the literature, we recently proposed criteria for the diagnosis of mast cell leukemia: (1) mast cells representing at least 10% of all circulating white blood cells; (2) atypical mast cell morphology; (3) diffuse bone marrow infiltration by mast cells; and (4) cytochemical and or ultrastructural features consistent with a mast cell origin (Travis et al., 1986). These patients presented with prominent constitutional signs and symptoms. The survival for patients with mast cell leukemia was the worst of all types of SMCD patients, with a mean survival of 5.2 months (range 2–9 months) (Travis et al., 1986).

Aggressive SMCD

Patients with aggressive SMCD comprise those with poor prognostic factors and a high score using the model derived by multivariate survival analysis (Travis et al., 1988b, 1989a) who do not have mast cell leukemia or a morphologically detectable associated hematological disorder. Some of these patients have a lymphoma-like course with massive lymph node involvement and lymphadenopathy. A group of patients that fits this description has been described from NIH as lymphadenopathic mastocytosis with eosinophilia (Meggs et al., 1985). The remaining patients may present with nonspecific constitutional signs and symptoms, such as fever, weight loss, and ascites.

VI. Chromosomal Abnormalities

We have previously found cytogenetic abnormalities in bone marrow specimens from 5 of 11 SMCD patients (Table 3) (Travis et al., 1986, 1988a). Four patients with associated hematological disorders had chromosomal changes typically seen in patients with dysplastic or neoplastic myeloid disorders (Travis et al., 1988a). This supports our observation that SMCD patients develop genuine dysplastic and neoplastic myeloid hematological disorders that are distinct from SMCD.

The fifth patient with an abnormal result had mast cell leukemia and an

Table 3 Chromosomal Abnormalities in Patients with SMCD

Type of SMCD	Chromosomal abnormality
Associated hematological disorder	
Refractory anemia with excess blasts in transformation	48,XY,+8,+11 [AA]
Chronic myelomonocytic leukemia	46,XY,del(13)(q12,q22) [AA]
Refractory anemia with excess blasts	15 metaphases: 51,XY,+6,+8,+10,+15,+19
	5 metaphases: 46,XY [AN]
Agnogenic myeloid metaplasia, cellular phase in blast crisis	4 metaphases: 45,XY,–7
	3 metaphases: 46,XY [AN]
Mast cell leukemia	46,XX,dir ins (10,16)(q2?2;q13q22) [AA]

Source: Data from Travis et al. (1986, 1988a).

insertion translocation involving chromosomes 10 and 16 (Travis et al., 1986). Whether this represents a specific marker for mast cell leukemia remains to be investigated in additional cases.

VII. Therapy for SMCD

There is no effective therapy for SMCD. Efforts to treat SMCD are directed primarily at controlling mast cell mediator–related symptoms. The most useful medications include antihistamines such as H_1 blockers, particularly diphenhydramine and chlorpheniramine, and H_2 antagonists such as cimetidine, cromolyn, and cyproheptadine (Frieri et al., 1985; Horan et al., 1990; Travis et al., 1988b). Patients who develop acute episodes of anaphylaxis with hypotensive shock should be treated with epinephrine administered intravenously (Travis, 1988b).

Patients with malignancies should receive chemotherapy or radiation therapy, according to the associated neoplasm. Chemotherapy has not been effective in treating mast cell leukemia (Travis et al., 1986). Splenectomy may have value in patients with associated hematological disorders or aggressive SMCD (Friedman et al., 1990).

Discussion

Dvorak: What happens to basophils in mast cell leukemia?

Travis: We did not identify basophil abnormalities in our case of mast cell leukemia.

Sullivan: What are the causes of death in the mastocytosis patients without neoplasia?

Travis: In the small number of our patients who died, one died of peptic ulcer–associated gastrointestinal hemorrhage, and another died of a myocardial infarction. The majority of patients died of complications related to an associated neoplasm and two patients died of anaphylaxis.

Kaliner: Can you speculate why in benign mastocytosis, which is associated with mast cell mediator release, there is no increase in eosinophil numbers?

Travis: Mast cell infiltrates in the tissues in patients with mastocytosis are frequently associated with eosinophils. Why the majority of patients with benign disease do not have marked peripheral eosinophilia is not known.

Galli: Are there specific chromosomal abnormalities in patients with mastocytosis?

Travis: We reported chromosomal abnormalities characteristic of myeloid disorders in four patients with mastocytosis with an associated hematological disorder, but no consistent abnormality was seen.

References

Bennett, J. M., Catovsky, D., Daniel, M-T., Flandrin, G., Galton, D. A. G., Gralnick, H. R., and Sultan, C. (1982). Proposals for the classification of the myelodysplastic syndromes. The French-American-British Cooperative Group. *Br. J. Haematol.* 51:189–199.

Bennett, J. M., Catovsky, D., Daniel, M. T., Flandrin, G., Galton, D. A. G., Gralnick, H. R., and Sultan C. (1985a). Proposed revised criteria for the classification of acute myeloid leukemia. A Report of the French-American-British Cooperative Group. *Ann. Intern. Med.* 103:620–629.

Bennett, J. M., Catovsky, D., Daniel, M-T., Flandrin, G., Galton, D. A. G., Gralnick, H. R., and Sultan, C. (1985b). Criteria for the diagnosis of acute leukemia of megakaryocyte lineage (M7). A report of the French-American-British Cooperative Group. *Ann. Intern. Med.* 103:460–462.

Boxer, M., Greenberger, P. A., and Patterson, R. (1987). Clinical summary and course of idiopathic anaphylaxis in 73 patients. *Arch. Intern. Med.* 147:269–272.

Brunning, R. D., McKenna, R. W., Rosai, J., Parkin, J. L., and Risdall, R. (1983). Systemic mastocytosis, extracutaneous manifestations. *Am. J. Surg. Pathol.* 7:425–438.

Dale, D. C., Guerry, D., Wewerka, J. R., Bull, J. M., and Chusid, M. J. (1979). Chronic neutropenia. *Medicine* 58:128–144.

Denburg, J. A., Richardson, M., Telizyn, S., and Bienenstock, J. (1983). Basophil/mast cell precursors in human peripheral blood. *Blood* 61:775–780.

Denburg, J. A., Telizyn, S., Ahlstedt, S., Olafsson, J. H., Roupe, G., and Bienenstock, J. (1986). Basophil/mast cell precursors in mast cell proliferative disorders. *Clin. Invest. Med.* 9:21–25.

Friedman, B. S., Steinberg, S. C., Meggs, W. J., Kaliner, M. A., Frieri, M., and Metcalfe, D. D. (1989). Analysis of plasma histamine levels in patients with mast cell disorders. *Am. J. Med.* 87:649–654.

Friedman, B., Darling, G., Norton, J., Hamby, L., and Metcalfe, D. (1990). Splenectomy in the management of systemic mast cell disease. *Surgery* 107:94–100.

Frieri, M., Alling, D. W., and Metcalfe, D. D. (1985). Comparison of the therapeutic efficacy of cromolyn sodium with that of combined chlorpheniramine and cimetidine in systemic mastocytosis, results of a double-blind clinical trial. *Am. J. Med.* 78:9–14.

Galli, S. J. (1987). New approaches for the analysis of mast cell maturation, heterogeneity, and function. *Fed. Proc.* 46:1906–1914.

Garriga, M. M., Friedman, M. M., and Metcalfe, D. D. (1988). A survey of the number and distribution of mast cells in the skin of patients with mast cell disorders. *J. Allergy Clin. Immunol.* 82:425–432.

Granerus, G., and Roupe, G. (1982). Increased urinary methylimidazoleacetic acid (MelmAA) as an indicator of systemic mastocytosis. *Agents Actions* 12:29–31.

Granerus, G., and Wass, U. (1984). Urinary excretion of histamine, methylhistamine (1-MeHi) and methylimidazoleacetic acid (MelmAA) in mastocytosis: comparison of new HPLC methods with other present methods. *Agents Actions* 14: 341–345.

Granerus, G., Olafsson, J. H., and Roupe, G. (1983). Studies on histamine metabolism in mastocytosis. *J. Invest. Dermatol.* 80:410–416.

Horny, H-P., Parwaresch, M. R., and Lennert, K. (1983). Klinisches Bild und Prognose generalisierter Mastoytosen. *Klin. Wochenschr.* 61:785–793.

Horny, H-P., Parwaresch, M. R., and Lennert, K. (1985). Bone marrow findings in systemic mastocytosis. *Hum. Pathol.* 16:808–814.

Horny, H-P., Parwaresch, M. R., Kaiserling, E., Muller, K., Olbermann, M., Mainzer, K., and Lennert, K. (1986). Mast cell sarcoma of the larynx. *J. Clin. Pathol.* 39:596–602.

Horny, H-P., Kaiserling, E., Campbell, M., Parwaresch, M. R., and Lennert, K. (1989). Liver findings in generalized mastocytosis. A clinicopathologic study. *Cancer* 63:532–538.

Horton, M. A., and O'Brien, H. A. W. (1983). Characterization of human mast cells in long-term culture. *Blood* 62:1251–1260.

Huang, T. Y., Yam, L. T., and Li, C. Y. (1987). Radiological features of systemic mast-cell disease. *Br. J. Radiol.* 60:765–770.

Ishizaka, T., Okudaira, H., Mauser, L. E., and Ishizaka, K. (1976). Development of rat mast cells *in vitro*. I. Differentiation of mast cells from thymus cells. *J. Immunol.* 116:747–754.

Johnson, W. C., and Helwig, E. B. (1961). Solitary mastocytosis (urticaria pigmentosa). *Arch. Dermatol.* 84:806–15.

Kettelhut B. U., Parker, R. I., Travis W. D., Metcalfe, D. D. (1989). Hematopathology of the bone marrow in pediatric cutaneous mastocytosis: a study of seventeen patients. *Am. J. Clin. Pathol.* 91:558–62.

Keyzer, J. J., de Monchy, J. G. R., van Doormaal, J. J., and van Voorst Vader, P. C. (1983). Improved diagnosis of mastocytosis by measurement of urinary histamine metabolites. *N. Engl. J. Med.* 309:1603–1605.

Laszlo, J. (1975). Myeloproliferative disorders (MPD): Myelofibrosis, myelosclerosis, extramedullary hematopoiesis, undifferentiated MPD, and hemorrhagic thrombocythemia. *Semin. Hematol.* 12:409–432.

Lennert, K., and Parwaresch, M. R. (1979). Mast cells and mast cell neoplasia: A review. *Histopathology* 3:349–365.

Meggs, W., Friedman, M. M., Kramer, N., and Metcalfe, D. D. (1985). Lymphadenopathic mastocytosis with eosinophilia. *Clin. Res.* 33:162A (abstract).

Metcalfe, D. D., Kaliner, M., and Donlon, M. A. (1981). The mast cell. *CRC Crit. Rev. Immunol.* 2:23–74.

Mihm, M. C., Clark, W. H., Reed, R. J., and Caruso, M. G. (1973). Mast cell infiltrates of the skin and the mastocytosis syndrome. *Hum. Pathol.* 4:231–239.

Mikhail, G. R., and Miller-Milinska, A. (1964). Mast cell population in human skin. *J. Invest. Dermatol.* 43:249–254.

Mutter, R. D., Tannenbaum, M., and Ultmann, J. E. (1963). Systemic mast cell disease. *Ann. Intern. Med.* 59:887–906.

Myers, J. (1960). Diagnosis: Urticaria pigmentosa. *Arch. Dermatol.* 81:199–200.

Nakano, T., Kanakura, Y., Nakahata, T., Matsuda, H., and Kitamura, Y. (1987). Genetically mast cell-deficient *W/Wv* mice as a tool for studies of differentiation and function of mast cells. *Fed. Proc.* 46:1920–1923. 1987.

Non-Hodgkin's Lymphoma Pathologic Classification Project (1982). National Cancer Institute sponsored study of classifications of non-Hodgkin's lymphomas. Summary and description of a working formulation for clinical usage. *Cancer* 49:2112–2135.

Norris, H. T., Zamcheck, N., and Gottleib, L. S. (1963). The presence and distribution of mast cells in the human gastrointestinal tract. *Gastroenterology* 44:448–455.

Olafsson, J. H. (1985). Cutaneous and systemic mastocytosis in adults. A clinical, histopathological and immunological evaluation in relation to histamine metabolism. *Acta Derm.-venereol.* 115(Suppl.):1–43.

Olafsson, J. H., Roupe, G., and Enerback, L. (1986). Dermal mast cells in mastocytosis: Fixation, distribution and quantitation. *Acta Derm. Venerol. (Stockh).* 66:16–22.

Parwaresch, M. R., Horny, H-P., and Lennert, K. (1985). Tissue mast cells in health and disease. *Pathol. Res. Pract.* 179:439–461.

Prokocimer, M., and Polliack, A. (1981). Increased bone marrow mast cells in preleukemic syndromes, acute leukemia, and lymphoproliferative disorders. *Am. J. Clin. Pathol.* 75:34–38.

Rosenbaum, R. C., Frieri, M., and Metcalfe, D. D. (1984). Patterns of skeletal scintigraphy and their relationship to plasma and urinary histamine levels in systemic mastocytosis. *J. Nucl. Med.* 25:859–864.

Sagher, F., and Even-Paz, Z. (1967). *Mastocytosis and the Mast Cell.* Chicago, Year Book Medical Publishers.

Sagher, F., Cohen, C., and Schoor, S. (1952). Concomitant bone changes in urticaria pigmentosa. *J. Invest. Dermatol.* 18:425–432.

Schwartz, L. B., Metcalfe, D. D., Miller, J. S., Earl, H. E., and Sullivan, T. (1987). Tryptase levels as an indicator of mast-cell activation in systemic anaphylaxis and mastocytosis. *N. Engl. J. Med.* 316:1622–1626.

Travis, W. D., and Li, C-Y. (1988). Pathology of the lymph node and spleen in systemic mastocytosis. *Modern Pathol.* 1:4–14.

Travis, W. D., and Pierre, R. V. (1985). Preleukemia/dysmyelopoietic syndrome. *Lab. Med.* 16:157–163.

Travis, W. D., Li, C-Y., and Su, W. P. D. (1985). Adult-onset urticaria pigmentosa and systemic mast cell disease. *Am. J. Clin. Pathol.* 84:710–714.

Travis, W. D., Li, C-Y., Hoagland, H. C., Travis, L. B., and Banks, P. M. (1986). Mast cell leukemia: report of a case and review of the literature. *Mayo Clin. Proc.* 61:957–966.

Travis, W. D., Li, C-Y., Yam, L. T., Bergstralh, E. J., and Swee, R. G. (1988a). Significance of systemic mast cell disease with associated hematologic disorders. *Cancer* 62:965–972.

Travis, W. D., Li, C-Y., Bergstralh, E. J., Yam, L. T., and Swee, R. G. (1988b). Systemic mast cell disease. Analysis of 58 cases and literature review. *Medicine* 67:345–368.

Travis, W. D., Li, C-Y., Bergstralh, E. J., Yam, L. T., and Swee, R. G. (1989a). *Medicine* 69:34 (erratum).

Travis, W. D., Li, C-Y., and Bergstralh, E. J. (1989b). Solid and hematologic malignancies in 60 patients with systemic mast cell disease. *Arch. Pathol. Lab. Med.* 113:365–368.

Webb, T. A., Li, C-Y., and Yam, L. T. (1982). Systemic mast cell disease: A clinical and hematopathologic study of 26 cases. *Cancer* 49:927–938.

Yam, L. T., Yam, C-F., and Li, C-Y., (1980). Eosinophilia in systemic mastocytosis. *Am. J. Clin. Pathol.* 73:48–54.

Yam, L. T., Chan, C. H., and Li, C-Y. (1986). Hepatic involvement in systemic mast cell disease. *Am. J. Med.* 80:819–826.

Yoo, D., and Lessin, L. S. (1982). Bone marrow mast cell content in preleukemic syndrome. *Am. J. Med.* 73:539–542.

31

Mast Cells, Stromal Cells, and Inflammation

JUDAH A. DENBURG, SUSETTA FINOTTO, JEAN S. MARSHALL, MANEL JORDANA, and JERRY DOLOVICH

McMaster University
Hamilton, Ontario, Canada

SHIN-ICHI KAWABORI

Asahikawa Medical School
Asahikawa, Hokkaido, Japan

JOSEPH H. BUTTERFIELD

Mayo Clinic
Rochester, Minnesota

I. Introduction

Mast cells are prominent in a variety of inflammatory reactions and have been shown to be one of the principal cellular components of allergic reactions in both animals and humans. It has been postulated that the role of mast cells in allergic or nonallergic inflammation relates to the presence and release of many preformed and synthesized mediators of inflammation with multiple biological effects. Numerous investigators have shown the histological presence of and measured mediator product release from mast cells, particularly in models of allergic inflammation after antigen challenge.

The role of the tissue microenvironment in the process of mast cell accumulation has received much attention in recent years. In this chapter, we shall highlight some information regarding the accumulation of inflammatory effector cells at sites of allergic and related nonallergic tissue inflammation, pointing out parallels among mechanisms leading to accumulation of basophils, eosinophils, or mast cells. Recent information on mast cells in human upper respiratory tract tissues, principally the nasal mucosa, will be discussed as a model for studying the relationship among mast cells, stromal cells, and inflammatory reactions in humans.

II. Mast Cells in Allergic-Type Inflammation

It is well known that in allergic rhinitis and nasal polyposis with chronic rhinitis, as well as various forms of chronic bronchitis and asthma, there is the continued presence and activation of mast cells and other granulocytes such as basophils and eosinophils (Gibson et al., 1989a,b; Gleich, 1990; Frigas and Gleich, 1986; Beasley et al., 1989; Kawabori et al., 1991; Otsuka et al., 1985). Within nasal mucosal tissues undergoing allergic-type inflammation, evidence has been provided relating the presence of mast cells, eosinophils, basophils, and their progenitors within the nasal mucosal layers or in circulation to symptoms and severity of illness (Bousquet et al., 1990; Dolovich et al., 1990; Gomez et al., 1987; Otsuka et al., 1985, 1986a,b,c, 1987; Gibson et al., 1990).

Following similar techniques used in the delineation of mast cell heterogeneity in the rat, we and others demonstrated the presence of subtypes of mast cells within the nasal mucosa by histochemical criteria (Otsuka et al., 1985; Gomez et al., 1987; Kawabori et al., 1991). The presence of a formaldehyde-blockable mast cell (i.e., one that loses its metachromatic staining after formaldehyde fixation) was shown to be closely associated with symptoms and signs of allergic rhinitis (Otsuka et al., 1985). Moreover, fluctuations in peripheral blood progenitors for metachromatic cells (basophils or a subtype of mast cell) and eosinophils related inversely to the presence of these formaldehyde-sensitive mast cells in nasal mucosal tissues (Otsuka et al., 1986a,b,c).

Although it has been difficult to demonstrate definitively the lineage relationship between the colony metachromatic cells grown from peripheral blood hemopoietic stem cells and mast cells in the tissues, the dynamic, reciprocal relationship between the two in the above studies suggested to us a feedback mechanism between the local tissue microenvironment in the nasal mucosa and the peripheral blood. A unique, low-frequency basophilic cell progenitor was found to be apparently enriched in nasal polyp tissues, giving rise to formaldehyde-sensitive metachromatic cells in colonies (Otsuka et al., 1987). In a parallel experiment in primates, parenteral administration of certain cytokines with hemopoietic colony-stimulating activities such as IL-3 and GM-CSF, some of which can be generated by cells within the respiratory mucosa (Ohnishi et al., 1988a,b, 1989; Ohtoshi et al., 1991a; Vancheri et al., 1991), can give rise to changes in circulating progenitor cells for metachromatic cells and eosinophils (Valent et al., 1989b,c; Mayer et al., 1989; Saito et al., 1988; Donahue et al., 1988). These same cytokines are clearly in vitro stimulators of basophil, eosinophil, and mast cell growth and differentiation as well as activation (Valent et al., 1989b,c; Mayer et al., 1989; Saito et al., 1988; Donahue et al., 1988; Hutt-Taylor et al., 1988; Denburg et al., 1983, 1985a,b,c, 1989a; Furitsu et al., 1989; Owen et al., 1987; Leary and Ogawa, 1984; Tadokoro et al., 1983; Ogawa et al., 1983; Kirschenbaum et al., 1989; Rothenberg et al., 1987a,b; Haak-

Frendscho et al., 1988). It is thus hypothesized that in vivo release of these cytokines systemically as well as locally determines the type and extent of inflammatory cell ingress and differentiation.

Further analysis of the subtypes of mast cells by histochemical and immunohistochemical techniques, using several combined staining reactions, has revealed a sequential change in mast cell phenotype within the layers of the nasal polyp mucosal tissue (Kawabori et al., 1991; Irani et al., 1986). This is shown in Figure 1. As can be seen, the stromal layer contained a chymase- and tryptase-positive mast cell, which also stained with chloroacetate esterase and was formaldehyde-resistant in its metachromatic staining properties. In the epithelial layer, however, the majority of mast cells did not contain chymase and did not stain with chloroacetate esterase; these cells were also, for the most part, formaldehyde-sensitive in their metachromatic staining reaction. The metachromatic cells in nasal mucosal secretions in allergic rhinitis, by contrast, are tryptase- and chymase-negative, chloroacetate esterase-negative, and formaldehyde-sensitive, characteristics that are consistent with the morphological evi-

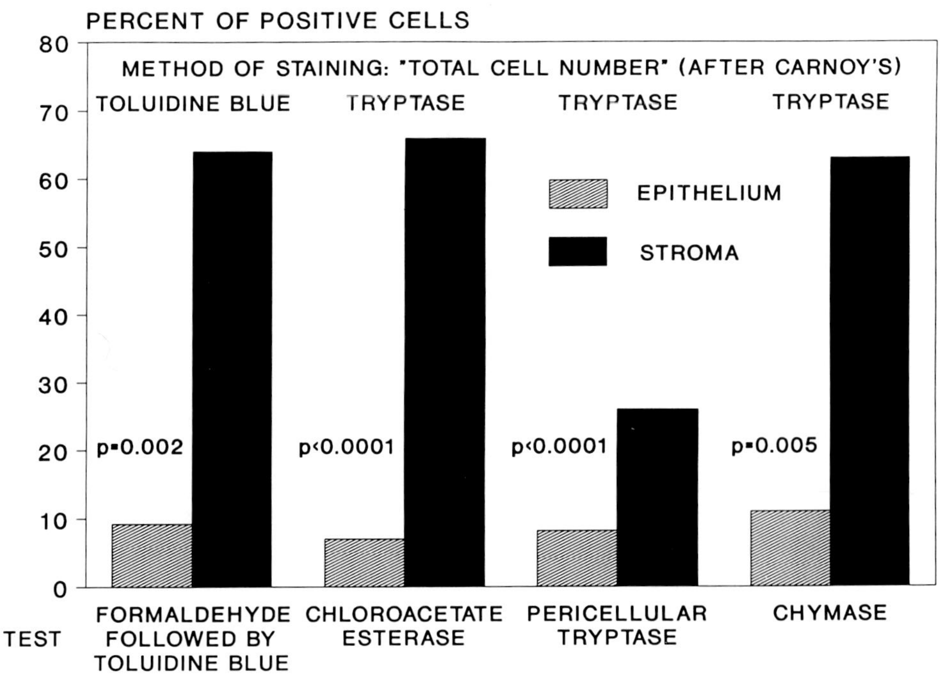

Figure 1 Subtypes of mast cells in human nasal polyp tissues by histochemical and immunohistochemical criteria.

dence for their designation as basophils (Irani et al., 1986; Bodger and Newton, 1987; Valent et al., 1989a; Stain et al., 1987). If one takes into account the studies of Enerbäck et al., (1986) showing an apparent transepithelial migration of mast cells during the course of natural allergen exposure using sequential biopsies, one can be led to postulate that the different mast cell subtypes present in nasal mucosal tissues such as the polyp represent different stages of maturation or activation of a progenitor for mast cells or for mast cells/basophils (Denburg et al., 1983, 1985a,b,c). The model of the nasal mucosal mast cell and its subtypes could thus be used to examine sources of mast cells in the human, by analogy to findings in experimental animal systems.

III. Sources and Lineages of Mast Cells

In the animal, either in graft-versus-host disease (Guy-Grand et al., 1984) or in nematode infestation (Denburg et al., 1980; Haig et al., 1982) there is clear-cut development of mucosa-associated mast cells in relation to immune stimulation and secretion of IL-3, but in the human this has been harder to pinpoint. The animal models reveal a progenitor-progeny kinetic relationship in that the mesenteric lymph nodes, bone marrow, and other tissues have varying numbers of progenitors for the mast cell at different points in time during the course of experimentally induced disease (Denburg et al., 1980; Schrader et al., 1981; Ihle et al., 1983). The closest approximation to this has been the finding of similar relationships between circulating granulocyte (basophil-eosinophil) progenitors and either natural or provoked allergen challenge in allergic individuals (Otsuka, 1986b,c; Gibson et al., 1990). While the basophil and the mucosal mast cell share some histochemical and immunohistochemical properties (Otsuka et al., 1986a; Denburg et al., 1986), the absence of tryptase is the distinguishing hallmark of the basophil and also of the metachromatic cell found in colonies from peripheral blood progenitors (Tsuda et al., 1991; Irani et al., 1986); in contrast, tryptase is present in virtually all mast cells that comprise the metachromatic cell population seen in the nasal mucosa and other parts of the respiratory tract, e.g., bronchial mucosa (Irani and Schwartz, 1989; Kawabori et al., 1991; and see Fig. 1).

Recent studies using fluorescence-activated cell sorting (FACS) analysis of a differentiating myeloid leukemic cell line, HL-60, in the presence of various cytokines, including IL-3, GM-CSF, IL-5, and nerve growth factor (NGF), the latter a cofactor in basophil/mast cell differentiation (Matsuda et al., 1988b; Tsuda et al., 1990, 1991), have revealed a remarkable uniformity in differentiation of the resulting histamine-containing, metachromatic cell lineage (Wong et al., 1990; Denburg et al., 1989b): the differentiated phenotype of the histamine-containing cell appears to be a tryptase-negative, BSP-1 (Bodger and Newton,

1987) and alcian blue–positive cell, most closely ascribable to the basophil lineage (Tsuda et al., 1991; Wong et al., 1990). However, intermediate stages of differentiation in this model suggest a transient, common precursor of the human basophil and mast cell, the latter distinguished by the presence of a mast cell–specific antigen, YB5B8 (Ashman et al., 1987; Wong et al., 1990). Indeed, in other recent studies reported in this volume, Ishizaka has shown that a newly described fibroblast-derived factor can promote mast cell differentiation of either tryptase (MC_T)- or tryptase/chymase (MC_{TC})-types in vitro (Furitsu et al., 1989). Moreover, Ogawa has recently observed tryptase-negative, large metachromatic cells in human cord blood cultures stimulated with stem cell factor (Ishizaka, T., personal communication), the ligand for the proto-oncogene, c-*kit* (Zsebo et al., 1990), which is also a mast cell growth factor in the rodent.

The above studies highlight the potential interrelationships in lineage of human mast cells and basophils. Whether the nasal polyp model outlined above can shed light on the basophil–mast cell lineage interrelationship in humans and the reason for the relationships between circulating basophil/eosinophil progenitors and mast cells in mucosal tissues of allergic individuals remains to be clarified. Information from our laboratory (Tanno et al., 1987; Denburg et al., 1991b) and recent experiments on interactions among IL-3, IL-5, and GM-CSF (Sillaber et al., 1991) have revealed that transforming growth factor-beta (TGF-β) and possibly a novel cytokine regulate reciprocal expression of basophils and eosinophils from a committed progenitor (Denburg et al., 1985a,c).

IV. Influence of the Tissue Microenvironment on Mast Cell Phenotype

Over the last few years, several investigators have examined phenotype switching in rodent mast cells and factors that influence this process (Levi-Schaffer et al., 1985; Serafin et al., 1987; Hamaguchi et al., 1987). Other investigators (Nakano et al., 1985; Sonoda et al., 1986) have developed the notion of bidirectional transdifferentiation of mast cells, directly linking the mucosal to connective tissue–type mast cell in lineage. Using mast cell–deficient W/W^v or Sl/Sl^d mice and marked mast cell granules from congenic beige *(bg)* mouse donors, the phenotype of the mast cell has been shown to be dependent on the local tissue microenvironment; e.g., a heparin-containing, connective tissue–type mast cell can arise from the mucosal type cell in the peritoneal microenvironment. Work by Levi-Schaffer et al. (1985) has focused on the fibroblast contribution to mast cell phenotype, demonstrating interactions between fibroblasts and mast cells in rodent systems; these studies extend the pioneering observations of Ginsburg (1963; Ginsburg and Lagunoff, 1967).

What effects fibroblasts and their factors have on human mast cell phenotype are not yet precisely known, although murine 3T3 fibroblasts release factor(s) that stimulate mast cell differentiation in humans (Furitsu et al., 1989; Kirschenbaum et al., 1989).

Recently Marshall et al. (1991) demonstrated that the mast cell population within the peritoneal cavity of the neonatal rat is morphologically and functionally distinct from its adult counterpart (see Table 1). Of particular interest is the low histamine content of this cell population and its reduced response to classic connective tissue–type, mast cell–specific secretagogues such as compound 48/80 (Marshall et al., 1990). This may explain why experimentally it has been possible to treat neonatal animals with relatively high doses of such agents without inducing anaphylaxis (Marshall et al., 1990). The majority of mast cells found within the peritoneal cavity of the 14-day-old neonatal rat have a lobulated or bilobed nuclear structure reminiscent of that observed within the basophils of other species. Similar nuclear morphology has been observed in the peritoneal mast cells of the adult rat and the intestinal mucosal mast cells of the rat following nematode parasite infection (Dvorak, 1983; Miller, 1971). However, basophils have not been well described in the rat, and the neonatal peritoneal mast cells contain granule-associated rat mast cell protease I (RMCPI), which is considered a specific marker for the connective tissue type of mast cell in the rat. The levels of the mucosal mast cell–specific protease RMCP-II were not increased in the neonatal mast cell population, suggesting that these neonatal peritoneal mast cells did not contain a substantial proportion of mast cells with a classic mucosal mast cell phenotype. Further studies of the maturation of mast cells during neonatal life and the role of various cytokines in this process should provide greater insight into the effects of microenvironment on mast cell development and function.

The neonatal rat has also provided a system in which one can examine the

Table 1 Comparison of Adult and Day 14 Neonatal Peritoneal Mast Cells

	Adult	Day 14 neonate
RMCP-I	+++	+++
RMCP-II	+	+
Histamine	15–20 pg/cell	1.5–2.5 pg/cell
Response to 48/80	+++	+
Response to NGF	+++	+
Response to substance P	++	++
Lobulated nuclei	Rare	Frequent

RMCP = rat mast cell protease; CTMC = connective tissue mast cells.

regulation of mast cell numbers within a variety of tissue sites. In early studies by Aloe and Levi-Montalcini (1977), 2.5S NGF, a substance known to be produced by a number of stromal cells, was shown to induce a mast cell hyperplasia. Our studies have extended these observations, as well as those on hemopoietic effects of NGF (Matsuda et al., 1988a,b; Tsuda et al., 1990, 1991) demonstrating that the NGF-induced CTMC hyperplasia is probably mediated by mast cell degranulation since this can be blocked by concurrent administration of the mast cell–stabilizing agent disodium cromoglycate and mimicked by the administration of mast cell degranulation products (Marshall et al., 1990). NGF appears to have a more direct effect on the development of RMCP-II-containing mucosal mast cells (Marshall et al., 1990). It is not yet clear to what extent these phenomena are limited to the microenvironments found within the neonatal animal; however, the ability of mast cell degranulation products to induce a mast cell hyperplasia has been observed in both neonatal and adult in vivo systems (Marshall et al., 1991). The recent demonstration of mast cell cytokine production in rodents (Wodnar-Filipowicz et al., 1989; Plaut et al., 1989) provides a mechanism whereby mast cells could potentially influence their own and other inflammatory cell differentiation and recruitment in allergic-type reactions. Indeed, production of tumor necrosis factor-alpha (TNF-α) by mast cells may be principally responsible for neutrophil ingress in IgE-dependent, mast cell–rich, late-phase skin reactions in mice (Wershil et al., 1991).

V. Hemopoietic Cytokines Produced by Respiratory Tract Structural Cells

Our attention has been focused on upper respiratory tract, allergic-type inflammation, using reconstructed tissue microenvironments from nasal mucosa in particular (Ohnishi et al., 1988a,b, 1989) and also from the bronchial mucosa (Jordana et al., 1989; Ohtoshi et al., 1991a,b; Vancheri et al., 1989, 1991; Denburg et al., 1989c, 1990b). Scrapings from the nasal epithelium were first shown to generate hemopoietic colony-stimulating factors for metachromatic cells and eosinophils (Ohnishi, 1988a,b, 1989). Primary pure cultures of nasal or bronchial structural cells, specifically epithelial cells and fibroblasts, have now been generated and their cytokine profiles assessed. These will now be discussed.

Nasal polyp, allergic rhinitis, or bronchial mucosal tissue–derived structural cells, either epithelial cells or fibroblasts, produce in vitro GM-CSF, IL-6, IL-8, and other as yet unidentified cytokines (Denburg et al., 1989c, 1990a,b; Ohtoshi et al., 1991a,b). It was shown by our group that nasal polyp structural cells, in contrast to those from normal nasal mucosa, were up-regulated in terms of cytokine production and responded better to proinflammatory stimuli such as

IL-1 and TNF-α in production of the above-mentioned cytokines (Denburg et al., 1989c, 1990a,b; Ohtoshi et al., 1991a,b). Expression of the genes for these cytokines was paralleled by increased protein product and varied according to clinical situations; the nasal polyp tissue structural cells represented a highly expressive, constitutively producing phenotype. Furthermore, IL-6, IL-8, and GM-CSF gene expression and production of protein could be down-regulated by corticosteroids in vitro (Ohtoshi et al., 1990), and antihistaminic drugs could block release of GM-CSF, TNF-α, and IL-1 from structural cells or alveolar macrophages (Denburg et al., 1990b, 1991a).

The influence of GM-CSF in particular on human basophil, and possibly mast cell, differentiation has been explored. Using both colony-forming assays in methylcellulose as well as differentiation of myeloid leukemic HL-60 cells to histamine-containing metachromatic cells, we have observed that the preponderant epithelial cell– or fibroblast-derived cytokine inducing this differentiation is GM-CSF (Ohtoshi et al., 1991a). A second factor that induces histamine production by HL-60 cells is present in T-cell supernatants and may be present in fibroblast-conditioned media, but has yet to be fully characterized (Denburg et al., 1991b, and unpublished data). The metachromatic cell phenotype differentiating in the HL-60 system under these conditions reveals a profile very similar to that of differentiating granulocytes, including basophils and eosinophils; tryptase is absent from these cells, which are also alcian blue–positive, safranin-negative, toluidine blue–positive, with sensitivity to formaldehyde (Wong et al., 1990; Tsuda et al., 1991). As stated earlier, there are phenotypically transitional forms between basophils and mast cells in these cultures (Table 2);

Table 2 Summary of FACS Analysis of Basophilic-Differentiating HL-60 Cells[a]

Phenotypic marker	Expression
CD15	↓
CD35	↑ ↑
CD11b	↑
CD25	↑
CD23	↑
BSP-1	↑ ↑
YB5.B8	↑

[a]See Hutt-Taylor et al. (1988).
Cf. Wong et al., 1990.
↓ = decreased, less than 10% of cells; ↑ = increased, less than 50% of cells; ↑ ↑ = increased, more than 50% of cells.

whether phenotype analysis can be used to show the existence in vivo of a transitional basophil/mast cell remains to be clarified.

With regard to effects on colony-forming cells, a full analysis of cytokines active in this process includes basophilic-differentiating effects of IL-3, IL-5, GM-CSF, and NGF as a synergizing cofactor (Matsuda et al., 1988a,b; Denburg et al., 1991b; Tsuda et al., 1991). In cord blood cultures, we and others have observed differentiation of basophils, eosinophils, and mast cells (Tanno et al., 1987; Saito et al., 1988; Ogawa et al., 1983; Furitsu et al., 1989; Kirschenbaum et al., 1989). Whether or not human mast cells, in addition to basophils and eosinophils, differentiate in cocultures of cord blood cells with up-regulated structural cells such as nasal polyp fibroblasts or epithelial cells remains to be determined.

VI. Human Mast Cell Phenotype: Influence of Airway Structural Cells

Recently, we have embarked on analysis of human mast cell phenotype, activation, and differentiation using reconstructed tissue microenvironments from the respiratory tract. Initial studies have revealed increased viability and attachment of rat peritoneal mast cells to human extracellular matrices and/or in the presence of respiratory tract tissue structural cell conditioned media (Finotto et al., unpublished). Recovery, viability, and attachment were increased in the presence of conditioned media and/or extracellular matrices, much in the same way as has been demonstrated for macrophages in this system (Jordana et al., unpublished).

To examine a physiological source of human mast cells relevant to the respiratory tract, we have embarked on cell separation and isolation of nasal polyp mast cells from the stromal and epithelial layers. Such mast cells show variations, in tissue sections, in histochemical and immunohistochemical properties (Kawabori et al., 1991; Dolovich et al., 1990). Indeed, on separation of the epithelial from stromal cell populations by density gradient differential centrifugation techniques, we have been able to isolate two populations of nasal polyp mucosal mast cells (Finotto et al., 1991). Table 3 shows the cell yields, recoveries, and compositions of these two populations. In preliminary studies, nasal stromal mast cells, primarily MC_{TC}-type, responded to anti-IgE with histamine release, while the epithelial population (primarily MC_T-type) did not (Finotto et al., 1991). Upon culture in the presence of conditioned media derived from nasal polyp structural cells, influences on mast cell phenotype have been observed (Table 4). A human mast cell leukemic line, HMC-1, aberrant though it is since it does not have IgE receptors (Butterfield et al., 1988), has been cocultured with respiratory tract structural cell-conditioned media; whereas

Discussion

Schleimer: Onishi, in your laboratory, has shown that colony formation is T-cell dependent. How much of the apparent increase in precursors in peripheral blood of challenged asthmatics or atopic subjects and in polyps is the result of changes in the T-cell compartment?
Denburg: The T-cell component serves to augment the phenomenon; however, Peter Gibson has used non-T, non-B cells and shown similar fluctuations in CFU-C.
Platts-Mills: What is the distribution of nerve fibers in nasal polyps?
Denburg: Kawabori, Jeffery, and Bienenstock have not been able to find nerve–mast cell associations in polyps. I do not know whether the polyp has any innervation.
Lichtenstein: What was the relationship between antigen challenge and cytokine levels?
Denburg: The relationship has yet to be worked out.
Platts-Mills: Do you use specific antigen in studies of polyps?
Denburg: Dolovich selects ragweed-only–positive patients on the basis of skin tests.

References

Aloe, L., and Levi-Montalcini, R. (1977). Mast cell increases in tissues of neonatal rats injected with nerve growth factor. *Brain Res.* 133:358–366.

Ashman, L. K., Gadd, S. J., Mayrhofer, G., Spargo, L. D. J., and Cole, S. R. (1987). A murine monoclonal antibody to an acute myeloid leukemia-associated antigen identifies tissue mast cells. In *Leucocyte Typing III,* Proceedings of the Third International Workshop and Conference on Human Leucocyte Differentiation Antigens. Edited by A. McMichel. London, Oxford University Press, pp. 726–731.

Beasley, R., Roche, W., Roberts, J. A., and Holgate, S. T. (1989). Cellular events in the bronchi in mild asthma and after bronchial provocation. *Am. Rev. Respir. Dis.* 139:806–817.

Bochner, B. S., Peachell, P. T., Brown, K. E., and Schleimer, R. P. (1988). Adherence of human basophils to cultured umbilical vein endothelial cells. *J. Clin. Invest.* 81:1355–1364.

Bodger, M. P., and Newton, L. A. (1987). The purification of human basophils: Their immunophenotype and cytochemistry. *Br. J. Haematol.* 67:281–284.

Bousquet, J., Chanez, P., Lacoste, J. Y., Barneon, G., Ghavanian, N., Enander, I., Verge, P., Ahlstedt, S., Simony-Lafontaine, J., Godard, P., Michel, F.-B. (1990). Eosinophilic inflammation in asthma. *N. Engl. J. Med.* 323:1033–1040.

Butterfield, J. H., Weiler, D., Dewald, G., and Gleich, G. J. (1988). Establishment of an immature mast cell line from a patient with mast cell leukemia. *Leuk. Res.* 12:345–355.

Denburg, J. A., Befus, A. D., and Bienenstock, J. (1980). Growth and differentiation in vitro of mast cells from mesenteric lymph nodes of *Nippostrongylus brasiliensis* infected rats. *Immunology* 41:195–202.

Denburg, J. A., Richardson, M., Telizyn, S., and Bienenstock, J. (1983). Basophil/mast cell precursors in human peripheral blood. *Blood* 61:775–780.

Denburg, J. A., Messner, H., Lim, B., Jamal, N., Telizyn, S., and Bienenstock, J. (1985a). Clonal origin of human basophil/mast cells from circulating multipotent hemopoietic progenitors. *Exp. Hematol.* 13:185–188.

Denburg, J. A., Telizyn, S., Belda, A., Dolovich, J., and Bienenstock, J. (1985b). Increased numbers of circulating basophil progenitors in atopic patients. *J. Allergy Clin. Immunol.* 76:466–472.

Denburg, J. A., Telizyn, S., Messner, H., Lim, B., Jamal, N., Ackerman, S. J., Gleich, G. J., and Bienenstock, J. (1985c). Heterogeneity of human peripheral blood eosinophil-type colonies: Evidence for a common basophil-eosinophil progenitor. *Blood* 66:312–318.

Denburg, J. A., Otsuka, H., Dolovich, J., Befus, A. D., and Bienenstock, J. (1986). Clinical relevance of basophil and mast cell growth and differentiation. In *Mast Cell Differentiation and Heterogeneity*. Edited by A. D. Befus, J. Bienenstock, and J. A. Denburg. New York, Raven Press, pp. 379–390.

Denburg, J. A., Dolovich, J., and Harnish, D. (1989a). Basophil/mast cell and eosinophil growth and differentiation factors in human allergic disease. *Clin. Exp. Allergy* 19:249–254.

Denburg, J. A., Hutt-Taylor, S. R., Dolovich, J., Switzer, J., and Harnish, D. G. (1989b). Factors influencing basophilic differentiation of HL-60 cells. *Int. Arch. Allergy Appl. Immunol.* 88:126–128.

Denburg, J. A., Jordana, M., Vancheri, C., Gauldie, J., Harnish, D. G., Ohtoshi, T., Tsuda, T., Gibson, P., Ruhno, J., Bienenstock, J., Hargreave, F. E., and Dolovich, J. (1989c). Locally derived hemopoietic cytokines for human basophils, mast cells and eosinophils in respiratory disease. In *Mast Cell and Basophil Differentiation and Function in Health and Disease*. Edited by S. Galli and K. F. Austen. New York, Raven Press, pp. 59–69.

Denburg, J. A., Dolovich, J., Ohtoshi, T., Cox, G., Gauldie, J., and Jordana, M. (1990a). The microenvironmental differentiation hypothesis of airway inflammation. *Am. J. Rhinol.* 4:29–32.

Denburg, J. A., Jordana, M., Gibson, P., Hargreave, F. H., Gauldie, J., and Dolovich, J. (1990b). Cellular and molecular basis of allergic airway inflammation. Allergy (supplement), *Pharmacia Allergy Research Foundation Award Book*, pp. 15–22.

Denburg, J. A., Gauldie, J., Dolovich, J., Ohtoshi, T., Cox, G., and Jordana, M. (1991a). Structural cell-derived cytokines in allergic inflammation. *Int. Arch. Allergy Appl. Immunol.* (in press).

Denburg, J. A., Silver, J. E., and Abrams, J. (1991b). Interleukin-5 is a human basophilopoietin: Induction of histamine content and basophilic differentiation of HL-60 cells and of peripheral blood basophil-eosinophil progenitors. *Blood* (in press).

Dolovich, J., Ohtoshi, T., Jordana, M., Gauldie, J., and Denburg, J. A. (1990). Nasal polyps: Local inductive microenvironment in the pathogenesis of the inflammation.

In *Rhinitis and Asthma—Similarities and Differences*. Edited by N. Mygind, U. Pipkorn, and R. Dahl. Copenhagen, Munksgaard, pp. 233–241.

Donahue, R. E., Seehra, J., Metzger, M., Lefebvre, D., Rock, B., Carbone, S., Nathan, D. G., Garnick, M., Sehgal, P. K., Laston, D., LaVallie, E., McMoy, J., Schiendel, P. F., Norton, C., Turner, D., Yang, Y., and Clark, S. C. (1988). Human IL-3 and GM-CSF act synergistically in stimulating hematopoiesis in primates. *Science* 241:1820–1823.

Dvorak, A. (1983). Ultrastructural criteria for the identification of mast cells and basophils in humans, guinea pig and mice. *Am. Rev. Respir. Dis.* 128:S49–S52.

Enerbäck, L., Pipkorn, U., and Granerus, G. (1986). Intraepithelial migration of nasal mucosal mast cells in hayfever. *Int. Arch. Allergy Appl. Immunol.* 80: 44–52.

Finotto, S., Marshall, J., Jordana, M., Dolovich, J., and Denburg, J. A. (1991). Isolation and functional studies of human nasal polyp mast cell populations. *J. Allergy Clin. Immunol.* (in press).

Frigas, E., and Gleich, G. J. (1986). The eosinophil and the pathophysiology of asthma. *J. Allergy Clin. Immunol.* 77:527–537.

Furitsu, T., Saito, H., Dvorak, A. M., Schwartz, L. B., Irani, A. M., Burdick, J. F., Ishizaka, K., and Ishizaka, T. (1989). Development of human mast cells in vitro. *Proc. Nat. Acad. Sci. USA* 86:10039–10043.

Gibson, P. G., Dolovich, J., Denburg, J., Ramsdale, E. H., and Hargreave, F. E. (1989a). Chronic cough: Eosinophilic bronchitis without asthma. *Lancet* 1:1346–1348.

Gibson, P. G., Girgis-Gabardo, A., Morris, M. M., Mattoli, S., Kay, J. M., Dolovich, J., Denburg, J., and Hargreave, F. E. (1989b). Cellular characteristics of sputum from patients with asthma and chronic bronchitis. *Thorax* 44:693–699.

Gibson, P. G., Dolovich, J., Girgis-Gabardo, A., Morris, M. M., Anderson, M., Hargreave, F. E., and Denburg, J. A. (1990). The inflammatory response in asthma exacerbation: Changes in circulation eosinophils, basophils and their progenitors. *Clin. Exp. Allergy* 20:661–668.

Ginsburg, H. (1963). The in vitro differentiation and culture of normal mast cells from mouse thymus. *Ann. NY Acad. Sci.* 103:20–39.

Ginsburg, H., and Lagunoff, D. (1967). The in vitro differentiation of mast cells: cultures of cells from immunized mouse lymph nodes and thoracic duct lymph on fibroblast monolayers. *J. Cell Biol.* 35:685–697.

Gleich, G. J. (1990). The eosinophil and bronchial asthma: Current understanding. *J. Allergy Clin. Immunol.* 83:422–436.

Gomez, E., Corrado, O. J., and Davies, R. T. (1987). Histochemical and functional characteristics of the human nasal mast cell. *Int. Arch. Allergy Appl. Immunol.* 83:52–56.

Guy-Grand, D., Dy, M., Luffau, L., and Vassalli, P. (1984). Gut mucosal mast cells: Origin, traffic, and differentiation. *J. Exp. Med.* 160:12–28.

Haak-Frendscho, M., Arai, M., Arai, K.-I., Baeza, M. L., Finn, A., and Kaplan, A. P. (1988). Human recombinant granulocyte-macrophage colony-stimulating factor and interleukin 3 cause basophil histamine release. *J. Clin. Invest.* 82:17–20.

Haig, D. M., McKee, T. A., Jarrett, E. E. E., Woodbury, R., and Miller, H. R. P.

(1982). Generation of mucosal mast cells is stimulated in vitro by factors derived from T-cells of helminth-infected rats. *Nature* 300:188–190.

Hamaguchi, Y., Kanakura, Y., Fukita, J., Takeda, S., Nakano, T., Tarui, S., Honjo, T., and Kitamura, Y. (1987). Interleukin 4 as an essential factor for in vitro clonal growth of murine connective tissue-type mast cells. *J. Exp. Med.* 165:268–273.

Hutt-Taylor, S. R., Harnish, D., Richardson, M., Ishizaka, T., and Denburg, J. A. (1988). Sodium butyrate and a T-lymphocyte cell line-derived differentiation factor induce basophilic differentiation of the human promyelocytic leukemia cell line HL-60. *Blood* 71:209–215.

Ihle, J. N., Keller, J., Oroszlan, S., Henderson, L. E., Copeland, T. D., Fitch, F., Prystowsky, M. B., Goldwasser, E., Schrader, J. W., Palaszynski, E., Dy, M., and Lebel, B. (1983). Biologic properties of homogeneous interleukin 3. 1. Demonstration of WEHI-3 growth factor activity, mast cell growth factor activity, P cell–stimulating factor activity, colony-stimulating factor activity and histamine-producing cell-stimulating factor activity. *J. Immunol.* 131:282–287.

Irani, A. A., and Schwartz, L. B. (1989). Mast cell heterogeneity. *Clin. Exp. Allergy* 19:143–155.

Irani, A. A., Schechter, N. M., Craig, S., DeBlois, M. D., and Schwartz, L. B. (1986). Two types of human mast cells that have distinct neutral protease compositions. *Proc. Natl. Acad. Sci. USA* 83:4464–4468.

Jordana, M., Vancheri, C., Ohtoshi, T., Harnish, D., Gauldie, J., Dolovich, J., and Denburg, J. A. (1989). Hemopoietic function of the microenvironment in chronic airway inflammation. *Agents Actions* 28(Suppl.):85–95.

Kawabori, S., Denburg, J. A., Schwartz, L. B., Irani, A. A., Wong, D., Jordana, G., Evans, S., and Dolovich, J. (1991). Histochemical and immunohistochemical characteristics of mast cells in nasal polyps. *Am. J. Respir. Cell. Mol. Biol.* (submitted).

Kirschenbaum, A. S., Goff, J. P., Dreskin, S. C., Irani, A.-M., Schwartz, L. B., and Metcalfe, D. D. (1989). IL-3-dependent growth of basophil-like cells and mast-like cells from human bone marrow. *J. Immunol.* 142:2424–2429.

Leary, A. G., and Ogawa, M. (1984). Identification of pure and mixed basophil colonies in culture of human peripheral blood and marrow cells. *Blood* 64:78–83.

Levi-Schaffer, F., Austen, K. F., Caulfield, J., Hein, A., Bloes, W. F., and Stevens, R. L. (1985). Fibroblasts maintain the phenotype and viability of the rat heparin-containing mast cell *in vitro*. *J. Immunol.* 135:3454–3462.

Lomas, A. M., Mulroney, C. M., and Schleimer, R. P. (1988). Studies of the adhesive interaction between purified human eosinophils and cultured vascular endothelial cells. *J. Immunol.* 140:1500–1505.

Marshall, J. S., Stead, R. H., McSharry, C., Nielsen, L., and Bienenstock, J. (1990). The role of mast cell degranulation products in mast cell hyperplasia. I. Mechanism of action of nerve growth factor. *J. Immunol.* 144:1886–1892.

Marshall, J. S., Kawabori, S., Nielsen, L., and Bienenstock, J. (1991). Neonatal rat peritoneal mast cells represent a morphologically and functionally distinct population from both intestinal mucosal mast cells and connective tissue mast cells in the adult rat (submitted).

Matsuda, H., Coughlin, M. D., Bienenstock, J., and Denburg, J. A. (1988a). Nerve growth factor promotes human hemopoietic colony growth and differentiation. *Proc. Natl. Acad. Sci. USA* 85:6508–6512.

Matsuda, H., Switzer, J., Coughlin, M. D., Bienenstock, J., and Denburg, J. A. (1988b). Human basophilic cell differentiation promoted by 2.5S nerve growth factor. *Int. Arch. Allergy Appl. Immunol.* 86:453–457.

Mayer, P., Valent, P., Schmidt, G., Liehl, E., and Bettelheim, P. (1989). The in vivo effects of recombinant human interleukin-3: Demonstration of basophil differentiation factor, histamine-producing activity, and priming of GM-CSF-responsive progenitors in nonhuman primates. *Blood* 74:613–621.

Miller, H. R. P. (1971). Immune reactions in mucous membranes. The differentiation of intestinal mast cells during helminth expulsion in the rat. *Lab. Invest.* 24: 339–347.

Nakano, T., Sonoda, T., Hayashi, C., Yamatodani, A., Kanayama, Y., Yamamura, T., Asai, H., Yonezawa, T., Kitamura, Y., and Galli, S. J. (1985). Fate of bone marrow-derived cultured mast cells after intracutaneous, intraperitoneal, and intravenous transfer into genetically mast cell-deficient W/W^v mice. Evidence that cultured mast cells can give rise to both connective tissue type and mucosal mast cells. *J. Exp. Med.* 162:1025–1043.

Ogawa, M., Nakahata, T., Leary, A. G., Sterk, A. R., Ishizaka, K., and Ishizaka, T. (1983). Suspension culture of human mast cells/basophils from umbilical cord blood mononuclear cells. *Proc. Natl. Acad. Sci. USA* 80:4494–4498.

Ohnishi, M., Ruhno, J., Bienenstock, J., Milner, R., Dolovich, J., and Denburg, J. A. (1988a). Human nasal polyp epithelial basophil/mast cell and eosinophil colony-stimulating activity. The effect is T-cell-dependent. *Am. Rev. Respir. Dis.* 138:560–564.

Ohnishi, M., Ruhno, J., Dolovich, J., and Denburg, J. A. (1988b). Allergic rhinitis nasal mucosal conditioned medium stimulates growth and differentiation of basophil/ mast cell and eosinophil progenitors from atopic blood. *J. Allergy Clin. Immunol.* 81:1149–1154.

Ohnishi, M., Ruhno, J., Bienenstock, J., Dolovich, J., and Denburg, J. A. (1989). Hematopoietic growth factor production by cultured cells of human nasal polyp epithelial scrapings: Kinetics, cell source and relationship to clinical status. *J. Allergy Clin. Immunol.* 83:1091–1100.

Ohtoshi, T., Xaubet, A., Andersson, B., Vanzeigleheim, M., Dolovich, J., Jordana, M., and Denburg, J. A. (1990). Nasal inflammation mediated by human structural cell-derived GM-CSF: Effect of budesonide. *J. Allergy Clin. Immunol.* 85:297a.

Ohtoshi, T., Tsuda, T., Vancheri, C., Abrams, J. S., Gauldie, J., Dolovich, J., and Denburg, J. A. (1991a). Human upper airway epithelial cell-derived granulocyte-macrophage colony-stimulating factor (GM-CSF) induces histamine-containing cell differentiation of human progenitor cells. *Int. Arch. Allergy Appl. Immunol.* (submitted).

Ohtoshi, T., Vancheri, C., Cox, G., Gauldie, J., Dolovich, J., Denburg, J. A., and Jordana, M. (1991b). Monocyte-macrophage differentiation induced by human upper airway epithelial cells. *Am. J. Resp. Cell. Mol. Biol.* (in press).

Otsuka, H., Denburg, J. A., Dolovich, J., Hitch, D., Lapp, P., Rajan, R. S., Bienenstock, J., and Befus, A. D. (1985). Heterogeneity of metachromatic cells in human nose: Significance of mucosal mast cells. *J. Allergy Clin. Immunol.* 76: 695–702.

Otsuka, H., Denburg, J. A., Befus, A. D., Hitch, D., Lapp, P., Rajan, R., Bienenstock, J., and Dolovich. J. (1986a). Effect of beclomethasone diproprionate on nasal metachromatic cell subpopulations. *Clin. Allergy* 16:589–595.

Otsuka, H., Dolovich, J., Befus, A. D., Bienenstock, J., and Denburg, J. A. (1986b). Peripheral blood basophils, basophil progenitors, and nasal metachromatic cells in allergic rhinitis. *Am. Rev. Respir. Dis.* 133:757–762.

Otsuka, H., Dolovich, J., Befus, A. D., Telizyn, S., Bienenstock, J., and Denburg, J. A. (1986c). Basophilic cell progenitors, nasal metachromatic cells and peripheral blood basophils in ragweed-allergic patients. *J. Allergy Clin. Immunol.* 78:365–371.

Otsuka, H., Dolovich, J., Richardson, M., Bienenstock, J., and Denburg, J. A. (1987). Metachromatic cell progenitors and specific growth and differentiation factors in human nasal mucosa and polyps. *Am. Rev. Respir. Dis.* 136:710–717.

Owen, W. F. Jr., Rothenberg, M. E., Silberstein, D. S., Gasson, J. C., Stevens, R. L., Austen, K. F., and Soberman, R. J. (1987). Regulation of human eosinophil viability, density and function by granulocyte/macrophage colony-stimulating factor in the presence of 3T3 fibroblasts. *J. Exp. Med.* 166:129–141.

Plaut, M., Pierce, J. H., Watson, C. J., Hanley-Hyde, J., Nordan, R. P., and Paul, W. E. (1989). Mast cell lines produce lymphokines in response to cross-linkage of Fc_ϵ RI or to calcium ionophores. *Nature* 339:64–67.

Rothenberg, M. E., Owen, W. F. Jr., Silberstein, D. S., Soberman, R. J., Austen, K. F., and Stevens, R. L. (1987a). Eosinophils co-cultured with endothelial cells have increased survival and functional properties. *Science* 237:645–647.

Rothenberg, M. E., Owen, W. F. Jr., Silberstein, D. S., Soberman, R. J., Sheffer, A. L., Austen, K. F., and Stevens, R. L. (1987b). Cytokine regulation of human eosinophil viability, density and function. *J. Exp. Med.* 166:129–141.

Saito, H., Hatake, K., Dvorak, A. M., Leiferman, K. M., Donnenberg, A. D., Arai, N., Ishizaka, K., and Ishizaka, T. (1988). Selective differentiation and proliferation of hematopoietic cells induced by recombinant human interleukins. *Proc. Nat. Acad. Sci. USA* 85:2288–2292.

Schrader, J. W., Lewis, S. J., Clark-Lewis, I., Culvenor, J. G. (1981). The persisting (P) cell: Histamine content, regulation by a T cell-derived factor, origin from a bone marrow precursor, and relationship to mast cells. *Proc. Natl. Acad. Sci. USA* 78:323–327.

Serafin, W. E., Dayton, E. T., Gravallese, P. M., Austen, K. F., Stevens, R. L. (1987). Carboxypeptidase A in mouse mast cells. Identification, characterization, and use as a differentiation marker. *J. Immunol.* 139:3771–3776.

Sillaber, C., Geissler, C., Eher, R., Kaltenbrunner, R., Lechner, K., Bettelheim, P., and Valent, P. (1991). Transforming growth factor-β1 promotes IL-3 dependent differentiation of human basophils but inhibits IL-3 dependent differentiation of human eosinophils. *J. Immunol.* (submitted).

Sonoda, S., Sonoda, T., Nakano, T., Kanayama, Y., Kanakura, Y., Asai, H., Yonezawa, T., and Kitamura, Y. (1986). Development of mucosal mast cell after injection of a single connective tissue-type mast cell in the stomach mucosa of genetically mast cell-deficient W/W^v mice. *J. Immunol.* 137:1319–1322.

Springer, T. (1990). Adhesion receptors of the immune system. *Nature* 346:425–434.

Stain, C., Stockinger, H., Scharf, M., Jäger, U., Gössinger, H., Lechner, K., and Bettelheim, P. (1987). Human blood basophils display a unique phenotype including activation-linked membrane structures. *Blood* 70:1872–1879.

Tadokoro, K., Stadler, B. M., and de Weck, A. L. (1983). Factor-dependent in vitro growth of human normal bone marrow-derived basophil-like cells. *J. Exp. Med.* 158:857–871.

Tanno, Y., Bienenstock, J., Richardson, M., Lee, T. G., Befus, A. D., and Denburg, J. (1987). Reciprocal regulation of human basophil and eosinophil differentiation by separate T-cell-derived factors. *Exp. Hematol.* 15:24–33.

Tsuda, T., Switzer, J., Bienenstock, J., and Denburg, J. A. (1990). Interactions of hemopoietic cytokines on differentiation of HL-60 cells: nerve growth factor is a basophilic lineage-specific co-factor. *Int. Arch. Allergy Appl. Immunol.* 91: 15–21.

Tsuda, T., Wong, D. A., Dolovich, J., Bienenstock, J., and Denburg, J. A. (1991). Synergistic effects of nerve growth factor and granulocyte-macrophage colony-stimulating factor on human basophilic cell differentiation. *Blood* (in press).

Valent, P., Ashman, L. K., Hinterberger, W., Eckersberger, F., Majdic, O., Lechner, K., and Bettelheim, P. (1989a). Mast cell typing: Demonstration of a distinct hematopoietic cell type and evidence for immunophenotypic relationship to mononuclear phagocytes. *Blood* 73:1778–1785.

Valent, P., Besemer, J., Muhm, M., Majdic, O., Lechner, K., and Bettelheim, P. (1989b). Interleukin-3 activates human blood basophils via high-affinity binding sites. *Proc. Natl. Acad. Sci. USA* 86:5542–5546.

Valent, P., Schmidt, G., Besemer, J., Mayer, P., Zenke, G., Liehl, E., Hinterbenger, W., Lechner, K., Maurer, D., and Bettelheim, P. (1989c). Interleukin-3 is a differentiation factor for human basophils. *Blood* 73:1763–1769.

Vancheri, C., Gauldie, J., Bienenstock, J., Cox, G., Scicchitano, R., Stanisz, A., and Jordana M. (1989). Human lung fibroblast-derived GM-CSF mediates eosinophil survival in vitro. *Am. J. Respir. Cell. Mol. Biol.* 1:289–295.

Vancheri, C., Ohtoshi, T., Cox, G., Abrams, J. S., Xaubet, A., Gauldie, J., Dolovich, J., Denburg, J. A., and Jordana, M. (1991). Neutrophilic differentiation induced by human upper airway fibroblast-derived granulocyte-macrophage colony-stimulating factor (GM-CSF). *Am. J. Resp. Cell. Mol. Biol.* 4:11–17.

Wershil, B. K., Wang, Z.-S., Gordon, J. R., and Galli, S. J. (1991). Recruitment of neutrophils during IgE-dependent cutaneous late phase reactions in the mouse is mast cell-dependent. Partial inhibition of the reaction with antiserum against tumour necrosis factor-alpha. *J. Clin. Invest.* 87:446–462.

Wodnar-Filipowicz, A., Heusser, C. H., and Morani, C. (1989). Production of the haemopoietic growth factors GM-CSF and interleukin-3 by mast cells in response to IgE receptor-mediated activation. *Nature* 339:150–152.

Wong, D. A., Kawabori, S., Switzer, J., Valent, P., Bettelheim, P., Dolovich, J., Ishizaka, T., Jordana, M., and Denburg, J. (1990). Characterization of histamine-containing basophilic cells induced by in vitro induction of HL-60 cell line. *J. Allergy Clin. Immunol.* 85:173 (abstract).

Zsebo, K. M., Williams, D. A., Geissler, E. N., Broudy, V. C., Martin, F. H., Atkins, H. L., Hsu, R.-Y., Birkett, N. C., Okino, K. H., Murdock, D. C., Jacobsen, F. W., Langley, K. E., Smith, K. A., Takeishi, T., Cattanach, B. M., Galli, S. J., and Suggs, S. V. (1990). Stem cell factor is encoded at the *S1* locus of the mouse and is the ligand for the c-*kit* tyrosine kinase receptor. *Cell* 63:213–224.

32

Adhesion Receptors and Their Relevance to the Biology of Mast Cells and Basophils

HELEN L. THOMPSON and DEAN D. METCALFE

National Institute of Allergy and Infectious Diseases
National Institutes of Health
Bethesda, Maryland

I. Introduction

The aphorism that cells of each lineage communicate during developmental localization and during the evolution of an inflammatory response is readily accepted. Cellular adhesion receptors comprise an important mechanism to facilitate transmission of signals within the microenvironment. Such signals can be mediated by interactions between cells and matrix molecules or through cell-to-cell contact. The establishment of families of adhesion receptors has shed some light on the interplay between these two adhesion processes and relationships between cells of diverse locations (Albelda and Buck, 1990). Many developments with regard to adhesion receptors and their ligands have been defined in the context of T cells and neutrophils and have delineated the complex procedures involved in determination of phenotype, circulation as nonadherent cells, and their role in the immune response (Springer, 1987).

In contrast, the cellular receptors governing the participation of mast cells and basophils in these respects are not well described, with the exception of the high-affinity IgE receptor. The development of human mast cells and basophils from pluripotent stem cells has been clarified with the determination of the CD34+ stem cell as their cell of origin (Kirshenbaum et al., 1989, 1991);

however, the cellular receptors that direct tissue localization in the case of mast cells and result in their egress from the bone marrow are largely undefined. Furthermore, investigations to examine effector molecules that direct mast cell and basophil migration during the immune response are just beginning. The purpose of this chapter is to review what is known concerning adhesion molecules and their ligands and how they direct the activities of T cells, neutrophils, eosinophils, keratinocytes, endothelial cells, and fibroblasts in development, immune reactions, and tumorigenesis, and to suggest how these molecules may then apply to future areas of research with regard to mast cells (and basophils) in view of the recent findings with regard to these two cell types.

Typically, adhesion receptors have been categorized into at least four groups, based on structural and behavioral characteristics. The immunoglobulin superfamily is recruited in cell-to-cell adhesion from MHC receptors and T-cell antigen recognition receptors important in inflammation to the calcium-independent N-CAMS or neural cellular adhesion molecules that come into play during embryogenesis. The integrin family is largely involved in cell-substrate interactions. The LECCAMS, or selectins, are molecules with a lectin terminus domain, and the cadherins are a family of receptors dependent on the presence of calcium; both selectins and cadherins are involved primarily in development but also provide cytoskeletal organization in mature individuals. In addition to these four groups are the lymph node homing receptors, which are derived from a number of different groups, including the selectins, a cartilage link protein family of molecules, and from the integrin family.

II. The Integrin Family

Cellular receptors of the integrin family are capable of mediating three types of receptor-ligand interactions: cell to substrate, heterophilic cell-to-cell adhesion, and a type of homophilic binding involving an intermediate recognition substrate. Cell-substrate interactions occur with a number of extracellular matrix proteins, including fibronectin, fibrinogen, laminin, many collagens, entactin, tenascin, thrombospondin, von Willebrand factor, and vitronectin (Hemler, 1990; Ruoslahti and Pierschbacher, 1987) (Table 1). Cell-to-cell adhesion is facilitated by the binding of integrins to cell membrane proteins, which are usually members of the immunoglobulin family. For example, the intercellular adhesion proteins ICAM-1 and ICAM-2 of the immunoglobulin family are the ligands for the leukocyte integrin LFA-1 (CD11a/CD18 or $\alpha_1\beta_2$) (Springer, 1987), and the counterreceptor for $\alpha_4\beta_1$ integrin is VCAM-1, which is also from the immunoglobulin superfamily (Elices et al., 1990).

Homologous binding between cells can be observed by the binding of platelets to one another through soluble multivalent mediator molecules acting as a bridge between the platelet integrin gp IIb/IIIa. The major ligands for this purpose are fibrinogen and von Willebrand factor; however, fibronectin and vitronectin have also been observed to function in this regard (Ginsberg et al., 1988).

Integrins are a family of membrane glycoproteins consisting of two subunits, α and β (Buck and Horwitz, 1987). Both α and β subunits affect ligand specificity (Buck et al., 1986). The cloning and amino acid analysis of each subunit has allowed for structural (Suzuki and Naitoh, 1990; Ignatius et al., 1990) and conformational analysis (Loftus et al., 1990; Vogel et al., 1990). The ligand binding site appears to be formed by sequences from both subunits. Integrins are associated with cytoskeletal actin filaments (Otey et al., 1990) via an indirect linkage to points where actin bundles terminate surrounded by a ring of vinculin and talin (Burridge et al., 1988). Talin association seems to be a widespread feature of integrins.

Although once thought to define specific subfamilies of integrins by associating only with α subunits of a particular category, the β subunits have since been observed to make multiple associations with other families. Similarly, α subunits, which were once thought to associate exclusively with one β subunit, also function in association with other β subunits, often changing in substrate specificity (Krissansen et al., 1990). This gives rise to a minimum of 16 different integrin receptors by various combinations of the 11 α and six β subunits that have been cloned to date (Hemler, 1990). The α_v subunit appears particularly adaptable, ranging from $\alpha_v\beta_3$, the classical vitronectin receptor, to $\alpha_v\beta_1$, with a single specificity for fibronectin (Vogel et al., 1990), and $\alpha_v\beta_5$, which no longer binds fibrinogen but binds vitronectin and fibronectin (Cheresh et al., 1989).

Ligand binding to integrins is facilitated by the formation of a ligand insertion site between the α subunit and a highly conserved region of the $\beta_{1\text{-}3}$ subunits—residues 109–171 (Kishimoto et al., 1989b). This region also binds to the Arg-Gly-Asp (RGD) active region of many of the integrin recognition substrates. In addition, integrins require Ca^{2+} or Mg^{2+} for function (Wardlaw et al., 1990), with the Asp residue of RGD binding one cation and a further five cations being located on the α-integrin subunit. Binding of integrins to ligands occurs at low affinity (10^{-6} M).

As originally described, integrins were divided into three subfamilies (β_1, β_2, β_3). The β_1 family of molecules were designated VLA (very late antigens) because VLA_1 and VLA_2 appear on lymphocytes 2–4 weeks after lymphocyte stimulation in vitro (Hemler, 1990). The classical fibronectin receptor ($\alpha_5\beta_1$), the $\alpha_v\beta_1$ fibronectin receptor, and the $\alpha_6\beta_1$ laminin receptor have unique ligands, while other receptors of this family express multiple specificities for collagen, laminin, and fibronectin. These receptors are found on nonhematopoietic cells and are in some cases primarily expressed on leukocytes. Their

Table 1 The Integrin Receptor Family

α Subunit	β Subunit	Ligands	RGD intervention
α_1 (VLA-1, CD49a)	β_1 (VLA-β, CD29)	Collagen I	–
		Collagen II	–
		Laminin	–
α_2 (VLA-2, CD49b)	β_1 (VLA-β, CD29)	Collagen I	–
		Collagen IV	–
		Laminin	–
α_3 (VLA-3, CD49c)	β_1 (VLA-β, CD29)	Fibronectin	–
		Laminin	–
		Collagen I	–
α_4 (VLA-4, CD49d)	β_1 (VLA-β, CD29)	Fibronectin	–
		(alternative region)	–
		VCAM	
α_5 (VLA-5, CD49e)	β_1 (VLA-β, CD29)	Fibronectin	+
α_6 (VLA-6, CD49f)	β_1 (VLA-β, CD29)	Laminin	–
α_V (CD51)	β_1 (VLA-β, CD29)	Fibronectin	+
α_L (LFA-1, CD11a)	β_2 (CD18)	ICAM-1	–
		ICAM-2	–
α_M (MAC-1, CD11b)	β_2 (CD18)	C3bi	+
		Fibrinogen	+
α_X (p150,95; CD11c)	β_2 (CD18)	Endothelial molecule	+
α_{IIB} (CD41)	β_3 (CD61)	Fibrinogen	+
		Fibronectin	+
		Vitronectin	+
		von Willebrand factor	+
α_V (CD51)	β_3 (CD61)	Vitronectin	–
		Fibrinogen	
		von Willebrand factor	–

Table 1 Continued

α Subunit	β Subunit	Ligands	RGD intervention
		Thrombospondin Osteopontin Bone sialoprotein I	–
α_6 (CD49f)	β_4	Laminin (basement membrane)	?
α_V (CD51)	β_5	Vitronectin Fibronectin	+ +
α_V (CD51)	β_6	?	?
α_4 (CD49d)	β_P	Peyer's patch Addressin	–

principal role is felt to be tissue organization of the muscle, nervous system, and underlying epithelia and endothelium.

Many of the β_1 integrins (in addition to β_3) recognize the RGD sequence in a prospective ligand; however, this is not resolute, as the $\alpha_4\beta_1$, (VLA_4) receptor binds to the variable region (CS-1) of fibronectin that does not contain an RGD sequence (Wayner et al., 1989; Guan and Hynes, 1990; Elices et al., 1990). As an example of the diversity of these receptors, the $\alpha_4\beta_1$ also binds to an inducible endothelial cell surface protein VCAM-1 or INCAM-110 through sites distinct from those involved in fibronectin binding (Elices et al., 1990). $\alpha_4\beta_1$ is expressed on resting lymphocytes, monocytes, and neural crest–derived cells.

The β_2 integrins are expressed exclusively on peripheral blood leukocytes. LFA-1, Mac-1, and gp150,95 all share the common β_2 subunit (Kishimoto et al., 1987). LFA-1 is expressed on most leukocytes, where it may be activated to mediate leukocyte-leukocyte interactions and leukocyte–endothelial cell interactions (Springer et al., 1987). LFA-1 is involved in a broad range of leukocyte functions, including T-helper and B-lymphocyte responses, natural killing, antibody-dependent cytotoxicity mediated by monocytes and granulocytes, and adherence of leukocytes to endothelial cells and fibroblasts. The ligands for LFA-1 are the ICAM receptors of the immunoglobulin family (Staunton et al., 1989a; Rothlein et al., 1986; Wawryk et al., 1989). Mac-1 and gp150,95 are found on neutrophils, monocytes, and some lymphocytes. Mac-1 also binds ICAMs and iC3b, but the ligands for gp150,95 have not been specifically determined. In spite of this, gp150,95 when immobilized to surfaces will act as an adhesion molecule binding a counterreceptor on stimulated endothelium (Stacker and Springer, 1991).

The most striking reflection of the role of adhesion molecules in vivo in leukocyte localization can be observed in patients with congenital leukocyte adhesion deficiency (LAD), which arises as a result of $\beta 2$ mutations (Kishimoto et al., 1989b; Anderson and Springer, 1987). In these patients, neutrophils fail to extravasate in response to chemoattractants and cannot bind to or cross endothelium, resulting in an inability to fight certain infections. Lymphocytes, however, by virtue of $\alpha_4\beta_1$ integrin, retain the ability to migrate across endothelium at inflammatory sites.

The main platelet integrin gpIIb/IIIa (α_{IIb}/β_3) and the vitronectin receptor (α_v/β_3) comprise the β_3 subfamily of integrins (Phillips et al., 1988). GpIIb/IIIa requires activation to bind to its primary ligands (fibrinogen). Lower-affinity binding is observed to von Willebrand factor and thrombospondin, as well as fibronectin. An RGD peptide can inhibit these interactions. An RGD-related sequence in the fibrinogen γ subunit, KDAGD, may form a structure that functions similarly to RGD and serves as a ligand for gpIIb/IIIa (Ginsberg et al., 1988).

The vitronectin receptor ($\alpha_v\beta_3$) recognizes vitronectin, fibronectin, thrombospondin, and von Willebrand factor and is also susceptible to RGD intervention. The $\alpha_v\beta_3$ integrin or a closely related integrin appears to bind osteoclasts to bone by interacting with an RGD-containing protein termed osteopontin (Reinholt et al., 1990). Furthermore, anti–vitronectin receptor antibodies can block the ability of macrophages to phagocytose neutrophils and lymphocytes that have undergone apoptosis (Savill et al., 1990).

Some integrins, as noted, are cell specific. For example, gpIIa/IIIb is expressed exclusively on megakaryocytes and platelets (Ginsberg et al., 1988), and LFA-1, Mac-1, and gp150,95 are found only on leukocytes (Springer, 1987). Furthermore, $\alpha_6\beta_4$ is specific for epithelial cells and their neoplastic counterparts (Kajiji et al., 1987). The β_4, β_5, and β_6 integrin subunits have recently been characterized (Shepopard et al., 1990; Suzuki and Naitoh, 1990; Hogervorst et al., 1990; Ramaswamy and Hemler, 1990). A novel α subunit, distinct from α_1–α_6 of the VLA family, has been shown to function with the β_1-integrin subunit to facilitate melanoma cell binding to laminin (Kramer et al., 1989).

III. The Immunoglobulin Family

Many of the receptors of the immunoglobulin family appear to cooperate with several other immunoglobulin surface molecules to exert an effective adhesion interaction. It is possible that these interactions occur through the immunoglobulin domains. For example, T-lymphocyte killing requires the active participation of no less than three immunoglobulin receptors and one integrin receptor, which recognize four different immunoglobulin receptors on the target cell CD3/TCR and CD8 to MHC-I, CD2 to LFA-3, and LFA-1 to ICAM-1 and ICAM-2 (Bieren et al., 1989; Martz, 1987; Kishimoto et al., 1989b; Haynes, 1984). Thus, as with all members of the immunoglobulin family, CD8 and CD4 receptors act as coreceptors of the T-cell receptor (TCR) CD3 for MHC-II and MHC-I molecules present on the surface of antigen-presenting cells and infected cells, respectively (Bieren et al., 1989; Swain, 1983). CD4 and CD8 receptors are ineffectual in the absence of antigen peptides or viral peptides presented by MHC-II and MHC-I complexes, respectively, but remain able to signal in synergy with the TCR to promote either proliferation of the helper T cell or cytotoxic killing of the target cell (Janeway, 1988; Kupfer and Singer, 1989; Salter et al., 1990). In addition, CD4 and CD8 receptors, by early association with the TCR, direct the subsequent differentiation of thymocytes into either cytotoxic (CD8+) or helper T-lymphocyte (CD4+) progeny (Janeway, 1988; von Boehmer, 1988).

Another T-cell receptor, CD2 or LFA-2, is a 40-kDa, single-chain glycoprotein found on all T lymphocytes (Table 2). Its counterpart, LFA-3, is a 50–77kDa glycoprotein found on many cell types, and both are members of the immunoglobulin superfamily (Bierer et al., 1989; Springer et al., 1987; Dustin et al., 1987). These heterocyclic cell adhesion molecules, in addition to the integrin LFA-1, help localize activated T cells to sites of antigen accumulation in the lymph nodes (Butcher, 1986). Both CD2 and LFA-3 are activated by what appears to be a reduction in surface charge known to be associated with sialic acid following the engagement of the MHC or activation with phorbol esters (Wigzell and Hayny, 1974). CD2 appears to transduce a signal that augments the signals from the TCR, but alone it is without effect (Bierer et al., 1989).

The counterreceptor for LFA-1 is ICAM-1, also a member of the immunoglobulin superfamily. It has five immunoglobulin domains (Simmons et al., 1988; Staunton et al., 1988). ICAM-1 can be expressed on a variety of cells and is either absent or present at very low levels on most cells in the absence of an immune response (Kishimoto et al., 1989b; Dustin et al., 1986, 1988). Besides LFA-1–ICAM-1 interactions being synergistic with the CD2–LFA-3 and MHC-I/MHC-II–CD4/CD8 interactions in cytotoxic T-cell and helper-T-cell interactions with target cells and antigen-presenting cells, ICAM-1 receptors mediate the initial interaction in the binding of leukocytes, eosinophils, and monocytes to endothelium in the localization of circulating cells in an inflammatory response. ICAM-1 receptors can be induced on endothelial, fibroblast, and epithelial cells in an inflammatory response by inflammatory mediators such as lipopolysaccharide, IFNγ, IL-1, and TNF (Springer et al., 1987; Kishimoto et al., 1989a; Dustin et al., 1988). The type of mediator release

Table 2 Cell-Cell Adhesion Molecules

Receptor	Family	Distribution	Ligand	Function
L-PAM-1	Integrin $\alpha 4m/\beta p$	Lymphocytes	?	Lymphocyte-EC adhesion
L-PAM-2/VLA-4	Integrin $\alpha 4/\beta 1$	Leukocytes, melanoma cells	VCAM-1, INCAM-110	Lymphocyte-EC adhesion Tumor-EC adhesion
CD11/CD18 (LEU-CAMs)	Integrins			Cell-cell adhesion
LFA-1 (CD11a)	α_L/β_2	All leukocytes	ICAM-1	Leukocyte-leukocyte adhesion Leukocyte-cell adhesion
MAC-1 (MO-1, CR3, CD11b)	α_m/β_2	Neutrophils, monocytes, some lymphocytes	iC3b, fibrinogen, factor X, ICAM-1, LPS	Cell-cell adhesion Phagocytosis Complement binding
gp150/95 (CR4, CD11c)	α_x/β_2	Granulocytes, monocytes	iC3b	Complement binding
ICAM-1	Ig superfamily	Many cells; induced by inflammation	LFA-1	Leukocyte adhesion
CD2 (LFA-2, OKT11)	Ig superfamily	All T cells	LFA-3	T cell adhesion
LFA-3	Ig superfamily	Widespread	CD2	T cell adhesion
EndoCAM, PECAM-1 (CD31)	Ig superfamily	EC, platelets, leukocytes	?	Initiation of EC-EC adhesion Platelet-monocyte adhesion

VCAM-1	Ig superfamily	Activated EC	VLA-4 (α_4/β_1)	Adhesion of WBCs to EC activated by IL-1 or TNF
Ca^{2+}-independent CAMs:	Ig Superfamily			Developmentally regulated cell-cell adhesion
N-CAM (D2, BSP-2)		Brain, muscle, heart, kidney	Homophilic binding	
Ng-CAM (L1, NILE)		Neural and glial cells	Homophilic binding (neural-neural) Heterophilic binding (neural-glial)	
MAG		Brain, oligodendrocytes Schwann cells	Homophilic binding (Schwann-Schwann)	
Fasciclin II		Grasshopper embryo segmental ganglia	Homophilic	
Ca^{2+}-dependent CAMs	Cadherins	Brain, muscle, lens	Homophilic binding	Developmentally regulated cell-cell adhesion
N-Cadherin (A-CAM, N-Cal-CAM)	Epithelium			
E-Cadherin (L-CAM, Arc-1, uvomorulin, cell CAM 120/180)		Placenta, epithelium, mesothelium		
P-Cadherin				

Table 2 Continued

Receptor	Family	Distribution	Ligand	Function
H-CAM (CD44, hermes antigen, ECMR III)	Cartilage link protein	Lymphocytes	Endothelial cell mucosal addressin	Homing RTR lymphocyte to HEV of peripheral LNs
LAM-1 (gp90^{MEL-14} [murine ab]; Leu-8 [human ab])	Lec-CAM	Lymphocytes	HEV carbohydrate?	Homing RTR lymphocyte to HEV of peripheral LNs
gp100^{MEL-14}	Lec-CAM	Neutrophils	Endothelial cell carbohydrate?	Initial adhesion of neutrophil to EC adjacent to inflammation
ELAM-1	Lec-CAM	Activated EC	?	Adhesion of WBCs to EC activated by LPS, IL-1, or TNF
GMP140 (PADGEM)	Lec-CAM	Platelets, neutrophils, monocytes, EC	?	Adhesion of activated platelets to monocytes and neutrophils Adhesion of WBCs to activated EC
CD36 (GPIV)	?	EC, platelets, monocytes	Thombospondin	Platelet-monocyte adhesion

Source: Abstracted with permission from Albelda and Buck, 1990.
Ig = Immunoglobulin

affects resident cells to differing extents and thus dictates varying patterns of cell localization via cell binding and subsequent tissue migration.

Although ICAM-1 expression is upregulated within 4 hr following cytokine stimulation and is maximal by 24 hr in the case of T cells, it is the crosslinking of the TCR causing a transient increase in the avidity of LFA-1 to ICAM-1 that results in an adhesive interaction between T cells and endothelium cells. The transient nature of this high avidity provides a mechanism for disengagement (Dustin et al., 1988).

The ICAM-2 receptor is a second ligand for LFA-1 and differs in tissue distribution from ICAM-1. ICAM-2 is basally expressed on endothelial cells and its expression is not increased by inflammatory mediators. ICAM-2 has two immunoglobulin domains. These are 35% identical to the N-terminal domains of ICAM-1 (Staunton et al., 1989a).

Another mechanism mediating leukocyte-endothelium interactions involves the immunoglobulin receptor VCAM, also induced on endothelial cells by inflammatory mediators with kinetics similar to ICAM-1 expression (Osborn et al., 1989). As mentioned earlier, the ligand for this receptor is the $\alpha_4\beta_1$ integrin found on lymphocytes but not neutrophils. This distribution may explain the presence of the former but not the latter cell at sites of inflammatory reactions in LAD patients. This receptor was also identified independently on melanoma cells, where it was given the nomenclature of INCAM-110 (Rice and Bevilacqua, 1989).

EndoCAM was recently described as an immunoglobulin receptor that may be involved in the junctional structures of endothelial cells found at the cell-cell borders of contiguous endothelial cells (Albelda et al., 1990; Newman et al., 1990). It may operate in homophilic binding interactions to a ligand that has not yet been identified. In addition, this 130-kDa glycoprotein is also presented on platelets and monocytes and may thus play a role in endothelial cell–monocyte interactions. EndoCAM may provide positioning cues necessary for angiogenesis or the establishment of a polarized, nonpermeable vascular lining.

Another subfamily of receptors within the immunoglobulin family consists of a group of cell surface glycoproteins important in the specification of interactions during development, maintenance, and regeneration of the nervous system. These adhesion molecules have distinct functions involving cells at different developmental stages, but, like other members of the immunoglobulin family, they may cooperate when expressed together (Keilhauer et al., 1985). These molecules, whose function is in developmentally regulated cell-cell adhesion, and which have C2-type immunoglobulin domains, are neuronal cell adhesion molecule (N-CAM) (Cunningham et al., 1987; Barthels et al., 1987; Hemperly et al., 1986), myelin-associated glycoprotein (MAG), a glial adhesion molecule (Arquint et al., 1987; Lai et al., 1987); L1, an axonal adhesion molecule (Moos et al., 1988) called NILE in mammals and G4 and NgCAM in chickens, and fasciclin II, an invertebrate adhesion molecule (Harrelson and Goodman, 1988). N-CAM, NgCAM, MAG, fasciclin II, and the cadherin family of receptors are named primary cell adhesion molecules because they appear early in development in tissues in all three germ layers, but they are also used later in histogenesis (Grumet et al., 1984). For example, NgCAM also functions as a secondary CAM, which appears later in development. In neural tissues, NgCAM is involved in neuron-neuron adhesion, neurite fasciculation, outgrowth of neurites, cerebellar granule migration, and interactions among epithelial cells of intestinal crypts. It is synthesized by neurons, not by glia, and is homophilic in neuron-neuron binding and heterophilic in neuron-glia binding (Grumet and Edelman, 1988).

N-CAM is expressed at sites of embryonic induction. N-CAM appears to exist in three alternatively spliced transcripts of a single N-CAM gene giving rise to different cytoplasmic domains, which interact differentially with cortical cytoskeletal elements, thus being subject to different forms of cell surface methylation (Rutishauser and Jessel, 1988; Edelman, 1988). N-CAM is also found in brain, heart, kidney, and muscle in the mature individual. In addition to multiple immunoglobulin repeats, these neural cell adhesion molecules, N-CAM, NgCAM/L1, MAG, and fasciclin II, also contain fibronectin type III repeats containing RGD sequences near their transmembrane domains and are regulated by sialation (Moss et al., 1988; Harrelson and Goodman, 1988). Polysialation of these receptors antagonizes their ability to promote adhesion. This sialation appears to decrease when these receptors are required during development (Hemperley et al., 1986).

MAG also exists in several isoforms as a result of alternate splicing. MAG mediates axonal-glial and glial-glial interactions in postnatal brain development, particularly in myelination (Lai et al., 1987; Arquint et al., 1987). As an example of the sequential activities of these receptors, MAG appears to take over Schwann cell–axon and Schwann cell–Schwann cell interactions initiated by NCAM and L1/neuron–glia cell adhesion molecules in the successive development of the peripheral nervous system. NCAM, NgCAM, MAG, and fasciclin II are calcium-independent receptors. This feature sets these receptors apart from another family of receptors also involved in developmentally regulated cell-cell adhesion, the cadherins, which are calcium-dependent adhesion molecules (Rutishauser and Jessel, 1988; Edelman, 1988).

IV. The Cadherin Family

Ultrastructural studies have revealed that cells are connected with multiple types of junctions, such as tight junctions, adherens junctions, gap junctions, and desmosomes. As mentioned above, the cadherins are a calcium-dependent (thus

CAD) family of integral membrane proteins and appear to be important constituents of adherens junctions affecting the alignment of cell layers (Takeichi, 1988). cDNA studies reveal they are 723–748 amino acids in length and share common sequences, ranging from 50 to 60% homology within a single species. These receptors have been divided into subfamilies based on immunological distinctions and tissue distributions, termed: E-cadherin [epithelial cadherin (Yoshida and Takeichi, 1982)] (also termed cell CAM 120/80, Arc-1, or L-CAM) (Gallin et al., 1983, 1985); N-cadherin [neural cadherin (Hatta and Takeichi, 1986)] [also termed A-CAM (Volk and Geiger, 1984) or N-cal-CAM (Bixby et al., 1987)], found in adult neural tissue and muscle; and P-cadherins, found primarily in placenta and epithelial cells but transiently expressed in other tissues during development (Nose et al., 1987; Nose and Takeichi, 1986). The role of calcium dependence of cadherin-mediated adhesion is not well understood; however, calcium is an essential ion for tissue association in all animal species. The calcium-dependent adherence mechanism has been defined as a mechanism whose components are exposed on cell surfaces, require Ca^{2+} for cell-cell binding action, and are protected by Ca^{2+} from proteolytic cleavage (Takcichi, 1988).

Cadherins bind by homophilic interactions at the extracellular domain. The presence of cadherins at cell-cell boundaries coincides with cortical actin bundles. This, in turn, suggests that cadherins may bind to vinculin at the cytoplasmic domain (Hirano et al., 1987).

Cadherin expression can be switched from one subclass to the other in relation to morphogenetic events. Cell layer separation during embryogenesis from the parent layer is associated with the termination or switching of cadherin subclasses. For example, such switching occurs during the formation of mesoderm, neural tube, the lens vesicle, the neural crest, and the differentiation of keratinocytes (Takeichi, 1988).

Heterotypic cells brought together during morphogenesis usually express identical cadherin subclasses for recognition. Thus, P-cadherin is expressed by both uterine decidual cells and extraembryonic cells in the formation of the placenta. Implantation does not occur if P-cadherin is not functional.

Finally, cadherin expression is associated with cell rearrangement in, for example, somite development when mesenchymal cells are converted into epithelial cells, or vice versa. If E-CAM is not expressed at the 2-day blastula, compaction and polarity are not established, and neither tight junctions nor gap junctions form (Damsky et al., 1983).

The expression of cadherins appears to be coordinated with that of other classes of cell-cell adhesion molecules. For example, the spatiotemporal pattern of expression of N-cadherin is similar to that of N-CAM, whose expression is also controlled to follow embryonic induction. This suggests the presence of a regulatory mechanism to coordinate expression of different classes of adhesion

receptor phenotypes, so that virgin T cells homogeneously express all classes of human homing receptors, Lam-1, CD44, and $\alpha 4$ integrin, and lack markers of tissue association (Picker et al., 1990b). Memory T cells heterogeneously express Lam-1 and higher but uniform levels of CD44 and $\alpha 4$-integrin and include the vast majority of T cells bearing MLA and CLA Ag. The bimodal expression of Lam-1 results from CLA Ag-positive cells, being predominantly high in expression of Lam-1 and β_1, whereas MLA Ag-positive cells lack Lam-1 and show low to intermediate expression of β_1 chains (Picker et al., 1990b).

The fact that virgin T cells uniformly express Lam-1 suggests that this entire population can extravasate in the peripheral lymph nodes, bestowing a wide and varied repertoire of antigen-specific T cells with access to the tissue. Memory cells deficient in Lam-1 are unable to enter the peripheral lymph node. However, because of their high expression of other adhesion molecules, memory cells preferentially extravasate at other sites.

CD44 and α_4 integrins show the same pattern of regulation on memory versus naïve T cells as LFA-3 and other adhesion molecules such as LFA-1 and CD2 (Springer et al., 1987). It thus appears that these molecules have a broad role in leukocyte adhesion, which does not favor the quantitative variation of these particular receptors in the genesis of a memory cell population of tissue-specific homing subsets. In spite of this, the elevated levels of these molecules on memory T cells may allow these cells to extravasate more rapidly in extralymphoid tissue sites compared to virgin T cells.

In accordance with this observation, T cells expressing high levels of adhesion molecules have been shown to have an increased ability to bind activated endothelium in vitro. They also make up the great majority of T cells recirculating through the afferent lymph nodes and comprise the great majority of T cells present in or recirculating through extralymphoid inflammatory sites. Compared to fully developed HEV, the endothelium of the vessels in extralymphoid sites probably expresses lower levels of the various endothelia ligands required for lymphocyte adhesion. Therefore, such endothelium may not be able to efficiently support the extravasation of virgin lymphocytes expressing low levels of adhesion molecules (Mackay et al., 1990). Lymphocyte homing thus appears to be regulated by the expression of an array of complementary adhesion molecules on each of the two participants: the homing receptors on recirculating lymphocytes and the addressins on particular organ HEVs or other structures distributed within an organism. Another specification for ELAM-1 has been described whereby ELAM-1 functions as the skin vascular addressin for CLA Ag-positive lymphocytes and thus provides a mechanism for selective homing of memory T lymphocytes, this time from the peripheral blood into the area of a chronic cutaneous inflammatory response. The local production of neutrophil and T-cell-specific activation and chemotactic factors then induces the diapedesis of these cells into the tissues (Picker et al., 1991; Shimizu et al., 1991).

A molecule similar to Lam-1 (termed $gp_{100}^{mel\text{-}14}$) has also been identified on neutrophils. It may have an additional role in neutrophil emigration at inflammatory sites by initiating adhesion to endothelial cells (Kishimoto et al., 1989a). $gp_{100}^{mel\text{-}14}$ is shed rapidly from the cell surface after stimulation with neutrophil chemoattractants. Thus, like ELAM-1, it may be involved only in the early steps of neutrophil-endothelial cell contact.

VI. Other Adhesion Molecules

Several other molecules exist that function as cell-cell or cell-substratum adhesion proteins. Platelet glycoprotein IV (CD36) is an 88-kDa glycoprotein found on endothelial cells, platelets, and leukocytes and binds to thrombospondin. This protein appears to function as a cell-cell receptor by crosslinking the thrombospondin on the surface of platelets and monocytes, in much the same way as CD44 binds hyaluronate (Miyake et al., 1990). *Plasmodium falciparum*–infected erythrocytes also bind to postcapillary endothelium via the CD36 receptor (Oquendo et al., 1989).

Proteoglycans also play an important role in cell adhesion. Interactions of proteoglycans with other substances can be mediated by the glycosaminoglycan component or the core protein (Schmidt et al., 1987). In addition to hyaluronate, the small fibroblast proteoglycan decorin binds to fibronectin and collagen via its core protein (Vogel et al., 1984). The membrane-intercalated proteoglycan syndecan binds to collagen and fibronectin through its heparan sulfate chains and mediates cell adhesion (Saunders and Bernfield, 1988). Cell adhesion to extracellular matrix through proteoglycans appears to be an auxiliary mechanism that complements the more specific integrin-mediated adhesion interactions (Ruoslahti, 1989).

A laminin-binding protein that is not a member of the integrin family has been identified on the surface of hepatocytes, neuronal cells, macrophages, and melanoma cells (Clement et al., 1990; von der Mark and Kuhl, 1985). The 1.1-kb cDNA codes for a 32-kDa glycoprotein (Wewer et al., 1986; Yow et al., 1988). A number of active sites, including RGD, YIGSR, and IKVAV within the laminin molecule, appear to mediate this binding (Graf et al., 1987; Iwamoto et al., 1987, 1988; Tashiro et al., 1989). A similar protein that recognizes the VGVPG site in elastin has also been identified. It is possible that many of these peptides play a role in chemotaxis and metastasis (Meacham et al., 1989).

Another non-integrin-binding protein for laminin is found on the cell surface of macrophages. It is identical to the Mac-2 antigen, or carbohydrate-binding protein 35. This protein functions as a galactose-specific lectin (Cherayil et al., 1989). Several reports have implicated galactose residues on laminin as important determinants of cell recognition (Runyan et al., 1988). Thus macrophage adhesion to laminin may be stabilized by this carbohydrate-protein interaction.

VII. Tumorigenesis

The metastatic spread of certain neoplasms has been associated with cell motility both at the primary site of growth and at the point of exit and entry of tumor cells into and out of the vasculature. This motility seems to be facilitated, in part, by a reduction both in the deposition of fibronectin, laminin, and collagens and in integrin receptor expression. Consequently, tumor cells are not limited in spreading by adhesion to their own matrix. In addition, some Rous sarcoma virus-transformed cells also exhibit phosphorylated β_1 integrins, which affects the efficiency of binding to cytoskeletal elements and extracellular ligands (Plantefaber and Hynes, 1989; Hirst et al., 1986).

There is, however, a dual role for fibronectin and integrin-mediated adherence in malignancy (Mould et al., 1990) whereby tumor cells preferentially migrate on extracellular matrix proteins. This is exemplified by the fact that RGD peptides can inhibit both the movement of human melanoma cells through amniotic basement membrane and the dissemination of intravenously injected melanoma tumor cells in mice lungs. Hence, there may be cyclical periods of integrin receptor expression in the process of tumorigenesis (Ruoslahti and Giancotti, 1989; Ruoslahti, 1990). Natural killer (NK) cells, natural cytotoxic (NC) cells, mononuclear phagocytes, monocytes, and macrophages are often found at sites of tumor. These cells have the unique capability of differentiating tumor cells from normal cells of the same type and selectively binding and lysing the tumor targets (Schwarz and Hiserodt, 1988). The molecules involved in the process of recognition are slowly becoming defined. In one model, the presence of cell surface laminin receptors on tumor cells (Laybourn et al., 1989; Schwarz and Hiserodt, 1988) is related to sensitivity to killing by NK cells or lysis by phagocytic cells. NK cells have been shown to express surface structures that are immunochemically cross-reactive with affinity-purified antilaminin antibody, facilitate tumor cell recognition, and are involved in activation of cytotoxicity. Furthermore, the expression of cell surface laminin and laminin receptors on both tumor cells and monocytes/macrophages may provide a mechanism for promoting tumor cell–monocyte/macrophage binding (Huard et al., 1985).

The dysfunctional utilization of cellular adhesion receptors may underlie various diseases (Isberg and Leong, 1990). ICAM-1 is also a receptor for rhinoviruses. Soluble pieces of ICAM-1 can inhibit viral entry into cells through competition with the binding of the virus to cell surface ICAM-1 (Staunton et al.,

1989b); RGD peptides inhibit entry of the foot-and-mouth disease virus (Fox et al., 1989). The transactivating protein, tat, of the human immunodeficiency virus also contains an RGD sequence and binds to cells in a RGD-dependent manner (Brake et al., 1990; Ensoli et al., 1990). *Leishmania* organisms can use the β_2 Mac-1 (CD11b/CD18) integrin to invade monocytes and macrophages, and *Plasmodium falciparum* utilizes the endothelial ICAM-1 receptor as a ligand (Berendt et al., 1989).

VIII. Inflammatory Responses

The sequence of events involved in responses of immediate hypersensitivity, late-phase responses, delayed hypersensitivity, and injury are highly dependent on the timely expression of cell adhesion receptors from many of these receptor families. Moreover, the production of soluble mediators in each of these events by cells resident in tissues, including dermal fibroblasts, endothelial cells, epidermal keratinocytes, melanocytes, mast cells, and alveoli macrophages, can affect decisively the functions and behavior of lymphocytes, neutrophils, eosinophils, and macrophages/monocytes because of their adhesion receptor repertoire.

The tissue response to injury comprises three overlapping phases: inflammation, formation of granulation tissue and matrix, and remodeling. The initial events of wound healing and coagulation include the binding of platelets to exposed matrix fibronectin via β_1 and β_3 integrins, including the $\alpha_2\beta_1$ collagen/laminin receptor, the $\alpha_5\beta_1$ fibronectin receptor, and the $\alpha_6\beta_1$ laminin receptor (Ginsberg et al., 1988). In fact, exposure to matrix peptide fragments, especially the RGD-containing fragments, has been shown to cause an enhancement of function in many cell types, including cytokine production. Thrombin is also generated via the coagulation cascade, which activates platelet gpIIb/IIIa and thereby promotes platelet aggregation via fibrin and fibrinogen. The ensuing granule release of TGF_β (Heino and Massague, 1989) and the synthesis of other primary cytokines such as $TNF\alpha$ and IL-1 may then induce the expression of ICAM-1, VCAM-1, and ELAM-1 on endothelial cells in the dermal plexus and around postcapillary venules. This in turn initiates leukocyte–endothelial cell binding in the evolution of an inflammatory response. During granulation tissue formation, fibroblasts proliferate and migrate into the wound space. The factors and receptors responsible for this latter event are not known; however, they undoubtedly involve members of the integrin family and the matrix components and soluble mediators produced by other cell types within the wound site.

Delayed hypersensitivity is a T-lymphocyte-mediated inflammatory reaction. It is responsible for a number of clinical phenomena, including contact dermatitis, classic allograft rejection reactions, graft-versus-host disease, granuloma formation, tumor immunity, bacterial or fungal infection, and cytopathic virus infection (Kirkpatrick, 1988). It has recently been suggested that the initiation of all these events results in a form of kinetic trauma in which keratinocytes, fibroblasts, melanocytes, and other sessile cells resident to the epidermis and dermis layers of skin respond with the release or *de novo* synthesis of epidermal IL-1α (Kupper, 1990). This is accompanied by the release of a host of proinflammatory molecules, including IL-6, TNFα, MIP-1α, TCA-3, and JE. Many of these are inducible cytokines produced as a result of the action of IL-1α on the nearby cells. Inducible cytokines, in addition to activating endothelial cells to express adhesion molecules, also act as potent chemoattractants for the directional migration of leukocytes toward the site of injury. There does not appear to be a mechanism for recruiting T cells into inflamed tissues based on their antigen specificity; however, memory T cells express elevated levels of LFA-1, LFA-3, CD44, CD29 (β_1 integrin), and VLA-4, -5, and -6 over naïve cells and may thus bind more readily to endothelium (Springer, 1987). Delayed hypersensitivity reactions are usually mediated by T lymphocytes of the CD4 helper phenotype (Poulter et al., 1983). In individuals not previously exposed to antigen or hapten, first contact leads to a naïve T cell bearing the appropriate TCR for the antigen, interacting with antigen-presenting cells such as Langerhans cells of the epidermis. Once activated in the lymph node environment, the naïve lymphocytes become longer-lived memory T cells, increase surface expression of adhesion receptors, and give rise to progeny also with elevated levels of adhesion molecules (Shimizu et al., 1990). Thus, on second exposure, memory T cells infiltrate more efficiently into the area of infection.

CD2 receptors engage with LFA-3 molecules on antigen-presenting cells. If there is no antigen recognition, the two cells disengage. Increased expression of LFA-1 and CD2 enhances sensitivity to antigen by stabilizing the interaction between lymphocytes and antigen-presenting cells. Eventually a recruited T cell encounters antigen in the proper molecular context and becomes activated to secrete cytokines. This process results in the chemotaxis of neutrophils, monocytes, activation of antigen-presenting cells to express MHC-II, activation of phagocytic cells, and enhancement of bactericidal activity.

Immediate hypersensitivity reactions are initiated by the crosslinking of high-affinity IgE receptors on the surface of sensitized tissue mast cells. This leads to the release of preformed and newly synthesized mediators, including leukotrienes, prostaglandins, proteases, proteoglycans, and histamine, which give rise to the symptoms of immediate hypersensitivity (Schwartz and Austen, 1988). Mast cell activations are also followed by the production of a variety of proinflammatory cytokines, such as MIP-1α, TCA3, TNF-α, IL-1, IL-6, TGF$_\beta$, and JE; and growth factor cytokines, such as IL-4, IL-3, and IL-5 (Plaut et al., 1989; Wodnar-Filipowicz et al., 1989; Burd et al., 1989; Takagi et al., 1989; Gordon and Galli, 1990).

A current hypothesis has developed regarding the immediate hypersensitivity reaction, the proinflammatory cytokine production therein, and the question of whether a late-phase reaction ensues. Immediate-type hypersensitivity reactions in the nose, skin, and lower airways, once thought to be isolated monophasic responses, are often followed in 3–24 hr by the gradual appearance of a more sustained inflammatory reaction. The intense cellular infiltrate is composed of mononuclear cells, neutrophils, eosinophils, and basophils. The proinflammatory molecules released during the immediate phase of the reaction appear responsible for the recruitment of cells, such that neutrophils and eosinophils bind to ELAM-1 and ICAM-1, expressed by endothelial cells through LFA-1 receptors and other complementary ligands.

The hypothesis about the genesis of this event relates to the division of mouse helper T cells into TH_1 and TH_2 subsets, whereby TH_1 cells are primarily responsible for the production of IFN-γ and TH_2 cells secrete IL-4, IL-5, and IL-6 (Coffman et al., 1988); hence, an infiltration of helper cells of the TH_2 subtype may stimulate IgE production by B cells, eosinophil differentiation, and B-cell immunoglobulin secretion according to the primary functions of cytokines IL-4, IL-5, and IL-6. In contrast, a TH_1 infiltrate and the subsequent IFN-γ secretion would dampen these responses and impede the development of a late-phase reaction. Furthermore, mast cells have been described as resembling the TH_2 subset of T cells in respect to their cytokine repertoire (Plaut et al., 1989) and may thus amplify a TH_2 subset response and enhance the late-phase reaction.

The mechanism for basophil recruitment is currently under investigation. Investigators have previously identified C5a, lymphokines, and serum from allergic donors as stimuli that are chemotactic for human basophils (Kay and Austen, 1972; Hirsch and Kalbfleisch, 1980; Ward et al., 1975; Lett-Brown et al., 1976). Recently, human basophils have been shown to adhere to human umbilical vein endothelial cells (HUVEC) following either stimulation of the HUVEC cells with IL-1, TNF-α, bacterial endotoxin, or TPA, or coincubation of basophils and HUVEC cells for 10 min with C5a, F-Met-Leu-Phe, calcium ionophore, PAF, TNF, or TPA (Bochner et al., 1988). This latter effect resulted from activation of the basophil and was determined, by the use of monoclonal antibodies, to be via an expression of β_2 integrin molecules (most likely binding to ICAM-1) and to be dependent on the presence of calcium ions (Bochner et al., 1989).

However, the activation of endothelial cell adhesion receptors ICAM-1, ELAM-1, and VCAM by cytokines TNF-α or IL-1 does not allow for the selective recruitment of specific cell types during certain responses. For example, delayed hypersensitivity is primarily a T-cell event, although some basophils have been detected at these sites (Kirkpatrick, 1988). This requires that ICAM-1 and VCAM be preferentially activated over ELAM-1, and during a late-phase response ELAM-1 and ICAM-1 molecules must come into play but with the preferential binding of eosinophils and basophils. This suggests that the circulating cells differentially adhere to endothelial cells as a result of some additional stimuli or that the primary tissue-based activation events of either mast cells or epidermal keratinocytes, melanocytes, and fibroblasts result in a modified array of proinflammatory molecules that act in concert to produce alternative modes of endothelial cell activation not yet described.

Consistent with the former hypothesis, IL-4 has been shown to act synergistically with IL-1β to promote lymphocyte adhesion to endothelium by induction of VCAM (Masinovsky et al., 1990). Furthermore, TNF can combine with either IL-4 or IFN-γ to selectively enhance endothelial cell adhesiveness for T cells via a VCAM-dependent mechanism (Thornhill et al., 1991). Hence, while IL-1 and TNF alone are unselective in terms of leukocyte adhesion to endothelial cells, the combination of TNF with IL-4 or IFN-γ may be of key importance in determining the recruitment of a lymphocyte-predominant infiltrate in immune-mediated inflammation and in initiating the transition from acute to chronic inflammation. Furthermore, GM-CSF has been shown to enhance PAF and F-Met-Leu-Phe–induced eosinophil expression of adherence molecules (CD11b) and increases F-Met-Leu-Phe–induced adherence to endothelial cells (Tomioka et al., 1991). Thus it is becoming more apparent that, while adhesion receptors expressed by endothelial cells are the result of widespread action by IL-1, TNF, and IFN-γ, the responses of leukocytes and T cells are tightly regulated by specific activating stimuli for the expression of adhesion receptors appropriate for a particular inflammatory response. Anti-IgE or antigen stimulation of basophils results in increased basophil adherence to human endothelial cells, increased expression of CD11b and CD11c, and decreased expression of Leu-8 antigen (Bochner and Sterbinsky, 1991). This effect on Leu-8 expression (Leu-8 is the monoclonal antibody that recognizes the human equivalent of the LAM-1 homing receptor) has been proposed as the mechanism whereby basophils, once attached to endothelium, may subsequently be released to migrate into tissues by the "clipping off" of this receptor. IL-3 treatment of basophils leads to a rapid, sustained increase in cell surface expression of CD11b (Mac 1) (Bochner et al., 1990a). Since neither of these responses was observed with neutrophils, it is possible that exposure of basophils to low concentrations of antigen in vivo and the local production of IL-3 during allergic reactions may selectively promote basophil activation, adhesion to endothelium, and recruitment to extravascular sites of inflammation (Bochner et al., 1990b).

In contrast to basophils, a surface receptor governing mast cell interactions with other cells has not been described; however, work has begun on defining mast cell–substrate receptors that presumably anchor the cells to their own matrix when present in tissues. Dog mastocytoma cells have been shown to adhere to tracheal epithelial cells in vitro; however, the cellular receptor for this interaction was not defined other than to exclude the involvement of β_2 integrins (Varsano et al., 1988). A 32-kDa laminin-binding protein has been identified on mast cell membranes, coded for by a cDNA of 1.1 kb (Thompson et al., 1989a). As mentioned earlier, this receptor is not a member of the receptor families described above and may be accompanied by additional receptor interactions with laminin that stabilize this contact. Mast cells chemotax and adhere to laminin substrate after antigen-mediated activation (Thompson et al., 1989b), and a peptide sequence found on the A chain of laminin, including the sequence IKVAV, has been shown to mediate these responses in the absence of stimulation (Thompson et al., 1991a). The adherence to laminin is observed in 20–30% of cultured mouse bone marrow mast cells and appears to be dependent on the presence of calcium ions (Thompson et al., 1990a). Thus, mast cell adherence to laminin appears to explain, in part, the distribution of mast cells in tissues. Mast cells are prominent on the undersurface of the endothelial cell membrane, which is known to be rich in laminin. Exposure of laminin, and its proteolytic degradation by stromolysin and other enzymes during wounding to smaller peptide fragments may promote the migration of mast cells into the wound site followed by their attachment. Mast cells have been shown to synthesize the components of basement membrane, including collagen IV, laminin, and heparin sulfate proteoglycan (Thompson et al., 1991b). This observation, coupled with the ability of laminin and the IKVAV laminin peptide to induce cytokine expression in mast cells without the need for degranulation, suggests a role for mast cells in wound repair in response to tissue injury.

As noted, fibroblasts migrate into a wound during the period of granulation tissue formation. The initial attraction for this response may be the synthesis of basement membrane type IV collagen by mast cells and the up-regulated expression of $\alpha_4\beta_1$ receptors on the fibroblast following activation with proinflammatory molecules. Electron microscopy of the mast cell–fibroblast interaction has shown that mast cells interdigitate with the fibroblast in culture. Hence, the observation that mast cells express laminin receptors may even explain the propensity of mast cells to attach to 3T3 fibroblasts, because 3T3 fibroblasts are known to synthesize laminin. In addition, mouse bone marrow cells, cultured for 1 week in the presence of IL-3 and sorted on the basis of IgE receptors, have subsequently been observed to adhere to laminin following activation (Thompson et al., 1990a). Some of these cells lack granules, but appear to represent mast cell precursors. The ability of mast cell precursors to adhere to laminin prior to the expression of phenotypic characteristics other than IgE receptors provides a mechanism to localize these cells in tissues. They may then develop their final phenotype dependent on the local tissue environment. The early appearance of high-affinity IgE receptors and laminin receptors during cell differentiation may be important for these cells to respond to IgE-mediated stimuli before granulation in the response to injury and inflammation (Thompson et al., 1990b). The physiological role of laminin receptors could thus in part be to mediate mast cell responses, including cytokine production, without inducing cellular degranulation. Mast cells have been observed as the primary cells to accumulate at tumor sites. One additional function of the mast cell may be defense against the metastatic spread of tumor cells by a process of recognition similar to that described earlier for macrophages: the ensuing engagement of mast cells with tumor cells resulting in cell activation with the release of cell granule contents.

Other mast cell adhesion receptors are currently being defined. These include an RGD-sensitive fibronectin receptor (Dastych et al., 1991) and a receptor for vitronectin (Bianchine and Metcalfe, 1991). The exact nature(s) of these receptors has yet to be determined, but since both are RGD sensitive, they may be the same integrin receptor $\alpha_v\beta_5$, which binds both substrates, or independent molecules, such as $\alpha_v\beta_3$ and $\alpha_5\beta_1$. Interestingly, attachment to vitronectin, unlike laminin and fibronectin, does not require cellular activation, also suggesting the possibility of distinct receptors. Fibronectin is a major constituent of the new matrix formation in wounds, and these receptors may then help to stabilize the mast cell in a clot while assisting in wound repair. The demonstration of surface antigens of both human lung and uterine mast cells by immunofluouscence and flow cytometry has provided further insight into possible adhesion interactions between mast cells and extracellular matrix or other cell types. Both human lung and uterine mast cells express surface antigens for ICAM-1 and are deficient in CD11a (LFA-1) and CD11b (Mac-1) (Guo et al., 1991). Uterine mast cells, in contrast to lung mast cells, also express both CD11c (gp150,95) and the $\beta 2$ subunit (CD18). Uterine mast cells also express the γ and β subunits of the classical vitronectin receptor (CD51 and CD61) $\alpha_v\beta_3$ and the VLA-4 ($\alpha_4\beta_1$) (CD49d and CD29), although the presence of these receptors on lung mast cells remains to be determined. A full summary of mast cell and basophil surface determinants is given in Table 3.

Table 3 Surface Determinants of Mast Cells and Basophils Determined by Flow Cytometry

	Resting	Activated	Negative for	Reference
Human basophils	CD9	CD11a→	CD1-8	Bochner et al., 1990a
	CD11a	CD11b ↑	CD10	Bochner and Sterbinksky, 1991
	CD11b	CD11c ↑	CD14	
	CD11c	CD35 ↑	CD15	
	CD13	Leu8 ↓	CD16 (Fc_γRIII)	Valent et al., 1989
	CD17		CD19	
	CD18		CD20	
	CD25 (IL2-R)		CD21	

Table 3 Continued

	Resting	Activated	Negative for	Reference
	CD32		CD23	
	CD33(gp67)		CD34	
	CD35(CR1)		CD36	
	CD38		CD64 ($Fc_\gamma RI$)	
	CD45		HLA-DR	
	CD54 (ICAM-1)			
	HLA-1			
	IgE ($Fc_\epsilon RI$)			
Human uterine mast cells	CD9		CD1-8	Guo et al., 1991
	CD11c (gp150, 95)		CD10	Valent et al., 1989
	CD18 (β_2)		CD11a (LFA-1)	
	CD29 (β_1)		CD11b (MAC-1)	
	CD33 (gp67)		CD13	
	CD43 (gp95)		CD14	
	CD45		CD15	
	CD49 (α_6)		CD16 ($Fc_\gamma RIII$)	
	CD49d (α_4)		CD17	
	CD51 (α_v)		CD19	
	CD54 (ICAM-1)		CD20	
	CD61 (β_3)		CD21	
	CDw32 ($Fc_\gamma RII$)		CD23	
	HLA-1		CD23 ($Fc_\epsilon RII$)	
	IgE ($Fc_\epsilon RI$)		CD24	
			CD25 (IL-2R)	
			CD32	
			CD34	
			CD35	
			CD36	
			CD38	
			CD64 ($Fc_\gamma RI$)	
Human lung mast cells	CD9		CD1-8	Guo et al., 1991
	CD33 (gp67)		CD10	Valent et al., 1989
	CD43 (gp95)		CD11b	
	CD45		CD11c	
	CD54 (ICAM-1)		CD13	
	HLA-1		CD14	
	IgE ($Fc_\epsilon RI$)		CD15	

Table 3 Continued

	Resting	Activated	Negative for	Reference
			CD17	
			CD19	
			CD20	
			CD21	
			CD23	
			CD24	
			CD25 (IL-2R)	
			CD38	
			CD34	
			CD32	
			CDw32 ($Fc_{\gamma}RII$)	
			CD35	
			CD36	
Bone marrow mast cells (mouse)	CD29[a] (β_1)			Bender et al., 1988
	CD49f(α_6)			
	DNL.4.4			
	G2			
	G12			
	$H2^k$			
	H11			Thompson et al., 1989a
	ICAM-2[a]			
	IgE ($Fc_{\epsilon}RI$)			Thompson and Metcalfe (unpublished observations)
	LBP (32 kDa[a])		ELAM-1[a]	
	Mac2[a]			

[a]Denotes mRNA expression.

The possibilities of further mast cell adhesion receptors are immense. The functional evaluation of many of the surface receptors, integrins, and ICAM receptors described above remains to be determined. These receptors have important consequences in stabilizing leukocyte and granulocyte presence following extravasation from the tissues during a late-phase or delayed hypersensitivity response. Other receptors that direct mast cell precursors to their tissue destination undoubtedly exist, and perhaps novel or previously described cell-to-cell adhesion receptors provide a basis for mast cell function in normal tissues.

References

Albelda, S. M., and Buck, C. (1990). Integrins and other cell adhesion molecules. *FASEB J.* 4:2868–2880.

Albelda, S. M., Oliver, P. D., Romer, L. H., and Buck, C. A. (1990). EndoCAM: A novel endothelial cell-cell adhesion molecule. *J. Cell Biol.* 110:1227–1237.

Anderson, D. C., and Springer, T. A. (1987). Leukocyte adhesion deficiency: An inherited defect in the Mac1, LFA-1, and p 150-95 glycoproteins. *Am. Rev. Med.* 38:175–194.

Arquint, M., Roder, J., Chia, L.-S., Down, J., Wilkinson, D., Bayley, H., Braun, P., and Dunn, R. (1987). Molecular cloning and primary structure of myelin-associated glycoprotein. *Proc. Natl. Acad. Sci. USA* 84:600–604.

Barthels, D., Santoni, M-J., Wille, W., Ruppert, C., Chaix, J-C., Hirsch, M-R., Fontecilla-Camps, J. C. and Goridis, C. (1987). Isolation and nucleotide sequence of mouse NCAM cDNA that codes for a Mr 79000 polypeptide without a membrane-spanning region. *EMBO J.* 6:907.

Bender, J. G., van Epps, D. E., and Stewart, C. C. (1988). Characterization of granulocytes and mast cells in cultures of mouse bone marrow stimulated with IL-3. *J. Cell. Physiol.* 135:71–78.

Berendt, A. R., Simmons, D. L., Tansey, J., Newbold, C. I., and Marsh, K. (1989). Intercellular adhesion molecule-1 is an endothelial cell adhesion receptor for plasmodium falciparum. *Nature (Lond.)* 341:57–59.

Berg, E. L., Goldstein, L. A., Jutila, M. A., Nakache, M., Picker, L. J., Streeter, P. R., Wu, N. W., Zhou, D., and Butcher, E. C. (1989). Homing receptors and vascular addressins: cell surface molecules that direct lymphocyte traffic. *Immunol. Rev.* 108:5.

Bevilacqua, M. P., Pober, J. S., Mendrick, D. L., Cotran, R. S., and Gimbrone, M. A. (1987). Identification of an inducible endothelial-leukocyte adhesion molecule. *Proc. Natl. Acad. Sci. USA* 84:9238.

Bevilacqua, M. P., Stengelin, S., Gimbrone, M. A., and Seed, B. (1989). Endothelial leukocyte adhesion molecule 1: An inducible receptor for neutrophils related to complement regulatory proteins and lectins. *Science* 243:1160–1165.

Bianchine, P., Burd, P. R. and Metcalfe, D. D. (1992). Unstimulated mast cell express as functional vitronectin receptor. *J. Allergy Clin. Immunol.,* in press.

Bierer, B. E., Sleckman, B. P., Ratnofsky, S. E., and Burakoff, S. J. (1989). The biologic roles of CD2, CD4, and CD8 in T cell activation. *Annu. Rev. Immunol.* 7:579–599.

Bixby, J., Pratt, J., Lilien, J., and Reichardt, L. (1987). Neurite outgrowth on muscle cell surfaces involves extracellular matrix receptors as well as Ca^{2+}-dependent and independent cell adhesion molecules. *Proc. Natl. Acad. Sci. USA* 84:2555–2559.

Bochner, B. S., and Sterbinsky, S. A. (1991). Altered expression of CD11 and Leu 8 during human basophil degranulation. *J. Allergy Clin. Immunol.* 87:302 #649 (abstract).

Bochner, B. S., Peachell, P. T., Brown, K. E., and Schleimer, R. P. (1988). Adherence of human basophils to cultured umbilical vein vascular endothelial cells. *J. Clin. Invest.* 81:1355–1363.

Bochner, B. S., MacGlashan, D. W., Jr., Marcotte, G. V., and Schleimer, R. P. (1989). IgE-dependent regulation of human basophil adherence to vascular endothelium. *J. Immunol.* 142:3180–3189.

Bochner, B. S., McKelvey, A. A., Sterbinsky, S. A., Schleimer, R. P., and MacGlashan, D. W., Jr. (1990a). Flow cytometric methods for analysis of human basophil (BASO) surface antigens and viability. *J. Allergy Clin. Immunol.* 85:171:112.

Bochner, B. S., McKelley, A. A., Sterbinsky, S. A., Hudreth, J. F. K., Derse, C. P., Klunk, D. A., Lichtenstein, L. M., and Schleimer, R. P. (1990b). IL-3 augments adhesiveness for endothelium and CD11b expression in human basophils not neutrophils. *J. Immunol.* 145:1832–1837.

Brake, D. A., Debouck, C., and Biesecker, G. (1990). Identification of an Arg-Gly-Asp (RGD) cell adhesion site in human immunodeficiency virus type I transactivation protein, tat. *J. Cell Biol.* 111:1275–1281.

Buck, C. A., and Horwitz, A. F. (1987). Cell surface receptors for extracellular matrix molecules. *Annu. Rev. Cell Biol.* 3:179–205.

Buck, C. A., Shea, E., Duggan, K., and Horwitz, A. F. (1986). Integrin (the CSAT antigen): Functionality requires oligomeric integrity. *J. Cell Biol.* 103:2421–2428.

Burd, P. R., Rogers, H. W., Gordon, J. R., Martin, C. A., Jayaraman, S., Wilson, S. D., Dvorak, A. M., Galli, S. J., and Dorf, M. E. (1989). Interleukin 3 dependent and independent mast cells stimulated with IgE express multiple cytokines. *J. Exp. Med.* 170:245–257.

Burridge, K., Fath, K., Kelly, T., Nuckolis, B., and Turner, C. (1988). Focal adhesions: Transmembrane junctions between the extracellular matrix and the cytoskeleton. *Annu. Rev. Cell Biol.* 4:487–525.

Butcher, E. C. (1986). The regulation of lymphocyte traffic. *Curr. Topics Microbiol. Immunol.* 128:85–122.

Butcher, E. C. (1990). Cellular and molecular mechanisms that direct leukocyte traffic. *Am. J. Pathol.* 136:3–11.

Cerf-Bensussan, N., Jarry, A., Brousse, N., Lisowska-Grospierre, B., Guy-Grand, D., and Griscelli, C. (1987). A monoclonal antibody (HML-1) defining a novel membrane molecule present on human intestinal k lymphocytes. *Eur. J. Immunol.* 17:1279.

Cherayil, B. J., Neiner, S. J., and Pillai, S. (1989). The Mac-2 antigen is a galactose specific lectin that binds IgE. *J. Exp. Med.* 170:1959–1972.

Cheresh, D., Smith, J., Cooper, H., and Quaranta, V. (1989). A novel vitronectin receptor integrin ($\alpha_v\beta_x$) is responsible for distinct adhesive properties of carcinoma cells. *Cell* 57:59–69.

Clement, B., Segui-Real, B., Savagner, P., Kleinman, H. K., and Yamada, Y. (1990). Hepatocyte attachment to laminin is mediated through multiple receptors. *J. Cell Biol.* 110:185–191.

Coffman, R. L., Seymour, B. W. P., Lebman, D. A., Hiraki, D. D., Christiansen, J. A., Schrader, B., Cherwinski, H., Sarelkowl, H. F. J., Finkelman, F. D., Bond, M. D., and Mosman, T. R. (1988). The role of helper T cell products in mouse B cell differentiation and isotype regulation. *Immunol. Rev.* 102:5–28.

Cunningham, B. A., Hemperly, J. J., Murray, B. A., Prediger, E. A., Brackenbury, R., and Edelman, G. M. (1987). Neural cell adhesion molecule: Structure, immunoglobulin-like domains, cell surface modulation, and alternative RNA splicing. *Science* 236:799.

Damsky, C. H., Richa, J., Solter, D., Knudsen, K., and Buck, C. A. (1983). Identification and purification of a cell surface glycoprotein mediating intercellular adhesion in embryonic and adult tissue. *Cell* 34:455–466.

Dastych, J., Costa, J. J., Thompson, H. L., and Metcalfe, D. D. (1991). Mast cell adhesion to fibronection. *Immunology* 73:478–484.

Drickamer, K. (1988). Two distinct classes of carbohydrate recognition domains in animal lectins. *J. Biol. Chem.* 263:9557–9560.

Dustin, M. L., Rothlein, R., Phan, A. K., Dinarello, C. A., and Springer, T. A. (1986). Induction by IL-1 and interferon-γ: tissue distribution, biochemistry and function of a natural adherence molecule (ICAM-1). *J. Immunol.* 137:245–254.

Dustin, M. L., Sanders, M. E., Shaw, S., and Springer, T. A. (1987). Purified lymphocyte function-associated antigen 3 binds to CD2 and mediates T-lymphocyte adhesion. *J. Exp. Med.* 165:677–692.

Dustin, M. L., Staunton, D. E., and Springer, T. A. (1988). Supergene families meet the immune system. *Immun. Today* 9:213–215.

Edelman, G. M. (1988). Morphoregulatory molecules. *Biochemistry* 27:3533–3543.

Elices, M. J., Osborn, L., Takada, Y., Crouse, C., Luhowsky, S., Hemler, M. E., and Lobb, R. R. (1990). VCAM-1 on activated endothelium interacts with the leukocyte integrin VLA-4 at a site distinct from the VLA-4/fibronectin binding site. *Cell* 60:577–584.

Ensoli, B., Barillari, G., Salahuddin, S. Z., Gallo, R. C., and Wong-Staal, F. (1990). Tat protein of HIV-1 stimulates growth of cells derived from Kaposi's sarcoma lesions of AIDS patients. *Nature (Lond.)* 345:84–86.

Fox, G. N., Parry, R., Barnett, P. V., McGinn, B., Rowlands, D. J., and Brown, F. (1989). The cell attachment site on foot-and-mouth disease virus includes the amino acid sequence RGD (arginine-glycine-aspartic acid). *J. Gen. Virol.* 70:625–637.

Gallatin, W. M., Wayner, E. A., Hoffman, P. A., St. John, T., Butcher, E. C., and Carter, W. G. (1989). Structural homology between lymphocyte receptors for high endothelium and class III extracellular matrix receptor. *Proc. Natl. Acad. Sci. USA* 86:4654–4658.

Gallin, W. J., Edelman, G. M., and Cunningham, D. A. (1983). Characterization of L-CAM, a major cell adhesion molecule from embryonic liver cells. *Proc. Natl. Acad. Sci. USA* 80:1038–1042.

Gallin, W. J., Prediger, E. A., Edelman, G. M., and Cunningham, B. A. (1985). Isolation of a cDNA clone for the liver cell adhesion molecule (L-CAM). *Proc. Natl. Acad. Sci. USA* 82:2809–2813.

Geng, J. G., Bevilacqua, M. S., Moore, K. L., Mctyre, T. M., Prescott, S. M., Kim, J. M., Bliss, G. A., Zimmerman, G. A., and McEver, R. P. (1990). Rapid neutrophil adhesion to activated endothelium mediated by GMP-140. *Nature (Lond.)* 343:757–760.

Gimbrone, M. A., Obin, M. S., Brock, A. F., Luis, E. A., Hass, P. E., Hebert, L. A., Yip, Y. K., Leung, D. W., Lowe, D. G., Kohr, W. J., Darbonne, W. C., Bechtol,

K. B., and Baker, J. B. (1989). Endothelial interleukin-8 A novel inhibitor of leukocyte endothelial interactions. *Science* 246:1601–1603.

Ginsberg, M. H., Loftus, J. C., and Plow, E. F. (1988). Cytoadhesins, integrins, and platelets. *Thromb. Haemostasis* 59:1–6.

Gordon, J. R., and Galli, S. J. (1990). Production of the haemostasis growth factor GM-CSF and interleukin 3 by mast cells in response to IgE receptor-mediated activation. *Nature* 346:274–276.

Graf, J., Iwamoto, Y., Sasaki, M., Martin, G. R., Kleinman, H. K., Robey, F. A., and Yamada, Y. (1987). Identification of an amino acid sequence in laminin mediating cell attachment, chemotaxis and receptor binding. *Cell* 48:989–996.

Grumet, M., and Edelman, G. M. (1988). Neuron-Glia cell adhesion molecule interacts with neurons and astroglia via different binding mechanisms. *J. Cell Biol.* 106:487–503.

Grumet, M., Hoffman, S., and Edelman, G. M. (1984). Two antigenically related neuronal cell cohesion molecules of different specificities mediate neuron-neuron and neuron-glia adhesion. *Proc. Natl. Acad. Sci. USA* 81:267–271.

Guan, J-L., and Hynes, R. O. (1990). Lymphoid cells recognize an alternatively spliced segment of fibronectin via the integrin receptor $\alpha_4\beta_1$. *Cell* 60:53–61.

Guo, C. B., Kagay-Sobotka, A., Lichtenstein, L. M., and Bochner, B. S. (1991). Unique phenotypic characteristics of human uterine mast cells (UMC). *J. Allergy Clin. Immunol.* 87:303–655.

Harrelson, A. L., and Goodman, C. S. (1988). Growth cone guidance in insects: Fasciclin II is a member of the immunoglobulin superfamily. *Science* 242:700–708.

Hatta, K., and Takeichi, M. (1986). Expression of N-cadherin adhesion molecule associated with early morphogenetic events in chick development. *Nature (Lond.)* 320:447–449.

Hatta, K., Takagi, S., Fujisawa, H., and Takeichi, M. (1987). Spatial and temporal expression pattern of N-cadherin cell adhesion molecules correlated with morphogenetic processes of chicken embryos. *Dev. Biol.* 120:215–227.

Haynes, B. F. (1984). The human thymic microenvironment. *Adv. Immun.* 36:87–142.

Heino, J., and Massague, J. (1989). Transforming growth factor-β switches the pattern of integrins expressed in MG-63 human osteosarcoma cells and causes a selective loss of cell adhesion to laminin. *J. Biol. Chem.* 264:21806–21811.

Hemler, M. E. (1990). VLA proteins in the integrin family: structures, functions, and their role on leukocytes. *Annu. Rev. Immunol.* 8:365–400.

Hemperly, J. J., Murray, B. A., Edelman, G. M., and Cunningham, B. A. (1986). Sequence of a cDNA clone encoding the polysialic acid-rich and cytoplasmic domains of the neural cell adhesion molecule NCAM. *Proc. Natl. Acad. Sci. USA* 83:3037–3041.

Hession, C., Osborn, L., Goff, D., Chi-Rosso, G., Vassallo, C., Pasek, M., Pittack, C., Tizard, R., Goetz, S., McCarthy, K., Hopple, S., and Lobb, R. (1990). Endothelial leukocyte adhesion molecule 1: Direct expression cloning and functional interactions. *Proc. Natl. Acad. Sci. USA* 87:1637–1642.

Hirano, S., Nose, A., Hatta, K., Kawakami, A., and Takeichi, M. (1987). Calcium-dependent cell-cell adhesion molecules (cadherins): Subclass-specificities and possible involvement of actin bundles. *J. Cell Biol.* 105:2501–2510.

Hirsch, S. R., and Kalbfleisch, J. H. (1980). Existence of basophil chemotaxis in subjects with hay fever. *J. Allergy Clin. Immunol.* 4:1523–1531.

Hirst, R., Horwitz, A., Buck, C., and Rohrschneider, L. (1986). Phosphorylation of the fibronectin receptor complex in cells transformed by oncogenes that encode tyrosine kinases. *Proc. Natl. Acad. Sci. USA* 83:6470–6474.

Hogervorst, F., Kuikman, L., von dem Borne, A. E. G., Jr., and Sonnenberg, A. (1990). Cloning and sequence analysis of beta-4 cDNA: An integrin subunit that contains a unique 118 kd cytoplasmic domain. *EMBO J.* 9:765–770.

Holzmann, B., and Weissman, I. L. (1989). Peyer's patch-specific lymphocyte homing receptors consist of a VLA-4 like α chain associated with either of two integrin β chains, one of which is novel. *EMBO J.* 8:1735–1741.

Huard, T. J., Banery, J. L., Wood, J. F. B., and Wicha, M. S. (1985). A potential role for the extracellular matrix glycoprotein laminin in macrophage–tumor cell interactions. *Int. J. Cancer* 36:511–517.

Ignatius, M. J., Large, T. H., Houde, M., Tawil, J. W., Burton, A., Esch, F., Carbonetto, S., and Reichardt, L. F. (1990). Molecular cloning of the rat integrin α_1-subunit: A receptor for laminin and collagen. *J. Cell Biol.* 111:709–720.

Isberg, R. R., and Leong, J. M. (1990). Multiple β_1 chain integrins are receptors for invasion, a protein that promotes bacterial penetration into mammalian cells. *Cell* 60:861–871.

Iwamoto, Y., Robey, F. A., Graf, J., Sasaki, M., Kleinman, H. K., Yamada, Y., and Martin, G. R. (1987). YIGSR, a synthetic laminin pentapeptide, inhibits experimental metastasis formation. *Science* 238:1132–1139.

Iwamoto, Y., Graf, J., Sasaki, M., Kleinman, H. K., Greatorex, D. R., Martin, G. R., Robey, F. A., and Yamada, Y. (1988). Synthetic pentapeptide from the B1 chain of laminin promotes B16-F10 melanoma cell migration. *J. Cell Physiol.* 134:287–293.

Janeway, C. A. (1988). T cell development accessories or co-receptors. *Nature* 335:208–210.

Kajiji, S., Tamura, R. N., and Quaranta, V. (1989). A novel integrin ($\alpha E\beta 4$) from human epithelial cells suggests a fourth family of integrin adhesion receptors. *EMBO J.* 8:673–680.

Kay, A. B., and Austen, K. F. (1972). Chemotaxis of human basophils. *Clin. Exp. Immunol.* 11:557–563.

Keilhauer, G., Faissner, A., and Schachner, M. (1985). Differential inhibition of neurone-neurone, neurone-astrocyte, and astrocyte-astrocyte adhesion by L1, L2, and NCAM antibodies. *Nature* 316:728–730.

Kirkpatrick, C. H. (1988). Delayed hypersensitivity. In *Immunological Diseases*, 11th ed. Edited by M. Samter, D. W. Talmage, M. M. Frank, K. F. Austen, and H. N. Claman. Boston, Little, Brown, pp. 157–202.

Kirshenbaum, A. S., Goff, J. P., Dreskin, S. C., Irani, A-M., Schwartz, L. B., and Metcalfe, D. D. (1989). IL-3-dependent growth of basophil-like cells and mastlike cells from human bone marrow. *J. Immunol.* 142:2424–2429.

Kirshenbaum, A. S., Kessler, S. W., Goff, J. P., and Metcalfe, D. D. (1991). Demonstration of the origin of human mast cells from CD34+ bone marrow progenitor cells. *J. Immunol.* 146:1410–1415.

Kishimoto, T. K., O'Connor, K., Lee, A., Roberts, T. M., and Springer, T. A. (1987). Cloning of the β subunit of the leukocyte adhesion proteins: Homology to an extracellular matrix receptor defines a novel supergene family. *Cell* 48:681–690.

Kishimoto, T. K., Jutila, M. A., Berg, E. L., and Butcher, E. C. (1989a). Neutrophil Mac-1 and Mel-14 adhesion proteins inversely regulated by chemotactic factors. *Science* 245:1238–1241.

Kishimoto, T. K., Larson, R. S., Corbi, A. L., Dustin, M. L., Staunton, D. E., and Springer, T. A. (1989b). The leukocyte integrins. *Adv. Immunol.* 46:149–182.

Kramer, R. H., McDonald, K. A., and Vu, M. P. (1989). Human melanoma cells express a novel integrin receptor for laminin. *J. Biol. Chem.* 264:15642–15649.

Krissansen, G. W., Elliott, M. J., Lucas, C. M., Stomski, F. C., Berndt, M. C., Cheresh, D. A., Lopez, A. F., and Burns, G. F. (1990). Identification of a novel integrin β subunit expressed on cultured monocytes (macrophages). *J. Biol. Chem.* 265:823–830.

Kupfer, A., and Singer, S. J. (1989). Cell biology of cytotoxic and helper T cell functions immunofluorence microscopic studies of single cells and cell couples. *Annu. Rev. Immunol.* 7:309–337.

Kupper, T. S. (1990). Immune and inflammatory processes in cutaneous tissues: Mechanisms and speculations. *J. Clin. Invest.* 86:1783–1789.

Lai, C., Brow, M. A., Nave, K-A., Novonha, A. B., Quarles, R. H., Bloom, F. E., Miner, R. J., and Sutcliffe, J. G. (1987). Two forms of 1B 236 myelin-associated glycoprotein, a cell adhesion molecule for postnatal neural development, are produced by alternative splicing. *Proc. Natl. Acad. Sci. USA* 84:4337–4341.

Larsen, E., Celli, A., Gilbert, G. E., Furie, B., Erban, J. K., Bonfanti, R., Wagner, D. D., and Furie, B. (1989). PADGEM protein: a receptor that mediates the interaction of activated platelets with neutrophils and monocytes. *Cell* 59: 305–312.

Laybourn, K. A., Hiserodt, J. C., and Varani, J. (1989). Laminin receptor expression on murine tumor cells: Correlation with sensitivity to natural cell-mediated cytotoxicity. *Int. J. Cancer* 43:737–742.

Lett-Brown, M. A., Boetcher, D. A., and Leonard, E. J. (1976). Chemotactic responses of normal human basophils to C5a and to lymphocyte-derived chemotactic factor. *J. Immunol.* 117:246–252.

Loftus, J. C., O'Toole, T. E., Plow, E. F., Glass, A., Frelinger, A. L., and Ginsberg, M. H. (1990). A beta 3 integrin mutation abolishes ligand binding and alters divalent cation dependent conformation. *Science* 249:915–918.

Mackay, C. R., Marston, W. L., and Dudler, L. (1990). Naïve and memory T cells show distinct pathways of lymphocyte recirculation. *J. Exp. Med.* 171:801–817.

Martz, E. (1987). LFA-1 and other accessory molecules functioning in adhesions of T and B lymphocytes. *Hum. Immun.* 18:3–37.

Masinovsky, B., Urdal, D., and Michael, W. (1990). IL-4 acts synergistically with IL-1β to promote lymphocyte adhesion to microvascular endothelium by induction of vascular cell adhesion molecule-1. *J. Immunol.* 145:2886–2895.

Meacham, R. P., Hinek, A., Griffin, G. L., Senior, R. M., and Liotta, L. A. (1989). The elastin receptor shows structural and functional similarities to the 67-kDa tumor cell laminin receptor. *J. Biol. Chem.* 264:16652–16657.

Miyake, K., Underhill, C. B., Lesley, J., and Kincade, P. W. (1990). Hyaluronate can function as a cell adhesion molecule and CD44 participates in hyaluronate recognition. *J. Exp. Med.* 172:69–75.

Moos, M., Tacke, R., Scherer, H., Teplow, D., Fruk, K., and Schachner, M. (1988). Neural adhesion molecule L1 as a member of the immunoglobulin superfamily with binding domains similar to fibronectin. *Nature* 334:701–703.

Mould, A. P., Wheldon, L. A., Komoriya, A., Wayner, E. A., Yamada, K. M., and Humphries, M. J. (1990). Affinity chromatographic isolation of the melanoma adhesion receptor for the IIICS region of fibronectin and its identification as the integrin $\alpha_4\beta_1$. *J. Biol. Chem.* 265:4020–4024.

Newman, P. J., Berndt, M. C., Gorsky, J., White, G. C., and Paddock, L. S., and Muller, W. A. (1990). PECAM-1 (CD31): Cloning and relation to adhesion molecules of the immunoglobulin gene superfamily. *Science* 247:1219–1222.

Nose, A., and Takeichi, M. (1986). A novel cadherin adhesion molecule: Its expression patterns associated with implantation and organogenesis of mouse embryos. *J. Cell Biol.* 103:2649–2658.

Nose, A., Nagafuchi, A., and Takeichi, M. (1987). Isolation of a placental cadherin cDNA: Identification of a novel gene family for cell-cell adhesion molecules. *EMBO J.* 6:3655–3661.

Oquendo, P., Hundt, E., Lawler, J., and Seed, B. (1989). CD36 directly mediates cytoadherence of plasmodium falciparum parasitized erythrocytes. *Cell* 58:95–101.

Osborn, L., Hession, C., Tizard, R., Vassallo, C., Luhowskyj, S., Chi-Rosso, G., and Lobb, R. (1989). Direct expression cloning of vascular cell adhesion molecule 1, a cytokine-induced endothelial protein that binds to lymphocytes. *Cell* 59:1203–1211.

Otey, C. A., Pavalko, F. M., and Burridge, K. (1990). An interaction between α-actinin and the β_1 integrin subunit in vitro. *J. Cell Biol.* 11:721–729.

Phillips, D. R., Charo, I. F., Parise, L. V., and Fitzgerald, L. A. (1988). The platelet membrane glycoprotein IIb-IIIa complex. *Blood* 71:831–843.

Picker, L. J., Michie, S. A., Rott, L. S., and Butcher, E. C. (1990a). A unique phenotype of skin-associated lymphocytes in humans: preferential expression of the HECA-452 epitope by benign and malignant T cells at cutaneous sites. *Am. J. Pathol.* 136:1053.

Picker, L. J., Terstappen, L. W. M. M., Rott, L. S., Streeter, P. R., Stein, H., and Butcher, E. C. (1990b). Differential expression of homing-associated adhesion molecules by T cell subsets in man. *J. Immunol.* 145:3247–3255.

Picker, L. J., Kishimoto, T. K., Smith, C. W., Warnock, R. A., and Butcher, E. C. (1991). ELAM-1 is an adhesion molecule for skin-homing T cells. *Nature* 349:796–799.

Plantefaber, L. C., and Hynes, R. O. (1989). Changes in integrin receptors on ontogenically transformed cells. *Cell* 56:281–290.

Plaut, M., Pierce, J. H., Watson, C. J., Hanley-Hyde, J., Nordan, R. P., and Paul, W. E. (1989). Mast cell lines produce lymphokines in response to cross-linkage of Fcϵ RI or to calcium ionophores. *Nature* 339:64–67.

Pober, J. S., Bevilacqua, M. P., Mendrick, D. L., Lapierre, L. A., Fiers, W., and Gimbrone, M. A. (1986a). Two distinct monokines, interleukin 1 and tumor necrosis factor, each independently induce the biosynthesis and transient expression of the same antigen on the surface of cultured human vascular endothelial cells. *J. Immunol.* 136:1680.

Pober, J. S., Gimbrone, M. A., Lapierre, L. A., Mendrick, D. L., Fiers, W., Rothlein, R., and Springer, T. A. (1986b). Overlapping patterns of activation of human endothelial cells by interleukin 1, tumour necrosis factor, and immune interferon. *J. Immunol.* 137:1893.

Poulter, L. W., Seymour, G. J., Duke, O, Janossy, G., and Panay, G. (1983). Immunohistological analysis of delayed-type hypersensitivity in man. *Cell. Immunol.* 74:385.

Ramaswamy, H., and Hemler, M. E. (1990). Cloning, primary structure and properties of a novel human integrin β subunit. *EMBO J.* 9:1561–1568.

Reinholt, F. P., Hultenby, K., Oldberg, A., and Heinegard, D. (1990). Osteopontin: a possible anchor of osoteoclasts to bone. *Proc. Natl. Acad. Sci. USA* 87:4473–4475.

Rice, E. G., and Bevilacqua, M. (1989). An inducible endothelial cell surface glycoprotein mediates melanoma adhesion. *Science* 246:1303–1306.

Rodriguez-Boulan, E., and Nelson, W. J. (1989). Morphogenesis of the polarized epithelial cell phenotype. *Science* 245:718–725.

Rothlein, R., Dustin, M. L., Martin, S. D., and Springer, T. A. (1986). A human intercellular adhesion molecule (ICAM-1) distinct from LFA-1. *J. Immunol.* 137:1270–1274.

Runyan, R. B., Versalovic, J., and Shur, R. D. (1988). Functionally distinct laminin receptors mediate cell adhesion and spreading: The requirement for surface galactosyl transferase in cell spreading. *J. Cell Biol.* 107:1863–1871.

Ruoslahti, E. (1989). Proteoglycans in cell regulation. *J. Biol. Chem.* 264:13369–13372.

Ruoslahti, E. (1990). Integrins. *J. Clin. Invest.* 87:1–5.

Ruoslahti, E., and Giancotti, F. G. (1989). Integrins and tumor cell dissemination. *Cancer Cells* 1:119–136.

Ruoslahti, E., and Pierschbacher, M. D. (1987). New perspectives in cell adhesion: RGD and integrins. *Science* 238:491–497.

Rutishauser, U., and Jessell, T. M. (1988). Cell adhesion molecules in vertebrate neural development. *Biol. Rev.* 68:819–857.

Savill, J., Dransfield, I., Hogg, N., and Haslett, C. (1990). Vitronectin receptor-mediated phagocytosis of cells undergoing apoptosis. *Nature (Lond.)* 343:170–173.

Salter, R. D., Benjamin, R. J., Wesley, P. K., Buxton, S. E., Gamet, T. P. J., Clayberger, C., Krensky, A. M., Novment, A. M., Littman, D. R., and Parham, P. (1990). A binding site for the T cell co-receptor CD8 on the α_3 domain of HLA-A2. *Nature* 345:41–46.

Saunders, S., and Bernfield, M. (1988). Cell surface proteoglycan binds mouse mammary epithelial cells to fibronectin and behaves as a receptor for interstitial matrix. *J. Cell Biol.* 106:423–430.

Schieferdecker, H. L., Ullrich, R., Weiss-Breckwoldt, A. N., Schwarting, R., Stein, H.,

Riecken, E-O., and Zeitz, M. (1990). The HML-1 antigen of intestinal lymphocytes is an activation antigen. *J. Immunol.* 144:2541.

Schmidt, G., Robenek, H., Harrach, B., Glössi, J., Nolte, V., Hormann, H., Richter, H., and Kresse, H. (1987). Interaction of small dermatan sulfate proteoglycan from fibroblasts with fibronectin. *J. Cell Biol.* 104:1683–1691.

Schwartz, L. B., and Austen, K. F. (1988). The mast cell and mediators of immediate hypersensitivity. In *Immunological Diseases*, 11th ed. Edited by M. Samter, D. W. Talmage, M. M. Frank, K. F. Austen, and H. L. Claman. Boston, Little, Brown, pp. 157–202.

Schwarz, E. R., and Hiserodt, J. C. (1988). The expression and functional involvement of laminin-like molecules in non-MHC restricted cytotoxicity by human leu-19^+/$CD3^-$ natural killer lymphocytes. *J. Immunol.* 141:3318–3323.

Shepopard, D., Rozzo, C., Starr, L., Quaranta, V., Erie, D. J., and Pytela, R. (1990). Complete amino acid sequence of a novel integrin β subunit (β_6) identified in epithelial cells using the polymerase chain reaction. *J. Biol. Chem.* 265:11502–11507.

Shimizu, Y., vanSeventor, G., Horgan, K., Horgan, Shaw, S. (1990). Regulated expression and binding of three VLA integrins receptors on T cells. *Nature (Lond.)* 345:250–252.

Shimizu, Y., Shaw, S., Graber, N., Gopai, T. V., Horgan, K. J., vanSeventer, G. A., and Newman, W. (1991). Activation of human memory T cells to adhesion molecule ELAM-1. *Nature* 349:799–802.

Simmons, D., Makgoba, M. W., and Seed, B. (1988), ICAM, an adhesion ligand of LFA-1, is homologous to the neural cell adhesion molecule NCAM. *Nature* 331:624–627.

Springer, T. A., Dustin, M. L., Kishimoto, T. K., and Marlin, S. (1987). The lymphocyte function-associated LFA-1, CD2, and LFA-3 molecules: Cell adhesion receptors of the immune system. *Annu. Rev. Immunol.* 5:223–252.

Stacker, S. A., and Springer, T. A. (1991). Leukocyte integrin P150, 95 (CD11c/CD18) functions as an adhesion molecule binding to a counter receptor on stimulated endothelium. *J. Immunol.* 146:648–655.

Staunton, D. E., Martin, S. D., Stratowa, C., Dustin, M. L., and Springer, T. A. (1988). Primary structure of ICAM-1 demonstrates interaction between members of the immunoglobulin and integrin supergene. *Cell* 52:925–933.

Staunton, D. E., Dustin, M. L., and Springer, T. A. (1989a). Functional cloning of ICAM-2, a cell adhesion ligand for LFA-1 homologous to ICAM-1. *Nature* 339:61–64.

Staunton, D. E., Merwizzi, V. J., Rothlein, R., Barton, R., Martin, S. D., and Springer, T. A. (1989b). A cell adhesion molecule ICAM-1 is the major surface receptor for rhinoviruses. *Cell* 56:849–853.

Stoolman, L. M. (1989). Adhesion molecules controlling lymphocyte migration. *Cell* 56:907–910.

Stoolman, L. M., and Rosen, S. D. (1983). Possible role of cell-surface carbohydrate-binding molecules in lymphocyte recirculation. *J. Cell Biol.* 96:722–730.

Suzuki, S., and Naitoh, Y. (1990). Amino acid sequence of a novel integrin β_4 subunit and primary expression of the mRNA in epithelial cells. *EMBO J.* 9:765–763.

Swain, S. L. (1983). T cell subsets the recognition of MHC class. *Immunol. Rev.* 74:129–142.

Takagi, M., Nakahata, T., Koike, K., Kobayashi, T., Tsuji, K., Kojima, S., Hirano, T., Miyajima, A., Aria, K-I., and Akabane, T. (1989). Stimulation of connective tissue-type mast cell proliferation by cross-linking of cell bound IgE. *J. Exp. Med.* 170:233–244.

Takeichi, M. (1988). The cadherins: cell-cell adhesion molecules controlling animal morphogenesis. *Development* 102:639–655.

Tashiro, K., Sephel, G. C., Weeks, B., Sasaki, M., Martin, G. R., Kleinman, H. K., and Yamada, Y. (1989). A synthetic peptide containing the IKVAV sequence from the A chain of laminin mediates cell attachment, migration, and neurite outgrowth. *J. Biol. Chem.* 264:16174–16183.

Thompson, H. L., Burbelo, P. D., Segui-Real, B., Yamada, Y., and Metcalfe, D. D. (1989a). Laminin promotes mast cell attachment. *J. Immunol.* 143:2323–2328.

Thompson, H. L., Burbelo, P. D., Yamada, Y., Kleinman, H. K., and Metcalfe, D. D. (1989b). Mast cells chemotax to laminin with enhancement after IgE-mediated activation. *J. Immunol.* 143:4188–4192.

Thompson, H. L., Burbelo, P. D., and Metcalfe, D. D. (1990a). Regulation of adhesion of mouse bone marrow-derived mast cells to laminin. *J. Immunol.* 145:3425–3431.

Thompson, H. L., Metcalfe, D. D., and Kinet, J-P. (1990b). Early expression of high-affinity receptor for immunoglobulin E (FcϵRI) during differentiation of mouse mast cells and human basophils. *J. Clin. Invest.* 85:1227–1233.

Thompson, H. L., Burbelo, P. D., Yamada, Y., Kleinman, H. K., and Metcalfe, D. D. (1991a). Identification of an amino acid sequence in the laminin A chain mediating mast cell attachment and spreading. *Immunology* 72:144–149.

Thompson, H. L., Burbelo, P. D., Gabriel, G., Yamada, Y., and Metcalfe, D. D. (1991b). Murine mast cells synthesize basement membrane components, a potential role in early fibrosis. *J. Clin. Invest.* 87:619–623.

Thornhill, M. H., Wellicome, S. M., Mahiouz, D. L., Jerry, S., Lanchbury, S., Kyan-Aung, U., and Haskard, D. O. (1991). Tumor necrosis factor combines with IL-4 or IFN-γ to selectively enhance endothelial cell adhesiveness for T cells: The contribution of vascular cell adhesion molecule-1-dependent and -independent binding mechanisms. *J. Immunol.* 146:592–598.

Tomioka, K., Bochner, B. S., Derse-Anthony, C., Lichtenstein, L. M., and Schleimer, R. P. (1991). GM-CSF enhances PAF- and FMLP-induced eosinophil expression of adherence molecules (CD11b) and increases FMLP-induced adherence to endothelial cells. *J. Allergy Clin. Immunol.* 871:303 #654 (abstract).

Valent, P., Ashman, L. K., Hinterberger, W., Eckersberger, F., Majdic, O., Lechnerk, and Bettelheim, P. (1989). Mast cell typing: demonstration of a distinct hematopoeitic cell type and evidence for immunophenotypic relationship to mononuclear phagocytes. *Blood* 73:1778–1785.

Varsano, S., Lazarus, S. C., Gold, W., and Nadel, J. (1988). Selective adhesion of mast cells to tracheal epithelial cell in vitro. *J. Immunol.* 140:2184–2194.

Vogel, B. E., Tarone, G., Giancotti, F. G., Gailit, J., and Ruoslahti, E. (1990). A novel fibronectin receptor with an unexpected subunit composition ($\alpha_v\beta_1$). *J. Biol. Chem.* 265:5934–5937.

Vogel, K. G., Paulson, M., and Heinegard, D. (1984). Specific inhibition of type I and type II collagen fibrillogenesis by the small proteoglycan of the tendon. *Biochem. J.* 223:587–597.

Volk, T., and Geiger, B. (1984). A 135kd membrane protein of intercellular adherent junctions. *EMBO J.* 3:2249–2260.

von Boehmer, H. (1988). The developmental biology of T lymphocytes. *Annu. Rev. Immunol.* 6:309–326.

von der Mark, K., and Kuhl, U. (1985). Laminin and its receptor. *Biochim. Biophys. Acta* 823:147–156.

Ward, P. A., Dvorak, H. F., Cohen, S., Yoshida, T., Data, R., and Selvaggio, D. (1975). Chemotaxis of basophils by lymphocyte-dependent and lymphocyte-independent mechanisms. *J. Immunol.* 4:1523–1531.

Wardlaw, A. J., Hibbs, M. L., Stacker, S. A., and Springer, T. A. (1990). Distinct mutations in two patients with leukocyte adhesion deficiency and their functional correlates. *J. Exp. Med.* 172:335–345.

Wawryk, S. O., Novotny, J. R., Wicks, I. P., Wilkinson, D., Maher, D., Salvaris, E., Welch, K., Fecondo, J., and Boyd, A. W. (1989). The role of the LFA-1/ICAM-1 interaction in human leukocyte homing and adhesion. *Immunol. Rev.* 108:135–161.

Wayner, E. A., Garcia-Pardo, A., Humphries, M. J., McDonald, J. A., and Carter, W. G. (1989). Identification and characterization of the lymphocyte adhesion receptor for an alternative cell attachment domain in plasma fibronectin. *J. Cell Biol.* 109:1321–1330.

Wewer, V. M., Liotta, L. A., Jaye, M., Ricca, G. A., Drohan, W. N., Claysmith, A. P., Rao, C. N., Wurth, P., Coligan, J. E., Albrechtsen, R., Mudryi, J. M., and Sobel, M. E. (1986). Altered levels of laminin receptor mRNA in various human carcinoma cells that have different abilities to bind laminin. *Proc. Natl. Acad. Sci. USA* 83:7137–7141.

Wigzell, H., and Hayny, P. (1974). Specific fractionation of immunocompetent cells. Application in the analysis of effector cells involved in cell mediated lysis. *Curr. Topics Microbiol. Immunol.* 67:1–42.

Wodnar-Filipowicz, A., Heusser, C., and Moroni, C. (1989). Production of the haemopoietic growth factors GM-CSF and interleukin-3 by mast cells in response to IgE receptor mediated activation. *Nature* 339:150–152.

Yednock, T. A., and Rosen, S. D. (1989). Lymphocyte homing. *Adv. Immunol.* 44:313–378.

Yednock, T. A., Stoolman, L. M., and Rosen, S. D. (1987). Phosphomannosyl-derivatized beads detect a receptor involved in lymphocyte homing. *J. Cell Biol.* 104:713–721.

Yoshida, C., and Takeichi, M. (1982). Teratocarcinoma cell adhesion: Identification of a cell surface protein involved in calcium-dependent cell aggregation. *Cell* 28:217–224.

Yow, H., Wong, J. M., Chen, H. S., Lee, C., Davis, S., Steele, G. D., and Chen, L. B. (1988). Increased mRNA expression of a laminin-binding protein in human colon carcinoma: Complete sequence of a full length cDNA encoding the protein. *Proc. Natl. Acad. Sci. USA* 85:6394–6442.

AUTHOR INDEX

Italic numbers give the page on which the complete reference is listed.

A

B

C

E

F

G

H

K

L

N

O

Q

R

T

U

V

X

Y

Z

SUBJECT INDEX

D

E

F

G

H

I

N

O

P

R

S

T

U

V

W

Z